Disorders
of the Cerebellum

Contemporary Neurology Series available:

Fred Plum, M.D., *Editor-in-Chief*
Fletcher H. McDowell, M.D., and J. Richard Baringer, M.D., *Editors*

Disorders
of the Cerebellum

SID GILMAN, M.D.

Professor and Chairman
Department of Neurology
The University of Michigan Medical School
Ann Arbor, Michigan

JAMES R. BLOEDEL, M.D., Ph.D.

Professor of Neurosurgery and Physiology
University of Minnesota Medical School
Minneapolis, Minnesota

RICHARD LECHTENBERG, M.D.

Assistant Professor of Neurology
State University of New York
Downstate Medical Center
Brooklyn, New York

 F. A. DAVIS COMPANY, PHILADELPHIA

Printed in the United States of America

Library of Congress Cataloging in Publication Data

Gilman, Sid.
    Disorders of the cerebellum.

    (Contemporary neurology series; 21)
    Includes bibliographies and index.
    1. Cerebellum—Diseases. I. Bloedel, James, joint author. II. Lechtenberg, Richard, joint author.
III. Title. IV. Series. [DNLM: 1. Cerebellar diseases. W1 CO769N v. 21 / WL320 G487d]
    RC386.2.G53   616.8   80–23393
    ISBN 0–8036–4150–8

Foreword

It is almost a hundred years since Ramon y Cajal made his brilliant analysis of the neuronal structure of the cerebellar cortex. The regular serried rows of thousands of large Purkinje cells, each with its climbing fibers, basket and granular cell terminals, have continued to fascinate anatomists, physiologists, and neurologists. The endless repetition of this stereotyped unique structure surely points to some very special aspect of nervous function. The elegant microelectrode analyses of the related synapses by Eccles, Ito, and others in recent years have greatly clarified the relations between the various components, and have defined the inhibitory function of the Purkinje cell effector pathway. More recently the new anatomic labeling methods have considerably expanded knowledge of the distribution of input pathways to cerebellar cortex and the output of the deep nuclei. The part played by the distinctive cerebellar units still defies analysis, though clearly they are important in almost all nervous functions. No longer can we characterize cerebellar activity as *coordination* except in some very broad sense.

The authors of this interesting text are each well qualified to address the anatomic, physiologic, and clinical aspects of cerebellar function. Drs. Gilman and Bloedel have carried out original investigations of cerebellar physiology in experimental animals for many years. Drs. Gilman and Lechtenberg have an extensive background in clinical studies of cerebellar symptomatology in a variety of conditions.

The book begins with a comprehensive review of cerebellar anatomy and physiology. Principles of localization are discussed and original data are presented from a large series of cases. There is a superb review of the genetically determined atrophies and metabolic disorders. The clinical characteristics of cerebellar tumors, abscesses, hemorrhages, and infarctions are well described and illustrative case reports are presented.

In the last few years there have been several efforts to use chronic stimulation by implanted cerebellar electrodes to modify the spasms and involuntary movements of cerebral palsy, or intractable epilepsy. A final chapter reviews potentialities and defects of this technique.

I strongly recommend this timely text.

D. Denny-Brown, M. D.
Putnam Professor of Neurology Emeritus
Harvard Medical School

Preface

More than two decades have elapsed since Dow and Moruzzi published their extensive review of the physiology and pathology of the cerebellum. Their book appeared during an epoch when cerebellar function was under intense investigation, chiefly with studies of the effects of stimulation or ablation of the cerebellum on posture and locomotion in experimental animals. Studies with microelectrode techniques had just begun. Since that time, knowledge of cerebellar physiology has advanced remarkably, particularly due to the application of microelectrode techniques to investigate cerebellar afferent and efferent pathways and the synaptic relations between various elements within the cerebellum. The introduction of techniques that permit fiber pathways to be traced has also furthered our understanding of cerebellar anatomy.

In the past 20 years there have been numerous advances in our knowledge of the localization of disease processes and clinical disorders affecting the cerebellum. Arteriography and pneumoencephalography have made it possible to gain further experience in the anatomic localization of focal disease processes. Several new classifications of degenerative disorders of the cerebellum and some biochemical disorders affecting cerebellar function have been identified. The development of computerized tomography has provided the single greatest advance for defining the location of focal disturbances in the cerebellum. The CT scan makes it possible to investigate cerebellar anatomy and disease processes, such as cerebellar hemorrhage, infarctions, or abscesses, without invasive procedures. This advance has demonstrated, for example, that cerebellar hemorrhages do not necessarily require immediate surgical intervention and that certain patients can be treated medically and improve without surgery. Positron emission tomography promises insights into metabolic disorders of the cerebellum.

The earlier ideas concerning the localization of disease processes in the cerebellum from bedside clinical examination were derived from studies that now are very old. Most of these cases did not have rigorous anatomic verification of the location of the pathology. It is now clear that disorders of the cerebellum can be localized only in the broadest and most general terms; specific point-to-point representations of body parts or discrete physiologic functions in the cerebellum apply only to the experimental animal under certain conditions.

This book provides an updated review of the anatomy and physiology of the cerebellum together with the principles of localization of cerebellar disorders and descriptions of the common disorders of the cerebellum. Chapters 1 through 9 review the anatomy and physiology of the cerebellum with strong emphasis on cerebellar function in terms of posture and movement. These chapters serve as the basis for Chapters 10 through 18, which discuss the clinical disorders of the cerebellum.

The clinical material came from the College of Physicians and Surgeons of Columbia University, The University of Michigan Medical School, and the Downstate Medical Center of the State University of New York. We are indebted to the many physicians who cared for the patients described, particularly to Drs. Philip Duffy and Samuel Hicks, and Ms. Constance D'Amato for the neuropathologic material; and to Drs. James Knake, Sharon Kreps, Joachim Seeger, and Michael Tenner for the neuroradiologic material.

Sid Gilman, M.D.
James R. Bloedel, M.D., Ph.D.
Richard Lechtenberg, M.D.

Contents

CHAPTER 1

Principles of Cerebellar Organization

The cerebellum is one of the three basic subdivisions of the brain which includes the cerebral hemispheres and the brainstem. Located behind and below the cerebral hemispheres, the cerebellum is separated from them by a membranous structure, the tentorium cerebelli. The cerebellum overlies the middle and posterior components of the brainstem, the pons and the medulla, and connects directly with these structures and with the third component of the brainstem, the mesencephalon. All major components of the central nervous system provide information to the cerebellum and it sends output projections to most of the same structures.

Although it probably does not initiate movements itself, the cerebellum participates with other central nervous system structures in the initiation of a wide variety of movements. It is needed to maintain the proper posture and balance for walking and running; to execute sequential movements for eating, dressing, and writing; to participate in rapidly alternating repetitive movements, such as when using a screwdriver or hammer, and complex smooth pursuit movements, such as following a moving target with the eyes and limbs when using a rifle; and to control certain properties of movements including trajectory, velocity, and acceleration.

This chapter provides a view of the anatomic and physiologic properties of the cerebellum and demonstrates how this view can assist the clinician in localizing pathologic processes within this structure. Comprehending the functions of the cerebellum makes it possible to understand the basis of the neurologic deficits resulting from its dysfunction. This understanding can be facilitated by considering the relationship between the cerebellum and the rest of the central nervous system within an evolutionary framework.

CEREBELLAR ORGANIZATION: AN EVOLUTIONARY VIEW

Phylogenetically early forms of animal life such as reptiles, amphibians, and other lower vertebrates have evolved a well-developed spinal cord and brainstem together with an unfoliated cerebellum. The cerebellum of these early vertebrates is homologous chiefly with the medial portions of the cerebellum of higher vertebrates. In contrast, early vertebrates have poor development of the cerebral cortex and portions of the cerebellum homologous with the lateral parts of the cerebellum of later vertebrates. Correspondingly, early vertebrates have adequate

1

neurophysiologic mechanisms for controlling stance and gait but only rudimentary development of finely coordinated distal limb movements. In later evolutionary forms, culminating in high primates and the human, remarkable developments in the coordination of distal limb movements make possible the use of the distal extremities in arboreal life and in the performance of manipulative tasks. Associated with these phylogenetic changes there is parallel development of the cerebral cortex and the cerebellum, particularly the lateral portions of the cerebellum. This development includes the foliation of the cerebellum together with the elaboration of the cerebellar hemispheres.

In the central nervous systems of early and later animal forms, neurons controlling the body musculature generally are represented anatomically from medial to lateral. The medial segments of musculature are represented in the medial portions of the central nervous system and the lateral segments are represented in the lateral portions. Thus, at the level of the spinal cord, anterior horn cells innervating muscles of the trunk generally are located medially in the ventral horn. Conversely, anterior horn cells innervating muscles of the limbs are located in more lateral portions of the ventral horn. This organization of functional units at the level of the spinal cord holds true in a broad sense at higher levels of the central nervous system. Thus, at the level of the cerebral hemispheres, medial structures such as the basal ganglia are involved in movements of the proximal musculature, while the more laterally located cerebral cortex is involved in movements of the distal extremities.

The same overall principles hold for the functions of regions within the cerebellum. Midline cerebellar structures, the vermis and midline nuclei, are related generally to activities of the midline musculature of the body. The vermal portions of the cerebellar cortex make synaptic connections with the fastigial nuclei, which connect with the reticular and vestibular neurons of the brainstem. These cells have extensive ascending projections to brainstem nuclei controlling extraocular movements and descending projections to anterior horn cells of the spinal cord through reticulospinal and vestibulospinal projections. Taken together, these projections govern the function of eye movements, orientation of the head in space, and coordination of stance and gait.

The more lateral portions of the cerebellum, the hemispheres, are concerned with movements of the distal extremities. These phylogenetically more recent components of the cerebellar cortex contain neurons projecting to the dentate nuclei which project into the ventrolateral nucleus of the thalamus. Nerve fibers from the ventrolateral nucleus ascend into the precentral area of the cerebral cortex, a region involved in movements of the limbs. Thus, the lateral parts of the cerebellum make connections with a portion of the motor system concerned with finely coordinated movements of the extremities.

The intermediate region of the cerebellum is involved in functions characteristic of both the midline and the lateral components. Intermediate portions of the cerebellar cortex have projections to the interposed nuclei which project to the red nucleus and the ventrolateral thalamic nucleus. Many neurons in the red nucleus contacted by fibers from the interposed nuclei serve as the origin of the rubrospinal tract. This tract projects to the spinal cord and makes synaptic connections with both medial and lateral groups of anterior horn cells. Thus, the rubrospinal tract affects anterior horn cells related both to proximal and distal limb musculature. This pathway has been implicated in several motor functions, including phasic movements, standing, and walking.

Based on these principles, a correlation can be made between certain neurologic signs and dysfunction of specific portions of the cerebellum. Lesions of midline portions of the cerebellum, including the anterior and posterior segments of the vermis, generally result in disorders of eye movements (nystagmus), abnormal postures of the head, and disturbances of stance and gait. The classic example of this kind of disorder is cerebellar degeneration secondary to alcoholism. This process involves the anterior vermal portions of the cerebellar cortex, largely preserving the structure and function of the cerebellar hemispheres. Patients with this disorder develop a severe disturbance of standing and walking with relatively preserved fine coordinated movements of the limbs. In contrast, disease of the cerebellar hemispheres has been correlated with severe disturbances of limb movements as well as disorders of stance, gait, and posture.

Evidence from recent anatomic and physiologic studies indicates that these principles of functional localization are correct only in broad general terms and that the neurologic clinician should be cautious in accepting them without qualification. This evidence includes the demonstration that: 1) the functions of the cerebral cortex are related to movement of proximal as well as distal musculature; 2) the basal ganglia may be involved in movements of distal as well as proximal musculature; 3) a projection exists from the cerebellar hemispheres through the descending limb of the brachium conjunctivum relating the cerebellar hemispheres to the spinal cord; and 4) several precerebellar nuclei project extensively to both medial and lateral portions of the cerebellum. These observations must be considered in any attempt to formulate principles of organization for the central nervous system. Indeed, some of these points may account for the poor localization of function within the cerebellum observed thus far.

SUBDIVISIONS OF THE CEREBELLUM

Several classifications have been used to define the anatomic components of the cerebellum which consist grossly of two large hemispheres and a midline structure termed the vermis (Fig. 1A). These classifications have been derived from anatomic, phylogenetic, embryologic and functional considerations.

General Anatomic Organization

Anatomically, the cerebellum consists of three major components — the anterior, posterior, and flocculonodular lobes (Fig. 1A and B). The landmarks segregating these lobes include the primary fissure, which separates the anterior lobe from the posterior lobe, and the postnodular fissure, which separates the posterior lobe from the flocculonodular lobe. The three lobes are further subdivided into a series of lobules (Figs. 1 and 2).[1, 35-37] In the vermis proceeding from rostral to caudal, the lobules are named lingula, central lobule, culmen, declive, folium, tuber, pyramis, uvula, and nodulus. The relationship between each of these components of the vermis and the lobules of the hemispheres is listed in Table 1. Although the names of the lobules continue to appear in the literature, these terms have been replaced by the numbering system introduced by Larsell[34, 35] which consists of Roman numerals applied to each of the folia in the vermis (Figs. 1 and 2). The hemispheric extensions of these folia are indicated by the prefix H fol-

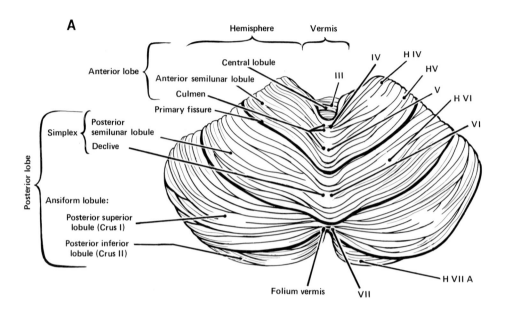

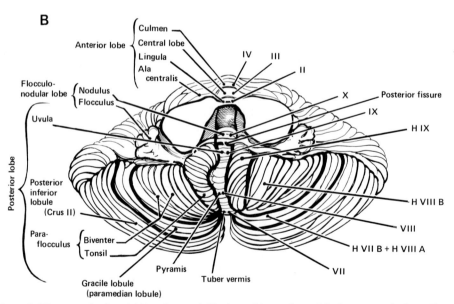

Figure 1. Diagrams of a dorsal (A) and ventral (B) view of the surface of the human cerebellum. These diagrams contain a synthesis of several types of nomenclature, including the names of the major lobes and lobules on the left and Larsell's numerical system on the right. Compare these diagrams with Table 1 for a rigorous correlation of the vermal and hemispheral components.

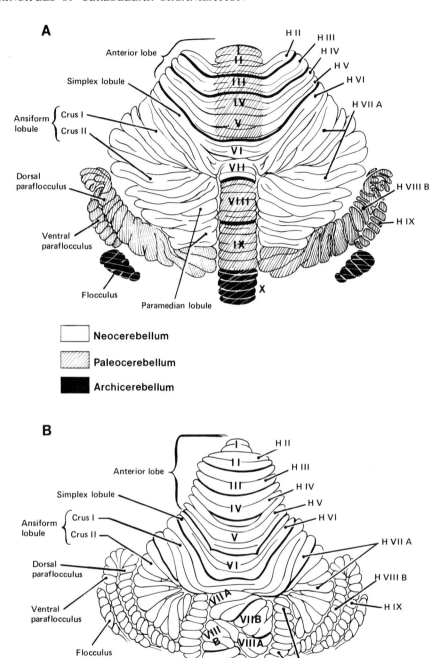

Figure 2. Diagrams of the monkey (A) and cat (B) cerebellar cortex. The cerebellum is shown "unfolded" to project the cerebellar cortex in a single plane. The components of the cerebellum comprising the neocerebellum, paleocerebellum, and archicerebellum are shown with shading in A. Note that a part of the vermis (lobules VI and VII) is actually a component of the neocerebellum.

Table 1. Components of the human cerebellum

Major Cerebellar Lobe	Hemisphere	Vermis
Anterior lobe	Ala centralis Anterior crescentic (semilunar) lobule	Lingula Central lobule Culmen
Posterior lobe	Posterior crescentic (semilunar) lobule Posterosuperior lobule Posteroinferior lobule Biventer Tonsilla	Declive Folium Tuber Pyramis Uvula
Flocculonodular lobe		Nodulus (flocculus)

lowed by the Roman numeral designation. Larsell's numerical system has been instrumental in providing a universal nomenclature with considerable phylogenetic consistency for each component of the cerebellum.

Comparative Anatomic Considerations

The terms archicerebellum, paleocerebellum, and neocerebellum have evolved from phylogenetic and embryologic studies. These studies originated with the examination of cerebellar embryogenesis by Comolli[9] and Edinger.[16] They proposed that the cerebellum can be divided into a paleocerebellum consisting of the midline vermal regions and a neocerebellum composed of the cerebellar hemispheres. Soon afterward, Bremer[2] pointed out the importance of the functional distinction between the paleocerebellum and the neocerebellum. Based on the effects of stimulating and ablating selected portions of these regions, he proposed that the paleocerebellum governs posture and movement through connections with brainstem structures and the neocerebellum governs these functions through connections with forebrain structures.

As cerebellar comparative anatomy became better understood, the flocculonodular lobe, phylogenetically the oldest component of the cerebellum, was viewed as a functionally distinct component of this structure. Hence, it was designated the archicerebellum.[13] Subsequent embryologic studies demonstrated that a zone between the cerebellar vermis and cerebellar hemispheres constitutes another distinct region of the cerebellum. This region, originally called the Zwischenstück,[22, 26, 28] subsequently has been designated the pars intermedia.

As described in the next section, the subdivisions of the cerebellum based on comparative anatomy match rather well the subdivisions based on the termination sites of afferent projections from the vestibular system, spinal cord, and forebrain — vestibulocerebellum, spinocerebellum, pontocerebellum. As more precise information became available concerning the anatomic and functional organization of these cerebellar afferent projections, the portions of the vermis in the posterior lobe receiving direct inputs from the pontine nuclei but not from the spinal cord were considered to be components of the neocerebellum.[17, 25, 34] These portions consist of the tuber, folium, and parts of the simplex. It has been difficult to classify the paramedian lobule into one of these subdivisions because its input and

6

output projections do not fit clearly into a single category. In current terminology, the archicerebellum is the flocculonodular lobe; the paleocerebellum consists of the vermis of the anterior lobe plus the pyramis, uvula, and paraflocculus; and the neocerebellum comprises the lateral parts of the cerebellum, including most of the hemispheres, and the middle portions of the vermis (see Fig. 2A).

Afferent and Efferent Organization

Other systems of nomenclature have been based on specific anatomic and physiologic characteristics of cerebellar afferent and efferent projections. One system is based on the sites of termination of the major afferent projections to the cerebellum, and, as mentioned above, this terminology overlaps with that derived from phylogenetic considerations. The vestibular afferents project heavily to the flocculonodular lobe (the archicerebellum) and thus the term "vestibulocerebellum" was applied to this lobe. Because the major afferent projections from the spinal cord terminate in the vermis (the paleocerebellum), the term "spinocerebellum" was given to this region. The projections from the pons terminate in the cerebellar hemispheres leading to the term "pontocerebellum" for the hemispheres.

The utility of dividing the cerebellum into three components based upon comparative anatomic considerations and afferent projection sites has decreased as anatomic and physiologic studies have shown that many cerebellar afferent and efferent projections are not confined to just one of these regions.[33] For example, the pontocerebellar projection, which classically is related to the lateral cerebellum, has been shown to terminate in both the paleocerebellum (the vermis) and the neocerebellum (the cerebellar hemispheres).[5, 24] Furthermore, vestibular afferents project to both the flocculonodular lobe and the vermis. As a consequence of these findings, it is no longer possible to divide the cerebellum strictly into the vestibulocerebellum, spinocerebellum, and pontocerebellum solely on the basis of afferent projections.[3] This classification is still used, however, because of its value in presenting experimental data and concepts concerning the predominant patterns of cerebellar organization.

Another system is based upon the organization of efferent projections from the cerebellar cortex to the deep cerebellar nuclei. In this classification the cerebellum is divided into three sagittal zones as is shown below.

SAGITTAL ZONES

Jansen and Brodal[28] made one of the initial contributions supporting the concept of sagittal zone organization in their studies of the projections from the cerebellar cortex to the cerebellar nuclei (Fig. 3A). They concluded that the cerebellum consists of three sagittal zones: 1) the midline zone, which contains cerebellar cortical neurons projecting to the fastigial nucleus; 2) the intermediate zone, including the paramedian lobule, which contains cortical neurons projecting to the interposed nuclei; and 3) the lateral zone, including the most lateral region of the anterior lobe and the lateral portions of crus I and II, which contains cortical neurons projecting to the dentate nucleus.[28] Contrary to prevailing views, cortical neurons of the paraflocculus were found to project to the parvocellular region of the dentate nucleus rather than to nuclei associated with the paleocerebellum. In addition, the cerebellar cortical neurons of the flocculus and nodulus were found

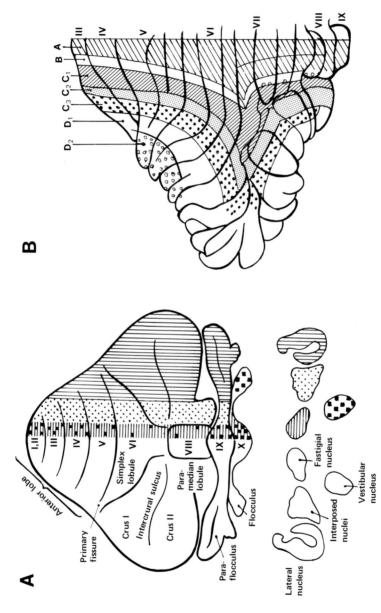

Figure 3. Diagrams of the zonal organization of the cerebellum. In the upper part of A, the cerebellum is divided into three sagittal zones, each of which connects with the deep cerebellar or vestibular nucleus shown in the lower part of A. This pattern of organization was obtained from studies of the projections of Purkinje cells onto the cerebellar nuclei in cats. B shows the results of recent studies of the zonal organization of cerebellar white matter in ferrets. Comparable but not identical zones have been shown in recent anatomic studies of the corticonuclear projections in cats. (A redrawn from Jansen and Brodal[28] and B redrawn from Voogd.[41] with permission.)

8

to project directly to the lateral vestibular (Deiters') nucleus in the brainstem rather than to one of the deep cerebellar nuclei.

Chambers and Sprague[7, 8] provided strong evidence supporting Jansen and Brodal's view that the cerebellum is organized functionally into longitudinally oriented sagittal zones. They showed that stimulation of the medial zone of the cerebellum evokes different patterns of movements in the extremities than those observed following stimulation of the intermediate zone. They also showed that neurologic deficits from lesions in the fastigial nucleus are different from those resulting from ablating the interposed or dentate nuclei. Their anatomic studies of the corticonuclear projection revealed a pattern of organization similar to that presented by Jansen and Brodal.

Eager's studies of the corticonuclear projection in cats[14] and monkeys[15] confirmed the sagittal organization of this projection but also suggested that there is more overlap between these zones than originally proposed. In the cat, cerebellar cortical lesions restricted to one of the sagittal zones of Jansen and Brodal caused degeneration in two and even three intracerebellar nuclei.[14] In the monkey, lesions of the paramedian lobule caused degeneration in all three cerebellar nuclei and lesions in the paravermal region of the anterior lobe led to degeneration in both the interposed and dentate nuclei.[15] Other investigators found a similar pattern of organization in the corticonuclear projections of birds[19, 23] and rats.[18] Despite this pattern of organization, however, stimulating the medial region of the cerebellum evoked different patterns of movement than stimulating the lateral region in these animals.[19]

Subsequent work in several species has substantiated the notion that the corticonuclear projection is organized into longitudinally oriented zones.[33, 40, 41] The predominance of each zone varies among different species, particularly with regard to the zones related to the cerebellar hemispheres.[30-33, 40, 41] In addition, the longitudinal organization of the cerebellum is much more complex than appreciated initially. Voogd[41] has found that there are at least seven longitudinal zones rather than three (Fig. 3B). Of these, the most medial zone in the vermis projects to the fastigial nucleus; the most lateral zone in the vermis projects to the lateral vestibular nucleus; the paravermal zone projects to the nucleus interpositus anterior and posterior; and the most lateral zone of the hemisphere projects to the dentate nucleus. In some regions such as the paramedian lobule the sagittal bands are very narrow. Consequently, small punctate lesions can interrupt cerebellar cortical axons projecting to more than one cerebellar nucleus. This may explain the discrepancies between the studies of Eager[14, 15] and those of other investigators. Voogd also showed that the strips in the hemispheres are not oriented strictly parallel to the sagittal plane. Rather, they are oriented perpendicular to the long axis of the folia (Fig. 3B).

The organization of corticonuclear projections has been clarified further with orthograde and retrograde labeling techniques for tracing neuronal pathways and refinements in degeneration techniques. These studies showed that corticonuclear fibers from the vermal regions of the anterior and posterior lobe in the cat clearly project only to the fastigial and the lateral vestibular nucleus.[10, 12] The corticonuclear projection to the fastigial nucleus originates in the cerebellar cortex medial to the region containing neurons projecting to the vestibular nuclei.[41] The corticonuclear projection from the vermis to the fastigial nucleus is organized topographically.[10, 20] In general, Purkinje cells in each lobule project to the closest location within the fastigial nucleus. The projection from the

9

paramedian lobule originates in very narrow zones. Fibers from the most lateral of these zones terminate in the dentate nucleus while those originating more medially terminate in the anterior and posterior interposed nuclei.[11] Cortico-nuclear fibers from crus II also terminate in these three cerebellar nuclei.[4] There is, however, no strict correlation between the laterality of the origin of a projection and the nucleus in which the projecting fibers terminate. This may relate to the fact that the folia of both crus I and II are not organized transversely to the caudal-rostral axis of the cerebellum. Similarly, there is no strict lon-

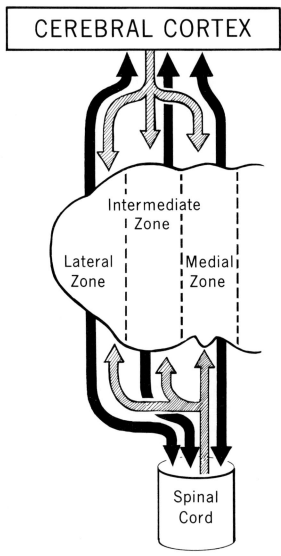

Figure 4. General organizational scheme of the afferent (shaded arrows) and efferent (solid arrows) projections of the three major cerebellar zones. All three zones, although morphologically distinct, are involved in interactions in the forebrain as well as in the brainstem and spinal cord.

10

gitudinal pattern for the zones from which the corticonuclear fibers in the hemispheres originate. Rather, these projections are oriented perpendicular to the direction of the folia in crus I and crus II.[40] Cerebellar cortical neurons in the flocculonodular lobe terminate within the vestibular fastigial nuclei and also within the ventral portions of the dentate nucleus, at least in the prosimian primate.[21]

The connections of a newly described projection to the cerebellar cortex, the nucleocortical fibers[38, 39] (see Chap. 2), have provided additional information regarding the sagittal organization of the cerebellum. These fibers originate in the deep cerebellar nuclei and terminate in the cerebellar cortex.[38, 39] In the cat, the organization of this projection correlates well with the organization of the corticonuclear fibers. The nucleocortical fibers from a given nucleus terminate in cerebellar cortical regions containing Purkinje cells that project back to the same cerebellar nucleus. In the monkey, however, the nucleocortical projections are not organized this way. Some nucleocortical fibers from the dentate nucleus, which is in the lateral zone, terminate in the cerebellar vermis.[38, 39] Consequently, the output of the lateral cerebellar nucleus can affect information processing in the most medial sagittal cerebellar cortical zone.

Other studies, reviewed in detail in Chapter 6, have addressed an important issue of cerebellar organization, namely the interaction of each cerebellar zone with other components of the central nervous system. All cerebellar zones, including the midline zone, have projections affecting neurons in forebrain structures as well as in the spinal cord. Even the most lateral cerebellar nucleus, the dentate nucleus, receives inputs from the flocculonodular lobe and projects to brainstem nuclei involved in eye movements, a function not often ascribed to the neocerebellum. Conversely, all cerebellar zones receive inputs either directly or indirectly from the spinal cord as well as from the forebrain. As a consequence, the interactions of each cerebellar zone cannot occur independently from those of other zones. It seems likely that both lateral and medial regions of the cerebellum are involved in posture as well as finely coordinated movements of the extremities, although the specific contribution of each cerebellar region to these different types of motor activity may be different. This overall pattern of organization is summarized in Figure 4.

REFERENCES

1. BOLK, L.: *Das Cerebellum der Saugetiere: Eine vergleichend anatomische Untersuchung.* Fischer-Verlag, Haarlem and Jena, 1906.

2. BREMER, F.: *Contribution à l'étude de la physiologie du cervelet: La fonction inhibitrice du paléocerebellum.* Arch. Int. Physiol. 19:189, 1922.

3. BRODAL, A.: *Cerebrocerebellar pathways. Anatomical data and some functional implications.* Acta Neurol. Scand. (Suppl.) 51:153, 1972.

4. BRODAL, A., AND COURVILLE, J.: *Cerebellar corticonuclear projection in the cat. Crus II: An experimental study with silver methods.* Brain Res. 50:1, 1973.

5. BRODAL, A., AND JANSEN, J.: *The ponto-cerebellar projection in the rabbit and cat. Experimental investigations.* J. Comp. Neurol. 84:31, 1946.

6. CARPENTER, M. B. AND STROMINGER, N. L.: *Cerebello-oculomotor fibers in the rhesus monkey.* J. Comp. Neurol. 123:211, 1964.

7. CHAMBERS, W. W., AND SPRAGUE, J. M.: *Functional localization in the cerebellum I. Organization in longitudinal cortico-nuclear zones and their contribution to the control of posture, both extrapyramidal and pyramidal.* J. Comp. Neurol. 103:105, 1955.

8. CHAMBERS, W. W., AND SPRAGUE, J. M.: *Functional localization in the cerebellum. II. Somatotopic organization in cortex and nuclei.* Arch. Neurol. Psychiat. 74:653, 1955.

9. COMOLLI, A.: *Per una nuova divisione del cervelletto dei mammiferi.* Arch. Ital. Anat. Embriol. 9: 247, 1910.

10. COURVILLE, J., AND DIAKIW, N.: *Cerebellar corticonuclear projection in the cat. The vermis of the anterior and posterior lobes.* Brain Res. 110:1, 1976.

11. COURVILLE, J., DIAKIW, N., AND BRODAL, A.: *Cerebellar corticonuclear projection in the cat. The paramedian lobule. An experimental study with silver methods.* Brain Res. 50:25, 1973.

12. COURVILLE, J., AND FARACO-CANTIN, F.: *Cerebellar corticonuclear projection demonstrated by the horseradish peroxidase method.* Neuroscience Abstr. 2, 1976, p. 108.

13. DOW, R. S.: *The electrical activity of the cerebellum and its functional significance.* J. Physiol. 94:67, 1938.

14. EAGER, R. P.: *Efferent cortico-nuclear pathways in the cerebellum of the cat.* J. Comp. Neurol. 120:81, 1963.

15. EAGER, R. P.: *Patterns and mode of termination of cerebellar corticonuclear pathways in the monkey (Macaca mulatta).* J. Comp. Neurol. 126:551, 1966.

16. EDINGER, L.: *Über die Einteilung des Cerebellums.* Anat. Anz. 35:319, 1909.

17. FULTON, J. F., AND DOW, R. S.: *The cerebellum: A summary of functional localization.* Yale J. Biol. Med. 10:89, 1937.

18. GOODMAN, D. C., HALLETT, R. E., AND WELCH, R. B.: *Patterns of localization in the cerebellar cortico-nuclear projections of the albino rat.* J. Comp. Neurol. 121:51, 1963.

19. GOODMAN, D. C., HOREL, J. A., AND FREEMAN, F. R.: *Functional localization in the cerebellum of the bird and its bearing on the evolution of cerebellar function.* J. Comp. Neurol. 123:45, 1964.

20. HAINES, D. E.: *Cerebellar cortical efferents of the posterior lobe vermis in a prosimian primate (Galago) and the tree shrew (Tupaia).* J. Comp. Neurol. 163:21, 1975.

21. HAINES, D. E.: *Cerebellar corticonuclear and corticovestibular fibers of the flocculonodular lobe in a prosimian primate.* J. Comp. Neurol. 174:607, 1977.

22. HAJASHI, M.: *Einige wichtige Tatsachen aus der ontogenetischen Entwicklung des menschlichen Kleinhirns, mit Demonstrationen.* Dtsch. Z. Nervenheilkd. 81:74, 1924.

23. HOREL, J. A., AND GOODMAN, D. C.: *Cerebellar corticonuclear projections of the bird (Anas domesticus).* Anat. Rec. 148:292, 1964.

24. INGVAR, S.: *Zur Phylo- und Ontogenese des Kleinhirns.* Folia Neuro-biol. (Leipzig) 11:205, 1918.

25. INGVAR, S.: *On cerebellar localization.* Brain 46:301, 1923.

26. JAKOB, A.: *Zum Problem der morphologischen und funktionellen Gliederung des Kleinhirns.* Dtsch. Z. Nervenheilkd. 105:217, 1928.

27. JAKOB, A.: *Das Kleinhirn,* in vonMöllendorf, W. (ed.): *Handbuch der Mikroskopischen Anatomie des Menschen.* Springer, Berlin, 1928, Vol. IV, pp. 674–916.

28. JANSEN, J., AND BRODAL, A.: *Experimental studies on the intrinsic fibers of the cerebellum. II. The corticonuclear projection.* J. Comp. Neurol. 73:267, 1940.

29. JANSEN, J., AND BRODAL, A.: *Experimental studies on the intrinsic fibers of the cerebellum. The corticonuclear projection in the rabbit and the monkey (Macacus rhesus).* Skr. Norske Vid.-Akad. Oslo (Avh.), I. Mat.-Naturv. Kl. No. 3, pp. 1–50, 1942.

30. KORNELIUSSEN, H. K.: *Cerebellar corticogenesis in Cetacea, with special reference to regional variations.* J. Hirnforsch. 9:151, 1967.

31. KORNELIUSSEN, H. K.: *Comments on the cerebellum and its division.* Brain Res. 8:229, 1968.

32. KORNELIUSSEN, H. K.: *On the ontogenetic development of the cerebellum (nuclei, fissures, and cortex) of the rat with special reference to regional variations in corticogenesis.* J. Hirnforsch. 10: 379, 1968.

33. KORNELIUSSEN, H. K.: *Histogenesis of the cerebellar cortex and cortical zones,* in Larsell, O., and Jansen, J. (eds.): *The comparative anatomy and histology of the cerebellum. The human cerebellum, cerebellar connections, and cerebellar cortex.* University of Minnesota Press, Minneapolis, 1972, pp. 164–174.

34. LARSELL, O.: *The cerebellum: A review and interpretation.* Arch. Neurol. Psychiat. 38:580, 1937.

35. LARSELL, O.: *The development of the cerebellum in man in relation to its comparative anatomy.* J. Comp. Neurol. 87:85, 1947.

36. LARSELL, O., AND JANSEN, J.: *The comparative anatomy and histology of the cerebellum: the human cerebellum, cerebellar connections, and cerebellar cortex.* University of Minnesota Press, Minneapolis, 1972.
37. SMITH, G. E.: *The primary subdivision of the mammalian cerebellum.* J. Anat. 36:381, 1902.
38. TOLBERT, D. L., BANTLI, H., AND BLOEDEL, J. R.: *The organization of the cerebellar nucleocortical projection in the monkey.* Anat. Rec. 190:562, 1978.
39. TOLBERT, D. L., BANTLI, H., AND BLOEDEL, J. R.: *Organizational features of the cat and monkey cerebellar nucleocortical projection.* J. Comp. Neurol. 182: 39, 1978.
40. VOOGD, J.: *The Cerebellum of the Cat. Structure and Fibre Connexions.* F. A. Davis, Philadelphia, 1964.
41. VOOGD, J.: *The importance of fibre connections in the comparative anatomy of the mammalian cerebellum,* in Llinas, R. (ed.): *Neurobiology of cerebellar evolution and development.* AMA, Chicago, 1969, pp. 493–514.

CHAPTER 2

Inputs to the Cerebellum:
Mossy Fiber Afferents

Large numbers of afferent projections carry information to the cerebellum from the peripheral nervous system and other parts of the central nervous system. In the past, these cerebellar afferent projections were divided into two types based on the morphologic characteristics of their terminal fibers. Recently, a third type has been described.[21] The first type, the mossy fibers, originates in many extracerebellar sites and terminates in the granular layer of the cerebellar cortex. The term "mossy fiber" was applied to these afferents because their terminals appeared moss-like on histologic examination. The second type, the climbing fibers, originates within a single nucleus, the inferior olive.[21] The term "climbing fiber" was derived from the characteristic way each fiber climbs along the dendritic tree of a Purkinje cell, forming multiple synapses as it entwines about the proximal and distal portions of the dendrites. The third type of cerebellar afferent, the aminergic fibers, has terminations that differ from those of both mossy fibers and climbing fibers.[21]

Mossy fiber afferents originate in the spinal cord, pontine nuclei, vestibular receptors and nuclei, trigeminal nuclei, reticular nuclei, and deep cerebellar nuclei. The spinocerebellar, pontocerebellar and reticulocerebellar pathways contain the largest number of projecting fibers. Afferents originating in the spinal cord project through the spinocerebellar pathways directly into the cerebellum. The spinocerebellar pathways convey information from spinal levels, though this information can be modified at the spinal level through the effects of descending projections. One component of these pathways, the dorsal spinocerebellar tract, enters the cerebellum through the inferior cerebellar peduncle. The other component, the ventral spinocerebellar tract, enters through the superior cerebellar peduncle. The afferents originating in the pontine nuclei project to the cerebellum in the pontocerebellar pathway which courses through the middle cerebellar peduncle. This projection conveys information mainly from the cerebral cortex through the corticopontine pathway. The reticular nuclei project information from the brainstem to the cerebellum, integrating information originating in a number of ascending and descending pathways. The reticulocerebellar afferents enter the cerebellum through the inferior and middle cerebellar peduncles.

SPINOCEREBELLAR PROJECTIONS

Dorsal Spinocerebellar Tract

Anatomic Characteristics

The dorsal spinocerebellar tract originates in neurons located in a long spinal nucleus termed Clarke's column or the nucleus dorsalis.[140, 204, 242, 264] This nucleus is located in the base of the posterior horn, extending from spinal segment T_1 to approximately L_4.[60, 131, 215, 235] The dorsal spinocerebellar tract ascends ipsilaterally along the dorsolateral part of the spinal cord and enters the cerebellum through the inferior cerebellar peduncle (Fig. 1B). The tract terminates in the anterior vermis and paravermis as well as in parts of the posterior vermis.[128, 235, 285] In the anterior vermis, the tract projects to lobules II to IV and a portion of lobule V. Posteriorly, there are projections to sublobules VIIIB and VIIIA, the paramedian lobule, and the dorsal paraflocculus (Fig. 1A).

The primary afferent fibers projecting to Clarke's column originate in dorsal roots extending from T_2 to S_1; projections from caudal cervical roots have been reported also.[22, 201] Many primary afferent fibers form synaptic junctions with the large cells of Clarke's column, the focal cells, contacting them on as many as 50 sites. In addition, some primary afferent fibers make synaptic connections with other afferent fibers, thereby forming axo-axonic synapses.[258] The demonstration of axo-axonic synapses in Clarke's column has led to the conclusion that the activity of some afferent terminals ending in this nucleus can affect the actions of other fibers projecting to the same nucleus. Axo-axonic synapses are thought to mediate primary afferent depolarization, which is a voltage change of the membranes of the terminal arborizations of primary afferent fibers.[261] As a consequence of this voltage change, there is a reduction in the release of transmitter when an action potential invades these terminals. This effect has been termed "presynaptic inhibition" and is distinguished from postsynaptic inhibition, which results from the direct action of a transmitter released by the presynaptic fiber on the membrane of the postsynaptic neuron. Presynaptic inhibition provides a method of controlling the actions of individual afferent terminals, whereas postsynaptic inhibition provides a mechanism for controlling the excitability of the neuron receiving input from the afferent terminals.

Collaterals of the dorsal spinocerebellar tract project to several extracerebellar structures (Fig. 2). Axons of some focal cells in Clarke's column form collaterals that terminate on other neurons within Clarke's column or in some other component of the spinal cord gray matter.[183, 215, 250, 272] Fibers in the dorsolateral fasciculus, probably from the dorsal spinocerebellar tract, contact neurons in brainstem nuclei x and z.[35, 40, 173, 174, 228] As shown electrophysiologically, these fibers monosynaptically activate neurons in nucleus z, a nucleus that mediates information from muscle proprioceptors to the forebrain. This information may be used in the perception of muscle length. Collaterals of the dorsal spinocerebellar tract probably contact neurons in one of the reticular nuclei projecting to the cerebellum, the lateral reticular nucleus,[20, 228] though the existence of this collateral projection is controversial.

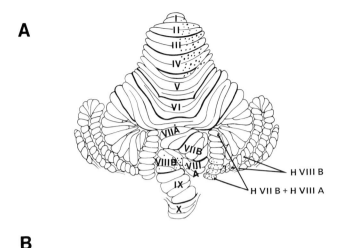

A

H VIII B

H VII B + H VIII A

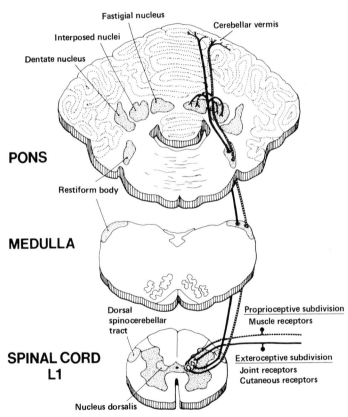

B

Fastigial nucleus

Interposed nuclei

Dentate nucleus

Cerebellar vermis

PONS

Restiform body

MEDULLA

Dorsal spinocerebellar tract

SPINAL CORD L1

Nucleus dorsalis

Proprioceptive subdivision
Muscle receptors

Exteroceptive subdivision
Joint receptors
Cutaneous receptors

Dorsal Spinocerebellar Tract

Figure 1. The organization of the dorsal spinocerebellar tract. A, Areas of termination in the cerebellar cortex are indicated by dots. Note that the pathway projects to both anterior and posterior lobes. B, The course of the dorsal spinocerebellar pathway. The cells of origin in Clarke's column are divided into exteroceptive and proprioceptive subdivisions. The fibers ascend ipsilaterally in the dorsolateral part of the spinal cord, entering the cerebellum through the restiform body, projecting to cerebellar nuclei and cerebellar cortex. (A, redrawn from Grant,[128] with permission.)

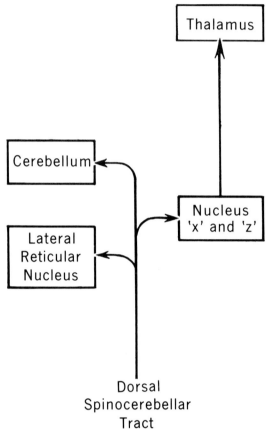

Figure 2. The projections of the dorsal spinocerebellar tract. This pathway terminates in the lateral reticular nucleus and in nuclei 'x' and 'z' in the brainstem. Although the projection to the lateral reticular nucleus has not been established with certainty, the existence of the projection is supported by both electrophysiologic and anatomic data.

Physiologic Properties

PROPRIOCEPTIVE SUBDIVISION. The dorsal spinocerebellar tract is divided into proprioceptive and exteroceptive subdivisions based upon the responses of neurons in Clarke's column to peripheral stimuli (see Fig. 1B).[215, 235] Neurons in the proprioceptive subdivision are activated by fibers of group Ia afferents (nerve fibers mediating information from muscle spindle primary afferents), group Ib afferents (nerve fibers from Golgi tendon organs), and group II afferents (nerve fibers from muscle spindle secondary afferents).[215, 235] Some neurons in the proprioceptive subdivision also receive polysynaptically mediated inputs from cutaneous afferents and from the more slowly conducting afferent fibers originating in muscle, the "flexor reflex afferents."[157, 166, 167] The flexor reflex afferents consist of the peripheral nerve fibers originating outside of the muscle spindle responsible for mediating the flexor reflex, which is a limb withdrawal movement from a noxious stimulus.

Activation of the proprioceptive afferents projecting to the proprioceptive subdivision leads to a large excitability change, even with stimulation of few peripheral fibers.[106, 108, 123, 185, 227] Spontaneously occurring excitatory postsynaptic potentials (EPSPs) have amplitudes as high as 5 mv and monosynaptically evoked EPSPs may have amplitudes of 65 mv.[96, 106, 108, 185] The large magnitude of these synaptic effects results from the extensive convergence of primary afferent fibers onto individual neurons in Clarke's column and on the multiple sites of synaptic contact between single afferent fibers and the dendrites of individual focal cells.[187 251, 258] The implication of these findings is that information carried by proprioceptive afferents can be transferred accurately to focal cells where additional integration occurs.

The initial electrophysiologic studies of neurons in Clarke's column, carried out with extracellular recording techniques, revealed little evidence of convergence among the different types of afferents.[235] Subsequent studies employing intracellular techniques, however, gave clear evidence of convergence. Convergence occurs both among different types of proprioceptive afferents and among afferent fibers originating in different muscle groups. Combinations of excitatory and inhibitory inputs can be evoked in neurons within the proprioceptive subdivision by stimulation of group Ia, Ib, and group II afferent fibers.[96] Some degree of reciprocal inhibition occurs among these segmental inputs. Thus, afferents from agonist and antagonist muscles can affect reciprocally the excitability of individual cells.[87, 96, 168-170] The convergence of excitatory and inhibitory inputs leads to complex patterns of integration in Clarke's column.

The cells of origin of the dorsal spinocerebellar tract have specific electrophysiologic properties which contribute to their responses to peripheral inputs. These cells have low thresholds as well as a characteristic after-hyperpolarization following an action potential.[107, 108, 185, 227] The after-hyperpolarization initially was ascribed to the action of an electrogenic pump,[185] but later was shown to result from increased membrane permeability to potassium.[134-138] Models of the behavior of these neurons have been constructed, based on combinations of two features: 1) the relationship between the number of quanta released presynaptically and the threshold of the cells[171, 172, 268, 269, 281] and 2) the characteristics of the after-hyperpolarization.[136] The models indicate how these features are important in determining the responses of these neurons to peripheral stimuli.

Neurons in the proprioceptive subdivision respond linearly to inputs consisting of small amplitudes of muscle stretch. When larger amplitudes (1 to 5 mm) of muscle stretch are used, however, nonlinear responses appear.[145] Some of these nonlinearities probably reflect nonlinearities in the responses of muscle spindles and the actions of segmental polysynaptic projections from muscle afferents to neurons in the proprioceptive division.[181]

Central nervous system pathways descending into the spinal cord affect the responses of neurons in Clarke's column to proprioceptive stimuli. Although the issue remains controversial,[19, 238] pathways originating in the cerebral cortex appear to affect the action of group I afferents on these neurons by both presynaptic and postsynaptic inhibitory mechanisms. The presynaptic inhibitory effects produced by stimulating the cerebral cortex occur only on the terminals of group Ib afferent fibers.[157, 158, 207, 213] The inhibitory effects of cerebral cortical stimulation disappear after lesions transecting the pyramids, indicating that the effects are mediated by the corticospinal tract. This conclusion presents an enigma, however, because some investigators have found that the corticospinal pathway exerts only a weak action on neurons in the proprioceptive subdivision.[183]

19

In summary, the proprioceptive subdivision of the dorsal spinocerebellar tract is much more than a relay pathway. Although it is capable of preserving information from the periphery and sending the information to the cerebellum, considerable integration can occur within its cells of origin. This integration reflects the pattern of convergence from peripheral inputs, synaptic interaction in Clarke's column, the electrophysiologic properties of the neurons, and the actions of descending pathways.

EXTEROCEPTIVE SUBDIVISION. A large group of neurons within Clarke's column responds preferentially to cutaneous (exteroceptive) inputs.[74, 75, 157, 179, 183, 214] These neurons have been designated the exteroceptive subdivision of the dorsal spinocerebellar tract.[214, 215, 235] They can be divided further into three groups based on their responses to input from different types of cutaneous afferents (see Fig. 1B).[192, 208, 215] These groups include those responsive to: 1) slowly adapting receptors on the footpad; 2) both phasic and tonic mechanoreceptors in hairy skin; and 3) both cutaneous and high threshold muscle inputs (flexor reflex afferents). Neurons responding preferentially to the activation of joint afferents have not been placed uniformly within either the proprioceptive or the exteroceptive subdivision.[179, 183, 186, 200] Because these neurons are activated also by cutaneous inputs, they have been included in the exteroceptive subdivision.[19]

Some dorsal spinocerebellar tract neurons responsive to stimulation of exteroceptive afferents are located outside of Clarke's column. Some responding preferentially to stimulation of flexor reflex afferents are located caudal to Clarke's column,[273] and some responding to stimulation of cutaneous and joint afferents are located lateral to Clarke's column in laminae IV and V of the dorsal horn.[186]

The receptive fields of neurons in the exteroceptive subdivision vary from a few square centimeters to a large region of the body surface. Some neurons have discontinuous receptive fields. The type of cutaneous stimuli to which a specific neuron responds in some cases depends upon the location in the receptive field at which the stimulus is applied.[215]

Similar to the neurons in the proprioceptive subdivision, those in the exteroceptive subdivision are highly sensitive to the effects of peripheral afferent inputs.[214, 216] The discharge of neurons in the exteroceptive subdivision usually replicates closely the discharge of the afferent fibers activated by the cutaneous stimulus.[214, 215] For example, neurons in Clarke's column activated by hair movement usually respond like the peripheral afferents with a single pulse or a short burst. The implication of this finding is that exteroceptive information carried in a peripheral afferent fiber can be transferred accurately to neurons in the exteroceptive subdivision.

Projections descending within the central nervous system, notably the corticospinal tract, affect the excitability of neurons in the exteroceptive subdivision of Clarke's column.[157, 183, 243] The effects of the corticospinal projection on neurons in this subdivision are generally stronger than those on neurons in the proprioceptive subdivision. The corticospinal pathway exerts both excitatory and inhibitory effects, including presynaptic inhibition,[157] and modifies the responses of neurons in the exteroceptive subdivision to inputs from the flexor reflex afferents. These modifications include effects on inhibitory interneurons activated by flexor reflex afferents which are not involved in reciprocal pathways and on interneurons mediating the excitatory segmental actions of flexor reflex afferents.[59, 154, 205, 207]

Projections descending from the brainstem can modify the behavior of neurons in the exteroceptive subdivision of Clarke's column.[140] One of these, the dorsal reticulospinal pathway, suppresses the effects of flexor reflex afferents and thereby reduces their actions on neurons in the exteroceptive subdivision.[153, 155, 235] An aminergic projection originating in the medial caudal brainstem also affects the action of flexor reflex afferents upon neurons in the exteroceptive subdivision.[88, 112-114, 140, 153, 154, 210] This projection, a component of the raphe-spinal pathway,[16, 88] descends through the dorsolateral fasciculus and affects the responses of neurons in Clarke's column to both high and low intensity cutaneous stimuli.[140] Thus, a descending pathway which affects the perception of noxious stimuli also affects the processing of information in cerebellar afferent pathways.

SUMMARY. The exteroceptive and the proprioceptive subdivisions of the dorsal spinocerebellar tract share two general features of the information processing that occurs in cerebellar afferent pathways. First, because of the strong synaptic coupling between the direct projections of primary afferent fibers and neurons in Clarke's column, the dorsal spinocerebellar tract can convey precise information to the cerebellum regarding the characteristics of stimuli applied to receptors in the skin, muscles, and joints. Second, the responses of neurons in Clarke's column can be modified by the combined actions of peripheral afferents and the descending central nervous system pathways involved in motor behavior.

Ventral Spinocerebellar Tract

Anatomic Characteristics

The ventral spinocerebellar tract originates chiefly in the spinal border cells, which are located in the lateral region of the ventral horn of lumbar segments L_3 to L_6.[53, 76, 116, 159, 209, 226, 267] The tract crosses the spinal cord and ascends in the contralateral ventrolateral fasciculus (Fig. 3B). In the brainstem the tract passes through the medulla and pons, entering the cerebellum through the superior cerebellar penduncle.[197] A projection through the inferior cerebellar peduncle has been reported,[226, 262] but this finding probably is artifactual, resulting from the interruption of dorsal spinocerebellar tract fibers which intermix with ventral spinocerebellar tract fibers in the spinal cord.

The ventral spinocerebellar tract enters the cerebellum, crosses, and terminates chiefly in the anterior lobe ipsilateral to the cells of origin of the projection.[65, 128, 282, 292] In both cat and monkey the projections are distributed predominantly to the paravermal region of lobules II to VI (Fig. 3A). There is a projection also to the paravermal region contralateral to the cells of origin, but this projection is much less dense than the ipsilateral projection. Posteriorly, fibers project to lobule VIII, particularly VIII B, and in the monkey to lobule IX as well.[282] In the cat,[128] fibers terminate in the dorsal paraflocculus and in the paramedian lobule.[128]

Physiologic Properties

RESPONSES TO PROPRIOCEPTIVE AND EXTEROCEPTIVE STIMULI. The spinal border cells giving rise to the ventral spinocerebellar tract respond to both exteroceptive and proprioceptive stimuli.[232-234] The initial studies of these neurons, based on extracellular recordings, showed that they receive monosynaptic projections only from group Ib afferent fibers.[234, 235] Subsequent intracellular recordings, however, revealed responses to group Ia afferents as well.[93, 211, 212] The input from many of these afferents is monosynaptic, but the postsynaptic potentials evoked by them often are too small to initiate action potentials. This is probably why the input from group Ia afferents was overlooked in earlier experiments. Each group

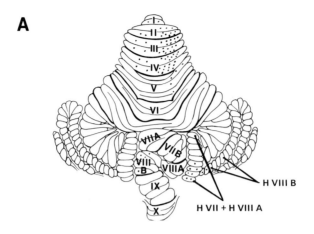

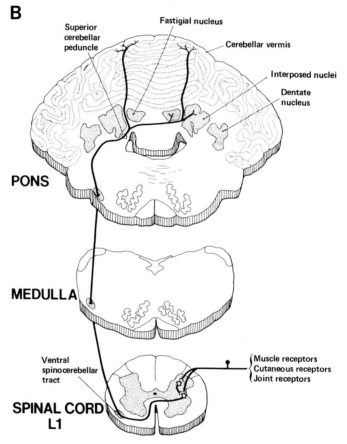

Ventral Spinocerebellar Tract

Figure 3. The organization of the ventral spinocerebellar tract. A, Areas of termination in the cerebellar cortex are indicated by dots. B, The course of the ventral spinocerebellar pathway. The cells of origin receive inputs from receptors in muscle, skin and joints. The pathway crosses both at the level of the spinal cord and in the cerebellar white matter after entering the cerebellum through the superior cerebellar peduncle. Note that this pathway terminates both in the cerebellar cortex and the cerebellar nuclei. (A, redrawn from Grant,[128] with permission.)

22

Ia and Ib afferent fiber contacts several pools of neurons. In general, the resulting convergence occurs among the afferents originating in functionally related groups of muscles.[198, 199, 212, 238]

Primary afferents projecting to spinal border cells also make connections with other pools of spinal neurons, including interneurons and alpha motoneurons. Thus, the actions of cutaneous and flexor reflex afferents on ventral spinocerebellar tract neurons are generally similar to their actions on alpha motoneurons.[105, 232, 233, 238] Both spinal border cells and alpha motoneurons are activated by flexor reflex afferents from the contralateral limb and from the periphery of the receptive field on the ipsilateral hindlimb. Stimulating the center of the receptive field inhibits both spinal border cells and alpha motoneurons.[105, 232, 233, 238] Some peripheral afferent fibers have parallel projections to spinal border cells and to certain pools of inhibitory interneurons. Thus, some ventral spinocerebellar tract neurons are activated monosynaptically and inhibited disynaptically by the same Ia and Ib afferent fibers.[211] The interneurons mediating this inhibition are the same as those which inhibit alpha motoneurons following activation of group I afferents. These properties indicate that ventral spinocerebellar tract neurons are organized so as to integrate exteroceptive and proprioceptive information from the periphery. In addition, the effects of these afferents are similar to those which they exert on some inhibitory interneurons and alpha motoneurons.

RESPONSES TO INPUTS FROM DESCENDING PATHWAYS. Several descending pathways have similar effects on neurons of the ventral spinocerebellar tract, alpha motoneurons, and some inhibitory interneurons. The rubrospinal and vestibulospinal projections activate monosynaptically both spinal border cells and alpha motoneurons.[11, 13] These two pathways also increase the amplitude of disynaptic inhibitory postsynaptic potentials evoked by Ia and Ib afferents on both types of neurons. In addition, these two pathways enhance the postsynaptic potentials evoked by flexor reflex afferents in both types of neurons.[12, 14] The corticospinal tract also has similar effects on spinal border cells and alpha motoneurons. These effects occur through actions on: 1) Ia inhibitory interneurons; 2) Ib reciprocal interneurons; and 3) inhibitory interneurons mediating the specific segmental effects of flexor reflex afferents.[59, 119, 154, 207, 213, 237]

Other pathways descending from the brainstem affect the excitability of the spinal border cells. One of these projections originates in the brainstem reticular formation and courses through the dorsolateral fasciculus of the spinal cord. This pathway suppresses tonically the actions of flexor reflex afferents on spinal border cells.[153, 155, 213, 234] A descending aminergic pathway, probably originating in the raphe nuclei, also affects the actions of the flexor reflex afferents on spinal border cells.[112, 153, 205, 234] This aminergic projection suppresses the excitability of interneurons receiving inputs from the flexor reflex afferents and also affects the excitability of some interneurons influenced by Ia and Ib afferents.[13, 114, 210, 213] The tonic inhibitory action of the aminergic projection can reduce the effects of inputs from flexor reflex afferents to ventral spinocerebellar neurons, leaving the action of proprioceptive inputs relatively unaffected. When the aminergic pathway is interrupted by severing the spinal cord, however, the ventral spinocerebellar tract neurons respond predominantly to cutaneous stimuli. Thus, the aminergic pathway appears to regulate the relative sensitivity of spinal border cells to inputs activated by exteroceptive or proprioceptive stimuli.

Three pathways descending from the brainstem facilitate the excitatory action of flexor reflex afferents on ventral spinocerebellar tract neurons.[13, 213] These pathways are the lateral vestibulospinal tract, a projection in the medial longitudinal fasciculus, and the rubrospinal tract. A fourth projection, which descends in the medial longitudinal fasciculus, has predominantly inhibitory effects on the actions of these afferents.[13, 15]

Descending projections modulate the excitability of ventral spinocerebellar tract neurons during locomotion. Even in deafferented preparations, these neurons show periodic excitability changes during walking, a characteristic not shared by neurons in Clarke's column.[6, 7]

LUNDBERG'S HYPOTHESIS. Lundberg[206] proposed that the ventral spinocerebellar tract neurons act as comparators between the action of the last order inhibitory interneurons and the excitatory input to them (Fig. 4). He based this proposal upon the finding that several peripheral inputs and descending pathways have similar effects on spinal border cells, inhibitory spinal interneurons, and alpha motoneurons. According to his hypothesis, peripheral afferents evoke changes in the

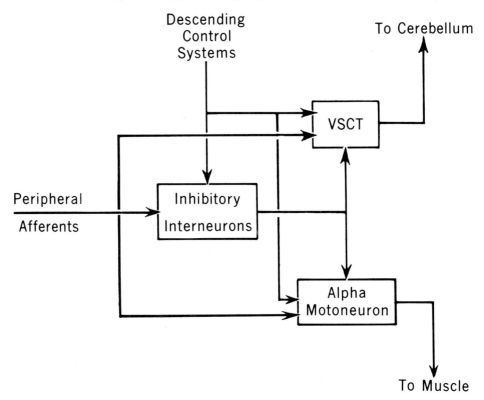

LUNDBERG'S HYPOTHESIS

Figure 4. Summary of Lundberg's hypothesis. The cells of origin of the ventral spinocerebellar tract receive inputs from primary afferent fibers and descending pathways as well as from interneurons. The interneurons receive inputs from the same primary afferent fibers and descending pathways. Alpha motoneurons receive inputs from the same primary afferent fibers, descending pathways, and interneurons. As a consequence of this organization, neurons of the ventral spinocerebellar tract can compare the combined excitatory and inhibitory actions of peripheral and descending inputs to spinal motoneurons, a comparison which reflects changes in the excitability of the inhibitory interneurons. VSCT = ventral spinocerebellar tract.

excitability of spinal border cells that depend upon and therefore reflect the excitability of spinal interneurons which receive the same inputs. Moreover, peripheral afferents evoke comparable responses in spinal border cells and alpha motoneurons because the inputs to these neurons are organized in parallel.

The same organizational pattern exists for the connections of many descending projections with spinal border cells, segmental interneurons, and alpha motoneurons. The synaptic effects upon these neurons of the rubrospinal, vestibulospinal, and corticospinal tracts are consistent with Lundberg's hypothesis. The actions of other descending projections have not been studied as completely. The available data indicate, however, that these pathways affect the actions of peripheral afferents on spinal border cells in a manner consistent with his proposal.

SUMMARY. The neurons giving rise to the ventral spinocerebellar tract integrate information from exteroceptive and proprioceptive peripheral inputs as well as from many descending pathways. The excitability changes occurring in these neurons reflect the action of the same inputs on pools of inhibitory interneurons and alpha motoneurons. The organization of these pathways supports Lundberg's hypothesis that the ventral spinocerebellar tract conveys information to the cerebellum about the excitability of these interneurons and the effects of many peripheral inputs to alpha motoneurons.

Spinocerebellar Tracts from the Cervical Cord

The dorsal and ventral spinocerebellar tracts, the two most extensively studied spinocerebellar pathways, mediate information only from the hindlimb. Another pair of spinocerebellar pathways transmits information from the forelimb. One pathway, the cuneocerebellar tract, is the forelimb equivalent of the dorsal spinocerebellar tract. The other, the rostral spinocerebellar tract, is analogous to the ventral spinocerebellar tract.

Cuneocerebellar Tract

The cuneocerebellar tract originates in neurons of the external cuneate nucleus and the main cuneate nucleus (Fig. 5B).[74, 127, 252] These nuclei receive afferents from dorsal roots C_1 to T_8 of the spinal cord. The cuneocerebellar pathway projects ipsilaterally through the inferior cerebellar peduncle to the pars intermedia and lateral vermis of lobules V to VI, and to lobule VIIIA and the pars posterior and anterior of the paramedian lobule in the posterior lobe (Fig. 5A). Projections from the rostral and caudal parts of the external cuneate nucleus and projections from the main cuneate nucleus terminate in different regions of the folia.[252] Fibers from the rostral part of the external cuneate nucleus terminate in the deep portions of the paramedian lobule and those from the caudal part of the external cuneate nucleus terminate within the anterior lobe. In contrast, fibers from the main cuneate nucleus terminate in the superficial folia of lobule V and the paramedian lobule.

Functionally, the cuneocerebellar tract can be divided into proprioceptive and exteroceptive subdivisions.[156] Most neurons in the proprioceptive subdivision are located within the external cuneate nucleus.[255] These neurons respond chiefly to activation of group Ia muscle afferents, though some respond to Ib and group II afferents also.[75, 255] Most neurons in the proprioceptive subdivision are activated monosynaptically by inputs from only one muscle nerve[75] and are inhibited by afferents in synergistic muscles.[75] Neurons of the exteroceptive subdivision are

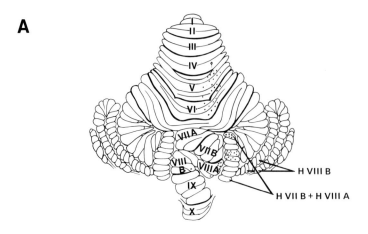

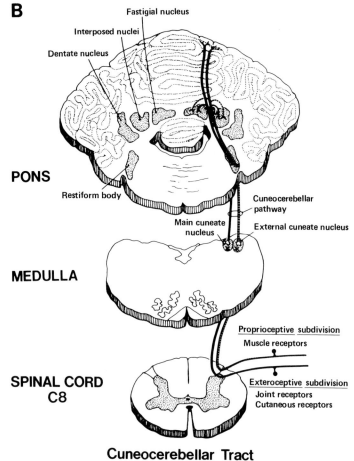

Cuneocerebellar Tract

Figure 5. The organization of the cuneocerebellar pathway. A, Areas of termination in the cerebellar cortex are indicated by dots. B, The course of the cuneocerebellar pathway. The cells of origin are organized into proprioceptive and exteroceptive subdivisions which receive inputs from different groups of peripheral receptors. The cells of origin of the exteroceptive division are located in the main cuneate nucleus and the cells of origin of the proprioceptive division are located in the external cuneate nucleus. The projection ascends in the dorsolateral part of the spinal cord, enters the cerebellum through the restiform body, and terminates within both cerebellar nuclei and cerebellar cortex. (A, redrawn from Grant,[127] with permission.)

located chiefly in the main cuneate nucleus[74] and respond exclusively to activation of cutaneous afferent fibers.[74, 75, 156] These neurons can be subdivided further based on their responses to the activation of hair receptors and to pressure.[156]

Some studies of the responses evoked from the cuneocerebellar tract indicate that proprioceptive and exteroceptive stimuli activate neurons in separate cerebellar cortical regions.[109] Other investigations, however, have shown that individual neurons in the anterior lobe can respond to both exteroceptive and proprioceptive stimuli applied to the forelimb, indicating that inputs from the two subdivisions can affect the same population of cerebellar neurons.[74, 75]

The only descending pathway that has been studied in relation to the cuneocerebellar projection is the one originating in the sensorimotor cortex.[75] Activation of this pathway by stimulating the sensorimotor cortex evokes different effects in the two subdivisions. The responses of neurons in the proprioceptive subdivision are suppressed while those of neurons in the exteroceptive subdivision show both excitatory and inhibitory effects.

Rostral Spinocerebellar Tract

The rostral spinocerebellar tract, the forelimb equivalent of the ventral spinocerebellar tract, originates in the nucleus centralis basalis of the cervical spinal cord.[149, 242] Unlike the ventral spinocerebellar tract, which crosses within the spinal cord, the rostral spinocerebellar pathway projects to the cerebellum ipsilaterally. Two-thirds of the fibers enter through the ipsilateral superior cerebellar peduncle and one-third enters through the inferior peduncle.[240] The rostral spinocerebellar tract terminates bilaterally in the pars intermedia and lateral vermis, mostly in lobules IV to VI.

Neurons of the rostral spinocerebellar tract respond to activation of Ib afferent and flexor reflex afferent fibers.[236, 240] There is extensive convergence of input from group I afferents originating in different muscles.

Other Spinocerebellar Projections

The use of intra-axonal tracing techniques and newer electrophysiologic methods has revealed additional spinocerebellar pathways. One pathway originates in the central cervical nucleus which extends from level C_1 to C_4 in the spinal cord.[85, 219, 264] The fibers in this pathway were thought initially to project contralaterally to the cerebellum,[85] but recent investigations have shown that the projection is bilateral.[264] A second pathway arises in neurons located caudal to the termination of Clarke's column.[264] This projection consists in part of spinocerebellar neurons that respond to the activation of exteroceptive afferents from the hindlimb. A third pathway from the rostral part of the nucleus gracilis to the anterior lobe was demonstrated in electrophysiologic studies.[8, 124, 125] Although initial anatomic studies did not confirm the existence of this pathway,[2, 142] recent studies have shown that the pathway does exist.[252]

PONTOCEREBELLAR AFFERENTS

Organization

Projections from the cerebral cortex to the pontine nuclei and from the pontine nuclei to the cerebellar cortex provide one of the main pathways by which the cerebral cortex can affect cerebellar neuronal activity. The pontocerebellar connections are organized topographically. Projections to the anterior lobe vermis originate in the dorsolateral and paramedian pontine nuclei, with a small projection originating in the ventral nucleus.[50, 150-152] Projections to the pars intermedia and lateral cortical regions arise in the peduncular and lateral nuclei and in portions of the dorsolateral and paramedian nuclei.[50, 150-152]

Large numbers of fibers project from the pontine nuclei to the cerebellar posterior lobe, terminating in lobules VI, VIIA and B, and VIIIA and B. This projection originates in four columns of cells located approximately in the dorsolateral, peduncular, lateral, and paramedian nuclei.[50, 152] Cell columns located somewhat more dorsally project to the anterior lobe. Projections to the hemispheral portions of the anterior and posterior lobes originate in the peduncular and lateral nuclei.[33] The peduncular nucleus projects also to the paramedian lobule. This projection originates in a region of the nucleus which receives a large input from the somatosensory cortex.[150, 152] Four other neuronal columns within the pontine nuclei project to the paraflocculus.[151] In addition, there is a projection from the paramedian pontine nucleus to the flocculus.[151]

Many pontocerebellar fibers terminate within the intracerebellar nuclei as well as the cerebellar cortex. Pontocerebellar fibers project to both the dentate and interposed nuclei in the cat and monkey.[18, 94, 150, 164, 263, 280] As a consequence, information transmitted from the cerebral cortex can affect neuronal excitability directly in both the cerebellar nuclei and the cerebellar cortex through the pontocerebellar projections.

Three features of the pontocerebellar projections are important in understanding the organization of these projections: 1) any single region of the pontine nuclei projects to several areas of the cerebellar cortex, demonstrating the feature of divergence; 2) each lobule of the cerebellar cortex receives inputs from several pontine nuclei, demonstrating the feature of convergence; and 3) pontocerebellar fibers project to regions of the cerebellar vermis in addition to the cerebellar hemispheres.

Inputs to the Pontine Nuclei

The major projections to the pontine nuclei originate within the cerebral cortex. In the cat, these projections generally terminate in medial and lateral columns of neurons, often including several pontine nuclei.[41-44, 197] In primates these columns are less distinct, consisting of a single dense column of neurons extending rostrocaudally through the pontine nuclei.[90] Collaterals of corticospinal tract fibers projecting to the spinal cord mediate some inputs from the cerebral cortex to the pontine nuclei.[3, 4, 180, 256]

The topography of the corticopontine projections is similar in cats[41-44] and monkeys.[90, 229, 271] The projection in cats is described here since it has been studied more completely. Projections from the primary sensorimotor cortex terminate in columns of pontine neurons which, in turn, project to the medial regions of the cerebellar cortex (Fig. 6).[41] Fibers from the primary motor cortex (MI) terminate in pontine nuclei that project chiefly to the cerebellar anterior lobe. Projections from the primary sensory cortex (SI) terminate in pontine neurons that project mainly to the cerebellar paramedian lobule. Fibers from the secondary sensory cortex (SII) project in part to a separate lateral column of neurons, but also converge with fibers projecting from SI onto neurons in the medial region of the

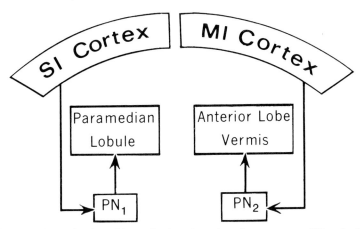

Figure 6. The general organization of the projections from the primary sensory (SI) and primary motor (MI) cortex to regions of the cerebellum. These two cortical regions terminate in nuclei of the pons which project to different regions of the cerebellar cortex. PN_1 and PN_2 represent two different regions of the pontine nuclei.

pontine nuclei.[41] There is less convergence of inputs from the primary and secondary sensory and primary motor cortex in cats than in monkeys.[257] In cats only about 25 percent of neurons in the pontine nuclei receive inputs from multiple regions of the cerebral cortex, while in monkeys over 50 percent of the neurons have this property.

Neurons in many cerebral cortical regions outside the primary sensorimotor cortex also project to the pontine nuclei.[43, 44, 47] Projections from the cerebral cortical association areas show greater overlap in the pontine nuclei than projections from the sensorimotor cortex.[225, 231, 259] In the cat, fibers from the proreate and orbital gyri also project to the pontine nuclei.[43, 44]

The visual and auditory systems have prominent projections to the pontine nuclei. Cerebral cortical areas 17, 18, and 19, which are visual receptive areas, project to these nuclei.[45, 46] These projections show little overlap with those from the primary sensorimotor cortex, but overlap among the three separate projections from the visual cortex does occur. The auditory area of the cerebral cortex sends projections to the dorsolateral region of the pontine nuclei. An extensive projection from the tectum mediating both visual and auditory information reaches the pontine nuclei through the tectopontine pathway.[175] This pathway originates in both the superior and inferior colliculi and projects to the dorsolateral region of the pontine nuclei, the region receiving inputs from both the auditory cortex[47] and the primary motor cortex. Thus, projections from the superior and inferior colliculi, the auditory cortex, and a portion of the sensorimotor cortex can influence neurons in the pontine nuclei which project to the cerebellar vermis (Fig. 7). In contrast, inputs from the visual cortex to the pontine nuclei affect neurons projecting to the cerebellar hemispheres.

Inputs from the basal ganglia to the pontine nuclei, particularly the caudate nucleus, have been described in electrophysiologic studies.[117, 118, 132, 133] These inputs have not been substantiated, however, and recent studies indicate that responses evoked by caudate nucleus stimulation may result from activation of collaterals from corticospinal neurons.[230]

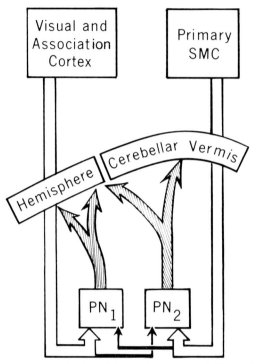

Figure 7. The general pattern of organization of the corticopontocerebellar projections. The input from the visual and association cortex reaches principally the cerebellar hemispheres. In contrast the input from the primary sensorimotor cortex (SMC) reaches principally the cerebellar vermis (see Fig. 6). PN_1 and PN_2 refer to two separate groups of nuclei within the pons.

Studies of the corticopontine projections have revealed several important organizational characteristics:[27] 1) fibers originating in more than one region of the cerebral cortex can project to a specific region within the pontine nuclei; 2) many cortical regions project to more than one region of the pontine nuclei, usually along several columns of neurons oriented in the rostral-caudal direction; and 3) although some overlap occurs in the termination of the corticopontine projections, these projections have a clear topographic organization, particularly those originating in the sensorimotor cortex. The properties of the cerebropontocerebellar projection, particularly the patterns of divergence and convergence, indicate that the pontine nuclei function as much more than relay nuclei, contributing strongly to the integrative processes occurring in the cerebropontocerebellar pathway.

VESTIBULOCEREBELLAR AFFERENTS

Fibers projecting from the vestibular system to the cerebellum arise in both the vestibular nerve and the vestibular nuclei (Fig. 8).[91, 162, 193-195, 249] The vestibular primary afferents reaching the cerebellum originate in the semicircular canals, the utricle, and saccule.[62, 121, 270] These fibers project ipsilaterally to the nodulus, uvula, and flocculus.[32, 56-58, 62] Recent studies indicate that the projections to the dorsal and ventral paraflocculus and lingula described originally do not exist.[182]

30

Secondary vestibular afferents arise in the vestibular nuclei and terminate bilaterally in approximately the same regions of cerebellum as the primary afferents (Fig. 8).[40, 56-58, 91, 184] In addition, secondary vestibular afferents project to almost the entire vermis.[184] These fibers originate throughout the medial and descending vestibular nuclei[40, 56-58, 91, 184] and in groups f and x of the vestibular nuclear complex.[35, 36, 40, 184] In cats and monkeys, primary and secondary vestibular afferents terminate within the cerebellum as mossy fibers.[30, 32, 40, 56-58, 91] A climbing fiber projection from the vestibular system has been demonstrated only in the frog.[146, 147, 202, 203]

Vestibular afferents also terminate within the intracerebellar nuclei (Fig. 8). Initial studies indicated that primary afferent fibers from the vestibular nerve project to the parvocellular part of the dentate nucleus[32, 62] but not to the fastigial nucleus.[32] More recent investigations indicate that the projection to the dentate nucleus does not exist.[182] Secondary afferent fibers from the vestibular nuclei project to the anterior and posterior interposed nuclei as well as the fastigial nucleus.[56-58, 91, 120]

Several important characteristics of the vestibulocerebellar projection should be pointed out. First, as mentioned above, in cats and monkeys all of the afferent fibers projecting from the vestibular nerve and nucleus terminate as mossy fibers.[28, 36] Second, the vestibulocerebellar projection originates within the descending and medial vestibular nuclei, both of which receive inputs from ascending spinal pathways as well as primary vestibular fibers.[28, 36, 182] Third, vestibulocerebellar fibers project not only to the "vestibulocerebellum" (the flocculonodular lobe), but also to other regions of the cerebellar cortex, including the portion of the posterior lobe receiving inputs from several other sensory modalities.

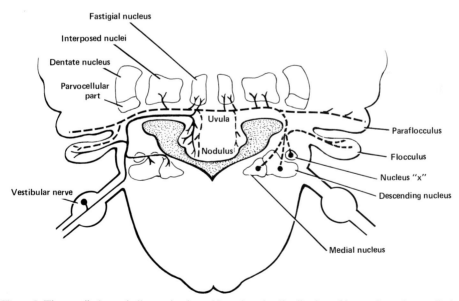

Figure 8. The vestibulocerebellar projections. Note that the distribution of inputs from the vestibular nuclei is much more extensive than from the vestibular nerve. The projection to the vermis of the anterior lobe is not shown in this diagram.

31

TRIGEMINOCEREBELLAR AFFERENTS

Projections from the trigeminal nuclei to the cerebellum mediate many of the responses evoked in the cerebellar cortex and intracerebellar nuclei by facial stimuli.[1, 263, 290] Trigeminocerebellar fibers originate in the principal sensory nucleus of V[111, 160, 196, 197, 241, 290, 291] and the mesencephalic nucleus.[60, 86, 89, 111, 196, 279] These fibers project to the cerebellum through the superior cerebellar peduncle[37, 86, 111] and terminate in lobules V and VI.[60]

RETICULOCEREBELLAR AFFERENTS

The reticulocerebellar pathways originate in nuclei of the brainstem reticular formation and terminate within the cerebellum as mossy fibers. At least two of the three precerebellar reticular nuclei receive inputs from both ascending and descending central nervous system pathways.

The Paramedian Reticular Nucleus

Located in the medial portion of the medulla,[25] the paramedian reticular nucleus receives inputs from a spinobulbar pathway and the dorsal column nuclei.[31, 39] Descending pathways also terminate in this nucleus. These consist of projections from the frontal and parietal areas of cerebral cortex, including the primary sensorimotor cortex and area 6, and from the vestibular nuclei and the fastigial nucleus.[31, 197, 266, 289]

Fibers from the paramedian reticular nucleus project to the ipsilateral anterior and posterior lobe vermis except for lobules VIIB and VIIIA.[39, 265] Less dense projections reach the simplex, crus I and II, paramedian lobules, flocculus, and paraflocculus. Fibers from the paramedian reticular nucleus also project to both the fastigial and interposed nuclei.[95] Neurons in the paramedian nucleus respond to activation of cutaneous mechanoreceptors.[93]

Lateral Reticular Nucleus

The lateral reticular nucleus consists of the pars principalis, which contains parvocellular and magnocellular components, and the pars subtrigeminalis.[286] The initial description of the projections from this nucleus[24, 26] included inputs to both the cerebellar hemispheres and vermis, but this description has been revised because the projection to the hemisphere could not be confirmed.[48, 66, 189, 220] Dense projections extend from the lateral reticular nucleus to lobules I to IV, VI, VIIB, VIIIA, and the paramedian lobules.[189, 220] The parvocellular component of the pars principalis projects to the caudal region of the paramedian lobule, and the magnocellular component projects predominantly to the caudal region of the anterior lobe and the rostral part of the paramedian lobule.[48] The pars subtrigeminalis projects chiefly to the same regions as the magnocellular component of the pars principalis.

Electrophysiologic studies have suggested that the projection from the lateral reticular nucleus to the cerebellar cortex affects selectively a population of granule cells that does not alter Purkinje cell excitability significantly.[5, 9] This finding was not supported by later studies showing that this reticulocerebellar projection can affect the excitability of Purkinje cells.[10, 20, 260] The current view is that the projection from the lateral reticular nucleus can affect the excitability of the same Purkinje cells affected by mossy fiber inputs to the cerebellar vermis from the spinal cord and pontine nuclei.

The lateral reticular nucleus projects to the intracerebellar nuclei, including the fastigial nucleus and the anterior and posterior interposed nuclei.[222] A projection to the dentate nucleus has been substantiated only in the rat.[111]

Spinal Projections to the Lateral Reticular Nucleus

Spinoreticular fibers ascending in the ventral quadrant of the spinal cord provide a major input to the lateral reticular nucleus (Fig. 9).[23, 55, 283] The cells of origin are located in Rexed laminae VI, VII, and VIII, both ipsilateral and contralateral to the nucleus in which they terminate.[5] This projection consists of several components, as defined electrophysiologically.[130, 209, 239] One of these, the bilateral ventral flexor reflex tract, projects from all spinal cord levels and is activated by polysynaptic reflex pathways from flexor reflex afferents.[209] The second pathway, the contralateral ventral flexor reflex tract, is activated by flexor reflex afferents arising in the contralateral hindlimb.[209] A third pathway, which projects from the cervical spinal cord to the lateral reticular nucleus, is activated by cutaneous and flexor reflex afferents in the forelimb.[68] This pathway, which is similar to the bilateral ventral flexor reflex tract, has been designated the ipsilateral forelimb tract.

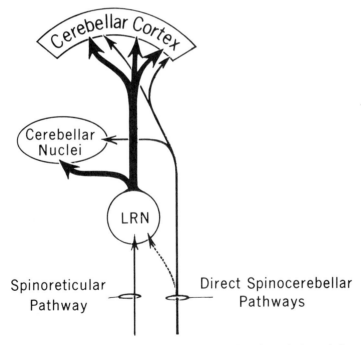

Figure 9. The relationship of the direct spinocerebellar and the spinoreticulocerebellar projections. Although this point is controversial, the direct spinocerebellar pathways probably project to nuclei in the spinoreticulocerebellar pathway. The density of inputs to the cerebellar nuclei from the reticulocerebellar projections is probably greater than the density of inputs from the direct spinocerebellar pathways. LRN = lateral reticular nucleus.

Another input to the lateral reticular nucleus is activated by both spinal and trigeminal afferents.[69] The brainstem neurons mediating this input have not been defined anatomically.

In addition to the spinoreticular fibers ascending in the ventral quadrant of the spinal cord, fibers in the dorsolateral fasciculus project to the lateral reticular nucleus (Fig. 9).[188, 228, 284] Electrophysiologic studies show that neurons in the lateral reticular nucleus can be activated through fibers in the dorsolateral region of the spinal cord.[54] Collaterals of the dorsal spinocerebellar tract probably mediate the responses,[54, 284] though this notion was challenged recently.[110] In the study providing the challenge, half the cells in the lateral reticular nucleus were activated by fibers in the dorsolateral fasciculus. Consequently, the possibility of a projection from the dorsal spinocerebellar tract to the lateral reticular nucleus remains viable.

The projections from the spinal cord to the lateral reticular nucleus show some degree of topographic organization.[67, 188, 217] Fibers from the cervical region terminate in the magnocellular portion of the pars principalis and fibers from the lumbar region terminate in the parvocellular portion. In addition, fibers from the ipsilateral dorsolateral fasciculus terminate in the parvocellular region.[188]

Neurons in the lateral reticular nucleus respond to the activation of low threshold cutaneous receptors in the hairy skin and footpad and to the activation of flexor reflex afferents.[178, 237, 253, 254] Receptive fields of varying sizes have been reported, including those involving more than one extremity. Activation of group I afferents in peripheral nerves also affects the activity of neurons in the lateral reticular nucleus.[54, 178] In addition, cells in this nucleus respond to inputs from macular receptors within the vestibular apparatus activated by changes of head position.[122, 147, 243, 244] The discharge rate of many neurons in the lateral reticular nucleus is modulated with considerable sensitivity in proportion to the degree of head tilt. These responses are mediated through a complex pathway involving a descending vestibulospinal pathway that activates an ascending spinoreticular projection.[79, 244, 247] The involvement of spinal neurons was demonstrated by the finding that macular stimulation of neuronal activity in the lateral reticular nucleus no longer occurs after transection of the cervical spinal cord. As might be expected by the number of stimulus modalities capable of modulating neuronal activity in the lateral reticular nucleus, many neurons responding to head tilt are activated also by peripheral cutaneous stimuli and neck muscle receptors.[79, 80, 244]

Projections Descending to the Lateral Reticular Nucleus

The two major projections descending to the lateral reticular nucleus originate in the cerebral cortex and the red nucleus. The projection from the cerebral cortex[49, 191, 225, 287] includes a large component from the primary sensorimotor cortex that terminates in the magnocellular region of the contralateral lateral reticular nucleus.[49] At least part of this pathway consists of collaterals from the pyramidal tract.[51, 190, 295] The projection from the red nucleus terminates within the magnocellular portion of the lateral reticular nucleus and is organized topographically.[77, 287] Neurons in the part of the red nucleus projecting to the cervical spinal cord terminate within the medial region of the lateral reticular nucleus, which is the region receiving inputs from the cervical spinal cord. Neurons in the part of the red nucleus projecting to the lumbar spinal cord terminate within the lateral region of the lateral reticular nucleus, the region receiving inputs from the lumbar cord.[246] Projections reach the lateral reticular nucleus also from the deep cerebellar nuclei, including the contralateral fastigial[176, 288] and interposed nuclei.[176]

Several descending projections affect the activity of neurons in the lateral reticular nucleus.[52, 176, 177] Some of the neurons affected by descending projections are activated also by ascending spinoreticular projections. The actions of descending pathways are mediated not only by fibers terminating directly in the nucleus but also by projections to the spinal cord that modify the segmental inputs to spinoreticular fibers. The vestibulospinal and pyramidal tracts,[130] for example, affect the segmental action of flexor reflex afferents on the cells of origin of the bilateral ventral flexor reflex tract, one of the major inputs to the lateral reticular nucleus.[205, 238]

Nucleus Reticularis Tegmenti Pontis

The nucleus reticularis tegmenti pontis projects to both the cerebellar vermis and the hemispheres[26, 33] and receives a major input from the intracerebellar nuclei through the brachium conjunctivum.[34, 38, 61, 285] It also receives inputs from several regions of the cerebral cortex, including the primary sensorimotor cortex, the secondary cortex, the proreate gyrus, and the orbital gyrus.[29] The nucleus reticularis tegmenti pontis is the only precerebellar reticular nucleus that does not receive projections from ascending spinal pathways.

Functions of the Reticulocerebellar Projections

The initial electrophysiologic studies of the reticulocerebellar projections led to the conclusion that these projections participate in cerebellar cortical function by providing a tonic "background" excitatory input to the cerebellar cortex and nuclei.[239] This conclusion now seems incorrect in view of the continuing demonstration of complex afferent and efferent connections between the cerebellum and the precerebellar reticular nuclei. For example, recent studies have shown interconnections between the interposed nuclei and the lateral reticular nucleus as well as a closed pathway between these two structures and the red nucleus.[176, 177]

The reticulocerebellar projections undoubtedly influence the spatial and temporal characteristics of responses evoked in the cerebellum. The spatial distribution of responses evoked in the cerebellar cortex reflects the characteristics of projections directly from the spinal cord and pontine nuclei and the projections from the precerebellar reticular nuclei, since all are activated by the same peripheral stimuli.[19, 20, 54, 72, 73, 84, 115, 178] For the same reason, the temporal characteristics of neuronal responses in the precerebellar reticular nuclei probably contribute to the time course of excitability changes in Purkinje cells. A causal relationship, however, has not been demonstrated experimentally.

The importance of the reticulocerebellar projections in motor behavior is indicated by the finding that lesions in the lateral reticular nucleus cause abnormalities of posture and movement.[78] These abnormalities have been attributed to the disruption of interactions between spinoreticulocerebellar projections, the fastigial nucleus, the cerebellar cortex, and the lateral reticular nucleus. This notion requires confirmation with other experimental paradigms, particularly those which assure that olivocerebellar fibers are not interrupted.

35

NUCLEOCORTICAL AFFERENTS

Most components of the central nervous system receive inputs from the nuclei to which they project. Until recently the cerebellar cortex had been viewed as one of the few central structures that is not organized according to this principle. In several early studies, however, degenerating fibers were found in the cerebellar cortex following deep cerebellar nuclear lesions, suggesting the existence of projections to the cerebellar cortex.[63, 70] Because afferent fibers projecting to the cerebellar cortex from outside the cerebellum course immediately adjacent to and through the intracerebellar nuclei and were probably interrupted by the lesions, these findings could not be accepted as proof of a nucleocortical projection. Moreover, many subsequent studies were thought to show that all afferent fibers to the cerebellar cortex, including climbing fibers, originate within extracerebellar nuclei. Early electrophysiologic studies provided an indication that nucleocortical fibers may exist by showing that neurons in the dentate nucleus respond antidromically to cerebellar cortical stimulation.[163] These findings were thought to result not from the activation of fibers terminating in the cerebellar cortex, but from the activation of nuclear neurons by current spreading from the stimulus site to the deep regions of the white matter where the axons of these cells course toward the cerebellar peduncles.[164]

The conclusive demonstration of a nucleocortical projection required the combination of electrophysiologic methods with the newly developed intra-axonal tracing techniques. These tracing techniques depend upon: 1) the uptake of substances (e.g., horseradish peroxidase) by nerve terminals and the retrograde transport of these substances to the cell body or 2) the uptake of substances (e.g., radioactive amino acids) by neuronal cell bodies and the orthograde transport of these substances to the nerve terminals. The injection of horseradish peroxidase into the cerebellar cortex results in retrograde labeling of neurons in the intracerebellar nuclei.[64, 126, 274, 275] In addition, the injection of radioactive amino acids into the intracerebellar nuclei labels fibers coursing to the granular layer of the cerebellar cortex (Fig. 10).[64, 274, 275] Thus, strong morphologic evidence has accumulated supporting the existence of a nucleocortical projection. Electrophysiologic studies carried out in conjunction with these morphologic experiments revealed that many neurons in the cerebellar nuclei can be activated antidromically both from the cerebellar surface and from the ascending limb of the brachium conjunctivum (Fig. 11). Thus, it appears that many nucleocortical fibers arise as collaterals of cerebellar output neurons.

The organization of the nucleocortical projections has been elucidated in both cats and monkeys. In cats the projection originates in all morphologic types of neurons within the intracerebellar nuclei,[126, 277] but in monkeys nucleocortical fibers originate chiefly in large cells.[64, 276, 277, 278] The topographic organization of the nucleocortical projection in cats differs from that in monkeys. In cats, nucleocortical fibers from a given intracerebellar nucleus project to the sagittal zone of the cerebellar cortex from which the nucleus receives its densest projection from Purkinje cells.[280] Although these projections have a clearly defined sagittal organization, some overlap occurs between adjacent zones. By contrast, in monkeys only the nucleocortical fibers originating in zones in the fastigial and interposed nuclei project to the corresponding zones of the cerebellar cortex. Fibers from the dentate nucleus project to the lateral sagittal zone and also to the more medial zones, including the cerebellar vermis.[64, 278]

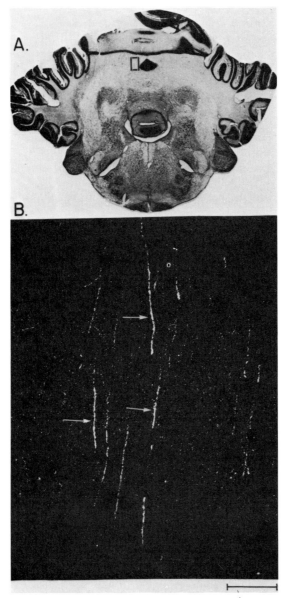

Figure 10. The demonstration of a projection from the cerebellar nuclei to the cerebellar cortex with autoradiographic techniques. In this experiment radioactive leucine was injected into the fastigial nucleus. This compound is known to be taken up by neuronal cell bodies and transported through the axons of these neurons to their sites of termination. The autoradiograph shown in B was taken from a region of the cerebellar white matter indicated in A with the square. The elements indicated with white arrows in B indicate the presence of fibers containing radioactive leucine coursing through this region of white matter. Radioactive leucine reduces the silver in the autoradiographic emulsion, indicating the course of the fibers containing the radioactive compound. (From Tolbert et al.,[275] with permission.)

37

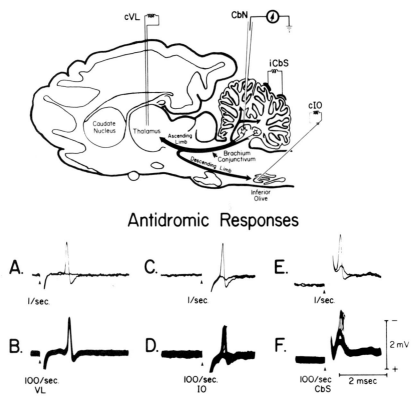

Figure 11. The electrophysiologic demonstration of the branching of nuclear neurons which contribute to the nucleocortical pathway. The records in A and B show the responses of a neuron in the dentate nucleus to antidromic stimulation of its axon in the thalamus. The responses of the same neuron to antidromic stimulation of its axon in the inferior olivary region are shown in C and D. The antidromic response of this neuron to stimulation of the cerebellar cortex is shown in E and F. CbN = cerebellar nuclei; cVL = contralateral ventrolateral thalamus; iCbS = ipsilateral cerebellar surface; cIO = contralateral inferior olive. (Adapted from Tolbert, D. L. et al.: *Multiple branching of cerebellar efferent projections in cats.* Exp. Brain Res. 31(3):305, 1978.)

The functions of the nucleocortical projections have not been determined. The nucleocortical fibers terminate within the granular layer and are classified as mossy fibers.[64, 275, 276] Since the nucleocortical projections have mossy fiber terminals, their actions probably are integrated together with the actions of other mossy fiber afferents in modulating the discharge of cerebellar cortical neurons. Because the nucleocortical fibers are collaterals of neurons projecting to extracerebellar nuclei, the nucleocortical fibers may provide a pathway by which information about cerebellar nuclear output can affect neuronal activity in the cerebellar cortex (Fig 12).

MOSSY FIBER INPUTS TO THE CEREBELLAR NUCLEI

Many mossy fiber projections terminate within the cerebellar cortex and also within the intracerebellar nuclei. These projections include pathways ascending directly from the spinal cord and from several brainstem nuclei. Inputs from spinocerebellar pathways terminate within both the fastigial and the interposed nu-

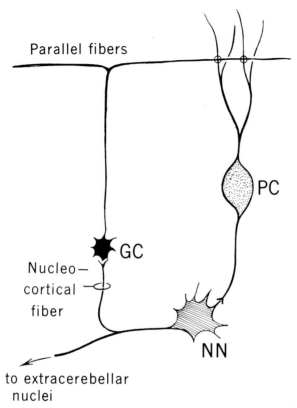

Figure 12. The organization of the nucleocortical pathway. Many nucleocortical fibers are collaterals of neurons in the cerebellar nuclei which also project to nuclei outside of the cerebellum. Available data indicate that these fibers terminate as mossy fibers within the granular layer of the cerebellar cortex. The circles in the dendritic tree of the Purkinje cell (PC) indicate sites of synaptic contact between parallel fibers and these neurons. NN = nuclear neuron; GC = granule cell.

clei.[71, 92, 94, 97-104, 144, 161, 165, 218, 221] There are no known direct spinocerebellar projections to the dentate nucleus.[161, 218, 221] In contrast to the spinocerebellar pathways, fibers from the trigeminal complex terminate within the fastigial, interposed, and dentate nuclei.[64, 111, 241, 279] Fibers projecting to the dentate nucleus originate within all of the trigeminal nuclei, but fibers terminating in the more medial cerebellar nuclei originate chiefly in the mesencephalic nucleus of the trigeminal complex. Several brainstem nuclei receiving inputs from spinobulbar fibers send projections to the deep cerebellar nuclei. These include the inferior olive, paramedian nuclei, and lateral reticular nucleus.

Brainstem nuclei mediate inputs from the cerebral cortex to the cerebellar nuclei. Neurons in the pontine nuclei project to both the dentate and interposed nuclei in the cat and monkey.[18, 64, 150, 164, 280] Neurons in the nucleus reticularis tegmenti pontis, which receive extensive inputs from descending pathways, project to the interposed and dentate nuclei.[17, 18, 64, 111] The red nucleus also receives inputs from descending projections and sends fibers to the intracerebellar nuclei. The rubrocerebellar projection[148] terminates exclusively within the anterior part of the contralateral interposed nucleus.[83]

REFERENCES

1. ADRIAN, E. D.: *Afferent areas in the cerebellum connected with the limbs.* Brain 66:289, 1943.

2. AFIFI, A. K., JABBUR, S. J., AND BAHUTH, N.: *Gracilocerebellar fiber connections in the cat.* Exp. Neurol. 31:465, 1971.

3. ALLEN, G. I., KORN, H., OSHIMA, T. ET AL.: *The mode of synaptic linkage in the cerebro-ponto-cerebellar pathway of the cat. II. Responses of single cells in the pontine nuclei.* Exp. Brain Res. 24:15, 1975.

4. ALLEN, G. I., OSHIMA, T., AND TOYAMA, K.: *The mode of synaptic linkage in the cerebro-ponto-cerebellar pathway investigated with intracellular recording from pontine nuclei cells of the cat.* EXP. BRAIN RES. 29:123, 1977.

5. ARSHAVSKY, Y. I., BERKINBLIT, M. B., AND FUKSON, O. I.: *Layer analysis of evoked potentials in the paramedian lobe of cerebellum cortex.* Fiziol. Zh. SSSR 55:429, 1969.

6. ARSHAVSKY, Y. I., BERKINBLIT, M. B., FUKSON, O. I. ET AL.: *Recording of neurons of the dorsal spinocerebellar tract during evoked locomotion.* Brain Res. 43:272, 1972.

7. ARSHAVSKY, Y. I., BERKINBLIT, M. B., FUKSON, O. I. ET AL.: *Origin and modulation of neurones of the ventral spinocerebellar tract during locomotion.* Brain Res. 43:276, 1972.

8. ARSHAVSKY, Y. I., BERKINBLIT, M. B., GELFAND, I. M. ET AL.: *Afferent connections and interaction of the cerebellar cortical neurons,* in Farnardjan, V. V. (ed.): *Structural and Functional Organization of the Cerebellum.* Nauka, Leningrad, 1971, pp. 40–47.

9. ARSHAVSKY, Y. I., BERKINBLIT, M. B., GELFAND, I. M. ET AL.: *Two types of granular cells in cerebellar cortex.* Neurofiziol 1:167, 1969.

10. AZZENA, G. B., AND OHNO, T.: *Influence of spino-reticulo-cerebellar pathway on Purkyně cells of paramedian lobule.* Exp. Brain Res. 17:63, 1973.

11. BALDISSERA, F., AND ROBERTS, W. J.: *Effects on the ventral spinocerebellar tract neurones from Deiters' nucleus and the medial longitudinal fascicle in the cat.* Acta Physiol. Scand. 93:228, 1975.

12. BALDISSERA, F., AND ROBERTS, W. J.: *Effects from the vestibulospinal tract on transmission from primary afferents to ventral spino-cerebellar tract neurones.* Acta Physiol. Scand. 96:217, 1976.

13. BALDISSERA, F., AND TEN BRUGGENCATE, G.: *Rubrospinal effects on spinal border cells.* Acta Physiol. Scand. (Suppl) 330:191, 1969.

14. BALDISSERA, F., AND TEN BRUGGENCATE, G.: *Rubrospinal effects on ventral spinocerebellar tract neurones.* Acta Physiol. Scand. 96:233, 1976.

15. BALDISSERA, F., AND WEIGHT, F.: *Descending monosynaptic connections to spinal border cells.* Acta Physiol. Scand. 76:28, 1969.

16. BASBAUM, A. I., CLANTON, C. H., AND FIELDS, H. L.: *Three bulbospinal pathways from the rostral medulla of the cat: an autoradiographic study of pain modulating systems.* J. Comp. Neurol. 178:209, 1978.

17. BEITZ, A. J.: *The topographical organization of the olivo-dentate and dentato-olivary pathways in the cat.* Brain Res. 115:311, 1976.

18. BISHOP, G. A., MCCREA, R. A., AND KITAL, S. T.: *Afferent projections to the nucleus interpositus anterior (NIA) and the lateral nucleus (LN) of the cat cerebellum.* Anat. Rec. 184:360, 1976.

19. BLOEDEL, J. R.: *Cerebellar afferent systems: A review,* in *Progress in Neurobiology,* Vol II, Part I. Pergamon Press, Oxford, England, 1973, pp. 1–68.

20. BLOEDEL, J. R., AND BURTON, J. E.: *Electrophysiological evidence for a mossy fiber input to the cerebellar cortex activated indirectly by collaterals of the spinocerebellar pathways.* J. Neurophysiol. 33:308, 1970.

21. BLOEDEL, J. R., AND COURVILLE, J.: *A review of cerebellar afferent systems,* in Handbook of Physiology. American Physiological Society, Bethesda, Md., 1981.

22. BOEHME, C. C.: *The neural structure of Clarke's nucleus of the spinal cord.* J. Comp. Neurol. 132:445, 1968.

23. BOHM, E.: *An electro-physiological study of the ascending spinal anterolateral fibre system connected to coarse cutaneous afferents. A spino-bulbo-cerebellar system.* Acta Physiol. Scand. (Suppl) 106:106, 1953.

24. BRODAL, A.: *The cerebellar connections of the nucleus reticularis lateralis (nucleus funiculi lateralis) in rabbit and cat. Experimental investigations.* Acta Psychiat. Scand. 18:171, 1943.

25. BRODAL, A.: *Reticulo-cerebellar connections in the cat. An experimental study.* J. Comp. Neurol. 98:113, 1953.

26. BRODAL, A.: *The Reticular Formation of the Brain Stem. Anatomical Aspects and Functional Correlations,* Vol. vii. Oliver and Boyd, Edinburgh, 1957, p. 87.

27. BRODAL, A.: *Cerebrocerebellar pathways. Anatomical data and some functional implications.* Acta Neurol. Scand. (Suppl) 51:153, 1972.

28. BRODAL, A.: *Vestibulocerebellar input in the cat: anatomy.* Prog. Brain Res. 37:315, 1972.

29. BRODAL, A., AND BRODAL, P.: *The organization of the nucleus reticularis tegmenti pontis in the cat in the light of experimental anatomical studies of its cerebral cortical afferents.* Exp. Brain Res. 13:90, 1971.

30. BRODAL, A., AND DRABLOS, P. A.: *Two types of mossy fiber terminals in the cerebellum and their regional distribution.* J. Comp. Neurol. 121:173, 1963.

31. BRODAL, A., AND GOGSTAD, A.: *Afferent connexions of the paramedian reticular nucleus of the medulla oblongata in the cat.* Acta Anat. (Basel) 30:133, 1957.

32. BRODAL, A., AND HØIVIK, B.: *Site and mode of termination of primary vestibulocerebellar fibres in the cat. An experimental study with silver impregnation methods.* Arch. Ital. Biol. 102:1, 1964.

33. BRODAL, A., AND JANSEN, J.: *The ponto-cerebellar projection in the rabbit and cat. Experimental investigations.* J. Comp. Neurol. 84:31, 1946.

34. BRODAL, A., LACERDA, A. M., DESTOMBES, J. ET AL.: *The pattern in the projection of the intracerebellar nuclei onto the nucleus reticularis tegmenti pontis in the cat. An experimental anatomical study.* Exp. Brain Res. 16:140, 1972.

35. BRODAL, A., AND POMPEIANO, O.: *The vestibular nuclei in the cat.* J. Anat. (London) 91:438, 1957.

36. BRODAL, A., POMPEIANO, O., AND WALBERG, F.: *The Vestibular Nuclei and Their Connections, Anatomy and Functional Correlations,* vol. VIII. Oliver and Boyd, Edinburgh, 1962, p. 193.

37. BRODAL, A., AND SAUGSTAD, L. F.: *Retrograde cellular changes in the mesencephalic trigeminal nucleus in the cat following cerebellar lesions.* Acta Morph. (Neer-Scand) 6:147, 1964–1966.

38. BRODAL, A., AND SZIKLA, G.: *The termination of the brachium conjunctivum descendens in the nucleus reticularis tegmenti pontis. An experimental anatomical study in the cat.* Brain Res. 39:337, 1972.

39. BRODAL, A., AND TORVIK, A.: *Cerebellar projections of paramedian reticular nucleus of medulla oblongata in cat.* J. Neurophysiol. 17:484, 1954.

40. BRODAL, A., AND TORVIK, A.: *Über den Ursprung der sekundären Vestibulo-cerebellaren Fasern bei der Katze. Eine experimentell-anatomische Studie.* Arch. Psychiatr. Neurol. 195:550, 1957.

41. BRODAL, P.: *The cortico-pontine projection in the cat: I. Demonstration of a somatotopically organized projection from the primary sensorimotor cortex.* Exp. Brain Res. 5:210, 1968.

42. BRODAL, P.: *The corticopontine projection in the cat. II. Demonstration of a somatotopically organized projection from the second somatosensory cortex.* Arch. Ital. Biol. 106:310, 1968.

43. BRODAL, P.: *The corticopontine projection in the cat. I. The projection from the proreate gyrus.* J. Comp. Neurol. 142:127, 1971.

44. BRODAL, P.: *The corticopontine projection in the cat. II. The projection from the orbital gyrus.* J. Comp. Neurol. 142:141, 1971.

45. BRODAL, P.: *The corticopontine projection from the visual cortex in the cat. II. The projection from areas 18 and 19.* Brain Res. 39:319, 1972.

46. BRODAL, P.: *The corticopontine projection from the visual cortex in the cat. I. The total projection and the projection from area 17.* Brain Res. 39:297, 1972.

47. BRODAL, P.: *The corticopontine projection in the cat. The projection from the auditory cortex.* Arch. Ital. Biol. 110:119, 1972.

48. BRODAL, P.: *Demonstration of a somatotopically organized projection onto the paramedian lobule and the anterior lobe from the lateral reticular nucleus. An experimental study with the horseradish peroxidase method.* Brain Res. 95:221, 1975.

49. BRODAL, P., MARŠALA, J., AND BRODAL, A.: *The cerebral cortical projection to the lateral reticular nucleus in the cat, with special reference to the sensorimotor cortical areas.* Brain Res. 6:252, 1967.

50. BRODAL, P., WALBERG, F.: *The pontine projection to the cerebellar anterior lobe. An experimen-*

tal study in the cat with retrograde transport of horseradish peroxidase. Exp. Brain Res. 29:233, 1977.

51. BRUCKMOSER, P., HEPP-REYMOND, M. C., AND WIESENDANGER, M.: *Cortical influence on the lateral reticular nucleus of the cat.* Brain Res. 15:556, 1969.

52. BRUCKMOSER, P., HEPP-REYMOND, M. C., AND WIESENDANGER, M.: *Effects of peripheral, rubral and fastigial stimulation on neurons of the lateral reticular nucleus of the cat.* Exp. Neurol. 27:388, 1970.

53. BURKE, R., LUNDBERG, A., AND WEIGHT, F.: *Spinal border cell origin of the ventral spinocerebellar tract.* Exp. Brain Res. 12:283, 1971.

54. BURTON, J. E., BLOEDEL, J. R., AND GREGORY, R. S.: *Electrophysiological evidence for an input to lateral reticular nucleus from collaterals of dorsal spinocerebellar and cuneocerebellar fibers.* J. Neurophysiol. 34:885, 1971.

55. BUSCH, H. F. M.: *An Anatomical Analysis of the White Matter in the Brain Stem of the Cat.* Van Gorcum, Assen, 1961.

56. CARPENTER, M. B.: *Fiber projections from the descending and lateral vestibular nuclei in the cat.* Am. J. Anat. 107:1, 1960.

57. CARPENTER, M. B.: *Experimental, anatomical, physiological studies of vestibular nerve and cerebellar connections,* in Rasmussen, G. L., and Windle, W. F. (eds.): *Neural Mechanisms of the Auditory and Vestibular Systems.* Charles C Thomas, Springfield, Ill., 1960, pp. 297–323.

58. CARPENTER, M. B., BARD, D. S., AND ALLING, F. A.: *Anatomical connections between the fastigial nuclei, the labyrinth and the vestibular nuclei in the cat.* J. Comp. Neurol. 111:1, 1959.

59. CARPENTER, D., ENGBERG, I., AND LUNDBERG, A.: *Differential supraspinal control of inhibitory and excitatory actions from the FRA to ascending spinal pathways.* Acta Physiol. Scand. 63: 103, 1965.

60. CARPENTER, M. B., AND HANNA, G. R.: *Fiber projections from the spinal trigeminal nucleus in the cat.* J. Comp. Neurol. 117:117, 1961.

61. CARPENTER, M. B., AND NOVA, H. R.: *Descending division of the brachium conjunctivum in the cat: a cerebello-reticular system.* J. Comp. Neurol. 114:295, 1960.

62. CARPENTER, M. B., STEIN, B. M., AND PETER, P.: *Primary vestibulocerebellar fibers in the monkey: Distribution of fibers arising from distinctive cell groups of the vestibular ganglia.* Am. J. Anat. 135:221, 1972.

63. CARREA, R. M. E., REISSIG, M., AND METTLER, F. A.: *The climbing fibers of the simian and feline cerebellum.* J. Comp. Neurol. 87:321, 1947.

64. CHAN-PALAY, V.: *Cerebellar Dentate Nucleus: Organization, Cytology, and Transmitters.* Springer-Verlag, New York, 1977.

65. CHANG, H. T., AND RUCH, T. C.: *The projection of the caudal segments of the spinal cord to the lingula in the spider monkey.* J. Anat. 83:304, 1949.

66. CLENDENIN, M., EKEROT, C. F., OSCARSSON, O. ET AL.: *The lateral reticular nucleus in the cat. I. Mossy fibre distribution in cerebellar cortex.* Exp. Brain Res. 21:473, 1974.

67. CLENDENIN, M., EKEROT, C. F., OSCARSSON, O. ET AL.: *The lateral reticular nucleus in the cat. II. Organization of component activated from bilateral ventral flexor reflex tract (bVFRT).* Exp. Brain Res. 21:487, 1974.

68. CLENDENIN, M., EKEROT, C. F., AND OSCARSSON, O.: *The lateral reticular nucleus in the cat. III. Organization of component activated from ipsilateral forelimb tract.* Exp. Brain Res. 21: 501, 1974.

69. CLENDENIN, M., EKEROT, C. F., AND OSCARSSON, O.: *The lateral reticular nucleus in the cat. IV. Activation from dorsal funiculus and trigeminal afferents.* Exp. Brain Res. 24:131, 1975.

70. COHEN, D., CHAMBERS, W. W., AND SPRAGUE, J. M.: *Experimental study of the efferent projections from the cerebellar nuclei to the brainstem of the cat.* J. Comp. Neurol. 109:233, 1958.

71. COLLIER, J., AND BUZZARD, E. F.: *The degenerations resulting from lesions of posterior nerve roots and from transverse lesions of the spinal cord in man.* A study of twenty cases. Brain 26:559, 1903.

72. COMBS, C. M.: *Electro-anatomical study of cerebellar localization. Stimulation of various afferents.* J. Neurophysiol. 17:123, 1954.

73. COMBS, C. M.: *Bulbar regions related to localized cerebellar afferent impulses.* J. Neurophysiol. 19:285, 1956.

74. COOKE, J. D., LARSON, B., OSCARSSON, O. ET AL.: *Origin and termination of cuneocerebellar tract.* Exp. Brain Res. 13:339, 1971.

75. COOKE, J. D., LARSON, B., OSCARSSON, O. ET AL.: *Organization of afferent connections to cuneocerebellar tract.* Exp. Brain Res. 13:359, 1971.

76. COOPER, S., AND SHERRINGTON, C. S.: *Gower's tract and spinal border cells.* Brain 63:123, 1940.

77. CORVAJA, N., GROFOVÁ, I., POMPEIANO, O. ET AL.: *The lateral reticular nucleus in the cat. I. An experimental anatomical study of its spinal and supraspinal afferent connections.* Neurosci. 2:537, 1977.

78. CORVAJA, N., GROFOVÁ, I., POMPEIANO, O. ET AL.: *The lateral reticular nucleus in the cat. II. Effects of lateral reticular lesions on posture and reflex movements.* Neurosci. 2:929, 1977.

79. COULTER, J. D., MERGNER, T., AND POMPEIANO, O.: *Effect of tilting on the responses of lateral reticular nucleus neurons to somatic afferent stimulation.* Arch. Ital. Biol. 115:294, 1977.

80. COULTER, J. D., MERGNER, T., AND POMPEIANO, O.: *Integration of afferent inputs from neck muscles and macular labyrinthine receptors within the lateral reticular nucleus.* Arch. Ital. Biol. 115:332, 1977.

81. COURVILLE, J.: *Rubrobulbar fibres to the facial nucleus and the lateral reticular nucleus (nucleus of the lateral funiculus). An experimental study in the cat with silver impregnation methods.* Brain Res. 1:317, 1966.

82. COURVILLE, J., AUGUSTINE, J. R., AND MARTEL, P.: *Projections from the inferior olive to the cerebellar nuclei in the cat demonstrated by retrograde transport of horseradish peroxidase.* Brain Res. 130:405, 1977.

83. COURVILLE, J., AND BRODAL, A.: *Rubro-cerebellar connections in the cat: An experimental study with silver impregnation methods.* J. Comp. Neurol. 126:471, 1966.

84. CRICHLOW, E. C., AND KENNEDY, T. T.: *Functional characteristics of neurons in the lateral reticular nucleus with reference to localized cerebellar potentials.* Exp. Neurol. 18:141, 1967.

85. CUMMINGS, J. F., AND PETRAS, J. M.: *The origin of spinocerebellar pathways. I. The nucleus cervicalis centralis of the cranial cervical spinal cord.* J. Comp. Neurol. 173:655, 1977.

86. CUPEDO, R. N. J.: *A trigeminal midbrain-cerebellar fiber connection in the rat.* J. Comp. Neurol. 124:61, 1965.

87. CURTIS, D. R., ECCLES, J. C., AND LUNDBERG, A.: *Intracellular recording from cells in Clarke's column.* Acta Physiol. Scand. 43:303, 1958.

88. DAHLSTRÖM, A., AND FUXE, K.: *Evidence for the existence of monoamine-containing neurons in the central nervous system. I. Demonstration of monoamines in the cell bodies of brain stem neurons.* Acta Physiol. Scand. (Suppl.) 232:1, 1964.

89. DARIAN-SMITH, I., AND PHILLIPS, G.: *Secondary neurones within a trigeminocerebellar projection to the anterior lobe of the cerebellum in the cat.* J. Physiol. (London) 170:53, 1964.

90. DHANARAJAN, P., RÜEGG, D. G., AND WIESENDANGER, M.: *An anatomical investigation of the corticopontine projection in primate (Saimiri sciureus). The projection from motor and somatosensory areas.* Neurosci. 2:913, 1977.

91. DOW, R. S.: *The fiber connections of the posterior parts of the cerebellum in the rat and cat.* J. Comp. Neurol. 63:527, 1936.

92. EBBESSON, S. O. E.: *Ascending axon degeneration following hemisection of the spinal cord in the tegu lizard (Tupinambis nigropunctatus).* Brain Res. 5:178, 1967.

93. ECCLES, J. C., HUBBARD, J. I., AND OSCARSSON, O.: *Intracellular recording from cells of the ventral spinocerebellar tract.* J. Physiol. (London) 158:486, 1961.

94. ECCLES, J. C., ITO, M., AND SZENTÁGOTHAI, J.: *The cerebellum as a neuronal machine.* Springer-Verlag, Berlin, 1967.

95. ECCLES, J. C., NICOLL, R. A., SCHWARZ, D. W. F. ET AL.: *Medial reticular and perihypoglossal neurons projecting to cerebellum.* J. Neurophysiol. 39:102, 1976.

96. ECCLES, J. C., OSCARSSON, O., AND WILLIS, W. D.: *Synaptic action of group I and II afferent fibres of muscle on the cells of the dorsal spinocerebellar tract.* J. Physiol. (London) 158:517, 1961.

97. ECCLES, J. C., ROSÉN, I., SCHEID, P., ET AL.: *Cutaneous afferent responses in interpositus neurons of the cat.* Brain Res. 42:207, 1972.

98. ECCLES, J. C., SABAH, N. H., AND TÁBOŘÍKOVÁ, H.: *Responses evoked in neurones of the fastigial nucleus by cutaneous mechanoreceptors.* Brain Res. 35:523, 1971.

43

99. ECCLES, J. C., SABAH, N. H., AND TÁBOŘÍKOVÁ, H.: *Excitatory and inhibitory responses of neurones of the cerebellar fastigial nucleus.* Exp. Brain Res. 19:61, 1974.

100. ECCLES, J. C., SABAH, N. H., AND TÁBOŘÍKOVÁ, H.: *The pathways responsible for excitation and inhibition of fastigial neurones.* Exp. Brain Res. 19:78, 1974.

101. ECCLES, J. C., RANTUCCI, T., SABAH, N. H. ET AL.: *Somatotopic studies on the cerebellar fastigial cells.* Exp. Brain Res. 19:100, 1974.

102. ECCLES, J. C., RANTUCCI, T., ROSÉN, I. ET AL.: *Somatotopic studies on cerebellar interpositus neurons.* J. Neurophysiol. 37:1449, 1974.

103. ECCLES, J. C., ROSÉN, I., SCHEID, P. ET AL.: *Temporal patterns of responses of interpositus neurons to peripheral afferent stimulation.* J. Neurophysiol. 37:1424, 1974.

104. ECCLES, J. C., ROSÉN, I., SCHEID, P. ET AL.: *Patterns of convergence onto interpositus neurons from peripheral afferents.* J. Neurophysiol. 37:1438, 1974.

105. ECCLES, R. M., AND LUNDBERG, A.: *Synaptic action in motoneurones by afferents which may evoke the flexion reflex.* Arch. Ital. Biol. 97:199, 1959.

106. EIDE, E., FEDINA, L., JANSEN, J. ET AL.: *Unitary excitatory postsynaptic potentials in Clarke's column neurones.* Nature (London) 215:1176, 1967.

107. EIDE, E., FEDINA, L., JANSEN, J. ET AL.: *Properties of Clarke's column neurones.* Acta Physiol. Scand. 77:125, 1969.

108. EIDE, E., FEDINA, L., JANSEN, J., ET AL.: *Unitary components in the activation of Clarke's column neurons.* Acta Physiol. Scand. 77:145, 1969.

109. EKEROT, C. F., AND LARSON, B.: *Differential termination of the exteroceptive and proprioceptive components of the cuneocerebellar tract.* Brain Res. 36:420, 1972.

110. EKEROT, C. F., AND OSCARSSON, O.: *The lateral reticular nucleus in the cat. V. Does collateral activation from the dorsal spinocerebellar tract occur?* Exp. Brain Res. 25:327, 1976.

111. ELLER, T., AND CHAN-PALAY, V.: *Afferents to the cerebellar lateral nucleus. Evidence from retrograde transport of horseradish peroxidase after pressure injections from micropipettes.* J. Comp. Neurol. 166:285, 1976.

112. ENGBERG, I., LUNDBERG, A., AND RYALL, R. W.: *Reticulospinal inhibition of transmission in reflex pathways.* J. Physiol. (London) 194:201, 1968.

113. ENGBERG, I., LUNDBERG, A. AND RYALL, R. W.: *Is the tonic decerebrate inhibition of reflex paths mediated by monoaminergic pathways?* Acta Physiol. Scand. 72:123, 1968.

114. ENGBERG, I., LUNDBERG, A., AND RYALL, R. W.: *Reticulospinal inhibition of interneurones.* J. Physiol. 194:225, 1968.

115. FARNARDJAN, V. V., AND KAZARIAN, L. L.: *Cerebellar evoked potentials in the unrestrained cat.* Fiziol. Zh. SSSR 56:1360, 1970.

116. FOERSTER, O., AND GAGEL, O.: *Die Vorderseitenstrangdurchschneidung beim Menschen.* Z. Neurol. Psychiat. 138:1, 1932.

117. FOX, M., AND WILLIAMS, T. D.: *Responses evoked in the cerebellar cortex by stimulation of the caudate nucleus in the cat.* J. Physiol. 198:435, 1968.

118. FOX, M., AND WILLIAMS, T. D.: *The caudate nucleus-cerebellar pathways: an electrophysiological study of their route through the midbrain.* Brain Res. 20:140, 1970.

119. FU, T. C., JANKOWSKA, E., AND TANAKA, R.: *Effects of volleys in cortico-spinal tract fibres on ventral spino-cerebellar tract cells in the cat.* Acta Physiol. Scand. 100:1, 1977.

120. FURUYA, N., KAWANO, K., AND SHIMAZU, H.: *Functional organization of vestibulofastigial projection in the horizontal semicircular canal system in the cat.* Exp. Brain Res. 24:75, 1975.

121. GACEK, R. R.: *The course and central termination of first order neurons supplying vestibular endorgans in the cat.* Acta Otolaryng. (Stockholm) (Suppl.) 254:1, 1969.

122. GHELARDUCCI, B., POMPEIANO, O., AND SPYER, K. M.: *Activity of precerebellar reticular neurones as a function of head position.* Arch. Ital. Biol. 112:98, 1974.

123. GHELARDUCCI, B., POMPEIANO, O., AND SPYER, K. M.: *Distribution of the neuronal responses to static tilts within cerebellar fastigial nucleus.* Arch. Ital. Biol. 112:126, 1974.

124. GORDON, G., AND HORROBIN, D.: *Antidromic and synaptic responses in the cat's gracile nucleus to cerebellar stimulation.* Brain Res. 5:419, 1967.

125. GORDON, G., AND SEED, W. A.: *An investigation of nucleus gracilis of the cat by antidromic stimulation.* J. Physiol. (London) 155:589, 1961.

126. GOULD, B. B., AND GRAYBIEL, A. M.: *Afferents to the cerebellar cortex in the cat: Evidence for an intrinsic pathway leading from the deep nuclei to the cortex.* Brain Res. 110:601, 1976.

127. GRANT, G.: *Projection of the external cuneate nucleus onto the cerebellum in the cat: An experimental study using silver methods.* Exp. Neurol. 5:179, 1962.

128. GRANT, G.: *Spinal course and somatotopically localized termination of the spinocerebellar tracts. An experimental study in the cat.* Acta Physiol. Scand. 56 (Suppl. 193):5–42, 1962.

129. GRANT, G.: *Demonstration of degenerating climbing fibres in the molecular layer of the cerebellum.* Brain Res. 22:236, 1970.

130. GRANT, G., OSCARSSON, O., AND ROSEN, I.: *Functional organization of the spinoreticulocerebellar path with identification of its spinal component.* Exp. Brain Res. 1:306, 1966.

131. GRANT, G., AND REXED, B.: *Dorsal spinal root afferents to Clarke's column.* Brain 81:567, 1958.

132. GRESTY, M. A., AND PAUL, D. H.: *Projection of the caudate nucleus on the anterior lobe of the cerebellum.* J. Physiol. (London) 204:81, 1969.

133. GRESTY, M. A., AND PAUL, D. H.: *Responses of fastigial nucleus neurones to stimulation of the caudate nucleus in the cat.* J. Physiol. 245:655, 1975.

134. GUSTAFSSON, B., LINDSTRÖM, S., AND TAKATA, M.: *A re-evaluation of the after hyperpolarization mechanism in dorsal spinocerebellar tract neurons.* Brain Res. 35:543, 1971.

135. GUSTAFSSON, B., LINDSTRÖM, S., AND TAKATA, M.: *Repetitive firing in dorsal spinocerebellar tract neurones.* Brain Res. 47:506, 1972.

136. GUSTAFSSON, B., LINDSTRÖM, S., AND TAKATA, M.: *Afterhyperpolarization mechanism in the dorsal spinocerebellar tract cells of the cat.* J. Physiol. 275:283, 1978.

137. GUSTAFSSON, B., LINDSTRÖM, S., AND ZANGGER, P.: *Firing behaviour of dorsal spinocerebellar tract neurones.* J. Physiol. 275:321, 1978.

138. GUSTAFSSON, B., AND ZANGGER, P.: *"Depression" of the afterhyperpolarization in dorsal spino-cerebellar tract neurones.* Brain Res. 72:320, 1974.

139. GUSTAFSSON, B., AND ZANGGER, P.: *Effect of repetitive activation on the afterhyperpolarization in dorsal spinocerebellar tract neurones.* J. Physiol. 275:303, 1978.

140. HAMES, E. G., EBNER, T. J., AND BLOEDEL, J. R.: *The dentato-rubro-spinal system in the cat.* Submitted for publication, 1980.

141. HAMES, E. G., TOLBERT, D. L., AND BLOEDEL, J. R.: *Evidence for a new spinocerebellar projection from the nucleus dorsalis (Clarke's column) in the cat.* Neurosci. Abstr. 4:65, 1978.

142. HAND, P. J.: *Lumbosacral dorsal root terminations in the nucleus gracilis of the cat. Some observations on terminal degeneration in other medullary sensory nuclei.* J. Comp. Neurol. 126:137, 1966.

143. HAND, P. J., AND LIU, C. N.: *Efferent projections of the nucleus gracilis.* Anat. Rev. 154:353, 1966.

144. HAZLETT, J. C., MARTIN, G. F., AND DOM, R.: *Spino-cerebellar fibers of the opossum (Didelphis marsupialis virginiana).* Brain Res. 33:257, 1971.

145. HIGGINS, D. C.: *Behavior of dorsal spinocerebellar neurons during sinusoidal muscle stretch.* Am. J. Physiol. 220:2032, 1971.

146. HILLMAN, D. E.: *Light and electron microscopical study of the relationships between the cerebellum and the vestibular organ of the frog.* Exp. Brain Res. 9:1, 1969.

147. HILLMAN, D. E.: *Vestibulocerebellar input in the frog: anatomy.* Prog. Brain Res. 37:329, 1972.

148. HINMAN, A., AND CARPENTER, M. B.: *Efferent fiber projections of the red nucleus in the cat.* J. Comp. Neurol. 113:61, 1959.

149. HIRAI, N., HONGO, T., KUDO, N. ET AL.: *Heterogeneous composition of the spinocerebellar tract originating from the cervical enlargement in the cat.* Brain Res. 109:387, 1976.

150. HODDEVIK, G. H.: *The pontocerebellar projection onto the paramedian lobule in the cat: An experimental study with the use of horseradish peroxidase as a tracer.* Brain Res. 95:291, 1975.

151. HODDEVIK, G. H.: *The pontine projection to the flocculonodular lobe and the paraflocculus studied by means of retrograde axonal transport of horseradish peroxidase in the rabbit.* Exp. Brain Res. 30:511, 1977.

152. HODDEVIK, G. H., BRODAL, A., KAWAMURA, K. ET AL.: *The pontine projection to the cerebellar vermal visual area studied by means of the retrograde axonal transport of horseradish peroxidase.* Brain Res. 123:209, 1977.

153. HOLMQVIST, B., AND LUNDBERG, A.: *On the organization of the supraspinal inhibitory control of interneurons of various spinal reflex arcs.* Arch. Ital. Biol. 97:340, 1959.

154. HOLMQVIST, B., AND LUNDBERG, A.: *Differential supraspinal control of synaptic actions evoked by volleys in the flexion reflex afferents in alpha motoneurones.* Acta Physiol. Scand. 54 (Suppl. 186):1, 1961.

155. HOLMQVIST, G., LUNDBERG, A., AND OSCARSSON, O.: *Supraspinal inhibitory control of transmission to three ascending spinal pathways influenced by the flexion reflex afferents.* Arch. Ital. Biol. 98:60, 1960.

156. HOLMQVIST, B., OSCARSSON, O., AND ROSÉN, I.: *Functional organization of the cuneocerebellar tract in the cat.* Acta Physiol. Scand. 58:216, 1963.

157. HONGO, T., AND OKADA, Y.: *Cortically evoked pre- and postsynaptic inhibition of impulse transmission to the dorsal spinocerebellar tract.* Exp. Brain Res. 3:163, 1967.

158. HONGO, T., OKADA, Y., AND SATO, M.: *Corticofugal influences on transmission to the dorsal spinocerebellar tract from hindlimb primary afferents.* Exp. Brain Res. 3:135, 1967.

159. HUBBARD, J. I., AND OSCARSSON, O.: *Localization of the cell bodies of the ventral spinocerebellar tract from hindlimb primary afferents.* J. Comp. Neurol. 118:119, 1962.

160. HYDE, J. B.: *A comparative study of certain trigeminal components in two soricid shrews, Blarina brevicauda and Sorex cinereus.* J. Comp. Neurol. 107:339, 1957.

161. IKEDA, M., AND MATSUSHITA, M.: *Electron microscopic observations on the spinal projections to the cerebellar nuclei in the cat and rabbit.* Experientia 29:1280, 1973.

162. INGVAR, S.: *Zur Phylo- und Ontogenese des Kleinhirns.* Folia Neurobiol. (Leipzig) 11:205, 1918.

163. ITO, M., YOSHIDA, M., AND OBATA, R.: *Monosynaptic inhibition of the intracellular nuclei induced from the cerebellar cortex.* Experientia 10:575, 1964.

164. ITO, M., YOSHIDA, M., OBATA, K. ET AL.: *Inhibitory control of intracerebellar nuclei by the Purkinje cell axons.* Exp. Brain Res. 20:64, 1970.

165. JAKOB, A.: *Das Kleinhirn,* in Mollendorff, W. V. (ed.): *Handbuch der mikroskopischen Anatomie des Menschen,* Vol. VI:1. Springer, Berlin, 1928, pp. 674–916.

166. JANKOWSKA, E., JUKES, M. G. M., AND LUND, S.: *On the presynaptic inhibition of transmission to the dorsal spinocerebellar tract.* J. Physiol. (London) 177:;19, 1965.

167. JANKOWSKA, E., JUKES, M. G. M., AND LUND, S.: *The pattern of presynaptic inhibition of transmission to the dorsal spinocerebellar tract of the cat.* J. Physiol. (London) 178:17, 1965.

168. JANSEN, J. K. S., NICOLAYSEN, K., AND RUDJORD, T.: *On the firing pattern of spinal neurones activated from the secondary endings of muscle spindles.* Acta Physiol. Scand. 70:188, 1967.

169. JANSEN, J. K. S., NICOLAYSEN, K., AND WALLØE, L.: *On the inhibition of transmission to the dorsal spinocerebellar tract by stretch of various ankle muscles of the cat.* Acta Physiol. Scand. 70:362, 1967.

170. JANSEN, J. K. S., NICOLAYSEN, K., AND WALLØE, L.: *The firing pattern of dorsal spinocerebellar tract neurones during inhibition.* Acta Physiol. Scand. 77:68, 1969.

171. JANSEN, J. K. S., AND WALLØE, L.: *Transmission of signals from muscle stretch receptors to the dorsal spinocerebellar tract,* in Fields, W. S., and Willis, W. D. (eds.):*The Cerebellum in Health and Disease.* Green, St. Louis, 1970, pp. 143–171.

172. JANSEN, J. K. S., AND WALLØE, L.: *Signal transmission between successive neurons in the dorsal spinocerebellar pathway,* in Schmitt, F. (ed.): *The Neurosciences: Second Study Program.* Rockefeller University Press, New York, 1970, pp. 617–629.

173. JOHANSSON, H., AND SILFVENIUS, H.: *Axon-collateral activation by dorsal spinocerebellar tract fibres of group I relay cells of nucleus z in the cat medulla oblongata.* J. Physiol. 265:341, 1977.

174. JOHANSSON, H., AND SILFVENIUS, H.: *Input from ipsilateral proprio- and exteroceptive hindlimb afferents to nucleus z of the cat medulla oblongata.* J. Physiol. 265:371, 1977.

175. KAWAMURA, K., AND BRODAL, A.: *The tectopontine projection in the cat: An experimental anatomical study with comments on pathways for teleceptive impulses to the cerebellum.* J. Comp. Neurol. 149:371, 1973.

176. KITAI, S. T., DeFRANCE, J. F., HATADA, K. ET AL.: *Electrophysiological properties of lateral reticular nucleus cells. II. Synaptic activation.* Exp. Brain Res. 21:419, 1974.

177. KITAI, S. T., HATADA, K., AND CASEY, W.: *Intracellular analysis of antidromically and synaptically activated lateral reticular neurons.* Brain Res. 43:629, 1972.

178. KITAI, S. T., KENNEDY, D. T., MORIN, F. ET AL.: *The lateral reticular nucleus of the medulla oblongata of the cat.* Exp. Neurol. 17:65, 1967.

179. KITAI, S. T., AND MORIN, F.: *Microelectrode study of dorsal spinocerebellar tract.* Am. J. Physiol. 203:799, 1962.

180. KITAI, S. T., OSHIMA, T., PROVINI, L. ET AL.: *Cerebro-cerebellar connections mediated by fast and slow conducting pyramidal tract fibres of the cat.* Brain Res. 15:267, 1969.

181. KNOX, C. K., KUBOTA, S., AND POPPELE, R. E.: *A determination of excitability changes in dorsal spinocerebellar tract neurons from spike-train analysis.* J. Neurophysiol. 40:626, 1977.

182. KORTE, G. E., AND MUGNAINI, E.: *The cerebellar projection of the vestibular nerve in the cat.* J. Comp. Neurol. 184:265, 1979.

183. KOSTYUK, P. G., AND ZADOROZHNY, A. G.: *Synaptic organization of the spinocerebellar pathways,* in Fanardjan, V. V. (ed.): *Structural and Functional Organization of the Cerebellum.* Nauka, Leningrad, 1971, pp. 28–34.

184. KOTCHABHAKDI, N., AND WALBERG, F.: *Cerebellar afferent projections from the vestibular nuclei in the cat: An experimental study with the method of retrograde axonal transport of horseradish peroxidase.* Exp. Brain Res. 31:591, 1978.

185. KUNO, M., AND MIYAHARA, J. T.: *Factors responsible for multiple discharge of neurons in Clarke's column.* J. Neurophysiol. 31:624, 1968.

186. KUNO, M., MUÑOZ-MARTINEZ, E. J., AND RANDIC, M.: *Sensory inputs to neurones in Clarke's column from muscle cutaneous and joint receptors.* J. Physiol. 228:327, 1973.

187. KUNO, M., MUÑOZ-MARTINEZ, E. J., AND RANDIC, M.: *Synaptic action on Clarke's column neurones in relation to afferent terminal size.* J. Physiol. 228:343, 1973.

188. KÜNZLE, H.: *The topographic organization of spinal afferents to the lateral reticular nucleus of the cat.* J. Comp. Neurol. 149:103, 1973.

189. KÜNZLE, H.: *Autoradiographic tracing of the cerebellar projections from the lateral reticular nucleus in the cat.* Exp. Brain Res. 22:255, 1975.

190. KÜNZLE, H., AND WIESENDANGER, M.: *Pyramidal connections to the lateral reticular nucleus in the cat: A degeneration study.* Acta Anat. (Basel) 88:105, 1974.

191. KUYPERS, H. G. J. M.: *An anatomical analysis of cortico-bulbar connexions to the pons and lower brain stem in the cat.* J. Anat. (London) 92:198, 1958.

192. LAPORTE, Y., LUNDBERG, A., AND OSCARSSON, O.: *Functional organization of the dorsal spinocerebellar tract in the cat. II. Single fibre recording in Flechsig's fasciculus on electrical stimulation of various peripheral nerves.* Acta Physiol. Scand. 36:188, 1956.

193. LARSELL, O.: *The development and morphology of the cerebellum in the opossum. II. Later development and adult.* J. Comp. Neurol. 63:251, 1936.

194. LARSELL, O.: *Cerebellum and corpus pontobulbare of the bat (Myotis).* J. Comp. Neurol. 64:275, 1936.

195. LARSELL, O.: *The development of the cerebellum in man in relation to its comparative anatomy.* J. Comp. Neurol. 87:85, 1947.

196. LARSELL, O.: *The cerebellum of myxinoids and petro-myzonts, including developmental stages in the lamprey.* J. Comp. Neurol. 86:395, 1947.

197. LARSELL, O., AND JANSEN, J.: *The Comparative Anatomy and Histology of the Cerebellum: The Human Cerebellum, Cerebellar Connections, and Cerebellar Cortex.* University of Minnesota Press, Minneapolis, 1972.

198. LINDSTRÖM, S., AND SCHOMBURG, E. D.: *Recurrent inhibition from motor axon collaterals of ventral spinocerebellar tract neurones.* Acta Physiol. Scand. 88:505, 1973.

199. LINDSTRÖM, S., AND SCHOMBURG, E. D.: *Group I inhibition in Ib excited ventral spinocerebellar tract neurones.* Acta Physiol. Scand. 90:166, 1974.

200. LINDSTRÖM, S., AND TAKATA, M.: *Monosynaptic excitation of dorsal spinocerebellar tract neurones from low threshold joint afferents.* Acta Physiol. Scand. 84:430, 1972.

201. LIU, C. N.: *Afferent nerves to Clarke's and the lateral cuneate nuclei in the cat.* Arch. Neurol. Psychiat. 75:67, 1956.

202. LLINÁS, R., AND PRECHT, W.: *Vestibulocerebellar input: physiology.* Prog. Brain Res. 37:341, 1972.

203. LLINÁS, R., PRECHT, W., AND KITAI, S. T.: *Climbing fibre activation of Purkinje cell following primary vestibular afferent stimulation in the frog.* Brain Res. 6:371, 1967.
204. LOEWY, A. D.: *A study of neuronal types in Clarke's column in the adult cat.* J. Comp. Neurol. 139:53, 1970.
205. LUNDBERG, A.: *Integration in the reflex pathway,* in Granit, R. (ed.): *Muscular Afferents and Motor Control.* Almqvist and Wiksell, Stockholm, 1966, pp. 275–305.
206. LUNDBERG, A.: *Function of the ventral spinocerebellar tract. A new hypothesis.* Exp. Brain Res. 12:317, 1971.
207. LUNDBERG, A., NORRSELL, U., AND VOORHOEVE, P.: *Effects from the sensorimotor cortex on ascending spinal pathways.* Acta Physiol. Scand. 59:462, 1963.
208. LUNDBERG, A., AND OSCARSSON, O.: *Functional organization of the dorsal spinocerebellar tract in the cat. VII. Identification of units by antidromic activation from the cerebellar cortex with recognition of five functional subdivisions.* Acta Physiol. Scand. 50:356, 1960.
209. LUNDBERG, A., AND OSCARSSON, O.: *Functional organization of the ventral spino-cerebellar tract in the cat. IV. Identification of units by antidromic activation from the cerebellar cortex.* Acta Physiol. Scand. 54:252, 1962.
210. LUNDBERG, A., AND VYKLICKY, L.: *Inhibition of transmission of primary afferents by electrical stimulation of the brain stem.* Arch. Ital. Biol. 104:86, 1966.
211. LUNDBERG, A., AND WEIGHT, F.: *Signaling of reciprocal Ia inhibition by the ventral spinocerebellar tract.* Brain Res. 23:109, 1970.
212. LUNDBERG, A., AND WEIGHT, F.: *Functional organization of connexions to the ventral spinocerebellar tract.* Exp. Brain Res. 12:295, 1971.
213. MAGNI, E., AND OSCARSSON, O.: *Cerebral control of transmission to the ventral spino-cerebellar tract.* Arch. Ital. Biol. 99:369, 1961.
214. MANN, M. D.: *Axons of dorsal spinocerebellar tract which respond to activity in cutaneous receptors.* J. Neurophysiol. 34:1035, 1971.
215. MANN, M. D.: *Clarke's column and the dorsal spinocerebellar tract. A review.* Brain Behav. Evol. 7:34, 1973.
216. MANN, M. D., AND TAPPER, D. N.: *Cutaneous subdivision of the dorsal spinocerebellar tract.* Physiologist 13:255, 1970.
217. MARTIN, G. F., BEATTIE, M. S., HUGHES, H. C. ET AL.: *The organization of reticulo-olivo-cerebellar circuits in the North American opossum.* Brain Res. 137:253, 1977.
218. MATSUSHITA, M., AND IKEDA, M.: *Spinal projections to the cerebellar nuclei in the cat.* Exp. Brain Res. 10:501, 1970.
219. MATSUSHITA, M., AND IKEDA, M.: *The central cervical nucleus as cell origin of a spinocerebellar tract arising from the cervical cord: A study in the cat using horseradish peroxidase.* Brain Res. 100:412, 1975.
220. MATSUSHITA, M., AND IKEDA, M.: *Projections from the lateral reticular nucleus to the cerebellar cortex and nuclei in the cat.* Exp. Brain Res. 24:403, 1976.
221. MATSUSHITA, M., AND UEYAMA, T.: *Projections from the spinal cord to the cerebellar nuclei in the rabbit and rat.* Exp. Neurol. 38:438, 1973.
222. MCCREA, R. A., BISHOP, G. A., AND KITAI, S. T.: *Electrophysiological horseradish peroxidase studies of precerebellar afferents to the nucleus interpositus anterior. II. Mossy fiber system.* Brain Res. 122:215, 1977.
223. MCINTYRE, A. K., AND MARK, R. F.: *Synaptic linkage between afferent fibres of the cat's hindlimb and ascending fibres in the dorsolateral funiculus.* J. Physiol. 153:306, 1960.
224. MIZUNO, N., MOCHIZUKI, K., AKIMOTO, C. ET AL.: *Pretectal projection to the inferior olive in the rabbit.* Exp. Neurol. 39:498, 1973.
225. MIZUNO, N., MOCHIZUKI, K., AKIMOTO, C. ET AL.: *Projections from the parietal cortex to the brain stem nuclei in the cat, with special reference to the parietal cerebrocerebellar system.* J. Comp. Neurol. 147:511, 1973.
226. MORIN, F., SCHWARTZ, H. G., AND O'LEARY, J. L.: *Experimental study of the spinothalamic and related tracts.* Acta Psychiat. Neurol. Scand. 26:371, 1951.
227. MUÑOZ-MARTINES, E. J.: *Effects of activity in single sensory fibres on the discharge patterns of dorsal spinocerebellar tract cells.* J. Physiol. 245:1, 1975.

48

228. NIJENSOHN, D. E., AND KERR, F. W.: *The ascending projections of the dorsolateral funiculus of the spinal cord in the primate.* J. Comp. Neurol. 161:459, 1975.

229. NYBY, O., AND JANSEN, J.: *An experimental investigation of the corticopontine projection in Macaca mulatta.* Skr. Norske. Vidensk-Akad, I. Mat.-Nat. Kl. 3:1, 1951.

230. OKA, H., AND JINNAL, K.: *Common projection of the motor cortex to the caudate nucleus and the cerebellum.* Exp. Brain Res. 31:31, 1978.

231. OKA, H., SASAKI, K., MATSUDA, Y. ET AL.: *Responses of pontocerebellar neurones to stimulation of the parietal association and the frontal motor cortices.* Brain Res. 93:399, 1975.

232. OSCARSSON, O.: *Functional organization of the ventral spino-cerebellar tract in the cat. II. Connections with muscle, joint, and skin nerve afferents and effects on adequate stimulation of various receptors.* Acta Physiol. Scand. 42(Suppl. 146):5, 1957.

233. OSCARSSON, O.: *Primary afferent collaterals and spinal relays of the dorsal and ventral spinocerebellar tracts.* Acta Physiol. Scand. 40:222, 1957.

234. OSCARSSON, O.: *Functional organization of the ventral spino-cerebellar tract in the cat. III. Supraspinal control of VSCT units of I-type.* Acta Physiol. Scand. 49:171, 1960.

235. OSCARSSON, O.: *Functional organization of the spino- and cuneocerebellar tracts.* Physiol. Rev. 45:495, 1965.

236. OSCARSSON, O.: *Integrative organization of the rostral spinocerebellar tract in the cat.* Acta Physiol. Scand. 64:154, 1965.

237. OSCARSSON, O.: *Functional significance of information channels from the spinal cord to the cerebellum,* in Yahr, M. D., and Purpura, D. P. (eds.): *Neurophysiological Basis of Normal and Abnormal Motor Activities.* Raven Press, New York, 1967, pp. 93–113.

238. OSCARSSON, O.: *Functional organization of spinocerebellar paths,* in Iggo, A. (ed.): *Handbook of Sensory Physiology,* Vol. II. *Somatosensory System.* Springer, Berlin, 1973, pp. 339–380.

239. OSCARSSON, O., AND ROSÉN, I.: *Response characteristics of reticulocerebellar neurones activated from spinal afferents.* Exp. Brain Res. 1:320, 1966.

240. OSCARSSON, O., AND UDDENBERG, N.: *Identification of a spinocerebellar tract activated from forelimb afferents in the cat.* Acta Physiol. Scand. 62:125, 1964.

241. PEARSON, A. A.: *The development and connections of the mesencephalic root of the trigeminal nerve in man.* J. Comp. Neurol. 90:1, 1949.

242. PETRAS, J. M., AND CUMMINGS, J. F.: *The origin of spinocerebellar pathways II. The nucleus centrobasalis of the cervical enlargement and the nucleus dorsalis of the thoracolumbar spinal cord.* J. Comp. Neurol. 173:693, 1977.

243. PIATIGORSKI, B. J., AND VASILENKO, D. A.: *Phonic and evoked activity of dorsal spino-cerebellar tract neurons and their supraspinal control,* in Fanardjan, V. V. (ed.): *Structural and Functional Organization of the Cerebellum.* Nauka, Lenningrad, 1971, pp. 34–39.

244. POMPEIANO, O.: *Macular input to neurons of the spino-reticulocerebellar pathway.* Brain Res. 95:351–368, 1975.

245. POMPEIANO, O.: *Macular influence on somatosensory transmission through the spinoreticulocerebellar pathway.* J. Physiol. (Paris) 73:387, 1977.

246. POMPEIANO, O., AND BRODAL, A.: *Experimental demonstration of a somatotopical origin of rubrospinal fibers in the cat.* J. Comp. Neurol. 108:225, 1957.

247. POMPEIANO, O., AND HOSHINO, K.: *Responses to static tilts of lateral reticular neurons mediated by contralateral labyrinthine receptors.* Arch. Ital. Biol. 115:211, 1977.

248. RAMON Y CAJAL, S.: *Histologie du système nerveux de l'homme et des vertébrés,* Vol. I. Maloine, Paris, 1909.

249. RAMON Y CAJAL, S.: *Histologie du système nerveux de l'homme et des vertébrés,* Vol. II. Maloine, Paris, 1911.

250. RÉTHELYI, M.: *Golgi architecture of Clarke's column.* Acta Morph. Hung. 16:311, 1968.

251. RÉTHELYI, M.: *Ultrastructural synaptology of Clarke's column.* Exp. Brain Res. 11:159, 1970.

252. RINVIK, E., AND WALBERG, F.: *Studies on the cerebellar projections from the main and external cuneate nuclei in the cat by means of retrograde axonal transport of horseradish peroxidase.* Brain Res. 95:371, 1975.

253. ROSÉN, I., AND SCHEID, P.: *Patterns of afferent input to the lateral reticular nucleus of the cat.* Exp. Brain Res. 18:242, 1973.

254. ROSÉN, I., AND SCHEID, P.: *Responses in the spino-reticulo-cerebellar pathway to stimulation of cutaneous mechanoreceptors.* Exp. Brain Res. 18:268, 1973.

255. ROSÉN, I., AND SJÖLUND, B.: *Natural stimulation of group I activated cells in the cuneate nuclei of the cat.* Acta Physiol. Scand. (Suppl.)330:189, 1969.

256. RÜEGG, D. G., SÉGUIN, J. J., AND WIESENDANGER, M.: *Effects of electrical stimulation of somatosensory and motor areas of the cerebral cortex on neurones of the pontine nuclei in squirrel monkeys.* Neurosci. 2:923, 1977.

257. RÜEGG, D. G., AND WIESENDANGER, M.: *Corticofugal effects from sensorimotor area I and somatosensory area II on neurones of the pontine nuclei in the cat.* J. Physiol. 247:745, 1975.

258. SAITO, K.: *The synaptology and cytology of the Clarke cell in nucleus dorsalis of the cat. An electron microscopic study.* J. Neurocytol. 3:179, 1974.

259. SASAKI, K., KAWAGUCHI, S., SHIMONO, T., ET AL.: *Electrophysiological studies of the pontine nuclei.* Brain Res. 20:425, 1970.

260. SASAKI, K., AND STRATA, P.: *Responses evoked in the cerebellar cortex by stimulating mossy fibre pathways to the cerebellum.* Exp. Brain Res. 3:95, 1967.

261. SCHMIDT, R. F.: *Control of the access of afferent activity to somatosensory pathways,* in Iggo, A. (ed.): *Handbook of Sensory Physiology.* Vol. II, Springer, Berlin, 1973, pp. 151 – 206.

262. SMITH, M. C.: *The anatomy of the spino-cerebellar fibers in man I. The course of fibers in the spinal cord and brain stem.* J. Comp. Neurol. 108:285, 1957.

263. SNIDER, R. S., AND STOWELL, A.: *Receiving areas of the tactile, auditory, and visual systems in the cerebellum.* J. Neurophysiol. 7:331, 1944.

264. SNYDER, R. L., FAULL, R. L. M., AND MEHLER, W. R.: *A comparative study of the neurons of origin of the spinocerebellar afferents in the rat, cat and squirrel monkey based on the retrograde transport of horseradish peroxidase.* J. Comp. Neurol. 181:833, 1978.

265. SOMANA, R., AND WALBERG, F.: *Cerebellar afferents from the paramedian reticular nucleus studied with retrograde transport of horseradish peroxidase.* Anat. Embryol. 154:353, 1978.

266. SOUSA-PINTO, A.: *The cortical projection onto the paramedian reticular and perihypoglossal nuclei (nucleus praepositus hypoglossi, nucleus intercalatus and nucleus of Roller) of the medulla oblongata of the cat. An experimental anatomical study.* Brain Res. 18:77, 1970.

267. SPRAGUE, J. M.: *Spinal border cells and their role in postural mechanism (Schiff-Sherrington phenomenon).* J. Neurophysiol. 16:464, 1953.

268. STEIN, R. B.: *A theoretical analysis of neuronal variability.* Biophys. J. 5:173, 1965.

269. STEIN, R. B.: *Some models of neuronal variability.* Biophys. J. 7:37, 1967.

270. STEIN, B. M., AND CARPENTER, M. B.: *Central projections of portions of the vestibular ganglia innervating specific parts of the labyrinth in the rhesus monkey.* Am. J. Anat. 120:281, 1967.

271. SUNDERLAND, S.: *The projection of the cerebral cortex on the pons and cerebellum in the macaque monkey.* J. Anat. (London) 74:201, 1940.

272. SZENTÁGOTHAI, J., AND ALBERT, A.: *The synaptology of Clarke's column.* Acta Morph. Hung. 5:43, 1955.

273. TAPPER, D. N., MANN, M. D., BROWN, P. B. ET AL.: *Cells of origin of the cutaneous subdivision of the dorsal spinocerebellar tract.* Brain Res. 85:59, 1975.

274. TOLBERT, D. L., BANTLI, H., AND BLOEDEL, J. R.: *A cerebellar nucleocortical projection in the cat.* Anat. Rec. 184:547, 1976.

275. TOLBERT, D. L., BANTLI, H., AND BLOEDEL, J. R.: *Anatomical and physiological evidence for a cerebellar nucleocortical projection in the cat.* Neurosci. 1:205, 1976.

276. TOLBERT, D. L., BANTLI, H., AND BLOEDEL, J. R.: *The topographical organization of the cat cerebellar nucleo-cortical projection.* Anat. Rec. 187:731, 1977.

277. TOLBERT, D. L., BANTLI, H., AND BLOEDEL, J. R.: *The organization of the cerebellar nucleo-cortical projection in the monkey.* Anat. Rec. 190:562, 1978.

278. TOLBERT, D. L., BANTLI, H., AND BLOEDEL, J. R.: *Organizational features of the cat and monkey cerebellar nucleocortical projection.* J. Comp. Neurol. 182:39, 1978.

279. TSANG, Y.: *The cerebellar connections of the mesencephalic nucleus of the trigeminus.* Sci. Sin. 7:867, 1961.

280. TSUKAHARA, N., KORN, H., AND STONE, J.: *Pontine relay from cerebral cortex to cerebellar cortex and nucleus interpositus.* Brain Res. 10:448, 1968.

281. TUCKWELL, H. C.: *Frequency of firing of Stein's model neuron with application to cells in the dorsal spino-cerebellar tract.* Brain Res. 116:323, 1976.

282. VACHANANDA, B.: *The major spinal afferent systems to the cerebellum and the cerebellar cortical nuclear connections in Macaca Mulatta.* J. Comp. Neurol. 112:303, 1959.

283. VAN BEUSEKOM, T. T.: *Fiber analysis of the anterior and lateral funiculi of the cord in the cat.* Eduard Ijdo N. V. Leiden, 143pp, 1955.

284. VERHAART, W. J. C.: *The lateral reticular nucleus of the medulla oblongata and the passing fibre systems of the lateral funiculus.* Acta Psychiat. Neurol. Scand. 32:211, 1957.

285. VOOGD, J.: *The Cerebellum of the Cat.* F. A. Davis Co., Philadelphia, 1964.

286. WALBERG, F.: *The lateral reticular nucleus of the medulla oblongata in mammals. A comparative-anatomical study.* J. Comp. Neurol. 96:283, 1952.

287. WALBERG, F.: *Descending connections to the lateral reticular nucleus. An experimental study in the cat.* J. Comp. Neurol. 109:363, 1958.

288. WALBERG, F., AND POMPEIANO, O.: *Fastigiofugal fibers to the lateral reticular nucleus: An experimental study in the cat.* Exp. Neurol. 2:40, 1960.

289. WALBERG, F., POMPEIANO, O., WESTRUM, L. E. ET AL.: *Fastigioreticular fibers in cat. An experimental study with silver methods.* J. Comp. Neurol. 119:187, 1962.

290. WHITLOCK, D. G.: *A neurohistological and neurophysiological study of afferent fiber tracts and receptive areas of the avian cerebellum.* J. Comp. Neurol. 97:567, 1952.

291. WOODBURNE. R. T.: *A phylogenetic consideration of the primary and secondary centers and connections of the trigeminal complex in a series of vertebrates.* J. Comp. Neurol. 65:403, 1936.

292. YOSS, R. E.: *Studies of the spinal cord. II. Topographic localization within the ventral spinocerebellar tract in the macaque.* J. Comp. Neurol. 99:613, 1953.

293. ZANGGER, P., AND WIESENDANGER, M.: *Excitation of lateral reticular nucleus neurones by collaterals of the pyramidal tract.* Exp. Brain Res. 17:144, 1973.

CHAPTER 3

Inputs to the Cerebellum: Climbing Fiber and Aminergic Afferents

CLIMBING FIBER PROJECTIONS

Origin and Course of Climbing Fibers

Ramon y Cajal described many of the remarkable morphologic characteristics of the climbing fibers almost a century ago.[110, 111] He identified the climbing fibers as a distinct cerebellar afferent projection with processes that ascend through the granular and Purkinje cell layers into the molecular cell layer and entwine the dendrites of Purkinje cells, appearing to "climb" along these neurons.

The origin of the climbing fibers has been controversial. Systematic investigation of this issue began with Brodal's studies showing that the inferior olive is the source of a topographically organized projection to the cerebellar cortex.[23] It was not until the subsequent degeneration studies of Szentágothai and Rajkovits,[128] however, that the inferior olive was recognized as a source of climbing fiber projections. Later investigations suggested that other sources of climbing fiber projections may exist. The pons seemed to be a likely source, because stimuli in this region evoked climbing fiber responses in the cerebellar cortex.[115, 116] Similar responses could be evoked by stimulation near the brachium conjunctivum.[12] Further support for the existence of extraolivary sources for climbing fibers came from studies showing responses in the cerebellar cortex evoked by climbing fibers in animals with chronic lesions of the olivocerebellar projection.[13, 14] Recent anatomic studies also have indicated that climbing fibers may originate in sites apart from the inferior olive. Injection of radioactive amino acids into the inferior olive labeled the terminals of climbing fibers organized in sagittal strips which were separated by other strips containing no labeled olivocerebellar fibers.[34, 37, 39, 59] The finding of strips without olivocerebellar projections was cited as evidence that the climbing fiber input to these bands originates within extraolivary sites.[43, 59]

Recent studies have shown that the climbing fiber input to all the strips originates in the olive. Suspecting that the earlier finding of unlabeled strips resulted from incomplete labeling of the inferior olive, Courville and Faraco-Cantin[38] attempted to label the entire inferior olive with radioactive amino acids. They found a distribution of labeled fibers and terminals consistent with the notion that all climbing fibers originate within the inferior olive.[44] Most of these fibers project in the inferior peduncle. Earlier studies showing that pontine stimulation evoked direct climbing fiber responses in the cerebellar cortex may be explained by the recent demonstration that the axons of some olivary neurons course in the pons before entering the cerebellum through the superior cerebellar peduncle.[38] Thus, olivocerebellar fibers enter the cerebellum through the inferior and superior cerebellar peduncles. In addition, some olivary neurons have fibers projecting to and terminating within the pons. These fibers probably are collaterals of fibers projecting from the inferior olive to the cerebellar cortex. Consequently, stimuli applied in the vicinity of the pontine nuclei may activate two types of climbing fibers originating in the olive: 1) axons of olivocerebellar neurons projecting rostrally before entering the cerebellum and 2) collaterals of the olivocerebellar pathway projecting to the pons. Based upon this compelling evidence, it seems certain now that the climbing fiber input to the cerebellum originates completely within the inferior olive in mammals. In lower vertebrates extraolivary sources of climbing fibers do exist.[83]

The Inferior Olive

The inferior olive consists of a lamellated structure with three major subdivisions: the dorsal accessory olive, principal olive, and medial accessory olive (Fig. 1A). All portions of this structure send fibers to the contralateral side of the cere-

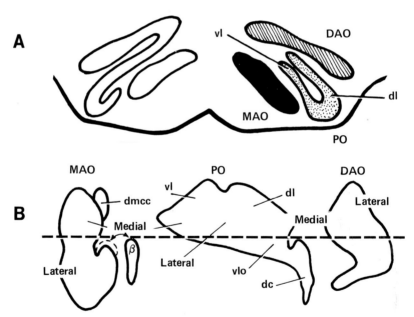

Figure 1. Diagrammatic representations of the inferior olive in the cat. A, A cross-section through the inferior olive at a point approximately midway through its rostrocaudal extent. The nucleus consists of folded sheets of neurons which can be divided topographically into three major regions: the dorsal accessory olive (DAO), the principal olive (PO), and the medial accessory olive (MAO). B, A horizontal view of the olive depicted as an unfolded nuclear mass divided into its three components. Each folded sheet is oriented in a caudal-rostral direction, and the dotted line indicates the section through which the upper diagram is taken (before the nucleus is unfolded). Abbreviations: dmcc = the dorsomedial cell column; β = subnucleus beta; vl = ventral lamella; dl = dorsal lamella; vlo = ventrolateral outgrowth; dc = dorsal cap. (Redrawn from Bloedel and Courville,[16] with permission.)

54

bellum. The description of the topographic relationships of the olivocerebellar and cerebello-olivary pathways requires a two dimensional representation of each major subdivision. This representation depicts the nuclear subgroups as unfolded sheets (Fig. 1B), making it possible to designate the origin and termination of various pathways in one diagram rather than several serial sections through the inferior olive.

The Organization of the Olivocerebellar Projection

Brodal's pioneering study of the olivocerebellar projection[23, 24] established some important principles concerning its organization: 1) small regions within the inferior olive project to discrete regions of the cerebellar cortex; 2) the olivocerebellar projection is completely crossed; and 3) projections from the olive reach all regions of the cerebellar cortex. Subsequent studies have shown that the olivocerebellar projection provides a highly organized topographic input to the cerebellar cortex (Fig. 2).[5, 16, 25, 27, 59, 60, 133] The fibers reaching the anterior lobe of the cerebellum originate in different regions of the inferior olive and project to different sagittal zones.[16, 59] In general, the projection to the medial regions of the cerebellar vermis arises in the medial accessory olive and the projection to the more lateral zones originates in the dorsal accessory olive.[29, 59, 133] The projection to lobule VI in the posterior lobe arises in the medial accessory olive and is oriented in a strip continuous with the one in the anterior lobe which receives fibers from the same olivary region. In contrast, the input to lobule VII comes from the subnucleus beta,[59] with some projections arising also in the lateral and medial regions of the medial accessory olive.[25] Climbing fibers originating in the subnucleus beta also project to sagittal zones of lobule VIII.

The climbing fiber input to the paramedian lobule is organized into sagittal zones. The most medial strip originates in the dorsal accessory olive, the middle strip in the medial accessory olive, and the lateral strip in the dorsal lamella of the principal olive.[27, 59] The climbing fiber projections to the uvula (lobule IX) arise in the subnucleus beta, the dorsal medial cell column, and two portions of the medial accessory olive.[25, 59] The projections to the flocculus originate in the dorsal cap and caudal pole of the principal olive. A projection from the medial accessory olive to the flocculonodular lobe has been identified also.[60, 64] The input to the nodulus comes from the dorsal cap, the dorsal medial cell column, and the medial accessory olive.[60, 64] Projections to the dorsal paraflocculus arise in the rostrolateral portion of the medial accessory olive and the projections to the ventral paraflocculus originate in the ventral portion of the principal olive. The olivary projections to the cerebellar hemispheres also terminate in strips which are oriented perpendicular to the direction of the folium (see Fig. 2).[59] Most of these projections originate in the rostral regions of each major subdivision of the inferior olive: the dorsal accessory olive, the medial accessory olive, and the principal olive.

The projections from specific regions of the inferior olive to the cerebellar nuclei are organized topographically. In general, fibers from a portion of the olive terminate in the cerebellar nucleus receiving Purkinje cell axons from the cerebellar cortical region to which the same climbing fibers project. Thus, the dentate nucleus receives its major olivary input from the principal olivary nucleus. The interposed nuclei receive fibers from the rostral halves of the dorsal and medial accessory olives. The fastigial nucleus receives fibers originating in the caudal region of the medial accessory olive, the dorsal cap of the principal olive, and a very

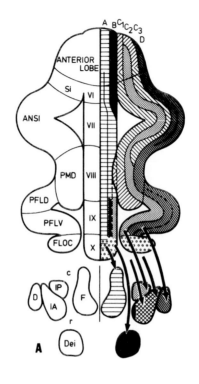

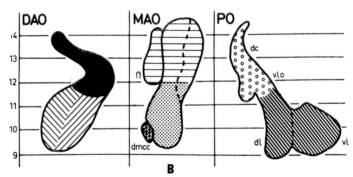

Figure 2. Organization of the olivocerebellar projections. A, Diagrammatic representation of the cerebellar cortex, shown unfolded, and the cerebellar nuclei. The strips A through D correspond to the zones from which specific portions of the corticonuclear projection originate (see Chap. 1). The general projections of each of these strips are indicated by the arrows. B, Diagrammatic representation of the olive shown unfolded. The locations of neurons in the inferior olive projecting to specific locations in the cerebellar cortex and cerebellar nuclei are indicated by the corresponding types of shading in the olive and cerebellum, respectively. Abbreviations: Si = simplex; ANSI = ansiform lobule; PMD = paramedian lobule; PFLD = dorsal paraflocculus; PFLV = ventral paraflocculus; FLOC = flocculus; F = fastigial nucleus; Dei = Deiters' nucleus; IP = posterior interposed nucleus; IA = anterior interposed nucleus; D = dentate nucleus; c = caudal; r = rostral; dmcc = dorsal medial cell column; β = subnucleus beta; dc = dorsal cap; vlo = ventrolateral outgrowth; dl = dorsal lamella; vl = ventral lamella; PO = principal olive; MAO = medial accessory olive; DAO = dorsal accessory olive. (From Groenewegen et al.,[60] with permission.)

56

small caudal portion of the dorsal accessory olive. Some projections to the fastigial nucleus have been reported also from the subnucleus beta and the dorsal medial cell column.

In summary, the olivocerebellar projection is organized topographically and projects throughout the cerebellum. Unlike the arrangement of mossy fiber pathways, there is no convergence of inputs from any two components of the olivocerebellar projection to a specific region of the cerebellar cortex.[16]

Projections to the Inferior Olive

Fibers projecting to the inferior olive originate in both ascending and descending central nervous system pathways and in the cerebellum (Fig. 3).[16] In the cat, direct spino-olivary fibers arise in the lumbar region of the spinal cord and project to the contralateral inferior olive. These fibers are located in the ventral fasciculus and the ventral part of the lateral fasciculus.[22, 28, 93] Some of the fibers are collaterals of neurons from ascending pathways that terminate in other central nuclei.[111, 117] In both cat and monkey, the direct spino-olivary fibers project to the caudal half of the medial accessory olive and major portions of the dorsal accessory olive.[89, 90] A small projection terminating in the subnucleus beta and the dorsal medial cell column and dorsal cap[28] was not verified in a subsequent study.[22]

The polysynaptic projections from the spinal cord to the inferior olive include pathways involving the dorsal column nuclei. The terminals of a crossed projection from the dorsal column nuclei to the inferior olive overlap with those of direct spino-olivary fibers in the medial and dorsal accessory olives.[22, 58] This projection is organized topographically. Projections from the gracile and cuneate nuclei terminate in portions of the inferior olive receiving spino-olivary fibers from the lumbar and cervical regions of the spinal cord, respectively. Several spino-olivary pathways have been identified on the basis of electrophysiologic criteria.[92, 104, 105] Only two of these, the direct spino-olivary projection and the projection via the dorsal column nuclei, correspond to pathways identified anatomically. The others are polysynaptic projections which may include parts of known ascending spinal pathways, or they may consist of pathways which have not been identified anatomically.

Several inputs to the inferior olive arise within medullary nuclei. A projection from the medial and descending vestibular nuclei terminates bilaterally in the dorsal medial cell column and subgroup beta.[114] Fibers from the trigeminal nuclei also terminate in the inferior olive.[30, 96, 127] Fibers from the spinal trigeminal nucleus project to the dorsal medial part of the ventral lamella in the contralateral inferior olive.[15, 22, 58] A small contralateral projection from the nucleus interpolaris reaches the caudal medial accessory olive. Neurons from portions of the reticular formation throughout the brainstem project ipsilaterally to the medial and dorsal accessory olives.[87] Other reticulo-olivary projections terminate bilaterally in the caudal half of the medial accessory olive and subnucleus beta.[136]

Aminergic afferent projections to the inferior olive originate in the raphe nuclei and locus ceruleus. A catecholaminergic projection has been found in both rat[53, 138] and cat.[69, 123] In the rat, this projection terminates in the dorsal lamella of the olive. In contrast, the serotonergic projection terminates in the caudal regions of the medial and dorsal accessory olives.[138] This projection, which has been demonstrated in the cat, originates in portions of the raphe nuclei in the pons and mesencephalon.[21]

Spinal Projections

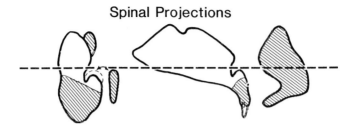

Cerebellar Projections

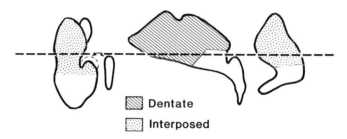

- ▨ Dentate
- ▦ Interposed

Cortico-olivary Projections

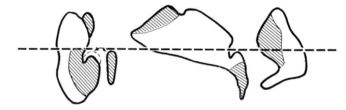

Descending Projections :
Subcortical Nuclei

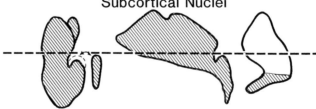

Figure 3. Organization of the major afferent projections to the inferior olive in the cat. The site of termination of each projection is shown in the four sections of the figure (summarized from Ref. 16). The dotted line indicates the same dorsoventral level as that shown in Figure 1. The spinal projections include those from the dorsal column nuclei. The projections from the cerebellar nuclei have been divided into the fibers from the dentate and interposed nuclei. The topographic organization of the projection from the fastigial nucleus in the cat is not shown because it has not been demonstrated adequately as yet. The inputs from the subcortical nuclei include the major descending projections originating outside the cerebral cortex.

Two important projections from brainstem structures to the inferior olive mediate the responses of olivary neurons to visual stimuli. In the rabbit a projection from the pretectum descends to the ipsilateral dorsal cap and subnucleus beta.[94, 95] This projection originates in the nucleus of the optic tract and the terminal nuclei of the accessory optic tract.[68, 130] A second pathway that can be activated by visual stimuli arises in the superior colliculus.[50, 56, 62, 99, 114] This pathway courses contralaterally and terminates in the medial accessory olive and subnucleus beta. The pathway terminates predominantly in the medial accessory olive of the cat and chiefly in subnucleus beta of the monkey.[62] The region of the medial accessory olive receiving these fibers projects to the portion of the posterior lobe vermis (lobules VI and VII) containing neurons that respond to stimuli of several modalities.

One of the largest inputs to the inferior olive originates in the mesencephalon and terminates in the rostral portion of the medial accessory olive, the ventral lamella of the principal olive, and the dorsal medial cell column.[91, 101, 134-136] One component arises in a continuous column of neurons in the central gray, including the nucleus parafascicularis and subparafascicularis, the nucleus of Darkschewitsch, the interstitial nucleus of Cajal, the nucleus of Edinger-Westphal, and the parvocellular portion of the red nucleus.[29, 40, 48, 63, 86, 114, 136] Another projection from the mesencephalon originating in the parvocellular portion of the red nucleus connects with the dorsal lamella of the ipsilateral principal olive.[40, 48, 114, 134]

The cerebellar nuclei provide a major input to the inferior olive, contacting neurons in almost all of its components.[34, 45, 88, 132] The fibers originate chiefly in small diameter neurons of the dentate and interposed nuclei[34, 131] and course to the contralateral olive through the crossed descending limb of the brachium conjunctivum.[57, 132] Fibers projecting from the anterior and posterior interposed nuclei terminate in the rostral part of the dorsal and medial accessory olives, respectively. Those from the dentate nucleus terminate in a large portion of the principal olive. A projection from the fastigial nucleus has been found only in the opposum.[45, 88] In this animal fibers from the fastigial nucleus project both ipsilaterally and contralaterally to the caudal portion of the medial accessory olive.[44, 88]

Fibers projecting to the olive from levels of the central nervous system rostral to the mesencephalon arise in the cerebral cortex and the caudate nucleus.[119, 194] As mentioned above, fibers from two thalamic nuclei, nucleus parafascicularis and subparafascicularis, also terminate in the olive. The fibers arising in the cerebral cortex are derived from many cortical regions, with a dense projection originating in the sensorimotor cortex.[126, 134] The fibers terminate in the contralateral olive, particularly within the ventral lamella of the principal olive, and also in the dorsorostral part of the dorsal accessory olive and the dorsomedial part of the rostral and medial accessory olive. There are small numbers of projections to the dorsal medial cell column and subnucleus beta, ventrolateral outgrowth, and the dorsal cap.

The pattern of organization of cortico-olivary fibers derived from anatomic studies is inconsistent with the pattern deduced from electrophysiologic studies.[16] Stimulation of the sensorimotor cortex activates a climbing fiber input to a region of the cerebellar cortex contralateral to the cortical stimulus.[4] Since the olivary fibers project to the contralateral side of the cerebellum, this finding indicates that the cortico-olivary projection is ipsilateral rather than contralateral, as demonstrated by anatomic studies. This problem has not been resolved, but it is possible that the predominant projections activated by stimulating the cerebral cortex consist of polysynaptic pathways involving neurons projecting from the mesencephalon rather than direct cortico-olivary fibers.[16]

In summary, the anatomic studies reveal an extensive pattern of projections from both ascending and descending central nervous system pathways to the inferior olive. These projections have considerable topographic organization, as shown by the reciprocal organizational pattern of the cerebello-olivary and olivocerebellar circuits. The direct projections from the cerebral cortex and the spinal cord do not overlap completely within the olive. Greater overlap exists between the projections of the ascending spinal pathways and the descending projections originating in the mesencephalon, pathways which corticofugal fibers undoubtedly activate. In addition, visual and vestibular stimuli activate inputs which include pathways originating in nuclei that are involved in the control of eye movements.[31]

Physiology of the Inferior Olive

The activation of inferior olivary neurons by any input results in a distinct, stereotyped response consisting of an initial action potential followed by a prolonged depolarization (Fig. 4).[7, 41, 81, 100, 118] The prolonged depolarization often is followed by regenerative responses of much smaller amplitude than the initial action potential.[6, 7, 100, 118] It has been proposed that these regenerative responses result from the action of recurrent collaterals of olivary neurons that reenter the inferior olive and activate other neurons in this structure.[4, 7, 46, 47] Alternatively, these regenerative responses may reflect the occurrence of dendritic spikes or membrane currents associated with the activation of these cells.

The activity of an olivary neuron can affect the excitability of a neighboring neuron as a consequence of the electrotonic coupling between their dendrites.[61, 75, 76, 82, 113, 125] This electrotonic coupling can result in graded depolarizations in neighboring olivary neurons that can be large enough to initiate an action potential.[81, 82] As a consequence of this arrangement, large populations of olivary cells with electrotonically coupled dendrites can be recruited from the activation of ascending or descending pathways. In accordance with this notion, Armstrong[4] suggested that neurons responding to a given input are located in longitudinal strips of neurons in the olive projecting to specific regions of the cerebellar cortex.

Following the excitatory response of olivary neurons, a hyperpolarization occurs, lasting approximately 100 msec.[4, 6, 41, 119] This hyperpolarization consists of an inhibitory postsynaptic potential (IPSP) whose duration in part determines the rate at which olivary neurons may discharge in response to the repetitive activation of any input.[82] The rate of discharge of olivary neurons is important in determining the rhythmicity of certain tremors. It has been hypothesized that the inhibitory input responsible for mediating this hyperpolarization may uncouple functionally the electrotonic interactions of the dendrites of olivary neurons, thereby regulating the degree to which electronic coupling occurs in response to various combinations of olivary inputs.[81, 82]

A one-to-one anatomic relationship exists between a given climbing fiber and the dendritic tree of a single Purkinje cell. As a result of this relationship, the responses of olivary neurons to peripheral stimuli can be assessed by recording either the responses of Purkinje cells to climbing fiber inputs or the responses of olivary neurons to various types of peripheral stimuli. Collectively, these studies demonstrate that olivary neurons respond to stimulation of all types of peripheral afferent fibers, including low threshold muscle and cutaneous afferents.[6, 7, 35, 36]

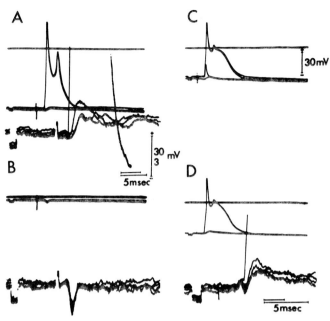

Figure 4. Electrophysiologic recordings of the responses of olivary neurons. Several superimposed responses were evoked antidromically by stimulating the cerebellum. The response in A was recorded at low gain (middle trace) to visualize the entire response and at high gain (lowest trace) to show the low amplitude short latency depolarization evoked via the electrotonic coupling of this cell with other olivary neurons. The stimulus strength was just at threshold for evoking the antidromic response of the cell. Thus, the small responses were evoked when the stimulus caused the activation of olivary neurons other than the one in which the electrode was located. The top line is the zero voltage reference for the DC recording in the middle trace. The records in B show the responses to the same stimulus with the electrode located just outside the cell body. The shift in the DC trace (middle trace) indicates the loss of the resting potential. Note that when the electrode was located outside the cell, only a small potential could be recorded. The records in C-D show the intracellularly recorded response of another olivary neuron. The responses of this cell have characteristics similar to those in A. The low voltage short latency responses evoked in the absence of the large action potential are again the consequence of the electrotonic coupling of this neuron with other cells in the inferior olive. Note the occurrence of secondary spikes on the slow depolarization observed immediately following the first action potential, a characteristic feature of the responses of these neurons to any input. (From Llinás et al.,[82] with permission.)

Some olivary neurons also respond to inputs from several different modalities.[6] The receptive fields of olivary neurons generally reflect the properties of the spino-olivary projections by which they are activated.[92, 105] Some neurons respond only to stimulation of very restricted receptive fields on a single limb, while others respond to stimulation either of the ipsilateral or the contralateral extremity.[4, 6, 7, 118, 119]

The olive is involved in motor behavior. Ablation of the olive results in deficits that resemble the effects of complete cerebellar ablation, including dysmetria, kinetic tremor, ataxia, and disorganization of movement.[32, 74, 98, 139] In addition, lesions of the cerebellar nuclei and the inferior olive have the same effects on the kinematic variables describing a ballistic movement.[124] The similarity in the deficits resulting from ablating either the inferior olive or the cerebellum may result from interrupting the interactions between these structures. The density of the

61

olivocerebellar and cerebello-olivary projections supports this view. Moreover, recent data suggest that the fibers of the descending limb of the brachium conjunctivum which project to the inferior olive also project to forebrain structures, including the thalamus.[131] Thus, the same output projections from the dentate and interposed nuclei affect nuclei of the forebrain which have been implicated in motor control and also affect the excitability of neurons in the inferior olive.

Pathways involving the inferior olive may participate in the generation of cerebellar tremor.[43] Following administration of the drug harmaline in monkeys,[77, 78, 96] a characteristic limb tremor occurs with a frequency similar to that of rhythmic neuronal discharge in the inferior olive, cerebellum, and several bulbar nuclei.[80, 84, 109] The rhythmic activity persists only in the inferior olive following ablation of the cerebellum and transection of the cervical spinal cord. Consequently, the inferior olive appears to generate the rhythmic activation of motor pathways responsible for the phasic movements characteristic of this tremor. In relating these studies to the physiologic action of the olivocerebellar projection, Llinás and Volkind[84] concluded that the output of the inferior olive generates the phasic movements associated with this tremor through its action on neurons in the cerebellar nuclei, because these structures also are necessary for the tremor to occur.

The inferior olive has been implicated in the regulation of slow eye movements through interactions with the cerebellum.[8-11] Studies of responses to visual stimuli recorded in the inferior olive and the effects of olivary lesions suggest that the olive participates in a control system that is needed to reduce the slip of images on the retina during low velocity eye movements.[11, 71]

Because the output of the inferior olive reaches the cerebellum, its function needs to be considered in the context of its action on cerebellar neurons. Several hypotheses have been presented. According to one view, the output of the inferior olive provides information to the cerebellum about patterns of convergence among the projections from ascending and descending pathways.[20, 54, 55, 104] In support of this hypothesis there is evidence that a spino-olivary pathway and a rubro-olivary pathway converge onto a single population of olivary neurons which projects to a localized region within the paramedian lobule of the cerebellum.[2, 3, 72, 73] This olivary projection can be activated both by the rubrospinal projections to fusimotor neurons innervating the hindlimb and by an ascending pathway that is activated by stimuli to the same hindlimb.[3]

Other hypotheses concerning the function of the inferior olive are based on assumptions regarding the actions of climbing fibers on the dendrites of Purkinje cells. These hypotheses have in common the notion that the climbing fiber afferents participate in processes necessary for motor learning to occur. One view is that the climbing fibers induce plastic changes in the cerebellar cortex. This is discussed further in Chapter 4. Another notion is that plastic changes occur in the inferior olive itself. Evidence for this idea stems from observations on the recovery from the motor deficits resulting from certain lesions of the central nervous system. Ablating the inferior olive of an experimental animal by administration of the drug 3-acetylpyridine renders the animal incapable of compensating for the effects of a unilateral labyrinthectomy.[85] In addition, ablation of the inferior olive following the compensation for the original vestibular deficit causes the neurologic abnormalities to reappear. The mechanisms underlying these observations are not known. Because compensation for unilateral vestibular lesions occurs even in the absence of the cerebellum,[112] the compensatory process probably does not involve interactions of the inferior olive with the deep cerebellar nuclei or the cerebellar cortex.

AMINERGIC AFFERENT PROJECTIONS

The aminergic afferent projections to the cerebellum have different morphologic characteristics than either the mossy or climbing fibers. Consequently, these fibers comprise a third type of cerebellar afferent projection. The aminergic afferent projections can be divided further into noradrenergic and serotonergic pathways on the basis of the transmitter substances which they produce and release.

The Noradrenergic Projection

The noradrenergic projection originates in the locus ceruleus and enters the cerebellum through the superior cerebellar peduncle.[1, 34, 48, 53, 70, 78, 97, 103, 106-108] Most of the morphologic studies of this projection have been performed in species

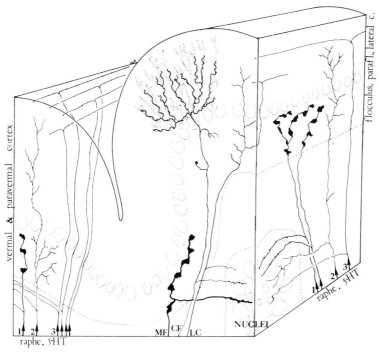

Figure 5. A diagram of the histologic characteristics of the aminergic projections to the cerebellum. Three types of terminal patterns have been observed for the serotonergic fibers from the raphe nuclei (inputs 1–3). The first type (1) terminates in the granular layer in a manner similar to that of mossy fibers. The second type (2) terminates as fine arborizations within the granular layer as well as within the molecular layer. In contrast, the terminals of the third type (3) course through the molecular layer where they bifurcate, forming fibers similar to parallel fibers. The aminergic fibers from the locus ceruleus (LC) also terminate within the granular layer and molecular layer. (From Chan-Palay,[33] with permission.) MF = mossy fiber; CF = climbing fiber.

other than primates and cats and therefore a discussion of its anatomic characteristics must be based on comparative studies. In the chicken, fibers of the projection course to the molecular layer where they are oriented in the direction of the parallel fibers.[97] In the rat,[34] these fibers branch extensively in the granular layer and also contact the somas and large dendrites of Purkinje cells (Fig. 5).[17, 70, 79, 107, 108] The noradrenergic afferent projection terminates also within the intracerebellar nuclei. Projections to the dentate nucleus and the posterior and anterior interposed nuclei have been demonstrated in the monkey.[34]

The actions of noradrenergic afferents on cerebellar neurons were investigated initially by observing the effect of iontophoretically applied norepinephrine on the spontaneous activity of Purkinje cells.[65, 67] This procedure results in a decreased rate of discharge of Purkinje cells. This effect occurs even in preparations in which the noradrenergic pathway has been destroyed previously by the administration of an agent, 6-hydroxydopamine, that destroys monoaminergic projections.[122] A decrease in spontaneous Purkinje cell activity results from the postsynaptic action of iontophoretically applied norepinephrine. These effects can be duplicated by injection of cyclic AMP.[122] These observations indicate that the suppressed excitability of Purkinje cells resulting from the release of norepinephrine is a consequence of the formation of cyclic AMP.

Iontophoretically applied norepinephrine evokes hyperpolarization of Purkinje cells without a change in membrane resistance.[66, 102, 121] Similar changes in the excitability of Purkinje cells occur upon stimulation of the locus ceruleus.[18, 66, 121] After destruction of the noradrenergic projection from the locus ceruleus by prior injection of 6-hydroxydopamine, stimulation of the locus ceruleus does not modify the excitability of the Purkinje cells. These studies demonstrate that the projection from the locus ceruleus to the cerebellum is responsible for the hyperpolarization of Purkinje cells observed after the iontophoretic application of norepinephrine.[66]

Additional studies have shown that the noradrenergic projections to the cerebellar cortex also modify the actions of both mossy and climbing fiber inputs to the cerebellar cortex.[52, 121] The actions of this pathway appear to result from the release of catecholamines from sites containing vesicles along the axons coursing through the intracerebellar nuclei and cerebellar cortex.[34] These specialized regions appear similar to presynaptic terminals; however, they do not contact other neurons.[34]

Serotonergic Projection

Serotonergic cerebellar afferents originate within the raphe nuclei[26, 33, 50, 51, 70, 120, 129] and project to all regions of the cerebellar cortex with the possible exception of lobule IV.[120, 129] Serotonergic afferents also reach the intracerebellar nuclei, but the density of this projection is controversial. Some investigators have reported a large input to these structures from the raphe nuclei in the rat and monkey;[34] however, others have observed a substantially smaller projection.[129] Studies employing horseradish peroxidase have demonstrated that raphecerebellar fibers originate in many of the raphe nuclei.[34, 120, 129] Only the nucleus linearis, nucleus intermedius, and possibly the nucleus linearis rostralis in the raphe nuclei do not contain neurons projecting to the cerebellum.[34, 120]

Serotonergic afferent fibers terminate within the cerebellum in three distinct patterns (see Fig. 5). One type of fiber within the granular layer of the cerebellar cortex has terminals similar to those of mossy fibers. A second type branches extensively through the molecular layer and bifurcates, forming a fiber system similar to but less dense than that of the parallel fibers. The terminals of the third group are distributed diffusely throughout the molecular and granular layers. Unlike the noradrenergic projection, the serotonergic fibers do not contact Purkinje cells directly.[19, 33, 34]

Few physiologic studies have been directed towards the serotonergic afferent projection. The iontophoretic administration of serotonin results in a decrease of Purkinje cell activity and an increase of granule cell activity.[19] Similar to noradrenergic fibers, serotonergic fibers contain specialized regions consisting of numerous synaptic vesicles. These structures do not contact postsynaptic neuronal sites.[34] These sites may mediate neurohumoral effects which regulate the actions of a fairly large number of neurons in their vicinity.[34]

REFERENCES

1. ANDEN, N. E., FUXE, K., AND UNGERSTEDT, U.: *Monoamine pathways to the cerebellum and cerebral cortex.* Experientia (Basel) 23:838, 1967.

2. APPELBERG, B.: *A rubro-olivary pathway. II. Simultaneous action on dynamic fusimotor neurones and the activity of the posterior lobe of the cerebellar cortex.* Exp. Brain Res. 3:382, 1967.

3. APPELBERG, B., AND JENESKOG, T.: *Parallel activation from the cat brain stem of hind limb dynamic fusimotor neurones and climbing fibres to the cerebellar paramedian lobule.* Brain Res. 58:229, 1973.

4. ARMSTRONG, D. M.: *Functional significance of connections of the inferior olive.* Physiol. Rev. 54:358, 1974.

5. ARMSTRONG, D. M., HARVEY, R. J., AND SCHILD, R. F.: *Topographical localization in the olivo-cerebellar projection: an electrophysiological study in the cat.* J. Comp. Neurol. 154:287, 1974.

6. ARMSTRONG, D. M., ECCLES, J. C., HARVEY, R. J. ET AL.: *Responses in the dorsal accessory olive of the cat to stimulation of the hind limb afferents.* J. Physiol. 194:125, 1968.

7. ARMSTRONG, D. M., AND HARVEY, R. J.: *Responses in the inferior olive to stimulation of the cerebellar and cerebral cortices in the cat.* J. Physiol. 187:553, 1966.

8. BARMACK, N. H.: *Visually evoked activity of neurons in the dorsal cap of the inferior olive and its relationship to the control of eye movement,* in Baker, R., and Berthoz, A. (eds.): *Control of Gaze by Brain Stem Neurons.* Raven Press, New York, 1977, pp. 361–370.

9. BARMACK, N. H., AND HESS, D. T.: *Multiple unit activity evoked in dorsal cap of inferior olive of the rabbit by visual stimulation.* J. Neurophysiol. 43:151, 1980.

10. BARMACK, N. H., AND HESS, D. T.: *Eye movements evoked by microstimulation of dorsal cap of inferior olive in the rabbit.* J. Neurophysiol. 43:165, 1980.

11. BARMACK, N. H., AND SIMPSON, J. I.: *Effects of microlesions of dorsal cap of inferior olive of rabbits on optokinetic and vestibulo-ocular reflexes.* J. Neurophysiol. 43:182, 1980.

12. BATINI, C., CORVISIER, J., DESTOMBES, J. ET AL.: *The climbing fibers of the cerebellar cortex, their origin and pathways in cat.* Exp. Brain Res. 26:407, 1976.

13. BATINI, C., AND PUMAIN, R.: *Activation of Purkinje neurons through climbing fibres after chronic lesions of the olivo-cerebellar pathway.* Experientia 24(2):914, 1968.

14. BATINI, C., AND PUMAIN, R.: *Données électrophysiologiques sur l'origine des fibres grimpantes.* Arch. Ital. Biol. 109:189, 1971.

15. BERKLEY, K. J., AND HAND, P. J.: *Projections to the inferior olive from the gracile, cuneate and trigeminal nuclei in the cat.* Anat. Rec. 184:359, 1976.

16. BLOEDEL, J. R., AND COURVILLE, J.: *A review of cerebellar afferent systems,* in *Handbook of Physiology.* American Physiological Society, Bethesda, Md., 1981.

17. BLOOM, F. E., HOFFER, B. J., AND SIGGINS, G. R.: *Studies on norepinephrine-containing afferents to Purkinje cells of rat cerebellum. I. Localization of the fibers and their synapses.* Brain Res. 25:501, 1971.

18. BLOOM, F. E., HOFFER, B. J., AND SIGGINS, G. R.: *Norepinephrine mediated cerebellar synapses: A model system for neuropsychopharmacology.* Biol. Psychiat. 4:157, 1972.

19. BLOOM, F. E., HOFFER, B. J., SIGGINS, G. R. ET AL.: *Effects of serotonin on central neurons: microiontophoretic administration.* Fed. Proc. 31:97, 1972.

20. BLOMFIELD, S., AND MARR, D.: *How the cerebellum may be used.* Nature 227:1224, 1970.

21. BOBILLIER, P., SEGUIN, S., PETITJEAN, F. ET AL.: *The raphe nuclei of the cat brain stem: A topographical atlas of their efferent projections as revealed by autoradiography.* Brain Res. 113:449, 1976.

22. BOESTEN, A. J. P., AND VOOGD, J.: *Projections of the dorsal column nuclei and the spinal cord on the inferior olive in the cat.* J. Comp. Neurol. 161:215, 1975.

23. BRODAL, A.: *Experimentelle Untersuchungen über die olivo-cerebellare Lokalisation.* Z. Neurol. Psychiat. 169:1, 1940.

24. BRODAL, A.: *Afferent cerebellar connections,* in Jansen, J., and Brodal, A. (eds.): *Aspects of Cerebellar Anatomy.* Johan Grundt Tanum, Oslo, 1954.

25. BRODAL, A.: *The olivocerebellar projection in the cat as studied with the method of retrograde axonal transport of horseradish peroxidase. II. The projection to the uvula.* J. Comp. Neurol. 166:417, 1976.

26. BRODAL, A., TABER, E., AND WALBERG, F.: *The raphe nuclei of the brain stem in the cat. II. Efferent projections.* J. Comp. Neurol. 114:239, 1960.

27. BRODAL, A., AND WALBERG, F.: *The olivocerebellar projection in the cat studied with the method of retrograde axonal transport of horseradish peroxidase. VI. The projection onto longitudinal zones of the paramedian lobule.* J. Comp. Neurol. 176:281, 1977.

28. BRODAL, A., WALBERG, F., AND BLACKSTAD, T.: *Termination of spinal afferents to inferior olive in cat.* J. Neurophysiol. 13:431, 1950.

29. BROWN, J. T., CHAN-PALAY, V., AND PALAY, S. L.: *A study of afferent input to the inferior olivary complex in the rat by retrograde axonal transport of horseradish peroxidase.* J. Comp. Neurol. 176:1, 1977.

30. CARPENTER, M. B., AND HANNA, G. R.: *Fiber projections from the spinal trigeminal nucleus in the cat.* J. Comp. Neurol. 117:117, 1961.

31. CARPENTER, M. B., HARBISON, J. W. AND PETER, P.: *Accessory oculomotor nuclei in the monkey: Projections and effects of discrete lesions.* J. Comp. Neurol. 140:131, 1970.

32. CARREA, R. M. E., REISSIG, M., AND METTLER, F. A.: *The climbing fibers of the simian and feline cerebellum.* J. Comp. Neurol. 87:321, 1947.

33. CHAN-PALAY, V.: *Fine structure of labelled axons in their cerebellar cortex and nuclei of rodents and primates after intraventricular infusions with tritiated serotonin.* Anat. Embryol. 148:235, 1975.

34. CHAN-PALAY, V.: *Cerebellar Dentate Nucleus: Organization, Cytology, and Transmitters.* Springer Verlag, New York, 1977.

35. CLENDENIN, M. A., SZUMSKI, A. J., AND ASTRUC, J.: *Proprioceptive influences on inferior olivary neurons during phasic reflex movement in the cat.* Exp. Neurol. 44:198, 1974.

36. COOK, J. R., AND WIESENDANGER, M.: *Input from trigeminal cutaneous afferents to neurones of the inferior olive in rats.* Exp. Brain Res. 26:193, 1976.

37. COURVILLE, J.: *Distribution of olivocerebellar fibers demonstrated by a radioautographic tracing method.* Brain Res. 95:253, 1975.

38. COURVILLE, J., AND FARACO-CANTIN, F.: *On the origin of the climbing fibers of the cerebellum. An experimental study in the cat with an autoradiographic tracing method.* Neurosci. 3:797, 1978.

39. COURVILLE, J., FARACO-CANTIN, F., AND DIAKIWAN, N.: *A functionally important feature of the distribution of the olivocerebellar climbing fibers.* Can. J. Physiol. Pharmacol. 52:1212, 1974.

40. COURVILLE, J., AND OTABE, S.: *The rubro-olivary projection in the macaque: An experimental study with silver impregnation methods.* J. Comp. Neurol. 158:479, 1974.

41. CRILL, W. E.: *Unitary multiple-spiked responses in cat inferior olive nucleus.* J. Neurophysiol. 33:199, 1970.

42. DAHLSTROM, A., AND FUXE, K.: *Evidence for the existence of monoamine-containing neurons in the central nervous system. I. Demonstration of monoamines in the cell bodies of brain stem neurons.* Acta. Physiol. Scand. 62(Suppl. 232):1, 1964.

43. DEMONTIGNY, C., AND LAMARRE, Y.: *Rhythmic activity induced by harmaline in the olivo-cerebello-bulbar system of the cat.* Brain Res. 53:81, 1973.

44. DESCLIN, J. C.: *Histological evidence supporting the inferior olive as the major source of cerebellar climbing fibers in the rat.* Brain Res. 77:365, 1974.

45. DOM, R., KING, J. S., AND MARTIN, G. F.: *Evidence for two direct cerebello-olivary connections.* Brain Res. 57:498, 1973.

46. ECCLES, J. C., LLINÁS, R., AND SASAKI, K.: *The excitatory synaptic action of climbing fibres on the Purkinje cells of the cerebellum.* J. Physiol. 182:268, 1966.

47. ECCLES, J. C., LLINÁS, R., SASAKI, K. ET AL.: *Interaction experiments on the responses evoked in Purkinje cells by climbing fibres.* J. Physiol. (London) 182:297, 1966.

48. EDWARDS, S. B.: *The ascending and descending projections of the red nucleus in the cat: an experimental study using an autoradiographic tracing method.* Brain Res. 48:45, 1972.

49. ELLER, T., AND CHAN-PALAY, V.: *Afferents to the cerebellar lateral nucleus: Evidence from retrograde transport of horseradish peroxidase after pressure injections through micropipettes.* J. Comp. Neurol. 166:285, 1976.

50. ESCOBAR, A., AND DECADENAS, M. J.: *On the connections between the superior colliculus and the inferior olivary nucleus. An experimental study in the cat.* Estud. Med. Biol. 25:281, 1968.

51. FRANKFURTER, A., WEBER, J. T., AND HARTING, J. K.: *Brain stem projections to lobule VII of the posterior vermis in the squirrel monkey as demonstrated by the retrograde axonal transport of tritiated horseradish peroxidase.* Brain Res. 124:135, 1977.

52. FREEDMAN, R., HOFFER, B. J., WOODWARD, D. J., AND PURO, D.: *Interaction of norepinephrine with cerebellar activity evoked by mossy and climbing fibers.* Exp. Neurol. 55:269, 1977.

53. FUXE, K.: *Evidence for the existence of monoamine neurons in the central nervous system. IV. Distribution of monoamine nerve terminals in central nervous system.* Acta. Physiol. Scand. 64(Suppl. 247):37, 1965.

54. GILBERT, P. F. C.: *A theory of memory that explains the function and structure of the cerebellum.* Brain Res. 70:1, 1974.

55. GILBERT, P. F. C.: *How the cerebellum could memorise movements.* Nature (London) 254:688, 1975.

56. GRAHAM, J.: *An autoradiographic study of the efferent connections of the superior colliculus in the cat.* J. Comp. Neurol. 173:629, 1977.

57. GRAYBIEL, A. M., NAUTA, H. J. W., LASEK, R. J. ET AL.: *A cerebello-olivary pathway in the cat: an experimental study using autoradiographic tracing techniques.* Brain Res. 58:205, 1973.

58. GROENEWEGEN, H. J., BOESTEN, A. J. P., AND VOOGD, J.: *The dorsal column nuclear projections to the nucleus ventralis posterior lateralis thalami and the inferior olive in the cat: An autoradiographic study.* J. Comp. Neurol. 162:505, 1975.

59. GROENEWEGEN, H. J., AND VOOGD, J.: *The parasagittal zonation within the olivocerebellar projection. I. Climbing fiber distribution in the vermis of cat cerebellum.* J. Comp. Neurol. 174:417, 1977.

60. GROENEWEGEN, H. J., VOOGD, J., AND FREEDMAN, S. L.: *The parasagittal zonation within the olivocerebellar projection. II. Climbing fiber distribution in the intermediate and hemispheric parts of cat cerebellum.* J. Comp. Neurol. 183:551, 1979.

61. GWYN, D. G., NICHOLSON, G. P., AND FLUMERFELT, B. A.: *The inferior olivary nucleus of the rat: A light and electron microscopic study.* J. Comp. Neurol. 174:489, 1977.

62. HARTING, J. K.: *Descending pathways from the superior colliculus: An autoradiographic analysis in the rhesus monkey (Macaca mulatta).* J. Comp. Neurol. 173:583, 1977.

63. HENKEL, C. K., LINAUTS, M., AND MARTIN, G. F.: *The origin of the annulo-olivary tract with notes on other mesencephalo-olivary pathways. A study by the horseradish peroxidase method.* Brain Res. 100:145, 1975.

64. HODDEVIK, G. H., AND BRODAL, A.: *The olivocerebellar projection studied with the method of retrograde axonal transport of horseradish peroxidase. V. The projections to the flocculonodular lobe and the paraflocculus in the rabbit.* J. Comp. Neurol. 176:269, 1977.

65. HOFFER, B. J., SIGGINS, G. R., AND BLOOM, F. E.: *Studies on norepinephrine-containing afferents to Purkinje cells of rat cerebellum. II. Sensitivity of Purkinje cells to norepinephrine and related substances administered by microiontophoresis.* Brain Res. 25:523, 1971.

66. HOFFER, B. J., SIGGINS, G. R., OLIVER, A. P. ET AL.: *Activation of the pathway from locus*

coeruleus to rat cerebellar Purkinje neurons: Pharmacological evidence of noradrenergic central inhibition. J. Pharmacol. Exp. Ther. 184:553, 1973.

67. HOFFER, B. J., SIGGINS, G. R., WOODWARD, D. J. ET AL.: *Spontaneous discharge of Purkinje neurons after destruction of catecholamine-containing afferents by 6-hydroxydopamine.* Brain Res. 30:425, 1971.

68. HOFFMAN, K. P., BEHREND, K., AND SCHOPPMANN, A.: *A direct afferent visual pathway from the nucleus of the optic tract to the inferior olive in the cat.* Brain Res. 115:150, 1976.

69. HOFFMAN, D. L., AND SLADEK, J. R.: *The distribution of catecholamine within the inferior olivary complex of the gerbil and rabbit.* J. Comp. Neurol. 151:101, 1973.

70. HOKFELT, T., AND FUXE, K.: *Cerebellar monoamine nerve terminals, a new type of afferent fiber to the cortex cerebelli.* Exp. Brain Res. 9:63, 1969.

71. ITO, M.: *Neural design of the cerebellar motor control system.* Brain Res. 40:81, 1972.

72. JENESKOG, T.: *Parallel activation of dynamic fusimotor neurones and climbing fibre system from cat brain stem. I. Effects from the rubral region.* Acta. Physiol. Scand. 91:223, 1974.

73. JENESKOG, T.: *Parallel activation of dynamic fusimotor neurones and the climbing fibre system from the cat brain stem. II. Effects from the inferior olivary region.* Acta. Physiol. Scand. 92:66, 1974.

74. KELLER, R.: *Über die Folgen von Verktzungen in der Gegend der unteren Olive in der Katze.* Arch. Anat. Entwickel. 23:177, 1901.

75. KING, J. S.: *The synaptic cluster (glomerulus) in the inferior olivary nucleus.* J. Comp. Neurol. 165:387, 1976.

76. KING, J. S., MARTIN, G. F., AND BOWMAN, M. H.: *The direct spinal area of the inferior olivary nucleus: An electron microscopic study.* Exp. Brain Res. 22:13, 1975.

77. LAMARRE, Y., DEMONTIGNY, C., DUMONT, M. ET AL.: *Harmaline-induced rhythm activity of cerebellar and lower brain stem neurons.* Brain Res. 32:246, 1971.

78. LAMARRE, Y., AND MERCIER, L.: *Neurophysiological studies of harmaline-induced tremor in the cat.* Can J. Physiol. Pharm. 49:1049, 1971.

79. LANDIS, S. C., SHOEMAKER, W. J., SCHLUMPF, M. ET AL.: *Catecholamines in mutant mouse cerebellum. Fluorescence microscopic and chemical studies.* Brain Res. 93:253, 1975.

80. LAROCHELLE, L., BEDARD, P., BOUCHER, R. ET AL.: *The rubro-olivo-cerebellorubral loop and postural tremor in the monkey.* J. Neurol. Sci. 11:53, 1970.

81. LLINÁS, R.: *The cerebellar cortex,* in Tower, D. (ed.): *The Nervous System. The Basic Neurosciences.* Raven Press, New York, Vol. 1; pp. 235–244, 1975.

82. LLINÁS, R., BAKER, R., AND SOTELO, C.: *Electronic coupling between neurons in cat inferior olive.* J. Neurophysiol. 37:560, 1974.

83. LLINÁS, R., PRECHT, W., AND KITAI, S. T.: *Climbing fibre activation of Purkinje cell following primary vestibular afferent stimulation in the frog.* Brain Res. 6:371, 1967.

84. LLINÁS, R., AND VOLKIND, R. A.: *The olivo-cerebellar system: Functional properties as revealed by harmaline-induced tremor.* Exp. Brain Res. 18:69, 1973.

85. LLINÁS, R., WALTON, K., AND HILLMAN, D. E.: *Inferior olive: its role in motor learning.* Science 190:1230, 1975.

86. LOEWY, A. D., AND SAPER, C. B.: *Edinger-Westphal nucleus: Projections to the brain stem and spinal cord in the cat.* Brain Res. 150:1, 1978.

87. MARTIN, G. F., BEATTIE, M. S., HUGHES, H. C. ET AL.: *The organization of reticulo-olivo-cerebellar circuits in the North American opossum.* Brain Res. 137:253, 1977.

88. MARTIN, G. F., HENKEL, C. K., AND KING, J. S.: *Cerebello-olivary fibers: Their origin, course and distribution in the North American opossum.* Exp. Brain Res. 24:219, 1976.

89. MEHLER, W. R.: *Some neurological species differences–a posteriori.* Ann. N.Y. Acad. Sciences 167:424, 1969.

90. MEHLER, W. R., FEFERMAN, M. E., AND NAUTA, W. J. H.: *Ascending axon degeneration following anterolateral cordotomy. An experimental study in the monkey.* Brain 83:718, 1960.

91. METTLER, F. A.: *The tegmento-olivary and central tegmental fasciculi.* J. Comp. Neurol. 80:149, 1944.

92. MILLER, S., AND OSCARSSON, O.: *Termination and functional organization of spino-olivo-cerebellar paths,* in Fields, W. S., and Willis, W. D. (eds.): *The Cerebellum in Health and Disease.* Green, St. Louis, 1970, pp. 172–200.

68

93. MIZUNO, N.: *An experimental study of the spino-olivary fibers in the rabbit and the cat.* J. Comp. Neurol. 127:267, 1966.

94. MIZUNO, N., MOCHIZUKI, K., AKIMOTO, C. ET AL.: *Pretectal projection to the inferior olive in the rabbit.* Exp. Neurol. 39:498, 1973.

95. MIZUNO, N., NAKAMURA, Y., AND IWAHORI, N.: *An electron microscope study of the dorsal cap of the inferior olive in the rabbit, with special reference to the pretecto-olivary fibers.* Brain Res. 77:385, 1974.

96. MOGAMI, H., KURODA, R., AND HAYAKAMA, T. ET AL.: *Ascending pathways from nucleus caudalis of spinal trigeminal nucleus in cat — With special reference to pain conducting pathways.* Med. J. Osaka Univ. 19:49, 1968.

97. MUGNAINI, E., AND DAHL, A. L.: *Mode of distribution of aminergic fibers in the cerebellar cortex of the chicken.* J. Comp. Neurol. 162:417, 1975.

98. MURPHY, M. G., AND O'LEARY, J. L.: *Neurological deficit in cats with lesions of the olivocerebellar system.* Arch. Neurol. 24:145, 1971.

99. NYBERG-HANSEN, R.: *The location and termination of tectospinal fibers in the cat.* Exp. Neurol. 9:212, 1964.

100. OCHI, R.: *Occurrence of postsynaptic potentials in the inferior olive neurones associated with their antidromic excitation.* Proc. Intern. Congr. Physiol. Sci. 23rd, Tokyo, 1965, p. 401.

101. OGAWA, T.: *The tractus tegmenti medialis and its connection with the inferior olive in the cat.* J. Comp. Neurol. 70:181, 1939.

102. OLIVER, A. P., SIGGINS, G. R., HOFFER, B. J. ET AL.: *Changes in transmembrane potential of Purkinje cells of rat cerebellum during microelectrophoretic administration of norepinephrine.* Fed. Proc. 29:251, 1970.

103. OLSON, L., AND FUXE, K.: *On the projections from the locus coeruleus noradrenaline neurons: The cerebellar innervation.* Brain Res. 28:165, 1971.

104. OSCARSSON, O.: *The sagittal organization of the cerebellar anterior lobe as revealed by the projection patterns of the climbing fiber system,* in Llinás, R. (ed.): *Neurobiology of Cerebellar Evolution and Development.* Am. Med. Assn. Educ. Res. Fdn. 1969, pp. 525–537.

105. OSCARSSON, O.: *Functional organization of spinocerebellar paths,* in Iggo, A. (ed.): *Handbook of Sensory Physiology. Vol. II, Somatosensory System.* Springer, Berlin, 1973, pp. 339–380.

106. PICKEL, V. M., KREBS, H., AND BLOOM, F. E.: *Proliferation of norepinephrine-containing axons in rat cerebellar cortex after peduncle lesions.* Brain Res. 59:169, 1973.

107. PICKEL, V. M., SEGAL, M., AND BLOOM, F. E.: *A radioautographic study of the efferent pathways of the nucleus locus coeruleus.* J. Comp. Neurol. 155:15, 1974.

108. PICKEL, V. M., SEGAL, M., AND BLOOM, F. E.: *Axonal proliferation following lesions of cerebellar peduncles. A combined fluorescence microscopic and radioautographic study.* J. Comp. Neurol. 155:43, 1974.

109. POIRIER, L. J., LAFLEUR, J., DeLEAN, J. ET AL.: *Physiopathology of the cerebellum in the monkey. Part 2. Motor disturbances associated with partial and complete destruction of cerebellar structures.* J. Neurol. Sci. 22:491, 1974.

110. RAMON Y CAJAL, S.: *Histologie du système nerveux de l'homme et des vertébrés, vol. I.* Maloine, Paris, 1909.

111. RAMON Y CAJAL, S.: *Histologie du système nerveux de l'homme et des vertébrés, vol. II.* Maloine, Paris, 1911.

112. ROBLES, S. S., AND ANDERSON, J. H.: *Compensation of vestibular deficits in the cat.* Brain Res. 147:183, 1978.

113. RUTHERFORD, J. G., AND GWYN, D. G.: *Gap junctions in the inferior olivary nucleus of the squirrel monkey.* Brain Res. 128:374, 1977.

114. SAINT-CYR, J., AND COURVILLE, J.: *Projection from the vestibular nuclei to the inferior olive in the cat: An autoradiographic and horseradish peroxidase study.* Brain Res. 165:189, 1979.

115. SASAKI, K., KAWAGUCHI, S., AND SHIMONO, T.: *Interfolial mossy fibre connections in the cat cerebellum.* Jap. J. Physiol. 19:110, 1969.

116. SASAKI, K., KAWAGUCHI, S., SHIMONO, T. ET AL.: *Responses evoked in the cerebellar cortex by the pontine stimulation.* Jap. J. Physiol. 19:95, 1969.

117. SCHEIBEL, M. E., AND SCHEIBEL, A. B.: *The inferior olive. A Golgi study.* J. Comp. Neurol. 102:77, 1955.

118. SEDGWICK, E. M., AND WILLIAMS, T. D.: *Afferent connexions to single units in the inferior olive of the cat.* Nature 212:1370, 1966.

119. SEDGWICK, E. M., AND WILLIAMS, T. D.: *Responses of single units in the inferior olive to stimulation of the limb nerves, peripheral skin receptors, cerebellum, caudate nucleus and motor cortex.* J. Physiol. 189:261, 1967.

120. SHINNAR, S., MACIEWICZ, R. J., AND SHOFER, R. J.: *A raphe projection of the cat cerebellar cortex.* Brain Res. 97:139, 1975.

121. SIGGINS, G. R., HOFFER, B. J., OLIVER, A. P. ET AL.: *Activation of a central noradrenergic projection to cerebellum.* Nature (London) 233:481, 1971.

122. SIGGINS, G. R., HOFFER, B. J., AND BLOOM, F. E.: *Studies of norepinephrine-containing afferents to Purkinje cells of rat cerebellum. III. Evidence for mediation of norepinephrine effects of 3'-5' adenosine monophosphate.* Brain Res. 25:535, 1971.

123. SLADEK, J. R., JR., AND BOWMAN, J. P.: *The distribution of catecholamines within the inferior olivary complex of the cat and rhesus monkey.* J. Comp. Neurol. 163:203, 1975.

124. SOECHTING, J. F., RANISH, N. A., PALMINTERI, R. ET AL.: *Changes in a motor pattern following cerebellar and olivary lesions in the squirrel monkey.* Brain Res. 105:21, 1976.

125. SOTELO, C., LLINAS, R., AND BAKER, R.: *Structural study of inferior olivary nucleus of the cat: Morphological correlates of electrotonic coupling.* J. Neurophysiol. 37:541, 1974.

126. SOUSA-PINTO, A., AND BRODAL, A.: *Demonstration of a somatotopical pattern in the cortico-olivary projection in the cat. An experimental anatomical study.* Exp. Brain Res. 8:364, 1969.

127. STEWART, W. A., AND KING, R. B.: *Fiber projections from the nucleus caudalis of the spinal trigeminal nucleus.* J. Comp. Neurol. 121:271, 1963.

128. SZENTÁGOTHAI, J., AND RAJKOVITS, K.: *Über den Ursprung der Kletterfasern des Kleinhirns.* Z. Anat. Entwicklungsgesch. 121:130, 1959.

129. TABER-PIERCE, E. A., HODDEVIK, G. H., AND WALBERG, F.: *The cerebellar projection from the raphe nuclei in the cat, as studied with the method of retrograde transport of horseradish peroxidase.* Anat. Embryol. 152:73, 1977.

130. TAKEDA, T., AND MAEKAWA, K.: *The origin of the pretecto-olivary tract. A study using the horseradish peroxidase method.* Brain Res. 117:319, 1976.

131. TOLBERT, D. L., BANTLI, H., AND BLOEDEL, J. R.: *Multiple branching of cerebellar efferent projections in cats.* Exp. Brain Res. 31:305, 1978.

132. TOLBERT, D. L., MASSOPUST, L. C., MURPHY, M. G. ET AL.: *The anatomical organization of the cerebello-olivary projection in the cat.* J. Comp. Neurol. 170:525, 1976.

133. VANGILDER, J. C., AND O'LEARY, J. L.: *Topical projection of the olivo-cerebellar system in the cat: An electrophysiological study.* J. Comp. Neurol. 140:69, 1970.

134. WALBERG, F.: *Descending connections to the inferior olive. An experimental study in the cat.* J. Comp. Neurol. 104:77, 1956.

135. WALBERG, F.: *Further studies on the descending connections to the inferior olive: reticulo-olivary fibers: An experimental study in the cat.* J. Comp. Neurol. 114:79, 1960.

136. WALBERG, F.: *Descending connections from the mesencephalon to the inferior olive: An experimental study in the cat.* Exp. Brain Res. 20:145, 1974.

137. WEBER, J. T., PARTLOW, G. O., AND HARTING, J. K.: *The projection of the superior colliculus upon the inferior olivary complex: An autoradiographic and horseradish peroxidase study.* Brain Res. 144:369, 1978.

138. WIKLUND, L., BJÖRKLUND, A., AND SJÖLUND, B.: *The indolaminergic innervation of the inferior olive. 1. Convergence with the direct spinal afferents in the areas projecting to the cerebellar anterior lobe.* Brain Res. 131:1, 1977.

139. WILSON, W. C., AND MAGOUN, H. W.: *The functional significance of the inferior olive in the cat.* J. Comp. Neurol. 83:69, 1945.

70

CHAPTER 4

Properties of the Cerebellar Cortex

ANATOMY OF THE CEREBELLAR CORTEX

The cerebellar cortex is a relatively uniform structure consisting of three distinct layers in all parts of the cerebellum: the molecular layer, the Purkinje cell layer, and the granular layer (Fig. 1). The molecular layer, the outermost of the three, contains two types of interneurons, the dendrites of the Purkinje and Golgi cells, parallel fibers, and several types of collateral fibers. The Purkinje cell layer contains the cell bodies of Purkinje cells. The granule cell layer, the deepest layer of the three, is composed of granule cells, Golgi cells, and numerous fibers. Functionally, the cerebellar cortex consists of a single type of output neuron, the Purkinje cell, and three afferent projections that can modify the activity of Purkinje cells either directly or through their actions on other cerebellar neurons. The mossy fibers provide input to Purkinje cells through the parallel fibers, which are the bifurcated axons of granule cells. The climbing fibers connect predominantly with the dendrites of Purkinje cells, but also with the three types of interneurons. The aminergic afferent pathways affect Purkinje cell activity through terminals in both the granule cell layer and the molecular layer.

The Mossy Fiber-Parallel Fiber Projection

As described in Chapter 2, the mossy fiber input to the cerebellum originates in many extracerebellar regions including the spinal cord, pontine nuclei, and precerebellar reticular nuclei. The fibers from these pathways enter the cerebellum through all three cerebellar peduncles, branching extensively before reaching the granular layer. As a result of this branching, some fibers terminate in both the anterior and posterior lobes. Upon entering the white matter of a single folium, the mossy fibers bifurcate further, coursing through the granular layer in a twisting, tortuous manner.[116, 125, 126] Mossy fibers contact granule cells in arborizations located along the fiber itself, at branch points, and at the terminals of each fiber.[116] Mossy fibers terminate in either simple or complex formations designated the mossy fiber rosettes (Fig. 2).[116]

At the rosettes, mossy fibers make synaptic contact with other elements which together form structures known as the cerebellar glomeruli (Fig. 2).[36, 73, 107, 116, 125] The glomeruli consist of mossy fiber rosettes, the claw-like dendrites of granule

71

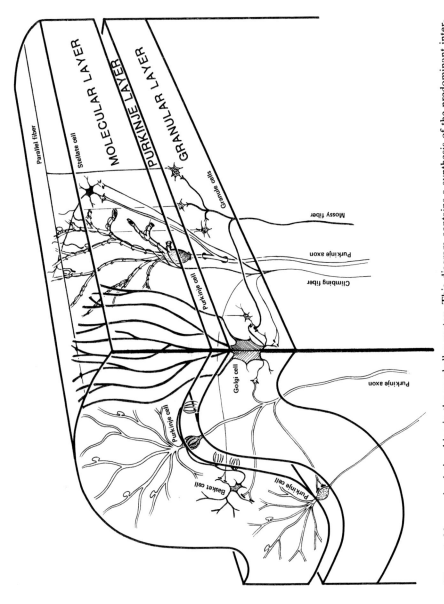

Figure 1. Neuronal relationships in the cerebellar cortex. This diagram contains a synthesis of the predominant interconnections in the monkey and cat. The diagram is oversimplified for clarity.

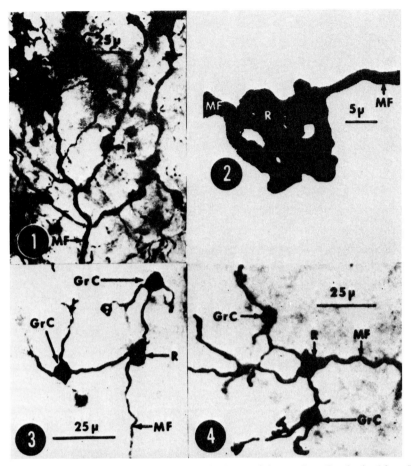

Figure 2. Connections of mossy fibers in the granular layer of the monkey (Synthesized from Fox et al.[50]). 1. The branch pattern of a mossy fiber (MF). Note the rosettes (R) which occur along the course of the branch. 2. The tortuous mossy fiber rosette (R) at a much higher magnification. 3. and 4. The multiple contacts of a rosette with several granule cells (GrC).

cells, and Golgi cell axons and dendrites. Contrary to previous reports,[79] mossy fibers do not synaptically contact the cell bodies of granule cells. Studies of glomerular ultrastructure have shown that, although some portions of the mossy fibers are contiguous with the bodies of granule cells,[116] no synaptic specializations are present at these sites.[116] Synaptic contact between the mossy fiber rosettes and granule cells occurs only at their dendrites.[13, 28, 50, 64, 66, 70, 81, 82, 94, 107, 115]

Groups of cerebellar glomeruli are organized into structures termed protoplasmic islets.[26, 107, 116, 125, 126] The individual glomeruli comprising a given protoplasmic islet often cannot be distinguished in anatomic sections, making it difficult to determine how many rosettes are contacted by the dendrites of a given granule cell. Consequently, the divergence occurring in the projection of a single mossy fiber cannot be measured accurately. Despite the limitations of these measurements, several rough estimates made from morphologic studies have provided important information. In the monkey, as many as 44 rosettes have been counted

73

on a single branch of a mossy fiber,[50] and in the cat each mossy fiber may have 16 to 20 rosettes.[36, 120] As many as 28 granule cells may contact a single rosette in each glomerulus.[120] The dendrites of each granule cell may contact as many as 6 glomeruli, each of which can be associated with a different mossy fiber.[36, 50, 120] These data lead to the conclusion that a single mossy fiber can contact as many as 400 to 600 granule cells in a given folium. This conclusion gives an indication of the degree of divergence occurring in the cerebellar cortex.

Granule cell axons course to the molecular layer where they bifurcate, forming parallel fibers that run longitudinally along the folium (see Fig. 1). The length of these fibers determines the distance over which mossy fibers and granule cells can affect cerebellar cortical neurons. This distance has proven to be important in theories of cerebellar cortical function. Studies of Golgi-impregnated tissue[36, 49, 50] as well as quantitative studies of the molecular layer[119, 120] have indicated that parallel fibers are 2 to 3 mm in length. Although these findings are consistent with some electrophysiologic findings,[36] they are inconsistent with Dow's[33] conclusion from early studies that the fibers are about 5 mm in length.

Recent investigations have demonstrated that Dow's estimate is substantially correct. Using a technique in which the lengths of degenerating fibers could be measured directly following discrete lesions of the cerebellar cortex, Brand and coworkers[19] showed that parallel fibers in cats extend 5 to 7 mm along the folium. Parallel fibers deep in the molecular layer are shorter, approximately 5 mm long, and parallel fibers located more superficially are about 7 mm long. Because these values come from direct measurements of fiber lengths which do not depend upon impregnation techniques, they provide the most accurate assessment available of parallel fiber length. Parallel fibers with different diameters are distributed differentially at various depths within the molecular layer.[49, 107, 116] This finding has not been substantiated in primates[50] and the situation in the human is unclear.

The spatial organization of elements within the molecular layer enhances both the convergence and the divergence of information conveyed from granule cells to Purkinje cells. The properties of convergence and divergence depend both on the relative numbers of cells in each population and the length of the parallel fibers. In the cat, there are approximately 1,770 granule cells for each Purkinje cell.[118] This ratio increases in higher phylogenetic species.[132] Owing to the length of the parallel fibers, however, each Purkinje cell receives parallel fiber inputs from an even larger number of granule cells, possibly up to 80,000.[120] Thus, there is a remarkable degree of convergence. The parallel fibers also contribute to the divergence that occurs in the molecular layer. Using an estimated length of 2 mm for parallel fibers and estimating the number of parallel fibers and the number of synapses between parallel fibers and Purkinje cells, Palkovits and others[120] concluded that each fiber contacts every fifth Purkinje cell whose dendrites it traverses, or approximately 45 Purkinje cells. In contrast, Brand and associates[19] argued that the distance between synaptic sites along a given parallel fiber indicates that it contacts every Purkinje cell along its course. This finding and the observation that the length of parallel fibers actually is 5 to 7 mm leads to the conclusion that a given parallel fiber may contact as many as 750 Purkinje cells.

The Purkinje Cells and Their Collaterals

The Purkinje cell is the only output neuron of the cerebellar cortex. It receives input from several elements, including parallel fibers, climbing fibers, stellate cells, and basket cells (see Fig. 1). The dendrites of Purkinje cells consist of a flattened array of processes extending about 300 microns perpendicular to the parallel fibers and only 3 to 18 microns in the direction of the parallel fibers.[19, 117] The spines on these dendrites are the sites of synaptic contact between the Purkinje cell and several of its inputs. The inputs from parallel fibers occur exclusively on these processes.[49, 50, 67] Purkinje cells are oriented in rows that deviate by approximately 11° from a direction perpendicular to the parallel fibers.[117] Thus, although Purkinje cells are aligned in rows, the rows are somewhat staggered. This orientation optimizes the degree to which the dendritic trees of adjacent Purkinje cells can be packed closely together.[20] These cells are packed in such a way that there is essentially no space between adjacent dendritic trees.

Purkinje cell axons form collaterals that project in two fiber systems, the infraganglionic and supraganglionic plexuses.[78, 107, 125] The axons enter the granular layer and bifurcate, forming collaterals that course back towards the Purkinje cell layer (see Fig. 1). While in the granular layer, these collaterals make contact with Golgi cells.[23, 36, 50, 71, 116] In the rat they also contact granule cells.[116] When they reach a depth just below the somas of Purkinje cells, the axon collaterals course transversely across the folium in the infraganglionic plexus. Here they continue to bifurcate and contact Purkinje cells, at least in some species, and possibly the interneurons termed Lugaro cells.[23, 50, 116] The fibers ascend to a level just above the Purkinje cell layer, where they extend longitudinally along the folium in the supraganglionic plexus and contact synaptically stellate cells and basket cells.[23, 50, 71, 83, 84, 86, 87] The extent of their branching, particularly within the supraganglionic plexus, is species dependent.[116] In addition, the density of these collaterals varies in different regions of the cerebellar cortex in man, monkey, and cat.[80] The collaterals in the supraganglionic plexus generally are more numerous in the vermis of the anterior lobe and less numerous in the hemispheres and vermis of the posterior lobe.

Cerebellar Interneurons

Parallel fibers contact three types of interneurons in the cerebellar cortex: 1) superficial stellate cells, 2) basket cells (deep stellate cells), and 3) Golgi cells (see Fig. 1). Another type of neuron whose interconnections are poorly understood, the Lugaro cell, can be classified as a fourth cerebellar cortical interneuron.[36, 47] Superficial stellate cells are located in the outer two-thirds of the molecular layer of the cerebellar cortex. They have dendritic trees oriented in the same direction as the dendrites of Purkinje cells, i.e., perpendicular to the parallel fibers.[36, 50, 116] In both cat[36] and rat,[116] the superficial stellate cells in the middle and outer thirds of the molecular layer are classified into two distinct cell groups based on their dendritic and axonal morphology. In the rat the dendrites of stellate cells in the middle third are oriented in a more planar fashion than those in the outer third. The axons from stellate cells in the middle third are often shorter than those in the outer third and contact the basilar dendrites and in some instances the somas of Purkinje cells.[116] In contrast, stellate cells in the outer third have axons that contact only the apical dendrites of Purkinje cells. Most of these longer axons from cells in the outer third extend about 400 microns across the folium;[50] however, some of them course up to 900 microns perpendicular to the direction of the parallel fibers.[36]

The basket cells are located in the molecular layer just superficial to the Purkinje cell layer (see Fig. 1). The dendrites of the basket cells receive synaptic contacts from parallel fibers and axon collaterals. The basket cell axons extend transversely across the folium for about 500 microns perpendicular to the direction of the parallel fibers.[36, 119] These axons ramify about 150 microns in each direction along their course. This characteristic pattern of branching, together with the 1:6 ratio of Purkinje cells to basket cells, led to the speculation that each basket cell can contact only 9 Purkinje cells and that each Purkinje cell is contacted by as many as 50 basket cells.[119]

Most synaptic contacts between basket cell axons and Purkinje cells consist of descending terminals which form a dense plexus in the shape of a basket around Purkinje cell bodies and axon hillock regions at several sites (see Fig. 1).[50, 66, 68, 106, 107, 116] In the rat, ascending terminals of basket cell axons contact the dendritic trees of Purkinje cells.[24, 116] The synapses formed by the descending terminals actually occupy a very small surface area of the Purkinje cell membrane.[107, 116] These terminals also course beyond the cell soma into the axon hillock region, forming the so-called pinceau. The anatomic characteristics of these terminals together with the low density of synapses has led to the speculation that electrical synaptic transmission can occur at this site.

A third type of interneuron, the Golgi cell, contains two dendritic ramifications, one in the granular layer, the other in the molecular layer (see Fig. 1). Within the molecular layer the Golgi cell dendrites form a hexagonal truncated pyramid overlapping little with the dendritic trees of adjacent Golgi cells.[36] Each dendritic tree of the Golgi cells spans a distance approximately equivalent to that of three Purkinje cell somas, consistent with the 1:3 ratio of Golgi cells to Purkinje cells.[118] Parallel fibers contact the dendrites of Golgi cells in the molecular layer, and mossy fibers contact the dendrites of Golgi cells in the granular layer.[23, 50, 70, 106, 107, 116] The axons of Golgi cells project to the cerebellar glomerulus where they contact granule cell dendrites.[36, 50, 70]

The connections of the Lugaro cells[47, 99] have been investigated less completely than those of other interneurons in the cerebellar cortex. Lugaro cells are fusiform neurons located just beneath the Purkinje cell layer.[99] These neurons have been found in several animals, including the rat, cat, monkey, and duck.[4, 47, 113, 116] The sources of inputs to Lugaro cells have not been resolved, though their dendrites have been observed in contact with the axonal terminals of basket cells, mossy fibers, Golgi cells, and Purkinje cells.[47, 50] The major inputs to Lugaro cells appear to come from collaterals of Purkinje cells.[4, 113, 116] Little is known about the efferent projections of Lugaro cells except that their axons make contact with basket cells.[47, 50]

Climbing Fibers

Climbing fibers pass from the cerebellar white matter to the molecular layer where they form multiple synaptic contacts with the dendritic arborizations of the Purkinje cells (see Fig. 1). Each Purkinje cell receives synaptic input from only one climbing fiber;[125] however, any single climbing fiber can bifurcate within the folium and project to more than one Purkinje cell.[45, 48] Because the inferior olive provides the sole source of climbing fibers,[14, 27] extensive branching of climbing fibers would be required to explain the large discrepancy between the number of olivary neurons and the number of Purkinje cells.[36, 100] In the cat there are at least 10 Purkinje cells for each inferior olivary neuron.

The initial electron microscopic studies of the junction between climbing fibers and Purkinje cells suggested that climbing fibers terminate on the smooth surface of the dendrites and not on dentritic spines.[50, 69] More recent evidence indicates, however, that climbing fibers terminate on many dendritic spines along the large dendritic trunks of Purkinje cells.[107, 116] The neuronal elements contacting synaptically the smooth region of the dendrite probably are the ascending axons of basket cells.[24]

In addition to projecting to Purkinje cell dendritic trees, climbing fiber collaterals contact other cerebellar cortical neurons. In one of the original descriptions of these collaterals, Scheibel and Scheibel[130] stated that they contact both stellate and basket cells in the cerebellar cortex of the cat. A similar set of collaterals was not found in morphologic studies of the monkey,[50] but electrophysiologic studies have given evidence for their existence in primates.[15] Terminals of climbing fibers also contact Golgi cells.[25, 69, 87, 116] The degree to which the climbing fibers terminate on various types of neurons depends to some degree upon the species studied. For example, a projection from the collaterals of climbing fibers to granule cells has been found only in the rat.[25, 116]

PHYSIOLOGY OF THE CEREBELLAR CORTEX

The contemporary era of cerebellar electrophysiology began with Adrian's[1, 2] recording of the "potential waves" on the cerebellar surface and the cerebellar responses to stimulating somatic afferents throughout the body. Subsequently, Dow[29-32] examined the cerebellar responses to peripheral stimuli and the effects of stimulating the cerebellar surface. He discovered that potentials could be evoked within the cerebellum by stimulating the cerebellar surface[33] and presented the first field recording from the depths of a cerebellar folium in response to cerebellar surface stimulation. Brookhart and coworkers[21] first recorded the discharge of single units within the cerebellar cortex. Although these investigators did not identify the neurons from which the recordings were made, it is clear now that they recorded the spontaneous activity of Purkinje cells. Subsequent studies have defined the responses of these neurons on the basis of their depth, their responses to climbing fiber stimulation, and the antidromic responses to stimulation in cerebellar white matter.[62, 63, 134, 136]

The contribution of Eccles and his colleagues towards the understanding of neuronal interactions in the cerebellar cortex represents one of the major advances in cerebellar cortical physiology. These investigators[5, 37-44, 50, 92] established in detail the excitatory and inhibitory actions of the individual types of cerebellar cortical neurons. The following description is based largely on their work.

The output neurons of the cerebellar cortex, the Purkinje cells, can be excited by both mossy fiber and climbing fiber inputs. The climbing fibers form direct excitatory synapses with the dendritic trees of Purkinje cells. In contrast, the excitatory mossy fiber input is mediated by the granule cells. The bifurcated axons of granule cells, the parallel fibers, provide an excitatory input to the dendritic spines of Purkinje cells. The parallel fibers also excite the three types of interneurons: the stellate cells, basket cells, and Golgi cells. The stellate cells and basket cells provide an inhibitory input to the dendrites and somas of Purkinje cells, respectively. Both parallel fibers and mossy fibers activate the Golgi cells, which inhibit the granule cells. The Purkinje cells have inhibitory effects upon neurons in the deep nuclei of the cerebellum and the vestibular nuclei. In addition, collaterals of the Purkinje cells inhibit the interneurons and the other Purkinje cells on which they terminate. In contrast, the collaterals of climbing fibers excite these interneurons.

Despite recent progress in our understanding of the synaptic effects of the neuronal elements in the cerebellar cortex, the functions of these elements remain unclear. Knowledge of the synaptic actions of cerebellar cortical neurons alone is insufficient to predict the response of a given cell to the activation of cerebellar afferent fibers because of the spatial orientation of the axons, dendrites, and collateral fibers in the cerebellar cortex. In addition, the temporal sequence of events and the relative levels of excitability in each group of cerebellar neurons can affect the responses to a given input.

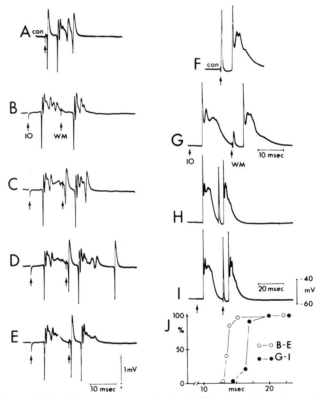

Figure 3. The characteristics of the responses evoked by climbing fibers from stimulating the cerebellar white matter (WM) and inferior olive (IO). The responses are recorded in Purkinje cells both extracellularly (A-E) and intracellularly (F-I). The control responses (con) in A and F consist of an antidromic action potential followed by a response evoked by climbing fibers after stimulation of the white matter in the vicinity of the fastigial nucleus. Note the similarity of the responses evoked by the climbing fiber activated from the white matter of the cerebellum and from the inferior olive. The extracellularly recorded responses evoked by stimulating the inferior olive consist of a large initial spike followed by several smaller action potentials. The intracellularly recorded responses to climbing fiber activation also have a large initial spike followed by a prolonged depolarization on which smaller amplitude regenerative responses occur. The interaction experiments in A-E and F-I demonstrate the inactivation of the spike generating mechanism during and after the large depolarization evoked by climbing fiber inputs. The graph in J shows the relationship between the amplitude of the antidromically evoked action potential in both sets of experiments and the interval between the stimuli applied to the inferior olive and the cerebellar white matter. (From Bloedel and Roberts,[17] with permission.)

78

The effect of climbing fiber input on the activity of Purkinje cells reflects the one-to-one morphologic relationship between these elements. After the initial studies of Schoepfle,[131] Granit and Phillips[62] demonstrated the all-or-nothing characteristics of the responses of Purkinje cells to a climbing fiber input in one of the first studies employing intracellular recording techniques in the cerebellum. The input from climbing fibers evokes a large depolarization which is associated with a train of action potentials (Fig. 3).[36, 96, 102, 103] Data from intracellular studies resulted in the speculation that the secondary spikes in the train are not propagated down the axons of Purkinje cells.[136] In subsequent experiments, however, the responses of Purkinje cell axons to climbing fiber inputs were recorded directly in the lateral vestibular (Deiters') nucleus. These responses consisted of a train of action potentials, indicating that at least some of the secondary spikes are propagated.[76]

The large depolarization of Purkinje cells evoked by climbing fiber inputs[36, 102, 103] results from an excitatory synaptic input distributed over extensive regions of Purkinje cell dendritic trees.[96] Simulation of this response with computer modeling revealed that the spike train resulting from the depolarization occurs initially in the somatic region of Purkinje cells and only secondarily invades their dendritic trees. The depolarization of the dendrites may evoke dendritic spikes.[102, 103] The presence of dendritic spikes has been demonstrated directly by recording these responses from Purkinje cells in the cerebellum of amphibians (alligators) and birds.[90, 91, 93, 95] Dendritic spikes have not been found in the intact cerebellar cortex of cats, however, indirect evidence of their existence came from studies showing a large increase in extracellular potassium evoked in the molecular layer by climbing fiber[135] or parallel fiber inputs.[112] Studies with agents that affect the membrane currents associated with these responses reveal that these action potentials may be produced by a regenerative calcium current.[98, 112] This conclusion is supported by recent studies of Purkinje cell responses recorded in vitro from cerebellar slices obtained from animals at different stages of cerebellar development. Calcium spikes can be recorded only when morphologically distinct dendrites have developed.[98]

THEORIES OF CEREBELLAR CORTICAL FUNCTION

Read-Out Theory

Several theories of cerebellar cortical function have been proposed, based primarily on the results of electrophysiologic studies of the cerebellar cortex. One of the first theories held that the cerebellar cortex may be conceptualized as a group of functional units 3 mm long and approximately 2 mm wide.[36] It was proposed that mossy fiber inputs to the cerebellar cortex would activate a pool of granule cells whose axons form a narrow beam of parallel fibers extending for a distance of 2 to 3 mm along a folium. These fibers in turn would activate rows of Purkinje cells and the dendrites of inhibitory interneurons located within the parallel fiber beam. Because of the lateral distribution of the long basket cell axons and their inhibitory action on Purkinje cells (Fig. 4), the activation of the parallel fiber beam would reduce the excitability of Purkinje cells lateral to the activated beam of parallel fibers. Moreover, the number of conducted action potentials evoked in Purkinje cells by the excitatory action of climbing fibers should reflect the level of excitability of these neurons. Electrophysiologic studies demonstrated that the

LOC

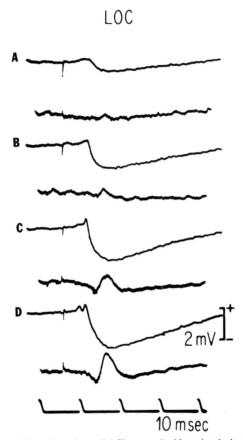

Figure 4. Responses of Purkinje cells and parallel fibers evoked by stimulating the cerebellar surface in cats anesthetized with sodium pentobarbital. In each of these four sets of records the upper trace consists of the response recorded intracellularly in a Purkinje cell and the lower trace shows the amplitude of the field potential evoked by the parallel fibers activated by the same stimulus. Progressively increasing stimuli (A-D) activate an increasing number of parallel fibers, as indicated by the increase in amplitude of the response to the stimulus. Within the Purkinje cell, a progressive increase in the amplitude of the inhibitory postsynaptic potential results from the action of the basket cells in response to the increased number of parallel fibers activated by the stimulus. The small excitatory response preceding each IPSP results from the excitatory action of parallel fibers on the dendrites of Purkinje cells. LOC = local surface stimulus. (From Eccles et al.,[41] with permission.)

number of secondary spikes in the response to a climbing fiber input can be reduced by the inhibitory action of interneurons on Purkinje cells. In addition, the number of spikes in the train can be varied by changing the amplitude of the inhibitory postsynaptic potentials evoked in the Purkinje cells. Hence the duration of the climbing fiber burst was thought to provide a mechanism whereby the excitability of Purkinje cells could be measured or "read-out." This conceptualization was termed the "read-out theory" of cerebellar cortical function.[36]

Several lines of evidence have indicated that the read-out theory does not explain adequately the neuronal interactions in the cerebellar cortex under functional conditions. As mentioned earlier, recent electrophysiologic studies[74] support the morphologic observations of Brand and others[19] and the early studies of

Dow[33] showing that parallel fibers extend for distances considerably longer than 3 mm, probably as long as 5 to 7 mm. Thus, the activation of a parallel fiber beam would affect the excitability of neurons in a larger region of the folium than proposed previously.[36]

A series of observations in unanesthetized decerebrate cats provided an additional challenge to the read-out theory. Bloedel and Roberts[16] demonstrated that the activation of a parallel fiber beam evokes interactions different from those observed in cats anesthetized with barbituates. Rather than a large inhibitory response in Purkinje cells, a marked increase in excitability of Purkinje cells occurs which is particularly apparent lateral to the parallel fiber beam. As a result, the surface stimulus actually may evoke a train of action potentials in the Purkinje cells (Fig. 5). A decrease in activity often follows this response,[16, 111] probably as a result of the actions of Golgi cells.

The findings of Bloedel and Roberts[16] in the decerebrate unanesthetized animal result from the effects of parallel fiber activation on the tonic inhibitory action of Purkinje axon collaterals on inhibitory interneurons. These effects depend upon the presence of spontaneous activity in Purkinje cells. The reduction of these effects can be correlated with a decrease in spontaneous activity of Purkinje cells resulting from barbiturate administration.[15] These findings, which have been substantiated in primates,[15] demonstrate the importance of the tonic level of neuronal excitability and the inhibitory effect of Purkinje cell axon collaterals[92, 97, 133] in determining the neuronal interactions within the cerebellar cortex.[16] Although other effects of barbiturates have been reported,[109] it appears certain that these drugs can reduce the excitatory action of mossy fibers in the cerebellar cortex.[60, 61] In addition, pentobarbital can reduce the excitability of neurons in the reticulocerebellar projection, a major mossy fiber input to the cerebellum (see Chapter 5).

Other hypotheses related to the read-out theory have been based on interactions of the effects produced by mossy and climbing fiber afferent projections. Oscarsson[114] found that inputs to the cerebellar anterior lobe from certain ascending spinocerebellar and spino-olivocerebellar pathways are oriented spatially in transverse and sagittal strips, respectively. Based on these findings, he proposed that mossy and climbing fiber inputs derived from different regions of the body surface activate matrices of Purkinje neurons determined by the overlap of these strips.[114] This proposal has not been supported by several studies reviewed in Chapter 5 showing that the responses evoked by mossy and climbing fiber inputs following natural peripheral stimuli are not distributed in a pattern of overlapping strips. On the contrary, these responses are not necessarily distributed to the same region of the cerebellar cortex. Consequently, a Purkinje cell may not be affected by both mossy and climbing fiber inputs following a given peripheral stimulus. This is particularly apparent in studies of the action of mossy and climbing fiber inputs to the flocculonodular lobe activated by stimuli which elicit the vestibulo-ocular reflex.

"Inactivation" Response to Climbing Fibers

Granit and Phillips[62] were among the first to comment on the inactivation of Purkinje cells that follows the marked depolarization resulting from climbing fiber inputs.[53] This feature was ignored in most hypotheses of cerebellar cortical function until the demonstration that climbing fiber inputs evoke not only the

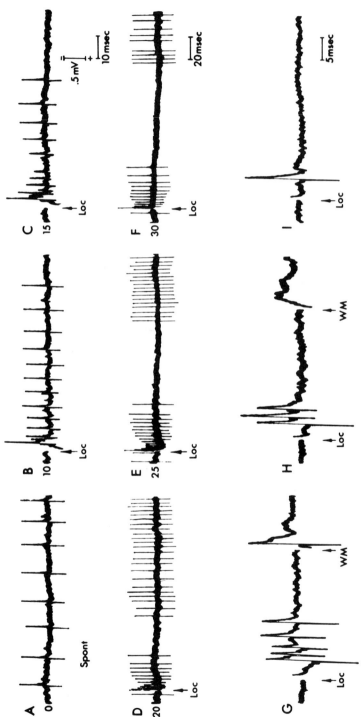

Figure 5. The responses of Purkinje cells, recorded extracellularly, to stimulation of the cerebellar surface in decerebrate unanesthetized cats. A. Spontaneous activity. B to F, Stimulation of the cerebellar surface (Loc) at increasing intensities (relative values at the left of each trace) evokes an initial excitatory response followed by a period of decreased Purkinje cell activity. The initial increase in excitability probably results from a combination of the excitatory action of parallel fibers on the dendrites of Purkinje cells and the reduced excitability of inhibitory interneurons by the axon collaterals of Purkinje cells. The period of reduced impulse activity probably results from the inhibitory actions of Golgi cells. G to I. Changes in neuronal interactions in the cerebellar cortex resulting from the progressive administration of sodium pentobarbital. G, The antidromic action potential of a Purkinje cell evoked by stimulating the white matter (WM) is not suppressed by stimulating the cerebellar surface (Loc), a stimulus which evokes a train of action potentials in this neuron. After the administration of 14 mg/kg of sodium pentobarbital (H) the antidromic invasion of this neuron is suppressed and a train of action potentials evoked by the surface stimulus is shorter. I, Administration of a slightly greater amount of anesthetic (21 mg/kg total) reduces further the train of action potentials evoked by the surface stimulus to a single action potential. The action of the anesthetic has changed the relative excitability of groups of cerebellar cortical neurons. Consequently, interactions evoked by stimulating parallel fibers are different in anesthetized and unanesthetized preparations. (From Bloedel and Roberts,[16] with permission.)

well known depolarization but also a hyperpolarization of Purkinje cells (Fig. 6).[17, 108, 110] The hyperpolarization is graded and can be evoked in the absence of the initial depolarization.[15, 17] As a result of the hyperpolarization, a period of reduced spike activity occurs which lasts considerably longer than the period of inactivation following the large depolarization.[17] The suppression of simple spike activity in Purkinje cells has been confirmed by several investigators.[22, 85, 127] Under some circumstances this suppression has a specific spatial distribution relative to that of the excitatory responses evoked by the same inputs.[127]

The marked suppression of activity accompanying the response to a climbing fiber input provides the basis for the "reset" hypothesis.[17, 65, 110] According to this view, rather than "reading out" the level of excitability of Purkinje cells, the climbing fiber input evokes episodic periods of suppressed impulse activity which

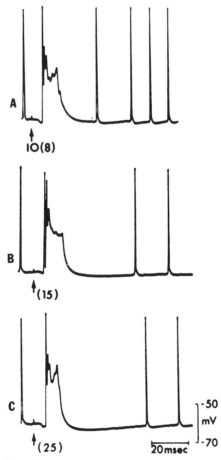

Figure 6. Activation of inhibitory interneurons in the cerebellar cortex by climbing fibers. The records in A to C were recorded intracellularly in a Purkinje cell while stimulating the inferior olive at three progressively increasing intensities. These intensities are indicated in relative units in parentheses. As the stimulus strength is increased, the excitatory response evoked by the climbing fiber does not change because of the 1:1 relationship between climbing fibers and Purkinje cells. As more olivocerebellar fibers are activated, however, hyperpolarization of the neuron occurs and is associated with a decrease in the spontaneous discharge rate of this cell. (From Bloedel and Roberts.[17] with permission.)

minimize transient instabilities resulting from neuronal interactions in the cerebellar cortex. A modification of this view suggests that the period of suppressed activity may produce a functionally important change in motor activity. This effect appears to determine the characteristics of eye movements evoked by synchronous climbing fiber inputs to the flocculus.[9, 10]

Temporal Patterning of Purkinje Cell Activity

Several studies have focused on the manner in which the cerebellar cortical circuitry determines the temporal relationship of neuronal activity among neighboring Purkinje cells in a given folium. Braitenberg[18] proposed that the cerebellar cortex functions as a type of biologic clock which determines the sequential activation of Purkinje cells on the basis of parallel fiber conduction velocities. He considered the generated time delays to be important in the control of motor behavior. This concept was tested experimentally by Freeman[51] who demonstrated that the sequential activation of Purkinje cells in the frog cerebellar cortex occurs in response to activation of a specific peripheral input. These findings have not been replicated in animal species with a foliated cerebellum in which the pattern of the spatial distribution of mossy fiber inputs differs from that of the frog.

Other investigators have examined the responses of multiple cerebellar cortical neurons by determining the cross correlation between the discharge of neighboring Purkinje cells.[11, 54] Gerstein and Perkel[54] demonstrated some correlation between the activity of two Purkinje cells in response to a click. In a more detailed study, Bell and Grimm[11] showed a positive correlation for the activity of neurons in three of five pairs of Purkinje cells. These correlations were found only for neurons located 50 to 100 microns apart and were not observed when the neurons were father apart. The lack of correlation over longer distances is consistent with the notion that the morphologic characteristics of the mossy fiber-granule cell projections assure little correlation of activity among neighboring parallel fibers and hence in the actions of the parallel fibers on the dendritic trees of individual Purkinje cells.[129] In a study by Bell and Kawasaki,[12] positive correlations over longer distances were observed only for the responses evoked by climbing fibers. Marked correlations over the longest distances were obtained when the recording electrodes were oriented in the sagittal plane of the cerebellum. In contrast, the climbing fiber responses of Purkinje cells in the longitudinal plane of the folium, that is, along the parallel fiber beam, could be observed only at distances less than 500 microns. In some cases they found suppression of the simple spike activity of a Purkinje cell located near another Purkinje cell responding to a climbing fiber input.[11]

The recent studies of Ebner and Bloedel[34] indicate that changes in the correlation of activity among neighboring Purkinje cells can occur in the cerebellar cortex following a peripheral stimulus, even in the absence of any evoked excitability changes in these neurons. These studies in the cat did not confirm the presence of a consistent sequential activation of Purkinje cells, either during spontaneous activity or during the application of natural peripheral stimuli. Owing to the extensive convergence of Purkinje cells onto neurons in the cerebellar nuclei, these changes in the correlation of the discharge of Purkinje cells provide an additional mechanism by which a peripheral input can alter the activity of efferent neurons projecting from the cerebellar nuclei.

Models of the Cerebellar Cortex

A number of proposals of cerebellar cortical function have focused on information processing in the mossy fiber – granule cell – parallel fiber projections. It has been suggested that these circuits function in a probabilistic manner in processing information from ascending and descending pathways. In support of this notion, Freeman[52] demonstrated that stimuli of many different modalities evoke similar Purkinje cell responses in the posterior lobe vermis when these responses are examined with poststimulus time histograms. The changes in cerebellar cortical neuronal discharge evoked by peripheral stimuli were thought to reflect increases and decreases in the probability of their discharge following different patterns of convergence from afferent pathways activated by combinations of peripheral stimuli.

Llinás[89] pointed out that any consideration of a probabilistic model of the cerebellar cortex must be made in the context of the spatial and temporal features of inputs to this structure. On this basis, the cerebellar cortex was thought to act probabilistically as a coincidence detector which enhances the spatial and temporal features of inputs to the granule cells in different cerebellar cortical regions. The results obtained from formal models of the probabilistic behavior of the cerebellar cortex indicate that the mossy fiber – parallel fiber afferents may act as pattern separators capable of enhancing both spatial and temporal patterns.[104] In a detailed probabilistic model of the granular layer of frog cerebellar cortex, Mittenthal and Leas[105] demonstrated that activating discrete pools of granule cells does not require a detailed specification of mossy fiber inputs to specific neurons in these pools. The spatial distribution of activity predicted from this model was similar to that predicted by another model in which a precise relationship between mossy fibers and granule cell populations was specified.[122]

In some models, the cerebellar cortex has been treated as a linear system with time delays to explain the dynamic behavior of neurons in the cerebellar cortex to time-variant inputs.[7, 8, 72] Analyses based on models of this type suggest that the dynamic behavior of Purkinje cells is determined by a parallel excitatory and feed-forward inhibitory system activated by excitatory inputs to the cerebellar cortex.[7, 8] In another model, the cerebellar cortex was considered to be a lead-lag compensator capable of matching its dynamics to that of a particular control system by varying the strength of the coefficients representing neuronal interactions among cerebellar cortical neurons.[72] These models show the value of conceptualizing cerebellar cortical functions on the basis of the way that cerebellar cortical neuronal populations process time-variant inputs rather than on the basis of responses evoked by the synchronous activation of a narrow beam of parallel fibers.[3] It is likely that peripheral inputs activate a more distributed group of parallel fibers than occurs in response to stimulating the cerebellar surface.[6]

Other models of cerebellar cortical function have simulated the cerebellar cortex with an assemblage of single units, each representing a cerebellar cortical neuron. These elements are distributed spatially so as to replicate the distribution of the various types of cerebellar neurons in the cerebellar cortex. An initial model of this type permitted visualization of the spatial distribution of neuronal responses following the activation of an input to a defined cerebellar cortical region.[121, 123, 124] This model was based on a cerebellar network containing parallel fibers 2 mm in length, without the collateral system of Purkinje cell axons. Despite these limitations, the model has provided some insights into the functions of Golgi cells and basket cells in determining the spatial and temporal characteristics of the Purkinje cell responses to a mossy fiber input. It was proposed that Golgi cells distribute spatially the activity of granule cells and increase the phasic component of the Purkinje cell responses to the mossy fiber inputs. The inclusion of basket cells in the circuit increased the spatial segregation of the Purkinje cells activated by a specific input. Only limited conclusions can be drawn from these studies, however, because the model did not take into account either the present view of a long parallel fiber length or the effects of Purkinje cell axon collaterals.

Recently, a simulation of the frog cerebellar cortex has been developed consisting of large numbers of neuronal components: 8,285 Purkinje cells, 1.68 million granule cells, and 16,820 mossy fibers.[122] In this model, activating a specified mossy fiber input with a divergent projection to many regions of the granular layer

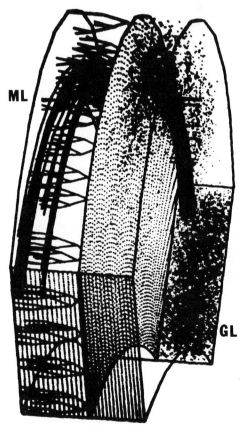

Figure 7. A computer simulation of the effects of mossy fiber inputs to the cerebellar cortex of the frog. The cortex is divided into two layers; the left is the molecular layer (ML) and the right is the granular layer (GL). The arborizations in the molecular layer represent the dendritic process of Purkinje cells. Mossy fiber input to a portion of the granular layer is represented by the dark bands of fibers entering this region. The dark bands in the molecular layer represent the parallel fibers activated as a consequence of the mossy fiber input to a restricted population of granule cells. Models of this type offer a neuroanatomic representation of neuronal interactions resulting from specific inputs to the cerebellar cortex. (From Pellionisz et al..[122] with permission.)

results in localized granule cell activation (Fig. 7). Simultaneously activating several mossy fiber afferent bundles still increases the activity of granule cells in localized populations despite the extensive divergence of each projection. These localized populations of granule cells in turn activate a localized population of Purkinje cells. The results obtained from this model indicate that localized responses can result from critical patterns of convergence on small granule cell populations despite the extensive branching of mossy fiber afferents.

Cerebellar Cortex and Motor Learning

Other theories of cerebellar cortical function are based on the premise that the synaptic relationship between parallel fibers and Purkinje cells can be modified during motor learning. Several studies have shown an inverse relationship between the simple spike activity of Purkinje cells evoked by mossy fibers and the complex responses evoked by climbing fibers.[11, 46, 55, 58, 59, 128] These findings contributed to the assumption that the action of climbing fibers on Purkinje cell dendrites can modify the effects of the granule cell – parallel fiber input to the same neurons. Marr[101] proposed originally that the coincident action of a climbing fiber input and a set of parallel fiber inputs onto the dendritic trees of the same Purkinje cell can modify the synaptic action of parallel fibers on the Purkinje cell. As a consequence, subsequent inputs from the same parallel fiber pattern would evoke a "learned" pattern of activity in the output of a given Purkinje cell. Another theory[3] held that the climbing fiber input reduces the excitatory synaptic action of a parallel fiber input to Purkinje cells due to the conditioning effect of the pause in the impulse activity following the excitatory component of the climbing fiber response. A later theory proposed by Gilbert[56, 57] held that the action of a synchronously activated group of climbing fibers can modify an entire population of neurons. Consequently, a functional unit of the cerebellar cortex could store a considerably greater number of patterns than expected from the theory proposed by Marr[101] which focused on the patterns retained by a single Purkinje cell. In Gilbert's theory, the number of action potentials evoked in Purkinje cells by climbing fibers determines the frequency with which these neurons respond to a mossy fiber input.

Eccles recently incorporated these theories into an instruction-selection hypothesis of motor learning.[35] This hypothesis is based upon the supposition that the action of one synaptic input can modify the action of another without an accompanying change in the morphology of the synapses. According to this view, the synaptic interactions between parallel fibers and Purkinje cells are altered by the action of the climbing fiber input to these neurons. Gilbert and Thach[59] have provided data indirectly supporting this theory. In these experiments a monkey was required to perform either a previously learned task to obtain a reward or to perform a novel movement which had not been rewarded previously. While the novel movement was performed there was an increase in the number of climbing fiber responses in single Purkinje cells. The number of simple spikes evoked by mossy fiber inputs during the same period was reduced. In support of Eccles' theory, the decrease in simple spike activity associated with the movement persisted despite the fact that the responses evoked by climbing fibers occurred with a progressively decreasing frequency as the movement was learned.

Undoubtedly this theory will need extensive testing before it can be refuted or accepted, but two reservations should be expressed at this time. First, as discussed in Chapter 5, the climbing fiber and mossy fiber inputs evoked by a peripheral stimulus need not affect the same population of Purkinje cells. Second, modifications of activity occurring in the cerebellar cortex during motor learning do not imply that the learning actually is taking place in the cerebellum.

REFERENCES

1. ADRIAN, E. D.: *Discharge frequencies in the cerebral and cerebellar cortex.* J. Physiol. 83:32, 1934.
2. ADRIAN, E. D.: *Afferent areas in the cerebellum connected with the limbs.* Brain 66:289, 1943.
3. ALBUS, J. S.: *A theory of cerebellar function.* Math. Biosci. 10:25, 1971.
4. ALTMAN, J.: *Postnatal development of the cerebellar cortex in the rat. III. Maturation of the components of the granular layer.* J. Comp. Neurol. 145:465, 1972.
5. ANDERSEN, P., ECCLES, J. C., AND VOORHOEVE, P. E.: *Postsynaptic inhibition of cerebellar Purkinje cells.* J. Neurophysiol. 27:1138, 1964.
6. BANTLI, H.: *Multi-electrode analysis of field potentials in the turtle cerebellum: An electrophysiological method for monitoring continuous spatial parameters.* Brain Res. 44:676, 1972.
7. BANTLI, H.: *Analysis of the dynamic behavior of neuron populations in the turtle cerebellum. I. General topological model.* Kybernetik 15:203, 1974.
8. BANTLI, H.: *Analysis of the dynamic behavior of neuron populations in the turtle cerebellum. II. Lumped circuit model.* Kybernetik 15:223, 1974.
9. BARMACK, N. H., AND HESS, D. T.: *Eye movements evoked by microstimulation of dorsal cap of inferior olive in the rabbit.* J. Neurophysiol. 43:165, 1980.
10. BARMACK, N. H., AND SIMPSON, J. I.: *Effects of microlesions of dorsal cap of inferior olive of rabbits on optokinetic and vestibuloocular reflexes.* J. Neurophysiol. 43:182, 1980.
11. BELL, C. C., AND GRIMM, R. J.: *Discharge properties of Purkinje cells recorded on single and double microelectrodes.* J. Neurophysiol. 32:1044, 1969.
12. BELL, C. C., AND KAWASAKI, T.: *Relations among climbing fiber responses of nearby Purkinje cells.* J. Neurophysiol. 35:155, 1972.
13. BIRCH-ANDERSEN, A., DAHL, V., AND OLSEN, S.: *Elektronenmikroskopische Untersuchungen über die Struktur der Kleinhirnrinde des Menschen,* in Jacob, H. (ed): *Proceedings, IVth International Congress of Neuropathology.* Thieme, Stuttgart, 1962, pp. 71–77.
14. BLOEDEL, J. R., AND COURVILLE, J.: *A review of cerebellar afferent systems,* in: *Handbook of Physiology.* American Physiological Society, Bethesda, Md., 1981.
15. BLOEDEL, J. R., GREGORY, R. S., AND MARTIN, S. H.: *Action of interneurons and axon collaterals in cerebellar cortex of a primate.* J. Neurophysiol. 35:847, 1972.
16. BLOEDEL, J. R., AND ROBERTS, W. J.: *Functional relationship among neurons of the cerebellar cortex in the absence of anesthesia.* J. Neurophysiol. 32:75, 1969.
17. BLOEDEL, J. R., AND ROBERTS, W. J.: *Action of climbing fibers in cerebellar cortex of the cat.* J. Neurophysiol. 34:17, 1971.
18. BRAITENBERG, V.: *Is the cerebellar cortex a biological clock in the millisecond range?* Prog. Brain Res. 25:334, 1967.
19. BRAND, S., DAHL, A. L., AND MUGNAINI, E.: *The length of parallel fibers in the cat cerebellar cortex. An experimental light and electron microscopic study.* Exp. Brain Res. 26:39, 1976.
20. BRAND, S., AND MUGNAINI, E.: *Fulminant Purkinje cell death following axotomy and its use for analysis of the dendritic arborization.* Exp. Brain Res. 26:105, 1976.
21. BROOKHART, J. M., MORUZZI, G., AND SNIDER, R. S.: *Spike discharges of single units in the cerebellar cortex.* J. Neurophysiol. 13:465, 1950.
22. BURG, D., AND RUBIA, F. J.: *Inhibition of cerebellar Purkinje cells by climbing fiber input.* Pflügers Arch. 337:367, 1972.
23. CHAN-PALAY, V.: *The recurrent collaterals of Purkinje cell axons: A correlated study of the rat's cerebellar cortex with electron microscopy and the Golgi method.* Z. Anat. Entwicklungsgesch. 134:200, 1971.

24. CHAN-PALAY, V., AND PALAY, S. L.: *Interrelations of basket cell axons and climbing fibers in the cerebellar cortex of the rat.* Z. Anat. Entwicklungsgesch. 132:191, 1970.

25. CHAN-PALAY, V., AND PALAY, S. L.: *Tendril and glomerular collaterals of climbing fibers in the granular layer of the rat's cerebellar cortex.* Z. Anat. Entwicklungsgesch. 133:247, 1971.

26. CHAN-PALAY, V., AND PALAY, S. L.: *The stellate cells of the rat's cerebellar cortex.* Z. Anat. Entwiclungsgesch. 136:224, 1972.

27. COURVILLE, J., AND FARACO-CANTIN, F.: *On the origin of the climbing fibers of the cerebellum. An experimental study in the cat with an autoradiographic tracing method.* Neurosci. 3:797, 1978.

28. DAHL, V., OLSEN, S., AND BIRCH-ANDERSEN, A.: *The fine structure of the granular layer in the human cerebellar cortex.* Acta Neurol. Scand. 38:81, 1962.

29. DOW, R. S.: *The electrical activity of the cerebellum and its functional significance.* J. Physiol. 94:67, 1938.

30. DOW, R. S.: *Cerebellar action potentials in response to stimulation of various afferent connections.* J. Neurophysiol. 2:543, 1939.

31. DOW, R. S.: *Cerebellar action potentials in response to stimulation of the cerebral cortex in monkeys and cats.* J. Neurophysiol. 5:121, 1942.

32. DOW, R. S.: *The evolution and anatomy of the cerebellum.* Biol. Rev. 17:179, 1942.

33. DOW, R. S.: *Action potentials of the cerebellar cortex in response to local electrical stimulation.* J. Neurophysiol. 12:245, 1949.

34. EBNER, T. J., AND BLOEDEL, J. R.: *Two modes of integration occurring in the cerebellar cortex.* Neurosci. Abstr. 4:64, 1978.

35. ECCLES, J. C.: *An instruction-selection theory of learning in the cerebellar cortex.* Brain Res. 127:327, 1977.

36. ECCLES, J. C., ITO, M., AND SZENTÁGOTHAI, J.: *The cerebellum as a neuronal machine.* Springer-Verlag, Berlin, 1967.

37. ECCLES, J. C., LLINÁS, R. AND SASAKI, K.: *Excitation of cerebellar Purkinje cells by the climbing fibres.* Nature (London) 203:245, 1964.

38. ECCLES, J. C., LLINÁS, R., AND SASKI, K.: *The action of antidromic impulses on the cerebellar Purkinje cells.* J. Physiol. (London) 182:316, 1966.

39. ECCLES, J. C., LLINÁS, R., AND SASAKI, K.: *The excitatory synaptic action of climbing fibres on the Purkinje cells of the cerebellum.* J. Physiol. (London) 182:268, 1966.

40. ECCLES, J. C., LLINÁS, R., AND SASAKI, K.: *The inhibitory interneurones within the cerebellar cortex.* Exp. Brain Res. 1:1, 1966.

41. ECCLES, J. C., LLINÁS, R., AND SASAKI, K.: *Intracellularly recorded responses of the cerebellar Purkinje cells.* Exp. Brain Res. 1:161, 1966.

42. ECCLES, J. C., LLINÁS, R., AND SASAKI, K.: *The mossy fibre-granule cell relay of the cerebellum and its inhibitory control by Golgi cells.* Exp. Brain Res. 1:82, 1966.

43. ECCLES, J. C., LLINÁS, R., AND SASAKI, K.: *Parallel fibre stimulation and the responses induced thereby in the Purkinje cells of the cerebellum.* Exp. Brain Res. 1:17, 1966.

44. ECCLES, J. C., LLINÁS, R., SASAKI, K. ET AL.: *Interaction experiments on the responses evoked in Purkinje cells by climbing fibres.* J. Physiol. (London) 182:297, 1966.

45. FABER, D. S., AND MURPHY, J. T.: *Axonal branching in the climbing fiber pathway to the cerebellum.* Brain Res. 15:262, 1969.

46. FERIN, M., GRIGORIAN, R. A., AND STRATA, P.: *Mossy and climbing fibre activation in the cat cerebellum by stimulation of the labyrinth.* Exp. Brain Res. 12:1, 1971.

47. FOX, C. A.: *The intermediate cells of Lugaro in the cerebellar cortex of the monkey.* J. Comp. Neurol. 112:39, 1959.

48. FOX, C. A., ANDRADE, A., AND SCHWYN, R. C.: *Climbing fiber branching in the granular layer,* in Llinas, R. (ed.): *Neurobiology of Cerebellar Evolution and Development.* AMA-ERF Institute for Biomedical Research, Chicago, 1969, pp. 603–611.

49. FOX, C. A., AND BARNARD, J. W.: *A quantitative study of the Purkinje cell dendritic branchlets and their relationship to afferent fibres.* J. Anat. (London) 91:299, 1957.

50. FOX, C. A., HILLMAN, D. E., SIEGESMUND, K. A. ET AL.: *The primate cerebellar cortex: A Gol-*

gi and electron microscopic study, in Fox, C. A., and Snider, R. S. (eds.): *Progress in Brain Research,* Vol. 25. Elsevier, New York, pp. 174–225, 1967.

51. FREEMAN, J. A.: *The cerebellum as a timing device: An experimental study in the frog,* in Llinás, R. (ed.): *Neurobiology of Cerebellar Evolution and Development.* AMA-ERF Institute for Biomedical Research, Chicago, 1969, pp. 397–420.

52. FREEMAN, J. A.: *Responses of cat cerebellar Purkinje cells to convergent inputs from cerebral cortex and peripheral sensory systems.* J. Neurophysiol. 33:697, 1970.

53. FUJITA, Y.: *Activity of dendrites of single Purkinje cells and its relationship to so-called inactivation response in rabbit cerebellum.* J. Neurophysiol. 31:131, 1968.

54. GERSTEIN, G. L., AND PERKEL, D. H.: *Simultaneously recorded trains of action potentials: analysis and functional interpretation.* Sci. 164:828, 1969.

55. GHELARDUCCI, B., ITO, M., AND YAGI, N.: *Impulse discharges from flocculus Purkinje cells of alert rabbits during visual stimulation combined with horizontal head rotation.* Brain Res. 87:66, 1975.

56. GILBERT, P. F. C.: *A theory of memory that explains the function and structure of the cerebellum.* Brain Res. 70:1, 1974.

57. GILBERT, P. F. C.: *How the cerebellum could memorise movements.* Nature (London) 254:688, 1975.

58. GILBERT, P. F. C.: *Simple spike frequency and the number of secondary spikes in the complex spike of the cerebellar Purkinje cell.* Brain Res. 114:334, 1976.

59. GILBERT, P. F. C., AND THACH, W. T.: *Purkinje cell activity during motor learning.* Brain Res. 128:309, 1977.

60. GORDON, M., RUBIA, F. J., AND STRATA, P.: *The effect of barbiturate anaesthesia on the transmission to the cerebellar cortex.* Brain Res. 43:677, 1972.

61. GORDON, M., RUBIA, F. J., AND STRATA, P.: *The effect of pentothal on the activity evoked in the cerebellar cortex.* Exp. Brain Res. 17:50, 1973.

62. GRANIT, R., AND PHILLIPS, C. G.: *Excitatory and inhibitory processes acting upon individual Purkinje cells of the cerebellum in cats.* J. Physiol. (London) 133:520, 1956.

63. GRANIT, R., AND PHILLIPS, C. G.: *Effect on Purkinje cells of surface stimulation of the cerebellum.* J. Physiol. (London) 135:73, 1957.

64. GRAY, E. G.: *The granule cells, mossy synapses and Purkinje spine synapses of the cerebellum: light and electron microscope observations.* J. Anat. (London) 95:345, 1961.

65. HARMON, L. D., KADO, R., AND LEWIS, E. R.: *Cerebellar modeling problems,* in Harmon, L. D. (ed.): *To Understand Brains.* Prentice-Hall, Englewood Cliffs, N.J. (in press).

66. HÁMORI, J.: *Identification in the cerebellar isles of Golgi II axon endings by aid of experimental degeneration,* in Titlbach, M. (ed.): *Electron Microscopy. Proceedings of the Third European Regional Conference held in Prague, Vol. B.* Czechoslovak Academy of Sciences, Prague, 1964, pp. 291–292.

67. HÁMORI, J., AND SZENTÁGOTHAI, J.: *The "crossing over" synapse. An electron microscope study of the molecular layer in the cerebellar cortex.* Acta Biol. Acad. Sci. Hung. 15:95, 1964.

68. HÁMORI, J., AND SZENTÁGOTHAI, J.: *The Purkinje cell baskets: Ultrastructure of an inhibitory synapse.* Acta Biol. Acad. Sc. Hung. 15:465, 1965.

69. HÁMORI, J., AND SZENTÁGOTHAI, J.: *Identification under the electron microscope of climbing fibers and their synaptic contacts.* Exp. Brain Res. 1:65, 1966.

70. HÁMORI, J., AND SZENTÁGOTHAI, J.: *Participation of Golgi neuron processes in the cerebellar glomeruli: An electron microscope study.* Exp. Brain Res. 2:35, 1966.

71. HÁMORI, J., AND SZENTÁGOTHAI, J.: *Identification of synapses formed in the cerebellar cortex by Purkinje axon collaterals: An electron microscope study.* Exp. Brain Res. 5:118, 1968.

72. HASSUL, M., AND DANIELS, P. D.: *Cerebellar dynamics: The mossy fiber input.* IEEE Transactions Biomed. Eng. 24:449, 1977.

73. HELD, H.: *Beiträge zur Struktur der Nervenzellen und ihrer Fortsätze III.* Arch. Anat. Entwick. (Suppl.) 273–312, 1897.

74. HOUK, J. C., AND WALSH, J. V.: *The length and organization of parallel fibers.* Proc. Int. Union Physiol. Sci. 776:1971.

75. ITO, M., OBATA, K., AND OCHI, P.: *The origin of cerebellar-induced inhibition of Deiters' neu-*

rones. II. Temporal correlation between the trans-synaptic activation of Purkinje cells and the inhibition of Deiters' neurones. Exp. Brain Res. 2:350, 1966.

76. ITO, M., AND SIMPSON, J. I.: *Discharges in Purkinje cell axons during climbing fiber activation.* Brain Res. 31:215, 1971.

77. ITO, M., YOSHIDA, M., OBATA, K. ET AL.: *Inhibitory control of intracerebellar nuclei by the Purkinje cell axons.* Exp. Brain Res. 10:64, 1970.

78. JAKOB, A.: *Zum Problem der morphologischen und funktionellen Gliederung des Kleinhirns.* Dtsch. Z. Nervenheilkd. 105:217, 1928.

79. JANSEN, J., AND BRODAL, A.: *Das Kleinhirn,* in Bargmann, W. (ed.): *Handbuch der Mikroskopischen Anatomie des Menschen.* Springer, Berlin, Vol. IV/8, 1958, pp. 101–103.

80. LANGE, W.: *Über regionale Unterschiede in der Myeloarchitektonik der Kleinhirnrinde, I. Der Plexus supraganglionaris.* Z. Zellforsch. 134:129, 1972.

81. LARRAMENDI, L. M. H.: *Analysis of synaptogenesis in the cerebellum of the mouse,* in Llinás, R. (ed.): *Neurobiology of Cerebellar Evolution and Development.* AMA-ERT Institute for Biomedical Research, Chicago, 1969, pp. 803–843.

82. LARRAMENDI, L. M. H.: *Morphological characteristics of extrinsic and intrinsic nerve terminals and their synapses in the cerebellar cortex of the mouse,* in Fields, W. S., and Willis, W. D., Jr. (eds.): *The Cerebellum in Health and Disease.* Warren H. Green, St. Louis, 1970, pp. 63–110.

83. LARRAMENDI, L. M. H., AND LEMKEY-JOHNSTON, N.: *The distribution of recurrent Purkinje collateral synapses on the mouse cerebellar cortex: An electron microscopic study.* J. Comp. Neurol. 138:451, 1970.

84. LARRAMENDI, L. M. H., AND VICTOR, T.: *Synapses on the Purkinje cell spines in the mouse. An electron microscopic study.* Brain Res. 5:15–30, 1967.

85. LATHAM, A., AND PAUL, D. H.: *Spontaneous activity of cerebellar Purkinje cells and their response to impulses in climbing fibres.* J. Physiol. 213:135, 1971.

86. LEMKEY-JOHNSTON, N., AND LARRAMENDI, L. M. H.: *Morphological characteristics of mouse stellate and basket cells and their neuroglial envelope: An electron microscopic study.* J. Comp. Neurol. 134:39, 1968.

87. LEMKEY-JOHNSTON, N., AND LARRAMENDI, L. M. H.: *Types and distribution of synapses upon basket and stellate cells of the mouse cerebellum: An electron miscropic study.* J. Comp. Neurol. 134:73, 1968.

88. LLINÁS, R.: *Functional aspects of interneuronal evolution in the cerebellar cortex,* in Brazier, M. A. (ed.): *The Interneuron.* University of California Press, Los Angeles, 1969, pp. 329–348.

89. LLINÁS, R.: *Neuronal operations in cerebellar transactions,* in Schmitt, F. O. (ed.): *The Neurosciences: Second Study Program.* Rockefeller University Press, New York, 1970, pp. 409–426.

90. LLINÁS, R.: *Eighteenth Bowditch Lecture: Motor aspects of cerebellar control.* Physiologist 17: 19, 1974.

91. LLINÁS, R.: *Electroresponsive properties of dendrites in central neurons,* in Kreutzberg, G. W. (ed.): Physiology and Pathology of Dendrites. Raven Press, New York, 1975, pp. 1–13.

92. LLINÁS, R., AND AYALA, G. F.: *Discussion of a paper by Oscarsson, O: Functional significance of information channels from the spinal cord to the cerebellum,* in Yahr, M. D., and Purpura, D. P. (eds.): *Neurophysiological Basis of Normal and Abnormal Motor Activities.* Raven Press, New York, 1967, pp. 113–115.

93. LLINÁS, R., AND HESS, R.: *Tetrodotoxin-resistant dendritic spikes in avian Purkinje cells.* Proc. Nat. Acad. Sci. (Wash) 73:2520, 1976.

94. LLINÁS, R., AND HILLMAN, D. E.: *Physiological and morphological organization of the cerebellar circuits in various vertebrates,* in Llinás, R. (ed.): *Neurobiology of Cerebellar Evolution and Development.* AMA-ERF Institute for Biomedical Research, Chicago, 1969, pp. 43–73.

95. LLINÁS, R., AND NICHOLSON, C.: *Electrophysiological properties of dendrites and somata in alligator Purkinje cells.* J. Neurophysiol. 34:532, 1971.

96. LLINÁS, R., AND NICHOLSON, C.: *Reversal properties of climbing fiber potential in cat Purkinje cells: an example of a distributed synapse.* J. Neurophysiol. 39:311, 1976.

97. LLINÁS, R., AND PRECHT, W.: *Recurrent facilitation by disinhibition in Purkinje cells of the cat cerebellum,* in: Llinás, R. (ed.): Neurobiology of Cerebellar Evolution and Development. AMA-ERF Institute for Biomedical Research, Chicago, 1969, pp. 619–627.

98. LLINÁS, R., AND SUGIMORI, M.: *Dendritic calcium spiking in mammalian Purkinje cells: in vitro study of its function and development.* Soc. Neurosci. Abstr. 4:66, 1978.

99. LUGARO, E.: *Sulle connessioni tra gli elementi nervosi della corteccia cerebellare con considerazioni generali sul significato fisiologico dei rapporti tra gli elementi nervosi.* Riv. Sper. Freniatr. 20:297, 1894.

100. MAGYAR, P., SZÉNCHENTY, B., AND PALKOVITS, M.: *A quantitative study of the olivocerebellar connections.* Acta Morph. Acad. Sci. Hung. 20:71, 1972.

101. MARR, D.: *A theory of cerebellar cortex.* J. Physiol. (London) 202:437, 1969.

102. MARTINEZ, F. E., CRILL, W. E., AND KENNEDY, T. T.: *Dendritic origin of climbing fiber responses in cat cerebellar Purkinje cells.* Fed. Proc. 29:324, 1970.

103. MARTINEZ, F. E., CRILL, W. E., AND KENNEDY, T. T.: *Electrogenesis of cerebellar Purkinje cell responses in cats.* J. Neurophysiol. 34:348, 1971.

104. MITTENTHAL, J. E.: *Reliability of pattern separation by the cerebellar mossy fiber-granule cell system.* Kybernetik 16:93, 1974.

105. MITTENTHAL, J. E., AND LEAS, D.: *A probabilistic model for the granular layer of frog cerebellar cortex.* Neurosci. 3:181, 1978.

106. MUGNAINI, E.: *Neurones as synaptic targets,* in: Andersen, P., and Jansen, J. K. S. (eds.): *Excitatory Synaptic Mechanisms.* University Press, Oslo, 1970, pp. 149–169.

107. MUGNAINI, E.: *The histology and cytology of the cerebellar cortex,* in Larsell, O., and Jansen, J. K. S. (eds.): *The Comparative Anatomy and Histology of the Cerebellum. The Human Cerebellum, Cerebellar Connections and Cerebellar Cortex.* University of Minnesota Press, Minneapolis, 1972, pp. 201–264.

108. MURPHY, J. T., AND SABAH, N. H.: *The inhibitory effect of climbing fiber activation on cerebellar Purkinje cells.* Brain Res. 19:486, 1970.

109. MURPHY, J. T., AND SABAH, N. H.: *Spontaneous firing of cerebellar Purkinje cells in decerebrate and barbiturate anesthetized cats.* Brain Res. 17:515, 1970.

110. MURPHY, J. T., AND SABAH, N. H.: *Cerebellar Purkinje cell responses to afferent inputs. I. Climbing fiber activation.* Brain Res. 25:449, 1971.

111. MURPHY, J. T., AND SABAH, N. H.: *Cerebellar Purkinje cell responses to afferent inputs II. Mossy fiber activation.* Brain Res. 25:469, 1971.

112. NICHOLSON, C., TEN BRUGGENCATE, G., AND SENEKOWITSCH, R.: *Large potassium signals and slow potentials evoked during aminopyridine or barium superfusion in cat cerebellum.* Brain Res. 113:606, 1976.

113. O'LEARY, J. L., PETTY, J., SMITH, J. M. ET AL.: *Cerebellar cortex of rat and other animals: A structural and ultrastructural study.* J. Comp. Neurol. 134:401, 1968.

114. OSCARSSON, O.: *The sagittal organization of the cerebellar anterior lobe as revealed by the projection patterns of the climbing fiber system,* in Llinas, R. (ed.): *Neurobiology of Cerebellar Evolution and Development.* AMA-ERF Institute for Biomedical Research, Chicago, 1969, pp. 525–537.

115. PALAY, S. L.: *The electron microscopy of the glomeruli cerebellosi,* in *Cytology of Nervous Tissue. Proceedings of the Anatomical Society of Great Britain and Ireland.* Taylor and Francis, London, 1961, pp. 82–84.

116. PALAY, S. L., AND CHAN-PALAY, V.: *Cerebellar cortex. Cytology and organization.* Springer-Verlag, Berlin, 1974.

117. PALKOVITS, M., MAGYAR, P., AND SZENTÁGOTHAI, J.: *Quantitative histological analysis of the cerebellar cortex in the cat. I. Number and arrangement in space of the Purkinje cells.* Brain Res. 32:1, 1971.

118. PALKOVITS, M., MAGYAR, P., AND SZENTÁGOTHAI, J.: *Quantitative histological analysis of the cerebellar cortex in the cat. II. Cell numbers and densities in the granular layer.* Brain Res. 32:15, 1971.

119. PALKOVITS, M., MAGYAR, P., AND SZENTÁGOTHAI, J.: *Quantitative histological analysis of the cerebellar cortex in the cat. III. Structural organization of the molecular layer.* Brain Res. 34:1, 1971.

120. PALKOVITS, M., MAGYAR, P., AND SZENTÁGOTHAI, J.: *Quantitative histological analysis of the cerebellar cortex in the cat. IV Mossy fiber-Purkinje cell numerical transfer.* Brain Res. 45:15, 1972.

121. PELLIONISZ, A.: *Computer simulation of the pattern transfer of large cerebellar neuronal fields.* Acta Biochim. Biophys. Acad. Sci. Hung. 5(1):71, 1970.

122. PELLIONISZ, A., LLINAS, R., AND PERKEL, D. H.: *A computer model of the cerebellar cortex of the frog.* Neurosci. 2:19, 1977.

123. PELLIONISZ, A., AND SZENTÁGOTHAI, J.: *Dynamic single unit simulation of a realistic cerebellar network model.* Brain Res. 49:83, 1973.

124. PELLIONISZ, A., AND SZENTÁGOTHAI, J.: *Dynamic single unit simulation of a realistic cerebellar network model. II. Purkinje cell activity within the basic circuit and modified by inhibitory systems.* Brain Res. 68:19, 1974.

125. RAMON Y CAJAL, S.: *Histologie du système nerveux de l'homme et des vertébrés, vol. II.* Maloine, Paris, 1911.

126. RAMON Y CAJAL, S.: *Sur les fibres mousseuses et quelques points douteux de la texture de l'écorce cérébelleuse.* Trab. Lab. Invest. Biol. (Madrid) 24:215, 1926.

127. RUBIA, F. J., HÖPPENER, U., AND LANGHOF, H.: *Lateral inhibition of Purkinje cells through climbing fiber afferents?* Brain Res. 70:153, 1974.

128. RUBIA, F. J., AND KOLB, F. P.: *Responses of cerebellar units to a passive movement in the decerebrate cat.* Exp. Brain Res. 31:387, 1978.

129. SABAH, N. H.: *Reliability of computation in the cerebellum.* Biophys. J. 11:429, 1971.

130. SCHEIBEL, M. E., AND SCHEIBEL, A. B.: *Observations on the intracortical relations of the climbing fibers of the cerebellum.* J. Comp. Neurol. 101:733, 1954.

131. SCHOEPFLE, G. M.: *Action potentials of the cerebellar cortex elicited by stimulation of olivo-cerebellar fibers.* Fed. Proc. 8:140, 1949.

132. SMOLJANINOV, V. V.: *Structural-functional models of certain biological systems,* in Gelfand. I. M., Gurfinkel, V. S., Fomin. S. V., et al. (eds.): *Several Characteristics in the Organization of the Cerebellum.* Izdatelstvo Nauka, Moscow, 1966, pp. 203–267, as cited in Palkovits. et al., 1971.

133. SNIDER, R. S., HIROTA, N., AND BAN, J. T.: *Function of Purkinje axon collaterals in isolated cerebellar folia.* Exp. Neurol. 20:285, 1968.

134. TALBOTT, R. E., TOWE, A. L., AND KENNEDY, T. T.: *Physiological and histological classification of cerebellar neurons in chloralose-anesthetized cats.* Exp. Neurol. 19:46, 1967.

135. TEN BRUGGENCATE, G. NICHOLSON, C., AND STÖCKLE, H.: *Climbing fiber evoked potassium release in cat cerebellum.* Pflügers Arch. 367:107, 1976.

136. THACH, W. T., JR.: *Somatosensory receptive fields of single units in cat cerebellar cortex.* J. Neurophysiol. 30:675, 1967.

CHAPTER 5

The Responses of Cerebellar Neurons

VESTIBULAR, VISUAL, AND AUDITORY STIMULI

Most types of natural peripheral stimuli affect the activity of large numbers of cerebellar neurons. In many instances, the responses to each stimulus modality have a characteristic time course and spatial distribution. Each stimulus activates inputs that show marked convergence because of the organization of both the cerebellar afferent projections and the cerebellar cortex. As a consequence, many cerebellar neurons respond to several types of peripheral stimuli. Even though this is the case, for the sake of clarity the responses evoked by each modality will be presented separately before certain features of spatial integration are discussed.

Vestibular Stimuli

Vestibular stimulation affects neuronal activity in a large cerebellar cortical region which extends considerably beyond the flocculonodular lobe, the classic location of the "vestibulocerebellum."[3, 16, 41, 50, 89, 158, 159, 163, 188] Responses appear in the nodulus, flocculus, uvula, lingula, lobus simplex, and lobules I through X of the vermis. This widespread distribution results in part from the vestibular nuclear projections to the lateral reticular nucleus,[116] a nucleus which projects to many parts of the cerebellar vermis and paravermis.[158]

Debate has arisen about the degree to which vestibular stimuli activate either mossy fiber or climbing fiber inputs to the cerebellum.[79, 156] Most recent findings indicate that the activation of receptors in either the semicircular canals or the maculae evokes responses mediated chiefly by mossy fibers, although responses mediated by climbing fibers have been observed.[123, 131, 132, 157, 158, 178] These studies show that the activity of a given Purkinje cell can be modulated by the activation of mossy fiber inputs in the absence of any response evoked by climbing fibers. The climbing fiber input to the flocculus is activated mostly by natural visual stimuli rather than vestibular stimuli.[157, 181]

The Purkinje cell responses to natural stimulation of the semicircular canals vary, depending upon whether the stimulus activates the ipsilateral or contralateral receptors.[30, 124, 158, 178] Some Purkinje cells increase in discharge rate only during the activation of ipsilateral receptors, while others respond only to the activation of the contralateral receptors. The activity of another group of Purkinje cells increases following the activation of either ipsilateral or contralateral receptors, and a final group shows a decrease of discharge rate to the same set of stimuli. Inputs from the different semicircular canals and macular receptors converge on single neurons to some degree, but most neurons respond only to the activation of one pair of receptors.[158] Consequently, a change in neuronal activity may reflect changes in head position occurring in one, two, or three dimensions of space, depending upon the convergence of inputs to a given neuron.[158] Vestibular inputs to the cerebellum converge with inputs activated by other afferents which are important in the control of eye and head position. Stimulating nerves originating in the deep tissues of the neck affect neuronal activity in lobules V and VI, the uvula, and the flocculonodular lobe.[29, 174, 193] Some of the afferents activated by these stimuli originate in nucleus x of the vestibular nuclear complex.[191-193] In general inputs to lobules V through VII show remarkable convergence, being activated by afferents from extraocular muscles, corticofugal projections, peripheral cutaneous receptors, and visual pathways.[24, 27, 29, 81, 175]

Many neurons of the fastigial nucleus respond to vestibular stimulation. The responses in the nuclei, unlike the responses in the cerebellar cortex, show strong convergence of afferents from more than one canal.[84] In the fastigial nucleus, as in the cerebellar cortex, static changes in position do not modify the activity of a high percentage of neurons.[84, 85, 87] Rather, their activity can be modulated (increased or decreased) by sinusoidal changes in head position. The harmonic distortion of these responses indicates that they are partly nonlinear,[84, 109] and their peak responses are a power function of the peak acceleration of the stimulus.[84]

Studies correlating the locations of neurons with their responses to vestibular stimuli have led to the conclusion that the projection from the fastigial nucleus to

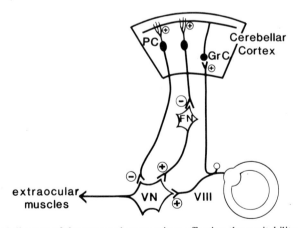

Figure 1. Simplified diagram of the neuronal connections affecting the excitability of neurons in the vestibular nuclei in response to natural vestibular stimuli. The direct cerebellar corticovestibular projection and the cerebellar corticofastigiovestibular projection act in parallel to modify the excitability of vestibular neurons responsible for regulating eye movements. The effects of the vestibular nuclei on eye movements are mediated by the extraocular nuclei and the reticular formation. PC = Purkinje cells; GrC = granule cells; FN = fastigial neuron; VN = vestibular neuron; VIII = 8th nerve.

96

the vestibular nuclei acts in parallel with the direct projection of Purkinje cells to the same nuclei.[83, 84, 109, 177] The organizational scheme resulting from these studies shows that receptors in the ipsilateral horizontal semicircular canal activate granule cells which excite Purkinje cells (Fig. 1). The Purkinje cells inhibit vestibular nuclear neurons directly and inhibit fastigial neurons which terminate on the same neurons in the vestibular nucleus. These vestibular neurons are activated also by the same vestibular stimulus.

Visual Stimuli

Neurons in many regions of the cerebellar cortex respond to visual stimuli, particularly in the posterior lobe.[74, 75, 105, 108, 112, 183] Two pontocerebellar projections mediate these responses—a corticopontocerebellar projection from the visual cortex[107] and a tectopontocerebellar projection from the superior colliculus.[104] Selective ablations of localized portions of these two pathways have marked but different effects on visual evoked responses.[107] The time course of the responses evoked by visual stimuli is altered by interrupting the corticopontocerebellar projection through lesions of the visual cortex or inactivation of the visual cortex by the application of potassium chloride.[134, 144] Even in the absence of this pathway in the decerebrate animal, a retinotopic pattern of responses to visual stimuli occurs in the posterior lobe of the cerebellum.[43] These responses, which are particularly sensitive to moving visual stimuli, involve the superior colliculus and are mediated by the tectopontocerebellar pathway, a mossy fiber input to the cerebellar cortex.

In the flocculus, climbing fibers mediate the neuronal responses to visual stimuli.[127, 128] This climbing fiber projection originates primarily in the dorsal cap of Kooy, a portion of the inferior olive. Dorsal cap neurons are activated by a projection from the accessory optic tract that responds selectively to visual stimuli.[127, 128] The climbing fiber input to the flocculus is directionally sensitive to visual stimuli moving at low velocities.[157, 180, 181] In contrast, vestibular stimuli evoke responses mediated chiefly by mossy fibers.[157]

Despite the fact that visual and vestibular stimuli activate separate inputs to the flocculus, the responses of Purkinje cells in this region to mossy fiber inputs evoked by vestibular stimuli can be modified by visual stimuli.[86] This can be demonstrated in the rabbit by examining this interaction during sinusoidal movements of the head. The modulation of Purkinje cell activity increases markedly when a slit of light is moved sinusoidally together with the animal's head. In contrast, when the animal's head is moved sinusoidally while the slit of light remains fixed, the depth of Purkinje cell modulation decreases. Movement of the visual stimulus alone, however, causes no change in the spontaneous simple spike activity of Purkinje cells, indicating that the mossy fiber inputs to the cerebellum activated by visual stimuli do not affect these Purkinje cells.

Observations in the awake monkey also show that visual stimuli can modify Purkinje cell activity in the flocculus evoked by modulating head position.[123] A considerably greater modulation of Purkinje cell discharge occurs when the monkey is required to fixate on a visual stimulus which moves together with the head than when compensatory eye movements occur during fixation on a motionless visual stimulus. These findings led to the hypothesis that the output of the flocculus, mediated by the inhibitory axons of Purkinje cells, suppresses the vestibulo-ocular reflex under certain behavioral conditions (Fig. 2). These effects on the activity of Purkinje cells are thought to reflect the combined action of two mossy fiber inputs, one signaling vestibular stimuli during head movement and the other signaling the velocity of eye movements.[123] The function of the climbing fiber input activated by visual stimuli in the vestibulo-ocular reflex has not been determined. It has been suggested that this input, which is activated by moving stimuli applied to the retina, is required for the stabilization of the retinal image during eye and head movement.[127, 128] Another proposal will be discussed in Chapter 9.

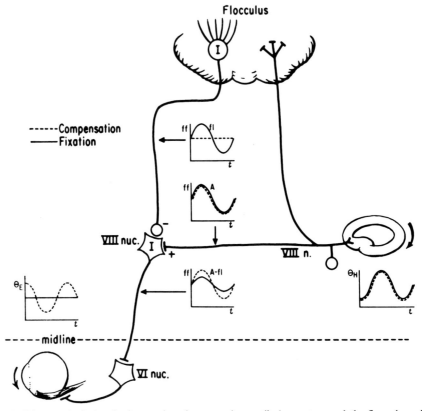

Figure 2. Diagram depicting the interactions between the vestibular system and the flocculus which regulate the gain of the vesibulo-ocular reflex. Graphs of the time variant responses to head movement under two conditions are shown next to the structures or neuronal components modified by the stimulus. The condition termed *compensation* indicates the compensating movement of the eye in response to movement of the head. The coordinated movement of the head and eyes is referred to as the vestibulo-ocular reflex. The condition termed *fixation* indicates the fixation of the animal or subject on a target which moves together with the movement of the head. This type of fixation requires the suppression of the vestibulo-ocular reflex. Note that the impulse activity of the Purkinje cell (I) in the flocculus is modulated only during the condition requiring fixation on a moving target. During this condition, there is a reduction in the modulation of the neuron projecting from the vestibular nucleus (VIII nuc.) to motoneurons in the abducens nucleus (VI nuc.). This effect together with the other interactions evoked by the vestibular stimulus results in a suppression of eye movement during fixation. t = time; ff = firing frequency; Θ_H = angular movement of the head; Θ_E = angular movement of the eye; fl = floccular Purkinje cell; A = afferent; A–fl = summed response to the afferent fiber and the floccular Purkinje cell. (From Lisberger and Fuchs,[123] with permission.)

98

Auditory Stimuli

The cerebellum processes auditory information through interactions in the cerebellar cortex and through actions on neurons in several nuclei of the auditory pathway. These include the cochlear nuclei, inferior colliculus, and superior olive.[93, 102, 184, 186]

The cerebellar regions responsive to auditory stimuli overlap considerably with those responsive to visual stimuli. These regions are limited essentially to the posterior lobe and include the lobulus simplex, tuber vermis, culmen, pyramis, medial crus I and crus II, paramedian lobules, and a portion of the paraflocculus.[40, 75, 183] The responses to auditory stimuli are evoked through cortical and subcortical pathways of the auditory system[140, 183] and are mediated mostly by mossy fibers.[179] In studies similar to those concerning the visual system, ablations of the auditory cortex caused marked changes in the responses evoked by auditory stimuli.[144] As in the visual system, subcortical projections are important also; the time course of the auditory responses in decerebrate animals is similar in intact animals anesthetized with alpha chloralose.[2] Components of these responses have been ascribed to projections involving the cochlear nuclei and projections from the inferior colliculus to the pontine nuclei.

The cerebellar responses to auditory stimuli may be important in adjusting the position of the body and head to the location of a sound. Neurons responding to auditory stimuli in lobules VI and VII show little specificity to stimuli differing only in frequency, but show marked sensitivity to the interaural time and intensity of two stimuli,[12] with the greatest sensitivity occuring for binaural stimuli of equal intensity.[2] Other neurons respond selectively to movement of the auditory stimulus.[12]

Input from the Perihypoglossal Nuclei

Cerebellar afferents were found to originate in the perihypoglossal nuclei more than 25 years ago.[35, 187] Physiologic interest in these afferents was aroused only with the recent demonstration that they can be activated by vestibular stimuli. The perihypoglossal nuclei consist of three subdivisions, all located in the medulla: the nucleus intercalatus, the nucleus praepositus hypoglossi, and the nucleus of Roller.[35, 187] All three nuclei project to the anterior lobe vermis and to the pyramis, uvula, and fastigial nucleus. Each projects to slightly different regions of the vermis.[114] Fibers from these nuclei also terminate in the vestibular projection areas of the cerebellum.[11, 114]

Neurons in the nucleus praepositus hypoglossi respond to vestibular, visual, and cervical afferent stimuli.[23, 31, 88] The inputs to this nucleus are organized in parallel with connections to the oculomotor neurons.[22, 28] Consequently, the excitatory and inhibitory actions of the afferents to the nucleus praepositus hypoglossi are similar to their actions on neurons in the oculomotor nuclei.

PERIPHERAL AND CORTICOFUGAL INPUTS

Proprioceptive Stimuli

The cerebellum has long been known as a structure important for processing proprioceptive information from the periphery. For this reason, many investigations have been concerned with the responses evoked in the cerebellum by stimulating muscle proprioceptive afferents. Stimulation of group Ia afferents (the large diameter primary afferents from muscle spindles) has surprisingly little effect on Purkinje cell activity.[95-97] Most neurons responding to naturally applied proprioceptive stimuli can be activated selectively by group Ib afferents (the large diameter fibers from Golgi tendon organs) or group II afferents (the smaller diameter secondary afferents from muscle spindles). The responses include changes in discharge rate due to both mossy and climbing fiber inputs activated by phasic (rapidly changing) and tonic (maintained) stimuli.[95-98, 145, 146]

Cerebellar neurons respond with considerable sensitivity to passive flexion or extension of a single joint.[18, 113, 166, 168, 185] Either phasic or tonic stimuli can modify cerebellar neuronal discharge through the action of both climbing fiber and mossy fiber afferents. In addition, Purkinje cells can be activated solely by either mossy fibers or climbing fibers in response to changes in the angle of a joint.

Cutaneous Stimuli

The influence of cutaneous inputs upon the cerebellum often is overlooked because of the lack of sensory deficits observed clinically in humans after large cerebellar lesions. Nevertheless, cutaneous stimuli activate many cerebellar afferent projections and evoke responses widely in the cerebellum.[50, 51] These responses can be elicited by low intensity phasic and tonic cutaneous stimuli via both mossy and climbing fibers.[55, 56, 65-69, 92, 94, 121, 122] Activation of pacinian corpuscles, rapidly and slowly adapting cutaneous receptors, and hair receptors can affect the discharge of cerebellar cortical neurons.[66] The same Purkinje cell often responds to activation of different types of peripheral cutaneous receptors, depending upon the site of stimulation within the receptive field. The Purkinje cell responses to a mossy fiber input generally adapt more rapidly than the responses of the mossy fibers themselves to the same stimuli.[66, 67]

Responses to climbing fiber inputs can be evoked not only by high intensity cutaneous stimuli as reported initially,[117, 139, 152] but also by low intensity cutaneous stimuli.[55, 56, 68, 121] Marked convergence occurs among the climbing fiber inputs responding to stimuli applied on different regions of the body surface.[121] The threshold required for activating a given Purkinje cell, however, can vary in different regions of the receptive field and, in some cases, in different regions of the same extremity. In addition, cutaneous stimuli can affect the activity of Purkinje cells which respond also to proprioceptive stimuli, demonstrating the convergence of inputs from these two different modalities.[47, 48, 52, 54-56, 141] As with other stimulus modalities, cutaneous stimuli can affect the activity of individual Purkinje cells through either mossy fiber or climbing fiber inputs in unanesthetized preparations.[121]

Spinal Input to the Lateral Cerebellum

Contrary to the previous notion that the lateral regions of the cerebellum interact only with forebrain structures, these regions respond to the activation of ascending spinal pathways.[106, 142, 143] Stimulation of forelimb and hindlimb afferents evokes responses in crus I and crus II of the cerebellum, and these responses can be obtained in both decerebrate and decorticate animals. Thus, the pathways mediating these responses are located in the spinal cord and brainstem. Both mossy fiber and climbing fiber projections to the lateral regions of the cerebellar cortex can be activated by electrical as well as natural peripheral stimuli.[25, 26] Characteristically the inputs to dentate neurons show extensive spatial convergence from many regions of the body surface, including the face (Fig. 3).

The pathways mediating the cerebellar responses to cutaneous stimuli are indirect, involving at least one brainstem precerebellar nucleus.[25] The spinal component of the pathway courses in the dorsal columns because interruption of the dorsal fasciculus abolishes the responses to stimuli below the lesion. The lateral reticular nucleus probably does not mediate the cerebellar responses to cutaneous stimuli; the projection from this nucleus to the dentate nucleus and cerebellar hemispheres has been questioned recently.[44, 115, 133] These responses may be mediated by spinopontocerebellar projections. One of these pathways is a direct spinopontine projection[38, 42, 147, 190] which has been confirmed recently with intraaxonal tracing techniques in monkeys.[167] Another spinopontocerebellar projection includes a pathway from the dorsal column nuclei to the pontine nuclei, possibly through collaterals of the medial lemniscus.[162, 190] The responses in the lateral parts of the cerebellum to spinal inputs described by Bantli and Bloedel[25] disappeared only when the dorsal columns were sectioned. Consequently, they are

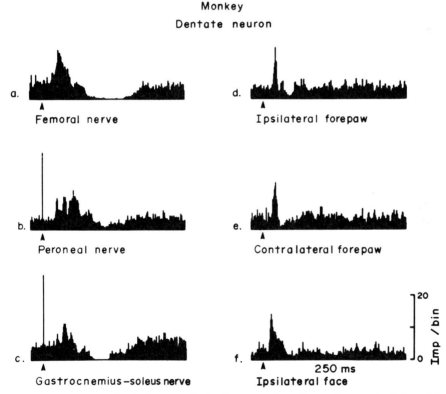

Figure 3. The responses of a single neuron in the dentate nucleus of a monkey to stimulation of three different peripheral nerves (a-c) and to stimulation of various regions of the body surface (d-f). The neuron can be activated from several sites, demonstrating the extensive convergence onto this neuron. Each record is a poststimulus time histogram constructed from the responses to 64 consecutive stimuli in each of the indicated stimulus sites. (From Bantli and Bloedel,[26] with permission.)

probably mediated by pathways involving the dorsal column nuclei rather than the direct spinopontine fibers. This conclusion is consistent with the finding that the input to the pontine nuclei from the dorsal column nuclei terminates in the peduncular pontine nucleus which projects to the cerebellar hemispheres, the region in which the responses were recorded.

Facial Stimuli

Stimulation of trigeminal cutaneous afferents evokes responses in the cerebellum to both mossy and climbing fiber inputs.[136, 137] The responses mediated by mossy fibers occur mainly in medial cerebellar regions. The responses mediated by climbing fibers appear in more lateral regions, including portions of the cerebellar hemispheres. The climbing fiber input can be activated by stimulating the superficial radial nerve as well as the cerebral cortex.[135-137]

Consistent with the notion that the cerebellum participates in the vestibulo-ocular reflex, the activation of mechanoreceptors in the extraocular muscles can evoke responses in cerebellar neurons.[21] Neurons in the trigeminal nuclei mediate these responses. The trigeminal neurons project to the cerebellum and are activated by passive stretch of the extraocular muscles.[13, 129, 130] Neuronal responses evoked from the extraocular muscles occur in cerebellar vermal lobules V, VI, and VII.[24, 27, 82, 175] Most commonly these responses are mediated by mossy fibers, although responses to climbing fibers also occur.[24, 27] The responses to climbing fiber inputs evoked from extraocular muscle afferents appear more laterally in the cerebellum than the responses to mossy fiber inputs.[24] The patterns of convergence of inputs to Purkinje cells from extraocular muscles on each side are consistent with the paired organization of muscle groups involved in conjugate ocular movements.[175]

Activation of Corticofugal Pathways

As mentioned earlier, pathways descending from the cerebral cortex can activate neurons in several nuclei which project to the cerebellum. Stimulation of the cerebral cortex evokes responses mediated by mossy and climbing fibers to specific regions of the cerebellar cortex.[6, 99, 100, 169-173] The initial studies of these responses revealed considerable overlap in their distribution, at least within the anterior lobe vermis and paravermis.[138, 160] Recent investigations have shown, however, that the distributions of the responses to mossy and climbing fiber inputs do not overlap completely.[149, 172, 173] Stimulation of a particular point on the sensorimotor cortex, for example, evokes responses to mossy fiber inputs in the anterior lobe vermis and the paramedian lobule. The same stimulus evokes responses to climbing fiber inputs in more lateral regions of the vermis, including lobules IV and V and the cerebellar hemisphere (Fig. 4).[149]

The cerebellar neuronal responses to stimulating different cerebral cortical regions show marked convergence. Single neurons respond to climbing fiber inputs activated by stimulating each somatosensory area, including SI, SII, and SIII.[164] The convergence of inputs activated by stimulating both the sensorimotor cortex and association cortex is less marked.[148, 149, 172, 173] Some Purkinje cells in the anterior lobe vermis responding to inputs evoked by stimulating the sensorimotor cortex also respond to the activation of spinal inputs.[119, 120, 138, 161, 164]

Pathways descending from the cerebral cortex can modify the responses of cer-

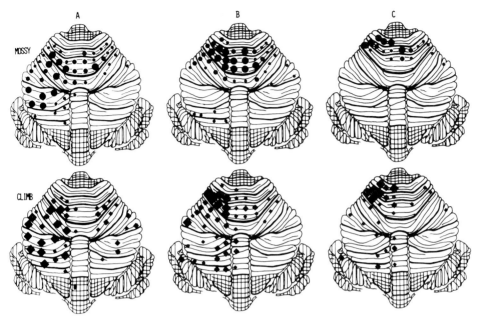

Figure 4. Distribution of responses to mossy fiber (upper row) and climbing fiber (lower row) inputs following stimulation of the lateral (A), intermediate (B), and medial (C) part of the precentral motor cortex. The amplitudes of the responses are indicated by the sizes of the dots. The shaded areas were not studied. There is a relationship but not a strict correspondence between the amplitudes and distributions of the responses evoked by mossy fibers and climbing fibers. Note the wide distribution of the responses evoked in the cerebellum from stimulating a single locus on the motor cortex. (From Sasaki et al.,[172] with permission.)

ebellar neurons to peripheral stimuli. Some of these modifications result from interactions in the cerebellar cortex evoked by converging corticopontocerebellar pathways. Other modifications result from interactions in the spinal cord and brainstem. Corticofugal pathways can affect the excitability of neurons projecting to the cerebellum from the spinal cord and brainstem and alter the responses of these neurons to peripheral stimuli. At least some of these pathways are organized topographically. Stimulating certain sensorimotor cortical regions suppresses selectively the responses evoked by cutaneous mechanical stimuli applied in the distribution of a specific peripheral nerve.[78]

Cerebellar Nuclear Responses to Peripheral Stimuli

Naturally applied peripheral cutaneous stimuli alter neuronal excitability in the fastigial, interposed, and dentate nuclei. Neurons in the fastigial nucleus respond to low intensity phasic and tonic cutaneous stimuli.[70, 71] Neurons responding to cutaneous stimulation of either the hindlimb or forelimb are located in specific regions of the nucleus, and some neurons respond to inputs from both locations.[17, 19, 61, 72] Natural peripheral cutaneous stimuli also affect neuronal excitability in the interposed nuclei.[62-64, 72] The responses in the interposed nuclei display less somatotopic organization than those in the fastigial nucleus.[60] Even in the interposed nuclei, however, there are groups of neurons responding selectively to afferents from either the forelimb or the hindlimb.[60] As mentioned earlier, neurons

103

in the dentate nucleus also respond to low intensity cutaneous stimuli.[25, 26] The inputs to these cells, however, show much more spatial convergence than the inputs to neurons in the other cerebellar nuclei.

The effect of stimulating proprioceptive afferents has been studied extensively only in the interposed nuclei. Neurons in this structure respond chiefly to the phasic component of muscle stretch.[125, 126] The responsive neurons are considerably more sensitive to activation of group II afferents than to either group Ia or Ib afferents.[103]

Debate has arisen concerning the relative contributions of direct spinocerebellar and indirect spinoreticulocerebellar projections in mediating neuronal responses from the periphery to the cerebellar nuclei. Measurements of response latencies in the interposed and fastigial nuclei led to the conclusion that the responses in these nuclei are mediated chiefly by indirect spinoreticulocerebellar projections involving the lateral reticular nucleus and that the responses in the cerebellar cortex are mediated principally by direct pathways.[62, 63, 70-72, 118] Although the inputs from reticulocerebellar projections may predominate under certain experimental conditions, this is not always the case. For example, a direct spinocerebellar projection mediates the neuronal responses to forelimb proprioceptive afferents within the interposed nuclei.[125, 126]

The time course of the neuronal responses in both the cerebellar cortex and nuclei undoubtedly reflects interactions between these structures. This conclusion is emphasized by the demonstration that cooling of the cerebellar cortex alters the responses of neurons in the cerebellar nuclei.[126] The characteristics of these interactions probably are determined by the actions of Purkinje cell axons and the nucleocortical projection.

Cerebellar Nuclear Responses to the Activation of Descending Pathways

Studies of the actions of descending pathways on neurons in the intracerebellar nuclei have focused either on their topographic organization or the patterns of convergence from cortical and spinal inputs onto individual neurons. Many cells within the interposed nuclei respond to stimulation of the nerves of the forelimbs and hindlimbs and to stimulation of the sensorimotor regions of the cerebral cortex.[5, 8, 9] Neurons in the anterior interposed nucleus respond chiefly to stimulation of hindlimb afferents and the primary sensorimotor cortex, supplementary motor cortex, and premotor cortex. In contrast, neurons in the posterior interposed nucleus respond chiefly to stimulation of forelimb afferents and the forelimb areas of the primary sensorimotor cortex and premotor cortex.

Inputs to the dentate nucleus activated by descending pathways are organized differently than the inputs to the interposed nuclei. The largest responses in the dentate nucleus are evoked from the premotor and supplementary motor cortex rather than the primary sensorimotor cortex.[10] The responses of neurons in the dentate nucleus to cerebral cortical stimulation show a topographic organization. Neurons responding to stimulation of the hindlimb region in the sensorimotor cortex are located anteriorly in the dentate nucleus and neurons responding to stimulation of the forelimb region are located more posteriorly. In one study, little convergence was found between the inputs activated from peripheral afferents and those activated from the cerebral cortex.[10] In this study the lack of input from spinal afferents could have resulted from the type of anesthetic used, because it has now been demonstrated that peripheral stimuli can affect neurons in the dentate nucleus in unanesthetized decerebrate animals and in animals anesthetized with alpha chloralose.[26] Consequently, studies of convergence between cortical and peripheral inputs should be repeated in these two types of preparations.

SPATIAL ORGANIZATION OF INPUTS TO THE CEREBELLAR CORTEX

Responses Evoked from Peripheral Afferents

Local stimulation of afferents from different regions of the body surface activates somatotopically organized inputs to small cerebellar cortical regions.[1, 183] Inputs activated from discrete regions of the primary sensorimotor cortex showed a comparable somatotopic organization.[90, 91, 182] These findings have led to the hypothesis that a complex representation of the body surface exists in the anterior lobe and a portion of the posterior lobe of the cerebellum. In support of this hypothesis, a series of anatomic and electrophysiologic studies revealed that individual spinocerebellar afferent pathways project to specific cerebellar cortical regions. The responses to mossy fiber inputs evoked through direct spinocerebellar pathways are distributed longitudinally in the same direction as parallel fibers.[150, 151] In contrast, the climbing fiber responses to stimulation of the olivocerebellar pathway appear along sagittally oriented strips of the cerebellar cortex.[14, 73, 139, 152-155]

The results of the foregoing lines of investigation have been taken as strong evidence for a somatotopic organization of cerebellar afferent projections, however, two important considerations have been overlooked. First, any peripheral stimulus activates many ascending spinal pathways. These pathways project directly to the cerebellum and also to the precerebellar reticular nuclei. Consequently, the distribution of cerebellar afferents responding to any peripheral stimulus reflects not only the distribution of one or two direct spinocerebellar pathways but also the widespread distribution of the reticulocerebellar projections.[32] The spatial distribution of the responses evoked by each individual cerebellar afferent projection responding to a hypothetical localized cutaneous stimulus has been plotted in diagrams of the anterior lobe. The responses cover a large area of the anterior lobe, and the existence of longitudinal or sagittal strips is not apparent.[32] Second, in many of the studies supporting the somatotopic organization of cerebellar afferents, sodium pentobarbital was employed as an anesthetic. This factor is important because pentobarbital depresses severely the reticulocerebellar projections activated by peripheral stimuli. In light of the widespread distribution of projections from the precerebellar reticular nuclei to the cerebellar cortex and the great sensitivity of these projections to barbiturates, the distribution of the responses evoked by peripheral stimuli undoubtedly was altered. The effects of anesthetic agents provide the basis for the difference between the observations of Adrian[1] and Snider and Stowell,[183] who utilized barbiturate anesthetics, and those of other investigators who employed preparations not anesthetized with sodium pentobarbital.[20, 45, 46, 50, 76, 77, 105] In the latter studies, stimuli to specific peripheral regions of the body evoked responses in widely distributed cerebellar cortical areas (see Fig. 6). These observations were made in many types of preparations, including decerebrate and unanesthetized animals.

Many subsequent investigations concerned with the somatotopic distribution of individual Purkinje cell responses have supported the conclusion that inputs to the cerebellar cortex show extensive spatial convergence. Even though the responses to climbing fiber inputs show a more pronounced somatotopic distribution than the responses to mossy fiber inputs, considerable overlap still occurs in the distribution of the responses to climbing fiber inputs evoked from forelimb and hindlimb afferents.[53, 57-59, 110] The distribution of responses to both types of inputs led to the proposal that stimulating different regions of the body evoked responses located in patchy mosaics and not a pattern of strips oriented sagittally and longitudinally across the surface of cerebellum (Fig. 5).[53, 57-59, 110, 111]

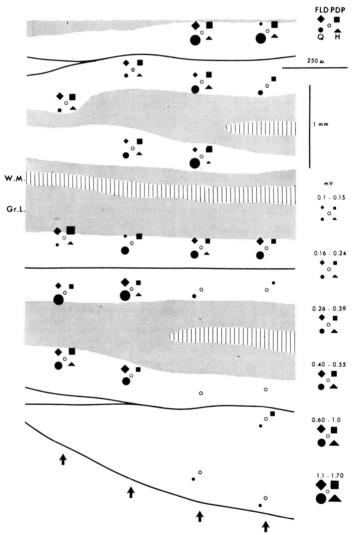

Figure 5. Responses evoked by climbing fiber inputs following stimulation of four different nerves innervating hindlimb muscles. The amplitude and distribution of responses to each nerve are shown on a diagram of the cerebellar cortex. The responses vary from place to place and have no clear somatotopic transition. Abbreviations: FLD = flexor digitorum longus; Q = quadriceps; H = hamstring; PDP = peroneal and deep peroneal; W.M. = white matter; Gr.L. = granular layer. (From Eccles et al.,[55] with permission.)

Studies in unanesthetized animals have supported strongly the lack of a strict somatotopic organization of inputs to the cerebellum.[94, 121, 122] In these preparations, cerebellar neurons have receptive fields distributed over wide regions of the body surface, often including more than one extremity. These large receptive fields characterize the responses of cerebellar neurons to either mossy or climbing fiber inputs. The administration of sodium pentobarbital in these animals results in a much more restricted distribution of field responses to peripheral stimuli. This finding illustrates the problem of interpreting the spatial distributions of responses in animals anesthetized with barbiturates.

A better localization of responses occurs in intact animals when the stimulus is confined to the stretch of a single muscle or movements about a single joint (Fig. 6). Stretch of single forelimb muscles in unanesthetized cats evokes responses to mossy fiber inputs in a restricted region of the ipsilateral pars intermedia in lobule V.[145, 146] Even with this focal stimulus, however, the distribution of the responses includes a total surface area which exceeds considerably both the size of the functional subunits proposed for restricted regions of a cerebellar folium[57] and the size predicted by the distribution of responses in anesthetized preparations.

The response to climbing fiber inputs evoked by peripheral stimuli also can be localized to a specific cerebellar cortical region in intact unanesthetized animals. Passive movement of the forepaw in the cat evokes climbing fiber responses oriented in a sagittal strip,[168] and electrical stimulation of the splanchnic nerve evokes responses located in a similar strip.[165] These strips, however, involve more than one folium and in some cases are as long as 9 mm. It has not been determined whether neurons in these strips also respond to inputs from other regions of the body. The conclusion is that, although responses to localized peripheral stimuli sometimes are confined to regions of the cerebellar cortex, the overall dis-

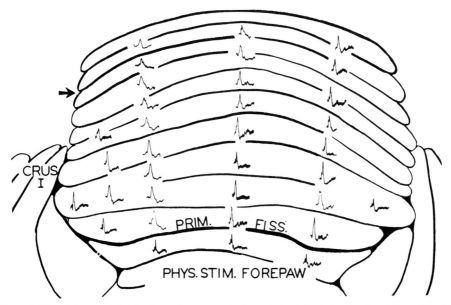

Figure 6. The widespread distribution of responses in the anterior lobe to tactile stimulation of the left forepaw in an unanesthetized decerebrate cat. (From Combs,[46] with permission.)

107

tribution of responses to different stimuli is not organized with a strict somatotopic pattern. Neurons with restricted receptive fields often are intermixed among neurons activated from other body regions. Furthermore, neurons in a region of the cortex containing other neurons responsive to the same stimulus may be activated by peripheral inputs of other modalities or by inputs from other regions of the body.

Responses Evoked from the Cerebral Cortex

Concepts regarding the somatotopic organization of cerebrocerebellar projections developed in parallel with those concerning the somatotopic distribution of responses to peripheral stimuli. Many studies employing animal preparations anesthetized with pentobarbital reveal a body representation in the cerebellar cortex related to the body representation found on the sensorimotor cortex.[90, 189] The responses to stimulation of the primary sensorimotor cortex appear mostly over the anterior lobe and part of the simplex. The responses to stimulation of the secondary somatosensory cortex appear in the paramedian lobule. Subsequent studies substantiated and further refined these observations.[6, 7, 172] Stimulating the forelimb region of the primary motor cortex in monkeys evokes responses to mossy fiber inputs mostly in the ansiparamedian lobule, caudal anterior lobe, and simplex. Stimulating the hindlimb cerebral cortical region evokes responses in the rostral anterior lobe. Even in these studies, however, Purkinje cells in lobules IVA and VA respond to stimulation throughout the sensorimotor cortex. Thus, although inputs from the cerebral cortex show a topographic distribution, the projections from different cortical regions converge onto Purkinje cell populations in the cerebellar cortex.

The responses to climbing fiber inputs evoked by stimulating forelimb and hindlimb regions of the sensorimotor cortex have a topographic distribution similar to that evoked by mossy fibers activated from the same cortical areas. Although the responses of Purkinje cells to climbing fiber inputs in some regions of the anterior lobe can be activated selectively from these cerebral cortical regions, many Purkinje cells in lobules II through IV of the pars intermedia can be activated by climbing fiber inputs following stimulation of several cerebral cortical regions.[164] In the lateral part of the vermis responses to the climbing fiber inputs are restricted to sagittal zones under certain experimental conditions.[138, 160, 161] In contrast, responses evoked in the pars intermedia in lobule V by stimulating the forelimb region are found more anteriorly while those evoked by stimulating the hindlimb area are observed posteriorly. Eccles[53] maintains, however, that these responses are not distributed in strips but in patches, similar to the somatotopic distribution of inputs from the periphery to the cerebellar cortex.

In preparations not anesthetized with barbiturates, cortical stimuli evoke responses in many locations within the cerebellar cortex.[99, 100] The distribution of these responses most likely reflects the combined pattern of inputs from the pontine nuclei, the nucleus reticularis tegmenti pontis, and the lateral reticular nucleus.[4, 15, 36] As observed in studies of ascending projections, the responses to stimulating the cerebral cortex mediated by the precerebellar reticular nuclei are highly sensitive to barbiturates. Thus, the variety of animal preparations in these studies may account for the inconsistencies in the distributions of responses to cerebral cortical stimulation.

108

Spatial Distribution of Responses to Peripheral and Cortical Stimuli

There is no doubt about the fact that neurons in certain cerebellar cortical regions can be activated preferentially by some peripheral and cerebral cortical stimuli. Nevertheless, the basic pattern of organization of the cerebellar afferents can be viewed as a convergence of inputs from stimuli of different modalities arising in different regions of the body surface and inputs from the cerebral cortex. The underlying basis for the spatial distribution of responses to inputs of these types can be ascribed to a combination of four factors, some of which have been commented upon earlier in this section.

First, any peripheral or cortical stimulus activates a number of cerebellar afferent projections, each of which affects cerebellar cortical neuronal activity in a characteristic distribution. Consequently, the cerebellar cortical region containing neurons affected by a peripheral stimulus reflects the distribution of several cerebellar afferent projections.

Second, stimuli activating several ascending spinal pathways affect Purkinje cell activity through direct spinocerebellar projections and also through indirect spinoreticulocerebellar projections. The pathways from the paramedian and lateral reticular nuclei terminate in a fairly large area of the vermis and paravermis in both the anterior and posterior lobes. Consequently, activation of reticulocerebellar projections from peripheral stimuli undoubtedly results in significant spatial divergence of afferent input to a wide region of the cerebellar cortex. This factor underlies the different results obtained in unanesthetized and anesthetized preparations, because reticulocerebellar projections are known to be sensitive to barbiturate anesthetics.[33, 49, 106] The importance of the indirect spinoreticulocerebellar projections is emphasized by the finding that stimulating a direct spinocerebellar pathway or peripheral afferents evokes a response with a "local component," showing a spatial distribution corresponding to the projection areas of direct spinocerebellar pathways, and a "diffuse component," distributed over a wide region of the cerebellar cortex.[20] This notion has been supported with data from unanesthetized intact animals.[113] Thus, the combined activation of direct and indirect spinocerebellar projections by peripheral stimuli affects markedly the distribution of neural responses to a given peripheral stimulus.

Third, the restricted distribution of responses resulting from stimuli applied to localized parts of the body surface often overlaps with the restricted distribution of responses evoked by stimulating other body regions. In addition, there can be overlap of the responses evoked by stimuli of different modalities. Responses in the anterior lobe evoked by passive stretch of single muscles in the forelimb, for example, occur in the same regions of the cerebellar cortex as responses to cutaneous stimulation of either the forelimb or the hindlimb.

Fourth, the intrinsic connections of the cerebellum act to increase the distribution of Purkinje cells responding to a particular mossy fiber input. Within the granular layer, the somatotopic organization of responses to mossy fiber inputs from stimulation of different regions of the body surface shows a very precise "fractured mosaic" representation of the body surface.[101, 176] In addition, mossy fiber inputs from spinal and pontine projections are segregated within separate regions of the anterior lobe.[189] Despite this organization of mossy fiber inputs, stimuli applied at several locations on the body surface and on the cerebral cortex can activate the same neurons, presumably because of the spatial convergence resulting from the intrinsic fiber systems of the cerebellar cortex. For example, parallel fibers extend as far as 7 mm along the folium.[34] As a consequence, the input activating any given granule cell can influence the excitability of Purkinje cell dendrites over at least this distance. In addition, basket and stellate cell axons extend for considerable distances lateral to their somas. The axon collaterals of Purkinje cells project in the infra- and supraganglionic plexuses, contacting neurons several folia away from the cells of origin of these collaterals. Finally, the terminals of mossy fibers and climbing fibers bifurcate and project to several regions of the same folium as well as to distant folia.

The anatomic characteristics of the cerebellar cortex are compatible with the notion that there is extensive spatial convergence onto individual Purkinje cells. Despite this fact, the spatial and temporal characteristics of each cerebellar afferent projection undoubtedly result in differences in the effect of a given peripheral stimulus on Purkinje cells in discrete regions of the cerebellar cortex. Electrophysiologic studies have shown, for example, that the temporal characteristics of the responses of spinoreticulocerebellar pathways differ from those of the direct spinocerebellar pathways.[32] Consequently, the varying overlap of cerebellar afferent pathways will contribute to the variability in the temporal characteristics of the responses of Purkinje cells in different regions of the cerebellar cortex.

REFERENCES

1. ADRIAN, E. D.: *Afferent areas in the cerebellum connected with the limbs.* Brain 66:289, 1943.
2. AITKIN, L. M., AND BOYD, J.: *Responses of single units in cerebellar vermis of the cat to monaural and binaural stimuli.* J. Neurophysiol. 38:418, 1975.
3. AJALA, G. F., AND POPPELE, R. E.: *Some problems in the central actions of vestibular inputs,* in Yahr, M. D., and Purpura, D. P. (eds.): *Neurophysiological Basis of Normal and Abnormal Motor Activities.* Raven Press, New York, 1967, pp. 141–154.
4. ALLEN, G. I., AZZENA, G. B., AND OHNO, T.: *Contribution of the cerebro-reticulo-cerebellar pathway to the early mossy fibre response in the cerebellar cortex.* Brain Res. 44:670, 1972.
5. ALLEN, G. I., AZZENA, G. B., AND OHNO, T.: *Responses of neurones of interpositus nucleus to stimulation of the sensorimotor motor cortex.* Brain Res. 45:585, 1972.
6. ALLEN, G. I., AZZENA, G. B., AND OHNO, T.: *Cerebellar Purkyně cell responses to inputs from sensorimotor cortex.* Exp. Brain Res. 20:239, 1974.
7. ALLEN, G. I., AZZENA, G. B., AND OHNO, T.: *Somatotopically organized inputs from fore- and hindlimb areas of sensorimotor cortex to cerebellar Purkyně cells.* Exp. Brain Res. 20:255, 1974.
8. ALLEN, G. I., GILBERT, P. F. C., MARINI, R. ET AL.: *Integration of cerebral and peripheral inputs by interpositus neurons in monkey.* Exp. Brain Res. 27:81, 1977.
9. ALLEN, G. I., GILBERT, P. F. C., AND YIN, T. C. T.: *Cerebral and peripheral inputs to interpositus neurons in monkey.* Brain Res. 105:337, 1976.
10. ALLEN, G. I., GILBERT, P. F. C., AND YIN, T. C. T.: *Convergence of cerebral inputs onto dentate neurons in monkey.* Exp. Brain Res. 32:151, 1978.
11. ALLEY, K., BAKER, R., AND SIMPSON, J. I.: *Afferents to the vestibulo-cerebellum and the origin of the visual climbing fibers in the rabbit.* Brain Res. 98:582, 1975.
12. ALTMAN, J. A., BECHTEREV, N. N., RADIONOVA, E. A. ET AL.: *Electrical responses of the auditory area of the cerebellar cortex to acoustic stimulation.* Exp. Brain Res. 26:285, 1976.
13. ALVARDO-MALLART, R. M., BATINI, C., BUISSERET, C. ET AL.: *Mesencephalic projections of the rectus lateralis muscle afferents in the cat.* Arch. Ital. Biol. 113:1, 1975.
14. ANDERSSON, G., AND OSCARSSON, O.: *Climbing fiber microzones in cerebellar vermis and their projection to different groups of cells in the lateral vestibular nucleus.* Exp. Brain Res. 32:565, 1978.
15. ANGAUT, P.: *Bases anatomo-fonctionnelles des interrelations cérébello-cérébrales.* J. Physiol. (Paris) 67:53A, 1973.

110

16. ARDUINI, A., AND POMPEIANO, O.: *Microelectrode analysis of units of the rostral portion of the nucleus fastigii.* Arch. Ital. Biol. 95:56, 1957.

17. ARMSTRONG, D. M., COGDELL, B., AND HARVEY, R. J.: *Responses of interpositus neurones to nerve stimulation in chloralose anaesthetized cats.* Brain Res. 55:461, 1973.

18. ARMSTRONG, D. M., COGDELL, B., AND HARVEY, R. J.: *Firing patterns of Purkinje cells in the cat cerebellum for different maintained positions of the limbs.* Brain Res. 50:452, 1973.

19. ARMSTRONG, D. M., COGDELL, B., AND HARVEY, R. J.: *Effects of afferent volleys from the limbs on the discharge patterns of interpositus neurones in cats anesthetized with α chloralose.* J. Physiol. 248:489, 1975.

20. ARSHAVSKYI, Y. I., BERKINBLIT, M. B., AND FUKSON, O. I.: *Layer analysis of evoked potentials in the paramedian lobe of cerebellum cortex.* Fiziol. Zh. SSSR 55:429, 1969.

21. BACH-Y-RITA, P., AND MURATA, K.: *Extraocular proprioceptive responses to the VI nerve of the cat.* Quart. J. Exp. Physiol. 49:408, 1964.

22. BAKER, R., AND BERTHOZ, A.: *Is the prepositus hypoglossi nucleus the source of another vestibulo-ocular pathway?* Brain Res. 86:121, 1975.

23. BAKER, R., GRESTY, M., AND BERTHOZ, A.: *Neuronal activity in the prepositus hypoglossi nucleus correlated with vertical and horizontal eye movement in the cat.* Brain Res. 101:366, 1976.

24. BAKER, R., PRECHT, W., AND LLINAS, R.: *Mossy and climbing fiber projections of extraocular muscle afferents to the cerebellum.* Brain Res. 38:440, 1972.

25. BANTLI, H., AND BLOEDEL, J. R.: *Indirect peripheral inputs to the neocerebellum.* Proc. Internatl. Union Physiol. Sci. 13:50, 1977.

26. BANTLI, H., AND BLOEDEL, J. R.: *Spinal input to the lateral cerebellum mediated by infratentorial structures.* Neurosci. 2:555, 1977.

27. BATINI, C., BUISSERET, P., AND KADO, R. T.: *Extraocular, proprioceptive and trigeminal projections to the Purkinje cells of the cerebellar cortex.* Arch. Ital. Biol. 112:1, 1974.

28. BERTHOZ, A., AND BAKER, R.: *Parallel processing in the vestibular control of eye movements.* Neurosci. 3:119, 1978.

29. BERTHOZ, A., AND LLINÁS, R.: *Afferent neck projection to the cat cerebellar cortex.* Exp. Brain Res. 20:385, 1974.

30. BLANKS, R. H. I., PRECHT, W., AND GIRETTI, M. L.: *Response characteristics and vestibular receptor convergence of frog cerebellar Purkinje cells. A natural stimulation study.* Exp. Brain Res. 27:181, 1977.

31. BLANKS, R. H. I., VOLKIND, R., PRECHT, W. ET AL.: *Responses of cat prepositus hypoglossi neurons to horizontal angular acceleration.* Neurosci. 2:391, 1977.

32. BLOEDEL, J. R.: *Cerebellar afferent systems: A review.* Prog. Neurobiol. 2:1, 1973.

33. BLOEDEL, J. R., AND BURTON, J. E.: *Electrophysiological evidence for a mossy fiber input to the cerebellar cortex activated indirectly by collaterals of spinocerebellar pathways.* J. Neurophysiol. 33:308, 1970.

34. BRAND, S., AND MUGNAINI, E.: *Fulminant Purkinje cell death following axotomy and its use in analysis of the dendritic arborization.* Exp. Brain Res. 26:105, 1976.

35. BRODAL, A.: *Experimental demonstration of cerebellar connexions from the perihypoglossal nuclei (nucleus intercalatus, nucleus praepositus hypoglossi, and nucleus of Roller) in the cat.* J. Anat. (London) 86:110, 1952.

36. BRODAL, A.: *Cerebrocerebellar pathways. Anatomical data and some functional implications.* Acta Neurol. Scand. (Suppl.) 51:153, 1972.

37. BRODAL, A.: *Vestibulocerebellar input in the cat: anatomy.* Prog. Brain Res. 37:315, 1972.

38. BRODAL, A., AND WALBERG, F.: *Ascending fibers in pyramidal tract of cat.* Arch. Neurol. Psychiat. (Chicago) 68:755, 1952.

39. BUCHTEL, H. A., IOSIF, G., MARCHESI, G. F., ET AL.: *Analysis of the activity evoked in the cerebellar cortex by stimulation of the visual pathways.* Exp. Brain Res. 15:278, 1972.

40. BUSER, P., AND FRANCHEL, H.: *Neurophysiologie. Existence d' un foyer de projection sensorielle acoustique au niveau du lobe ansiforme du cervelet chez le chat.* C. R. Acad. Sci. (Paris) 251:791, 1960.

41. CAMIS, M.: *Le correnti d'azione nel cervelletto per eccitamento del laberintino.* Arch. Sci. Biol. 1:92, 1919–1920.

42. CHOROSCHKO, W. K.: *Sekundäre Degenerationen in aufsteigender Richtung bei Rückenmarks-verletzungen.* Monatsschr. Psychiat. Neurol. 26:534, 1909.

43. CLARKE, P. G. H.: *The organization of visual processing in the pigeon cerebellum.* J. Physiol. 243:267, 1974.

44. CLENDENIN, M., EKEROT, C. F., OSCARSSON, O. ET AL.: *The lateral reticular nucleus in the cat. I. Mossy fibre distribution in cerebellar cortex.* Exp. Brain Res. 21:473, 1974.

45. COFFEY, G. L., GODWIN-AUSTEN, R. B., MACGILLIVRAY, B. B., ET AL.: *The form and distribution of the surface evoked responses in cerebellar cortex from intercostal nerves in the cat.* J. Physiol. 212:129, 1971.

46. COMBS, C. M.: *Electro-anatomical study of cerebellar localization. Stimulation of various afferents.* J. Neurophysiol. 17:123, 1954.

47. COOKE, J. D., LARSON, B., OSCARSSON, O. ET AL.: *Origin and termination of cuneocerebellar tract.* Exp. Brain Res. 13:339, 1971.

48. COOKE, J. D., LARSON, B., OSCARSSON, O. ET AL.: *Origin of afferent connections to cuneocere-bellar tract.* Exp. Brain Res. 13:359, 1971.

49. CRICHLOW, E. C., AND KENNEDY, T. T.: *Functional characteristics of neurons in the lateral reticular nucleus with reference to localized cerebellar potentials.* Exp. Neurol. 18:141, 1967.

50. DOW, R. S.: *Cerebellar action potentials in response to stimulation of various afferent connections.* J. Neurophysiol. 2:543, 1939.

51. DOW, R. S., AND ANDERSON, R.: *Cerebellar action potentials in response to stimulation of proprioceptors and exteroceptors in the rat.* J. Neurophysiol. 5:363, 1942.

52. ECCLES, J. C.: *The development of the cerebellum of vertebrates in relation to the control of movement.* Naturwissenschaften 56:525, 1969.

53. ECCLES, J. C.: *The topography of the mossy and climbing fiber inputs to the anterior lobe of the cerebellum,* in Fields, W. S., and Willis, W. D. (eds.): *The Cerebellum in Health and Disease.* Warren H. Green Inc., St. Louis, 1970, pp. 231–262.

54. ECCLES, J. C., FABER, D. S., MURPHY, J. T. ET AL.: *Afferent volleys in limb nerves influencing impulse discharges in cerebellar cortex. I. In mossy fibers and granule cells.* Exp. Brain Res. 13: 15, 1971.

55. ECCLES, J. C., FABER, D. S., MURPHY, J. T. ET AL.: *Afferent volleys in limb nerves influencing impulse discharges in cerebellar cortex. II. In Purkyně cells.* Exp. Brain Res. 13:36, 1971.

56. ECCLES, J. C., FABER, D. S., MURPHY, J. T. ET AL.: *Investigations on integration of mossy fiber inputs to Purkyně cells in the anterior lobe.* Exp. Brain Res. 13:54, 1971.

57. ECCLES, J. C., ITO, M., AND SZENTÁGOTHAI, J.: *The cerebellum as a neuronal machine.* Springer-Verlag, Berlin, 1967.

58. ECCLES, J. C., PROVINI, L., STRATA, P. ET AL.: *Analysis of electrical potentials evoked in the cerebellar anterior lobe by stimulation of hindlimb and forelimb nerves.* Exp. Brain Res. 6:171, 1968.

59. ECCLES, J. C., PROVINI, L., STRATA, P. ET AL.: *Topographical investigations on the climbing fiber inputs from forelimb and hindlimb afferents to the cerebellar anterior lobe.* Exp. Brain Res. 6:195, 1968.

60. ECCLES, J. C., RANTUCCI, T., ROSÉN, I. ET AL.: *Somatotopic studies on cerebellar interpositus neurons,* J. Neurophysiol. 37:1449, 1974.

61. ECCLES, J. C., RANTUCCI, T., SABAH, N. H. ET AL.: *Somatotopic studies on cerebellar fastigial cells.* Exp. Brain Res. 19:100, 1974.

62. ECCLES, J. C., ROSÉN, I., SCHEID, P. ET AL.: *Cutaneous afferent responses in interpositus neurones of the cat.* Brain Res. 42:207, 211, 1972.

63. ECCLES, J. C., ROSÉN, I., SCHEID, P. ET AL.: *Temporal patterns of responses of interpositus neurons to peripheral afferent stimulation.* J. Neurophysiol. 37:1424, 1974.

64. ECCLES, J. C., ROSÉN, I., SCHEID, P. ET AL.: *Patterns of convergence onto interpositus neurons from peripheral afferents.* J. Neurophysiol. 37:1438, 1974.

65. ECCLES, J. C., SABAH, N. H., SCHMIDT, R. F. ET AL.: *Cerebellar Purkyně cell responses to cutaneous mechanoreceptors.* Brain Res. 30:419, 1971.

66. ECCLES, J. C., SABAH, N. H., SCHMIDT, R. F. ET AL.: *Cutaneous mechanoreceptors influencing impulse discharges in cerebellar cortex. I. In mossy fibers.* Exp. Brain Res. 15:245, 1972.

67. ECCLES, J. C., SABAH, N. H., SCHMIDT, R. F. ET AL.: *Cutaneous mechanoreceptors influencing impulse discharges in cerebellar cortex. II. In Purkyně cells by mossy fiber input.* Exp. Brain Res. 15:261, 1972.

68. ECCLES, J. C., SABAH, N. H., SCHMIDT, R. F. ET AL.: *Cutaneous mechanoreceptors influencing impulse discharges in cerebellar cortex. III. In Purkyně cells by climbing fiber input.* Exp. Brain Res. 15:484, 1972.

69. ECCLES, J. C., SABAH, N. H. SCHMIDT, R. F. ET AL.: *Integration by Purkyně cells of mossy and climbing fiber inputs from cutaneous mechanoreceptors.* Exp. Brain Res. 15:498, 1972.

70. ECCLES, J. C., SABAH, N. H., AND TÁBOŘÍKOVÁ, H.: *Responses evoked in neurones of the fastigial nucleus by cutaneous mechanoreceptors.* Brain Res. 35:523, 1971.

71. ECCLES, J. C., SABAH, N. H., AND TÁBOŘÍKOVÁ, H.: *Excitatory and inhibitory responses of neurones of the cerebellar fastigial nucleus.* Exp. Brain Res. 19:61, 1974.

72. ECCLES, J. C., SABAH, N. H., AND TÁBOŘÍKOVÁ, H.: *The pathways responsible for excitation and inhibition of fastigial neurones.* Exp. Brain Res. 19:78, 1974.

73. EKEROT, C. F., AND LARSON, B.: *Correlation between sagittal projection zones of climbing and mossy fibre paths in cat cerebellar anterior lobe.* Brain Res. 64:446, 1973.

74. FADIGA, E., VON BERGER, G. P., AND PUPILLI, G. C.: *Ricerche electrofisiologiche intorno alle vie percorse dagl' impulsi cerebellipeti di origine visiva.* Arch. Sci. Biol. (Bologna) 43:245, 1959.

75. FADIGA, E., AND PUPILLI, G. C.: *Teleceptive components of the cerebellar function.* Physiol. Rev. 44:432, 1964.

76. FANARDJAN, V. V., AND KAZARIAN, L. L.: *Cerebellar evoked potentials in the unrestrained cat.* Fiziol. Zh. SSSR 56:1360, 1970.

77. FANARDJAN, V. V., AND KAZARIAN, L. L.: *Localized and diffuse afferent projections to the cerebellar cortex.* Fiziol. Zh. SSSR 56:1523, 1970.

78. FENNELL, E., AND ROWE, M. J.: *Sensorimotor cortical influences on the climbing fibre input to cerebellar Purkyně cells.* Brain Res. 60:263, 1973.

79. FERIN, M., GRIGORIAN, R. A., AND STRATA, P.: *Purkinje cell activation by stimulation of the labyrinth.* Pflügers Arch. 321:253, 1970.

80. FERIN, M., GRIGORIAN, R. A., AND STRATA, P.: *Mossy and climbing fibre activation in the cat cerebellum by stimulation of the labyrinth.* Exp. Brain Res. 12:1, 1971.

81. FREEMAN, J. A.: *Responses of cat cerebellar Purkinje cells to convergent inputs from cerebral cortex and peripheral sensory systems.* J. Neurophysiol. 33:697, 1970.

82. FUCHS, A. F., AND KORNHUBER, H. H.: *Extraocular muscle afferents to the cerebellum of the cat.* J. Physiol. (London) 200:713, 1969.

83. FURUYA, N., KAWANO, K., AND SHIMAZU, H.: *Functional organization of vestibulofastigial projection in the horizontal semicircular canal system in the cat.* Exp. Brain Res. 24:75, 1975.

84. GARDNER, E. P., AND FUCHS, A. F.: *Single-unit responses to natural vestibular stimuli and eye movements in deep cerebellar nuclei of the alert Rhesus monkey.* J. Neurophysiol. 38:627, 1975.

85. GHELARDUCCI, B.: *Responses of the cerebellar fastigial neurones to tilt.* Pflügers Arch. 344:195, 1973.

86. GHELARDUCCI, B., ITO, M., AND YAGI, N.: *Impulse discharges from flocculus Purkinje cells of alert rabbits during visual stimulation combined with horizontal head rotation.* Brain Res. 87:66, 1975.

87. GHELARDUCCI, B., POMPEIANO, O., AND SPYER, K. M.: *Distribution of neuronal responses to static tilts within the cerebellar fastigial nucleus.* Arch. Ital. Biol. 112:126, 1974.

88. GRESTY, M., AND BAKER, R.: *Neurons with visual receptive field eye movement and neck displacement sensitivity within and around the nucleus prepositus hypoglossi in the alert cat.* Exp. Brain Res. 24:429, 1976.

89. GRIGORIAN, R. A., AND KRISTI, E. M.: *Reaction of neurones of nuclei of cat cerebellum to adequate stimulation of vestibular apparatus.* Dokl. Akad. Nauk SSSR 188:249, 1969.

90. HAMPSON, J. L.: *Relationships between cat cerebral and cerebellar cortices.* J. Neurophysiol. 12:37, 1949.

91. HAMPSON, J. L., HARRISON, C. R., AND WOOLSEY, C. M.: *Cerebro-cerebellar projections and the somatotopic localization of motor function in the cerebellum,* in Research Publications of the Association for Research in Nervous and Mental Disease 30:299, 1952.

92. HARVEY, R. J., PORTER, R., AND RAWSON, J. A.: *The natural discharge of Purkinje cells in paravermal regions of lobules V and VI of the monkey's cerebellum.* J. Physiol. 271:515, 1977.

93. HIROKANE, A., MIZUNO, S., AND NOZU, H.: *Cerebellar influences of the functioning of the auditory nuclei of the brain stems of cats.* Seishin Shinkei 66:86 (Cited in Teramoto and Snider, 1966).

94. HISS, E., LEICHT, R., AND SCHMIDT, R. F.: *Cutaneous receptive fields of cerebellar Purkinje cells of unanesthetized cats.* Exp. Brain Res. 27:319, 1977.

95. IOSIF, G., POMPEIANO, O., STRATA, P. ET AL.: *The effect of stimulation of spindle receptors and Golgi tendon organs on the cerebellar anterior lobe. I. Field potentials induced by sinusoidal stretch or contraction of hindlimb extensor muscles.* Arch. Ital. Biol. 110:476, 1972.

96. IOSIF, G., POMPEIANO, O., STRATA, P. ET AL.: *The effect of stimulation of spindle receptors and Golgi tendon organs on the cerebellar anterior lobe. II. Responses of Purkinje cells to sinusoidal stretch or contraction of hindlimb extensor muscles.* Arch. Ital. Biol. 110:502, 1972.

97. ISHIKAWA, K., KAWAGUCHI, S., AND ROWE, M. J.: *Actions of afferent impulses from muscle receptors in cerebellar Purkyně cells. I. Responses to muscle vibration.* Exp. and Brain Res. 15: 177, 1972.

98. ISHIKAWA, K., KAWAGUCHI, S., AND ROWE, M. J.: *Actions of afferent impulses from muscle receptors on cerebellar Purkyně cells. II. Responses to muscle contraction: Effects mediated via the climbing fiber pathway.* Exp. Brain Res. 16:104, 1972.

99. JANSEN, J., JR.: *Afferent impulses to the cerebellar hemispheres from the cerebral cortex and certain subcortical nuclei.* Acta Physiol. Scand. 41(Suppl 143):1, 1957.

100. JANSEN, J., JR., AND FANGEL, C.: *Observations on cerebrocerebellar evoked potentials in the cat.* Exp. Neurol. 3:160, 1961.

101. JOSEPH, J. W., SHAMBES, G. M., GIBSON, J. M. ET AL.: *Tactile projections to granule cells in caudal vermis of the rat's cerebellum.* Brain Behav. Evol. 15:141, 1978.

102. JUNGERT, S.: *Auditory pathways in the brain stem. A neurophysiological study.* Acta Otolaryngol. (Suppl.)138:1, 1958.

103. KAWAGUCHI, S., AND ONO, T.: *Responses of interpositus neurones to inputs from muscle receptors.* Exp. Brain Res. 21:375, 1974.

104. KAWAMURA, K., AND BRODAL, A.: *The tectopontine projection in the cat: An experimental anatomical study with comments on pathways for teleceptive impulses to the cerebellum.* J. Comp. Neurol. 149:371, 1973.

105. KAZARIAN, L. L.: *Some properties of the evoked potentials of the normal cat's cerebellar cortex to peripheral stimulations,* in Fanardjan, V. V. (ed.): *Structural and FunctionalOrganization of the Cerebellum.* Nauka, Leningrad, 1971, pp. 86–89.

106. KENNEDY, T. T., GRIMM, R. J., AND TOWE, A. L.: *The role of cerebral cortex in evoked somatosensory activity in cat cerebellum.* Exp. Neurol. 14:13, 1966.

107. KHAMARE, B. S., AND COMBS, C. M.: *Duality in retinocerebellar projections in the rabbit.* Exp. Neurol. 48:610, 1975.

108. KHANBABIAN, M. V.: *On the cerebellum neurones response to visual stimulation.* Fiziol. Zh. SSSR 56:339, 1970.

109. KIMM, J., HASSUL, M., AND COGDELL, B.: *Fastigial neuronal responses to sinusoidal horizontal rotation.* Exp. Neurol. 50:579, 1976.

110. KITAI, S. T., TÁBOŘÍKOVÁ, H., TSUKAHARA, N. ET AL.: *Discriminative patterns for cutaneous inputs to the cerebellar anterior lobe.* Fed. Proc. 27:518, 1968.

111. KITAI, S. T., TÁBOŘÍKOVÁ, H., TSUKAHARA, N. ET AL.: *The distribution to the cerebellar anterior lobe of the climbing and mossy fiber inputs from the plantar and palmar cutaneous afferents.* Exp. Brain Res. 7:1, 1969.

112. KOELLA, W. P.: *Some functional properties of optically evoked potentials in cerebellar cortex of cat.* J. Neurophysiol. 22:61, 1959.

113. KONORSKI, J., AND TARNECKI, R.: *Purkinje cells in the cerebellum: Their responses to postural stimuli in cats.* Proc. Nat. Acad. Sci. 65:892, 1970.

114. KOTCHABHAKDI, N. HODDEVIK, G. H., AND WALBERG, F.: *Cerebellar afferent projections from the perihypoglossal nuclei: An experimental study with the method of retrograde axonal transport of horseradish peroxidase.* Exp. Brain Res. 31:13, 1978.

115. KÜNZLE, H.: *Autoradiographic tracing of the cerebellar projections from the lateral reticular nucleus in the cat.* Exp. Brain Res. 22:255, 1975.

116. LADPLI, R., AND BRODAL, A.: *Experimental studies of commissural and reticular formation projections from the vestibular nuclei in the cat.* Brain Res. 8:65, 1968.

117. LARSON, B., MILLER, S., AND OSCARSSON, O.: *Termination and functional organization of the dorsolateral spino-olivocerebellar path.* J. Physiol. 203:611, 1969.

118. LATHAM, A., PAUL, D. H., AND POTTS, A. J.: *Responses of fastigial nucleus neurones to stimulation of a peripheral nerve.* J. Physiol. (London) 206:15P, 1970.

119. LEICHT, R., ROWE, M. J., AND SCHMIDT, R. F.: *Inhibition of cerebellar climbing fibre activity by stimulation of precruciate cortex.* Brain Res. 43:640, 1972.

120. LEICHT, R. ROWE, M. J., AND SCHMIDT, R. F.: *Cortical and peripheral modification of cerebellar climbing fibre activity arising from cutaneous mechanoreceptors.* J. Physiol. 228:619, 1973.

121. LEICHT, R., ROWE, M. J., AND SCHMIDT, R. F.: *Mossy and climbing fiber inputs from cutaneous mechanoreceptors to cerebellar Purkyně cells in unanesthetized cats.* Exp. Brain Res. 27:459, 1977.

122. LEICHT, R., AND SCHMIDT, R. F.: *Somatotopic studies on the vermal cortex of the cerebellar anterior lobe of unanesthetized cat.* Exp. Brain Res. 27:479, 1977.

123. LISBERGER, S. G., AND FUCHS, A. F.: *Response of flocculus Purkinje cells to adequate vestibular stimulation in the alert monkey: fixation vs. compensatory eye movements.* Brain Res. 69: 347, 1974.

124. LLINÁS, R., PRECHT, W., AND CLARKE, M.: *Cerebellar Purkinje cell responses to physiological stimulation of the vestibular system in the frog.* Exp. Brain Res. 13:408, 1971.

125. MACKAY, W. A., AND MURPHY, J. T.: *Activation of anterior interpositus neurons by forelimb muscle stretch.* Brain Res. 56:335, 1973.

126. MACKAY, W. A., AND MURPHY, J. T.: *Responses of interpositus neurons to passive muscle stretch.* J. Neurophysiol. 37:1410, 1974.

127. MAEKAWA, K., AND SIMPSON, J. I.: *Climbing fiber activation of Purkinje cells in the flocculus by impulses transferred through the visual pathway.* Brain Res. 39:245, 1972.

128. MAEKAWA, K., AND SIMPSON, J. I.: *Climbing fiber responses evoked in vestibulocerebellum of rabbit from visual system.* J. Neurophysiol. 36:649, 1973.

129. MANNI, E., PALMIERI, G., AND MARINI, R.: *Central pathway of the extraocular muscle proprioception.* Exp. Neurol. 42:181, 1974.

130. MANNI, E., PALMIERI, G., MARINI, R. ET AL.: *Trigeminal influences on extensor muscles of the neck.* Exp. Neurol. 47:330, 1975.

131. MARINI, G., PROVINI, L., AND ROSINA, A.: *Macular input to the cerebellar nodulus.* Brain Res. 99:367, 1975.

132. MARINI, G., PROVINI, L., AND ROSINA, A.: *Gravity responses of Purkinje cells in the nodulus.* Exp. Brain Res. 24:311, 1976.

133. MATSUSHITA, M., AND IKEDA, M.: *Projections from the lateral reticular nucleus to the cerebellar cortex and nuclei in the cat.* Exp. Brain Res. 24:403, 1976.

134. MEULDERS, M., AND COLLE, J.: *Influence du cortex visuel sur l'activité evoqúée dans les voies optiques sous-corticales.* Electroencephal. Clin. Neurophysiol. 20:475, 1966.

135. MILES, T. S., COOKE, J. D., AND WIESENDANGER, M.: *Localization in the cerebellar hemisphere of climbing-fiber responses evoked from the trigeminal nerve in the cat.* Can. J. Physiol. Pharmacol. 52:1147, 1974.

136. MILES, T. S., AND WIESENDANGER, M.: *Climbing fibre inputs to cerebellar Purkinje cells from trigeminal cutaneous afferents and the SI face area of the cerebral cortex in the cat.* J. Physiol. 245:425, 1975.

137. MILES, T. S., AND WIESENDANGER, M.: *Organization of climbing fibre projections to the cerebellar cortex from trigeminal cutaneous afferents and from the SI face area of the cerebral cortex in the cat.* J. Physiol. 245:409, 1975.

138. MILLER, S., NEZLINA, N., AND OSCARSSON, O.: *Projection and convergence patterns in climbing fibre paths to cerebellar anterior lobe activated from cerebral cortex and the spinal cord.* Brain Res. 14:230, 1969.

139. MILLER, S., AND OSCARSSON, O.: *Termination and functional organization of spino-olivocere-*

bellar paths, in Fields, W. S., and Willis, W. D. (eds.): *The Cerebellum in Health and Disease.* Green, St. Louis, 1970, pp. 172–200.

140. MISRAHY, G. A., SPRADLEY, J. F., BERAN, A. V. ET AL.: *Acoustic cerebellar pathway in cats.* J. Neurophysiol. 24:159, 1961.

141. MORIN, F., AND GARDNER, E. D.: *Spinal pathways for cerebellar projections in the monkey Macaca mulatta.* Am. J. Physiol. 174:155, 1953.

142. MORIN, F., KITAI, S. T., AND DEMIRJIAN, C.: *Peripheral afferents to neocerebellum.* Fed. Proc. 22:458, 1963.

143. MORIN, F., KITAI, S. T., FERNANDO, O. ET AL.: *Peripheral projections to the neo-cerebellum.* Anat. Rec. 145:263, 1963.

144. MUNSON, J. B.: *Cortical modulation of cerebellar teleceptive input: some new considerations.* Brain Res. 7:474, 1968.

145. MURPHY, J. T., MACKAY, W. A., AND JOHNSON, F.: *Differences between cerebellar mossy and climbing fibre responses to natural stimulation of forelimb muscle proprioceptors.* Brain Res. 55: 263, 1973.

146. MURPHY, J. T., MACKAY, W. A., AND JOHNSON, F.: *Responses of cerebellar cortical neurons to dynamic proprioceptive inputs from forelimb muscles.* J. Neurophysiol. 36:711, 1973.

147. NATHAN, P. W., AND SMITH, M. C.: *Spino-cortical fibres in man.* J. Neurol. Neurosurg. Psychiat. 18:181, 1955.

148. OKA, H., SASAKI, K., MATSUDA, Y. ET AL.: *Responses of pontocerebellar neurones to stimulation of the parietal association and the frontal motor cortices.* Brain Res. 93:399, 1975.

149. OKA, H., YASUDA, T., JINNAI, K. ET AL.: *Reexamination of cerebellar responses to stimulation of sensorimotor areas of the cerebral cortex.* Brain Res. 118:312, 1976.

150. OSCARSSON, O.: *Functional organization of the spino- and cuneocerebellar tracts.* Physiol. Rev. 45:495, 1965.

151. OSCARSSON, O.: *Functional significance of information channels from the spinal cord to the cerebellum,* in Yahr, M. D., and Purpura, D. P. (eds.): *Neurophysiological Basis of Normal and Abnormal Motor Activities.* Raven Press, New York, 1967, pp. 93–113.

152. OSCARSSON, O.: *The sagittal organization of the cerebellar anterior lobe as revealed by the projection patterns of the climbing fiber system,* in Llinas, R.(ed.): *Neurobiology of Cerebellar Evolution and Development.* AMA-ERF Institute for Biomedical Research, Chicago, 1969, pp. 525–537.

153. OSCARSSON, O., AND SJÖLUND, B.: *The ventral spino-olivocerebellar system in the cat. I. Identification of five paths and their termination in the cerebellar anterior lobe.* Exp. Brain Res. 28: 469, 1977.

154. OSCARSSON, O., AND SJÖLUND, B.: *The ventral spino-olivocerebellar system in the cat. II. Termination zones in the cerebellar posterior lobe.* Exp. Brain Res. 28:487, 1977.

155. OSCARSSON, O., AND SJÖLUND, B.: *The ventral spino-olivocerebellar system in the cat. III. Functional characteristics of the five paths.* Exp. Brain Res. 28:505, 1977.

156. PRECHT, W., AND LLINÁS, R.: *Functional organization of the vestibular afferents to the cerebellar cortex of frog and cat.* Exp. Brain Res. 9:30, 1969.

157. PRECHT, W., SIMPSON, J. I., AND LLINÁS, R.: *Responses of Purkinje cells in rabbit nodulus and uvula to natural vestibular and visual stimuli.* Pflügers Arch. 367:1, 1976.

158. PRECHT, W., VOLKIND, R., AND BLANKS, R. H. I.: *Functional organization of the vestibular input to the anterior and posterior cerebellar vermis of cat.* Exp. Brain Res. 27:143, 1977.

159. PRICE, J. B., AND SPEIGEL, E. A.: *Vestibulocerebral pathways. A contribution to the central mechanism of vertigo.* Arch. Otolaryngol. 26:658, 1937.

160. PROVINI, L., REDMAN, S., AND STRATA, P.: *Somatotopic organization of mossy and climbing fibres to the anterior lobe of cerebellum activated by the sensorimotor cortex.* Brain Res. 6:378, 1967.

161. PROVINI, L., REDMAN, S., AND STRATA, P.: *Mossy and climbing fibre organization on the anterior lobe of the cerebellum activated by forelimb and hindlimb areas of the sensorimotor cortex.* Exp. Brain Res. 6:216, 1968.

162. RAMON Y CAJAL, S.: *Histologie du système nerveux de l'homme et des vertébrés,* vol. 1. Paris, Maloine, 1909.

163. RIVA-SANSEVERINO, E., AND URBANO, A.: *Electrical activity of paraflocculus and other cerebellar lobuli following vestibular rotatory stimulation in the cat.* Arch. Sci. Biol. 49:83, 1965.

164. ROWE, M. J.: *Cerebral cortical areas associated with the activation of climbing fibre input to cerebellar Purkinje cells.* Arch. Ital. Biol. 115:79, 1977.

165. RUBIA, F. J., HÖPPENER, U., AND LANGHOF, H.: *Lateral inhibition of Purkinje cells through climbing fiber afferents.* Brain Res. 70:153, 1974.

166. RUBIA, F. J., AND KOLB, F. P.: *Responses of cerebellar units to a passive movement in the decerebrate cat.* Exp. Brain Res. 31:387, 1978.

167. RUEGG, D. G., ELDRED, E., AND WIESENDANGER, M.: *Spinal projection to the dorsolateral nucleus of the caudal basilar pons in the cat.* J. Comp. Neurol. 179:383, 1978.

168. RUSHMER, D. S., ROBERTS, W. J., AND AUGTER, G. K.: *Climbing fiber responses of cerebellar Purkinje cells to passive movement of the cat forepaw.* Brain Res. 106:1, 1976.

169. SASAKI, K., KAWAGUCHI, S., AND SHIMONO, T.: *Interfolial mossy fibre connections in the cat cerebellum.* Jap. J. Physiol. 19:110, 1969.

170. SASAKI, K., KAWAGUCHI, S., SHIMONO, T., ET AL.: *Electrophysiological studies of the cortical pontocerebellar pathway.* J. Physiol. Soc. Jap. 30:678, 1968.

171. SASAKI, K., KAWAGUCHI, S., SHIMONO, T. ET AL.: *Responses evoked in the cerebellar cortex by the pontine stimulation.* Jap. J. Physiol. 19:95, 1969.

172. SASAKI, K., OKA, H., KAWAGUCHI, S. ET AL.: *Mossy fibre and climbing fibre responses produced in the cerebellar cortex by stimulation of the cerebral cortex in monkeys.* Exp. Brain Res. 29:419, 1977.

173. SASAKI, K., OKA, H., MATSUDA, Y. ET AL.: *Electrophysiological studies of the projections from the parietal association area to the cerebellar cortex.* Exp. Brain Res. 23:91, 1975.

174. SCHWARZ, D. W. F., AND MILNE, A. C.: *Somatosensory representation in the vestibulocerebellum.* Brain Res. 102:181, 1976.

175. SCHWARZ, D. W. F., AND TOMLINSON, R. D.: *Neuronal responses to eye muscle stretch in cerebellar lobule VI of the cat.* Exp. Brain Res. 27:101, 1977.

176. SHAMBES, G. M., GIBSON, J. M., AND WELKER, W.: *Fractured somatotopy in granule cell tactile areas of rat cerebellar hemispheres revealed by micromapping.* Brain Behav. Evol. 15:94, 1978.

177. SHIMAZU, H., AND SMITH, C. M.: *Cerebellar and labyrinthine influences on single vestibular neurons identified by natural stimuli.* Exp. J. Neurophysiol. 34:493, 1971.

178. SHINODA, Y., AND YOSHIDA, K.: *Neural pathways from the vestibular labyrinths to the flocculus in the cat.* Exp. Brain Res. 22:97, 1975.

179. SHOFER, R. J., AND NAHVI, M. J.: *Firing patterns induced by sound in single units of the cerebellar cortex.* Exp. Brain Res. 8:327, 1969.

180. SIMPSON, J. I., AND ALLEY, K. E.: *Visual climbing fiber input to rabbit vestibulocerebellum: a source of direction-specific information.* Brain Res. 82:302, 1974.

181. SIMPSON, J. I., PRECHT, W., AND LLINAS, R.: *Sensory separation in climbing and mossy fiber inputs to cat vestibulocerebellum.* Pflugers Arch. 351:183, 1974.

182. SNIDER, R. S., AND ELDRED, E.: *Cerebro-cerebellar relationships in the monkey.* J. Neurophysiol. 15:27, 1952.

183. SNIDER, R. S., AND STOWELL, A.: *Receiving areas of the tactile, auditory and visual systems in the cerebellum.* J. Neurophysiol. 7:331, 1944.

184. STERIADE, M., AND STOUPEL, N.: *Contribution à l'étude des relations entre l'aire auditive du cervelet et l'écorce cérébrale chez le chat.* Electroencephal. Clin. Neurophysiol. 12:119, 1960.

185. TARNECKI, R., AND KONORSKI, J.: *Patterns of responses of Purkinje cells in cats to passive displacements of limbs, squeezing and touching.* Acta Neurobiol. Exp. 30:95, 1970.

186. TERAMOTO, S., AND SNIDER, R. S.: *Modification of auditory responses by cerebellar stimulation.* Exp. Neurol. 16:191, 1966.

187. TORVIK, A., AND BRODAL, A.: *The cerebellar projection of the peri-hypoglossal nuclei (nucleus intercalatus, nucleus praepositus hypoglossi and nucleus of Roller) in the cat.* J. Neuropath. 13:515, 1954.

188. VENTZEL, M. D., GAZENKO, O. G., GRIGORIAN, R. A., ET AL.: *Analysis of the electrical reactions of the cerebellum of cats to an adequate vestibular excitation by motion.* Izv. Akad. Nauk. SSSR 4:545, 1969.

189. VOOGD, J., BROERE, G., AND VANROSSUM, J.: *The medio-lateral distribution of the spinocerebellar projection in the anterior lobe and the simplex lobule in the cat and a comparison with some other afferent systems.* Psychiatr. Neurol. Neurochir. 72:137, 1969.

190. WALBERG, F., AND BRODAL, A.: *Spino-pontine fibers in the cat. An experimental study.* J. Comp. Neurol. 99:251, 1953.

191. WILSON, V. J., MAEDA, M., AND FRANCK, J. I.: *Inhibitory interaction between labyrinthine, visual and neck inputs to the cat flocculus.* Brain Res. 96:357, 1975.

192. WILSON, V. J., MAEDA, M., AND FRANCK, J. I.: *Input from neck afferents to the cat flocculus.* Brain Res. 89:133, 1975.

193. WILSON, V. J., MAEDA, M., FRANCK, J. I. ET AL.: *Mossy fiber neck and second-order labyrinthine projections to cat flocculus.* J. Neurophysiol. 39:301, 1976.

CHAPTER 6

Cerebellar Descending and Ascending Projections

DESCENDING PROJECTIONS

Pathways Descending from the Midline Zone of the Cerebellum

Pathways from the Fastigial Nucleus

The midline regions of the cerebellum contain two types of output pathways: projections from the fastigial nucleus to the brainstem and projections of Purkinje cells in the cerebellar cortex to the vestibular nuclei. The fibers from each fastigial nucleus form two pathways to the brainstem, one crossed and the other uncrossed. Studies of these fastigiobulbar projections with traditional anatomic degeneration techniques have been difficult technically because lesions of one fastigial nucleus can interrupt fibers in the crossed projection originating in the contralateral fastigial nucleus as well as fibers leaving the lesioned nucleus.[134] Because of this problem, some of the results obtained with degeneration techniques[39, 65, 77, 110, 137] are at variance with the findings in autoradiographic studies.[16] The following description, which will include results of both types, probably will require revision as more data become available from studies with orthograde and retrograde labeling techniques.

The crossed and uncrossed fastigiobulbar pathways were thought initially to originate in caudal and rostral parts of the fastigial nucleus, respectively (Fig. 1A).[4, 33, 39, 77, 110, 125, 132] Recent studies with autoradiographic methods in monkeys indicate, however, that the crossed and uncrossed projections originate in both the rostral and caudal portions of the fastigial nuclei (Fig. 1B).[16] Only the origin of the crossed projection to the reticular formation is restricted to the rostral portion of the fastigial nucleus.[16]

CROSSED FASTIGIAL PROJECTIONS. The crossed projection from the fastigial nucleus, the so-called uncinate fasciculus or hook bundle of Russell, crosses the midline and passes above the rostral end of the contralateral fastigial nucleus. The fibers then pass ventrolaterally around the dorsal and lateral portion of the brachium conjunctivum and descend just medial to the restiform body before entering the medulla.[77, 110, 111] Degeneration studies indicate that these fibers terminate in the superior and medial vestibular nuclei, the ventral half of the lateral nucleus,

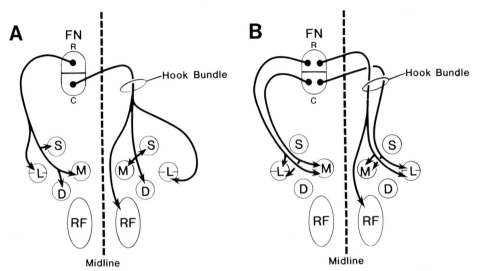

Figure 1. A, The fastigiobulbar projections as determined by degeneration studies in cats. The rostral portion of the fastigial nucleus projects to all of the ipsilateral vestibular nuclei and is restricted to the dorsal half of the lateral vestibular nucleus. The caudal portion of the fastigial nucleus projects across the midline and also terminates in all of the vestibular nuclei, including the ventral portion of the lateral vestibular nucleus. The input to the reticular formation from the fastigial nucleus is entirely crossed. **B,** The projection of the fastigial nucleus as determined by autoradiographic studies in monkeys. These projections differ from those in A in two respects. First, both the rostral and caudal poles of the fastigial nucleus contribute to the ipsilateral and contralateral projections. Second, the fastigiovestibular fibers terminate principally in the medial and lateral vestibular nuclei. Note also that the projection to the reticular formation originates in the contralateral rostral fastigial nucleus. FN = Fastigial nucleus R = rostral; C = caudal; S = superior vestibular nucleus; L = lateral vestibular nucleus; M = medial vestibular nucleus; D = descending vestibular nucleus; RF = reticular formation.

and the ventrolateral portion of the descending nucleus (Fig. 1A). Fibers terminate also in nuclear groups f and x.[25, 137] In addition, a small projection to the nucleus parasolitarius has been demonstrated.[137] Recent autoradiographic studies in monkeys indicate that some of these findings may have resulted from interrupting fibers from the opposite fastigial nucleus passing through the site of the lesion, because no evidence of crossed projections to the superior vestibular nucleus could be found (Fig. 1B).[16] The pathway to the medial and lateral nuclei was substantiated.

Crossed projections from the fastigial nucleus reach many nuclei within the reticular formation. The most dense of these pathways terminates in the medial nucleus gigantocellularis, the dorsal paramedian nucleus, and the magnocellular portion of the lateral reticular nucleus.[16, 33, 132, 136, 137] Although not yet confirmed by autoradiographic studies, crossed projections have been described from the fastigial nucleus to the perihypoglossal nuclei,[39] the nucleus reticularis tegmenti pontis, and portions of the pontine reticular nuclei.[1, 137]

A projection from the fastigial nucleus to the contralateral dorsolateral pontine nuclei was found recently.[16] This projection enables the output of the midline cerebellar regions to affect information processing within the corticopontocerebellar pathway. Strong evidence also has emerged supporting the existence of a direct fastigiospinal tract.[1, 16, 68, 125, 132] This pathway has been demonstrated with retrograde and orthograde tracing techniques as well as degeneration methods and has been described in rats, cats, and monkeys.

UNCROSSED FASTIGIAL PROJECTIONS. Previous investigations of the uncrossed fastigiobulbar pathway in the cat revealed that fibers projecting ipsilaterally to the brainstem originate in the rostral portion of the fastigial nucleus (Fig. 1A).[39, 137] Autoradiographic studies in the monkey, however, show that these fibers originate throughout the fastigial nucleus and terminate in the vestibular nuclei.[16] Studies with degeneration techniques indicate that the ipsilateral fastigiovestibular projection terminates in the same vestibular nuclei as the contralateral projection, but in somewhat different locations. Similar experiments show that projections from the ipsilateral and contralateral fastigial nucleus to the lateral vestibular (Deiters') nucleus are organized topographically (Fig. 1A, Fig. 2).[23, 108] Fibers from the forelimb and hindlimb regions of the ipsilateral fastigial nucleus terminate in the corresponding part of the dorsal half of Deiters' nucleus. In contrast,

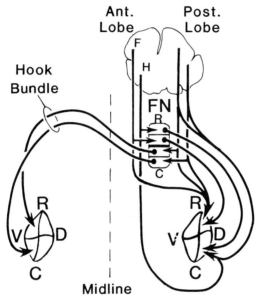

Figure 2. The relationship of the corticofastigiovestibular projection and the direct corticovestibular fibers. The hindlimb region of the anterior lobe projects to the anterior (rostral) portion of the rostral fastigial nucleus which in turn projects to the hindlimb (caudal) portion of the ipsilateral lateral vestibular nucleus. A comparable projection exists from the forelimb (posterior) region of the anterior lobe to the forelimb (caudal) part of the rostral fastigial nucleus and the forelimb (rostral) region of the ipsilateral lateral vestibular nucleus. The caudal-most pole of the fastigial nucleus contains a second hindlimb region which projects somatotopically to the hindlimb region of the contralateral lateral vestibular nucleus. A comparable projection from the forelimb (rostral) part of the caudal fastigial nucleus terminates in the forelimb region of the contralateral lateral vestibular nucleus. The direct fibers from the cerebellar cortex all terminate in the dorsal half of the ipsilateral lateral vestibular nucleus. The projection from the anterior lobe to the vestibular nucleus is organized topographically, with the projection from the hindlimb (anterior) region terminating in the caudal half of the dorsal part of this nucleus while the projection from the forelimb (posterior) region terminates in the rostral half. The projections from the posterior lobe to both the fastigial and vestibular nuclei show less topographic organization than the projections from the anterior lobe. FN = fastigial nucleus; V = ventral; D = dorsal; C = caudal; R = rostral; Ant. Lobe = anterior lobe of the cerebellum; Post. Lobe = posterior lobe of the cerebellum; F = forelimb area; H = hindlimb area.

121

fibers projecting from the equivalent regions of the contralateral fastigial nucleus terminate in the corresponding ventral parts of Deiters' nucleus.[23, 108] Recent autoradiographic studies in monkeys reveal a different topographic pattern; fibers from both the ipsilateral and contralateral fastigial nucleus terminate in the same regions of the lateral and medial vestibular nucleus and do not terminate within the superior vestibular nucleus (Fig. 1B).[16]

The organization of the uncrossed projections from the fastigial nucleus to the reticular formation is unclear. Indeed, even their existence has been questioned, at least in monkeys.[16] In the cat this projection clearly is less dense than that of the crossed fastigioreticular projection.[137] It is unclear whether the uncrossed projections described in the cat will be confirmed with autoradiographic studies.

The reticular neurons contacted by fibers from the fastigial nuclei have a variety of afferent and efferent connections.[57, 58, 75] Many of the reticulospinal neurons activated monosynaptically or polysynaptically from the fastigial nucleus have fast (90 to 150 meters/sec) conduction velocities. Many of these reticulospinal neurons are activated also by ascending afferent pathways responsive to cutaneous stimuli.[57]

Corticovestibular Projections

In both the rat and the cat, Purkinje cells in the cerebellar vermis project directly to the vestibular nuclei.[1, 52, 53, 78, 79, 111, 135] Although some controversy still exists, it appears certain that the predominant number of these fibers originate in the cerebellar vermis and not in the intermediate or lateral zones of the cerebellar cortex.[1, 70, 111, 132] A few of these fibers originate in the posterior lobe,[52, 54, 135] but most come from regions of the anterior and flocculonodular lobes.[53, 55, 132, 135] Fibers from the posterior lobe also terminate in the cochlear nucleus.[69]

PROJECTIONS FROM THE ANTERIOR LOBE. Studies with degeneration techniques in the cat indicate that the projection from the cerebellar anterior lobe to the vestibular nuclei is organized somatotopically (Fig. 2).[134] The forelimb and hindlimb regions of the dorsal part of Deiters' nucleus receive fibers from the corresponding regions of both the anterior lobe vermis and the ipsilateral rostral fastigial nucleus. In contrast, the ventral half receives fibers only from the contralateral fastigial nucleus. As a consequence, only the dorsal half of Deiters' nucleus receives two parallel cerebellar projections, one from the cerebellar anterior lobe and the other from the rostral part of the ipsilateral fastigial nucleus. As mentioned earlier, these conclusions may need to be revised when autoradiographic methods are used to substantiate these connections in the cat.

Inputs from the periphery to cells in Deiters' nucleus are organized topographically with respect to the corticovestibular projection. Neurons responsive to a specific peripheral stimulus are inhibited by Purkinje cells whose activity is affected by the same afferents.[27-29]

The physiologic actions of Purkinje cells projecting directly to Deiters' nucleus have been studied extensively by Ito and his colleagues.[50, 74, 76, 102] These studies demonstrated that the output of Purkinje cells is inhibitory and gave a basis for understanding the profound extensor hypertonus occurring immediately after removal of the cerebellar anterior lobe in cats. Because Purkinje cells are active spontaneously in the unanesthetized animal, removal of the cerebellar anterior lobe decreases the tonic inhibitory action of Purkinje cells on neurons of the descending vestibulospinal tract. This results in an increase in the tonic excitatory action of the vestibulospinal tract on alpha motoneurons (Chap. 7).

PROJECTIONS FROM THE FLOCCULONODULAR LOBE AND UVULA. Many Purkinje cells in the flocculonodular lobe project directly to the vestibular nuclei.[10, 52, 53, 132] This projection constitutes the major output pathway of the flocculonodular lobe, because only a small number of fibers from the nodulus terminate in the fastigial nucleus.[134] The projections from the flocculus consist of two groups of fibers, one terminating in the superior and medial vestibular nuclei and the other in portions of all four vestibular nuclei as well as cell group f (Fig. 2). Projections from the nodulus and uvula pass through the ipsilateral fastigial nucleus and possibly the medial regions of nucleus interpositus before coursing to the ipsilateral vestibular nuclear complex. Fibers from the uvula project chiefly to the superior vestibular nucleus and the descending nucleus as well as to nuclear group x. A few fibers terminate in the lateral vestibular nucleus, however, no projection to the medial vestibular nucleus has been described. The nodulus also projects to the superior, medial, and descending vestibular nuclei and to groups f and x. Thus, the flocculonodular lobule sends few fibers to the lateral vestibular nucleus. The majority of fibers in this projection terminates in other regions of the vestibular complex.[134]

Spinal Actions of Projections Descending from the Midline Zone of the Cerebellum

The output projections of the cerebellar vermis affect neuronal activity in the spinal cord. The actions of these projections on proprioceptive reflexes are reviewed in Chapters 7 and 8. These projections also affect the excitability of the terminals of primary afferent fibers in the spinal cord. Stimulation of the fastigial nucleus evokes a negative dorsal root potential in the lumbar region of the spinal cord,[30, 43] indicating depolarization of the primary afferent fibers.[119] This depolarization is restricted to the terminals of group I afferent fibers of both extensor and flexor muscles in the hindlimb and to the terminals of cutaneous afferents on the contralateral side of the body. In contrast, stimulation of the anterior lobe vermis evokes a positive dorsal root potential ipsilaterally in the spinal cord,[31] indicating reduced excitability of primary afferent fibers. Stimulation of the lateral part of the anterior lobe evokes the opposite effect, a negative dorsal root potential.[31, 32] These effects are mediated by the action of the fastigial nucleus on neurons in the descending and medial vestibular complex.[32, 106] This view is supported by the fact that primary afferent depolarization similar to that resulting from cerebellar stimulation can be evoked by stimulating the vestibular nuclei and the eighth cranial nerve.[32, 42, 45] In addition, stimulating the cerebellar anterior lobe suppresses the negative dorsal root potential evoked by stimulating the eighth nerve,[31] while ablation of the anterior lobe increases this negative dorsal root potential. Furthermore, stimulating the anterior lobe of the cerebellum affects dorsal root potentials evoked from the vestibular nerve, but does not affect the dorsal root potential evoked from peripheral nerves.[31] These findings indicate that the cerebellar effects on dorsal root potentials result from interactions within the vestibular nuclei.

Some of the effects of fastigial stimulation on the terminals of primary afferent fibers in the cat are thought to be mediated by the action of the crossed fastigioreticular projection on the cells of origin of reticulospinal pathways.[44, 45] In part this conclusion stems from the finding that stimulation of the contralateral fastigial nucleus depresses the excitability of the monosynaptic reflex, while stimulation of the ipsilateral eighth nerve increases its excitability.[15, 44, 45]

The cerebellar vermis influences the excitability of spinal reflexes through several segmental mechanisms. These include the activation of descending excitatory pathways which affect the excitability of alpha and gamma motoneurons. Changes in the excitability of primary afferent terminals originating in muscles and cutaneous tissue also are involved. These effects are mediated by both vestibulospinal and reticulospinal projections.

Pathways Descending from the Lateral Zones of the Cerebellum

Descending Limb of the Brachium Conjunctivum

The importance of the projections from the fastigial nucleus to the cells of origin of bulbospinal pathways is well recognized. It is not commonly appreciated, however, that the output pathways from the dentate and interposed nuclei also can affect the activity of neurons projecting from the brainstem to the spinal cord. In part these effects are mediated by the descending limb of the brachium conjunctivum, a structure known anatomically since the studies of Ramon y Cajal,[109] but recognized only recently as an important projection by which the lateral cerebellum affects the excitability of spinal reflexes.

The existence of the descending limb of the brachium conjunctivum is well accepted, but details of its origin, extent, and termination are still debated. Its fibers are known to originate in both the dentate and interposed nuclei.[24, 34, 36, 38, 39, 95, 128, 132] Fibers from the dentate nucleus course mainly in the lateral third of the brachium conjunctivum and cross in the ventral part of the decussation en route to various brainstem nuclei.[36, 38, 39, 98, 110, 128, 132] Ramon y Cajal[109] showed that many individual fibers in the descending limb of the brachium conjunctivum pass caudally after branching at right angles from fibers projecting in the ascending limb of the brachium conjunctivum. The branching of the same fiber into both the ascending and descending components of the brachium conjunctivum has been confirmed anatomically[36, 132] and electrophysiologically.[13, 127] Thus, many dentate neurons project both to the contralateral thalamus and to nuclei in the medulla. Some neurons in the dentate nucleus contribute collaterals to the ascending and descending limbs of the brachium conjunctivum and also project to the cerebellar cortex through the nucleocortical projection.[127]

The ipsilateral descending limb, also called the direct dentatobulbar descending projection, was described by Ramon y Cajal. Although it has been found in the rat, guinea pig,[1, 37, 62, 94] and shark,[56] Mehler[94] concluded that the projection does not exist in higher vertebrates such as the cat, monkey, and human. Because the initial description of this projection was based on degeneration studies, the lesions used to cause degeneration may have interrupted the uncinate fasciculus, causing degeneration of the crossed fastigiobulbar pathway rather than an ipsilateral dentatobulbar pathway. Three studies indicate, however, that fibers from the dentate nucleus do contribute to an ipsilateral descending limb.[14, 38, 65] Flood and Jansen[65] found that all neurons in the dentate nuclei show retrograde changes after lesions of the superior cerebellar peduncles, but lesions within the decussation of the

124

brachium conjunctivum fail to produce retrograde changes in many neurons. This indicated that some dentate neurons project ipsilaterally to the brainstem. Subsequently, Bantli and Bloedel[14] demonstrated that stimulating the dentate nucleus activates neurons ipsilaterally in the ventromedial reticular formation. In addition, recent anatomic studies in monkeys with autoradiographic techniques show an ipsilateral projection from the dentate nucleus to the spinal nucleus V, the periaqueductal gray, the nucleus raphe dorsalis, and the pontine reticular formation.[38]

Fibers in the descending limb of the brachium conjunctivum terminate in nuclei extending from the nucleus reticularis tegmenti pontis to the inferior olive (Fig. 3) and possibly down into the spinal cord. The nucleus reticularis tegmenti pontis receives one of the main projections of the descending limb.[24, 26, 34, 38, 39, 95, 98, 132] In the cat this projection originates in both the caudal region of the dentate nucleus and the component of this nucleus termed the subnucleus parvocellularis lateralis of Flood and Jansen.[64]

The descending limb of the brachium conjunctivum also contains a direct projection from the dentate and interposed nuclei to the inferior olive. This pathway has been demonstrated with ortho- and retrograde labeling techniques[20, 38, 71, 85, 86, 128] and in degeneration studies.[1, 17, 35, 36, 39, 82, 95, 110, 132] The cerebello-olivary projection originates in a specific subpopulation of small neurons in the dentate and interposed nuclei.[38, 126, 128] Many of these neurons are located within the subnucleus parvocellularis, the region receiving an extensive input from the paraflocculus.[24] Fibers from the ventrolateral part of the dentate nucleus project to the dorsal laminae of the contralateral principal olivary nucleus. Fibers from the dorsomedial area of the dentate nucleus project to the con-

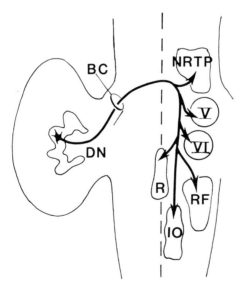

Figure 3. The crossed descending limb of the brachium conjunctivum. This pathway originates in both the dentate and interposed nuclei, however, for simplicity only the projection from the dentate nucleus is shown. The pathway courses through the brachium conjunctivum (BC) and terminates in several brainstem nuclei. These include the nucleus reticularis tegmentum pontis (NRTP), trigeminal nuclei (V), abducens nucleus (VI), raphe nuclei (R), reticular formation (RF), and inferior olive (IO). Although the existence of an ipsilateral descending limb has been debated, it has been demonstrated in monkeys with autoradiographic techniques (see text).

125

tralateral ventral laminae of the olive. These projections are distinct from those of the medial and dorsal accessory olivary nuclei, respectively.

The topographic characteristics of the dentato-olivary projection in the monkey differ from those in the cat.[38] In the monkey, the lateral to medial portions of the dentate nucleus are represented in the ventral to dorsal axis of the principal olivary nucleus. This pattern is different from that in the human, as shown by studies of dentate lesions.[82] Thus, the topology of the dentato-olivary projection may vary considerably throughout phylogeny.[38]

The descending limb of the brachium conjunctivum in monkeys and cats terminates in the motor nucleus of the trigeminal nerve[38, 109] and in the abducens nucleus.[36, 109] Fibers from the descending limb also terminate in the medial reticular formation,[36, 39, 94, 95] the nucleus giganticellularis,[98] and the paramedian reticular formation, where they overlap with projections from the fastigial nucleus.[34, 94, 95, 132] Terminations of the descending limb of the brachium conjunctivum also have been found in the raphe dorsalis, raphe superior centralis,[38] and the nucleus raphe pontis and magnus.[98]

The question of whether the descending limb terminates directly within the spinal cord is controversial. Ramon y Cajal[109] found that the crossed descending limb can be followed at least to the level of the cervical spinal cord. Several investigators have confirmed this finding. Achenbach and Goodman[1] found fibers from the cerebellar nuclei extending into the ventral horn of the cervical spinal cord in the rat. Projections to the spinal cord also have been reported in the monkey,[36, 110] cat,[96, 124, 132] guinea pig,[94] and shark.[56] The studies of Orioli and his colleagues supported the existence of a direct projection from the dentate nucleus to the spinal cord in the cat.[103, 104] In these studies, stimuli in the brachium conjunctivum or dentate nucleus evoked short latency responses in the lumbar region of the spinal cord in the decerebrate cat. The latencies of these responses, 2.5 to 3 msec, indicated that the stimuli activated a rapidly conducting pathway. On the basis of their control experiments, they thought that these responses could not be evoked by the antidromic activation of spinocerebellar pathways or by the activation of a dentatorubrospinal projection.

Contrary to these findings, many investigators have not found spinal terminals of this projection in cats and monkeys despite the use of many neuroanatomic methods.[34, 38, 39, 94, 95] Larsell and Jansen[83] concluded that the finding of degenerating fibers in the cervical region of the spinal cord results from disturbances of the vascular supply to the cord caused by a dentate lesion. They concluded that fibers from the descending limb do not extend caudal to the inferior olive. Orioli's electrophysiologic findings[103] could have resulted from stimulation of fibers from the fastigial nucleus in the uncinate fasciculus rather than a portion of the descending branch of the brachium conjunctivum from the dentate nucleus. In addition, the response recorded in the lumbar region of the spinal cord could have been evoked transsynaptically through a portion of the dentatoreticulospinal pathway. Bantli and Bloedel[14] demonstrated that rapidly conducting reticulospinal neurons receive monosynaptic connections from neurons in the descending limb projecting from the dentate nucleus. The activation of a component of the rubrospinal tract also has been demonstrated recently.[22] These projections involving the reticulospinal and rubrospinal tracts undoubtedly contribute to the effects of dentate stimulation on the excitability of spinal reflexes in decerebrate animals.[22]

Cerebellorubral Projections

The historic work of Massion and Albe-Fessard[88] demonstrated that the excitability of single neurons in the red nucleus can be altered by the output of the cerebellum. The pathway mediating these effects, the cerebellorubral projection, originates in the cerebellar nuclei and not in the cerebellar cortex as suggested in an early investigation.[115] This projection consists of fibers from the interposed and dentate nuclei which course through the brachium conjunctivum to the contralateral red nucleus.[36-38, 66, 87, 132] These fibers terminate in both the parvo- and magnocellular portions of the red nucleus in the cat, monkey, and rat.[36, 38, 63]

In the cat, degeneration studies indicate that the projections from the dentate nucleus are restricted to the rostral one-third of the red nucleus,[46, 112] and projections from the interposed nuclei terminate in the caudal two-thirds.[112] These regions of the red nucleus correspond approximately to the parvocellular and magnocellular divisions, respectively. Thus, the dentate nucleus projects mainly to the parvocellular part of the red nucleus and the interposed nuclei project to the magnocellular part. A comparable organization of the cerebellorubral projection has been reported in the monkey,[67] rat,[37] and opposum.[80] Recently, however, studies employing orthograde labeling techniques have demonstrated a projection from the dentate nucleus to both the rostral and caudal components of the red nucleus in monkeys (Fig. 4).[38]

Projections from the anterior interposed nucleus to the red nucleus are organized somatotopically.[8, 46, 47] Neurons along a medial to lateral gradient in the interposed nuclei project along a caudal to rostral gradient in the magnocellular part of the red nucleus.[45] The neurons along this gradient in the red nucleus project to specific populations of motoneurons in the cat.[105] The projection to the red nucleus from the posterior interposed nucleus is much smaller than that originating in the anterior interposed nucleus. Most fibers originating in the caudal region of the posterior interposed nucleus terminate medial to the red nucleus. Neurons in its rostral part project to approximately the medial one-half of the nucleus.[6] These projections are summarized in Figure 4.

Neuroanatomic studies in cats indicate that the interpositorubral projection should affect the excitability of spinal neurons through the rubrospinal tract. The existence of a rubrospinal tract in primates, however, has been highly controversial. Recently, neuroanatomic studies have confirmed the existence of a rubrospinal tract in both cats and monkeys.[59, 73, 97, 105] These findings support the observation that stimulation of the interposed nuclei in monkeys can evoke excitatory postsynaptic potentials (EPSPs) in spinal motoneurons at a latency consistent with the conduction velocity of the rubrospinal tract.[120] Stimulation of the magnocellular part of the red nucleus also affects neuronal activity in several brainstem nuclei contralateral to the side of stimulation, including the cuneate and gracile nuclei.[59, 73] The collaterals projecting to these nuclei arise from fibers coursing to the spinal cord. This projection has been called the crossed rubrobulbospinal projection.[73]

A large number of fibers from the dentate nucleus project to the parvocellular part of the red nucleus, the origin of the rubro-olivary tract.[48, 97, 105, 133] The projection from the dentate nucleus to the red nucleus does not form part of a dentatorubrothalamic projection; refined degeneration techniques and intra-axonal tracing methods have shown that a rubrothalamic projection from the rostral red nucleus

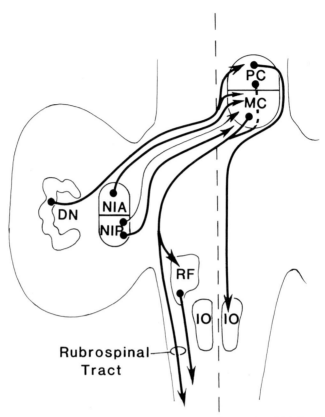

Figure 4. The cerebellorubral projections. The connections designated by thick lines indicate the predominant projections. Note that the nucleus interpositus posterior has only a small projection to the magnocellular part of the red nucleus. The dashed line from the cell body in the parvocellular part of the red nucleus indicates a proposed projection from this region of the red nucleus into the rubrospinal tract on the basis of the recent electrophysiologic studies cited in the text. The projection from the dentate nucleus to the magnocellular part of the red nucleus was demonstrated in monkeys recently. DN = dentate nucleus; NIA = nucleus interpositus anterior; NIP = nucleus interpositus posterior; PC = parvocellular part of the red nucleus; MC = magnocellular part of the red nucleus; RF = reticular formation; IO = inferior olive.

does not exist.[59, 73, 105] These studies indicate that few dentatorubral fibers terminate in the magnocellular region of the red nucleus, the origin of the rubrospinal tract. Based on the argument that few rubrospinal neurons originate in the rostral part of the red nucleus, it has been assumed that dentatorubral connections do not activate rubrospinal fibers. This, however, may be an oversimplification. In a recent study, neurons projecting from the rostral part of the red nucleus to the medulla and spinal cord could be activated by inputs from the cerebellum.[5] Furthermore, Chan-Palay[38] has shown that some dentate fibers in monkeys terminate in the magnocellular portion of the red nucleus where many rubrospinal fibers originate. The existence of a dentatorubrospinal pathway also is consistent with the recent findings of Bloedel and coworkers[22] showing that stimulation in the dentate nucleus evokes a response in a rapidly conducting descending projection that can be interrupted by a lesion of the contralateral red nucleus.

The pathways to the red nucleus from the cerebral cortex and the cerebellum are involved in trophic modifications of central nervous system function occurring during motor learning and during the compensatory processes required for recovery from a central lesion. In one series of experiments, degeneration of cerebello-rubral projections was produced by lesions of the interposed nuclei. This resulted in the redistribution of synapses from the corticorubral pathway, as indicated by changes in the characteristics of the postsynaptic potentials evoked by stimulating the cerebral cortex.[99, 100] These findings have been interpreted as reflecting a sprouting of the corticorubral projection onto the more proximal dendritic sites vacated by degeneration of the cerebellorubral projections. Changes in the distribution of synapses from the cerebellorubral and corticorubral projections can be induced also without selective degeneration of one of these pathways. The crossed innervation of forelimb nerves alters the rise time of the EPSP evoked by stimulating the corticorubral projection in the cat, a finding suggesting that a reorganization of synaptic inputs onto cells in the red nucleus has occurred.[129] Thus, the cerebellorubral projections may be one of the output projections of the cerebellum that can undergo trophic modification due to alterations in learned patterns of motor behavior.

Spinal Actions of Descending Projections from the Lateral Zones of the Cerebellum

Until recently, little information was available concerning the spinal actions of dentatobulbospinal projections. The effects of dentate output projections on spinal reflexes now have been examined in decerebrate unanesthetized cats.[21, 22, 93] Stimulation in the dentate nucleus affects the excitability of both cutaneous and proprioceptive reflexes evoked by natural mechanical stimuli. These stimuli also modify the dynamic characteristics of the stretch reflex.[93] Both the amplitude of the reflex and its phase relative to the peripheral stimulus are altered. The large effects on cutaneous reflexes evoked by the dentatobulbospinal projections indicate that these pathways influence the processing of exteroceptive as well as proprioceptive information. In part the changes in the cutaneous reflexes may be due to the action of the dentate efferent projections on the responses of dorsal horn neurons activated selectively by low threshold cutaneous afferents.[21]

ASCENDING PROJECTIONS

All of the cerebellar nuclei contribute to projections reaching forebrain structures. In addition to the well known ascending fibers from the interposed and dentate nuclei, projections ascending from the fastigial nucleus can affect neuronal activity in the thalamus and cerebral cortex.

Projections from the Fastigial Nucleus

Projections ascending from the fastigial nucleus course to forebrain nuclei through the ascending branch of the uncinate fasciculus and the superior cerebellar peduncle.[9, 65, 83, 91] In cats the projection is bilateral, although the crossed projection is more dense. In monkeys the entire ascending projection is crossed.[16]

The fastigial nucleus projects through the ascending limb of the uncinate fasciculus to specific ventral thalamic nuclei in the cat[9, 12] and to the ventral posterolateral nucleus in the monkey.[16] The fastigial nucleus projects also to the midline thalamic nuclei, including the intralaminar nuclei,[81] centrum medianum, and zona inserta.[9, 33] Fibers projecting to the centrum medianum may not actually terminate there.[9] Recent studies with autoradiographic tracing techniques have failed to confirm this projection in monkeys.[16] Fibers ascending from the fastigial nucleus terminate also in the superior colliculus, the nucleus of the posterior commissure,[16] and in the ectosylvian gyrus, the portion of the cerebral cortex in the cat homologous to SII in primates.[72]

The fastigial nucleus can affect neuronal activity in the cerebral cortex through these ascending projections.[114, 117] In the monkey, fastigial stimulation evokes responses in the hindlimb region of area 4 and in area 5 through the deep thalamocortical projections.[117] Responses are evoked bilaterally despite the use of barbiturate anesthesia. The responses are localized to the motor cortical region corresponding to the proximal axial musculature, a distribution similar to that evoked from the dentate nucleus.

Projections from the Dentate and Interposed Nuclei

The projections ascending from the dentate and interposed nuclei course through the superior peduncle[82] and enter principally the contralateral ascending limb of the brachium conjunctivum. The projections may enter an ipsilateral ascending limb also (Fig. 5),[36, 38, 65] but its existence is controversial. In support of bilateral output projections, several anatomic studies have demonstrated degenerating fibers distributed bilaterally after lesions in the dentate and interposed nuclei.[36, 65, 101] Other studies, however, have shown only a crossed projection ascending from the brachium conjunctivum.[35] Whiteside and Snider[139] found that stimulating the dentate and interposed nuclei evokes potentials bilaterally in the cerebral cortex. Although similar findings have been presented,[60, 61, 84] other studies have failed to confirm these observations.[11, 40, 41, 116-118] The discrepancies between these studies may be related to differences in the preparations employed. In experiments in which the responses appeared only contralaterally, the preparations usually were anesthetized with sodium pentobarbital. In contrast, bilateral responses were observed in studies of unanesthetized animals.[60, 61] Thus the sensitivity to barbiturate anesthesia of the projections mediating the bilaterally distributed responses probably contributes to the distribution of the responses.

The bilateral cerebral cortical distribution of responses evoked from the dentate and interposed nuclei may be mediated by projections to the midline thalamic nuclei and to regions of the rostral brainstem which, in turn, project bilaterally to diencephalic structures and the cerebral cortex (Fig. 5).[38, 39, 49, 121] The dentate and interposed nuclei project to the centrum medianum, parafascicular complex, intralaminar nuclei[39, 49, 95] and the periventricular gray matter.[110] Some responses in the ipsilateral thalamus and cerebral cortex, of course, may be mediated by a small ipsilateral[36, 38, 65] ascending branch of the brachium conjunctivum. The bilateral distribution of these responses also may result from interactions between the ipsilateral and contralateral specific thalamic nuclei.[18]

Contrary to the early reports, fibers in the crossed ascending limb do not terminate on neurons in the parvocellular portion of the red nucleus. Moreover, as discussed earlier, a rubrothalamic projection does not exist. Recent studies have demonstrated that the parvocellular portion of the red nucleus projects to the inferior olive and not to the thalamus. Thus, the pathways from the interposed and

130

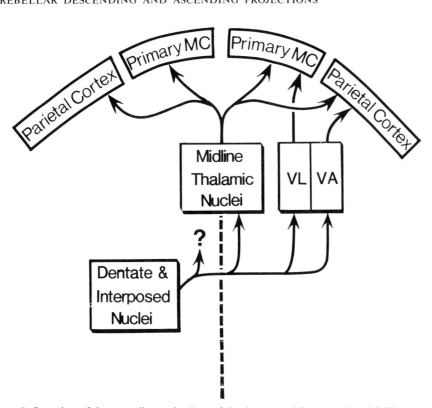

Figure 5. Overview of the ascending projections of the dentate and interposed nuclei. These projections terminate in the contralateral midline and specific thalamic nuclei. Terminations have been found in the specific thalamic nuclei outside of the ventrolateral and ventral anterior nuclei, however, VL and VA are the predominant sites of termination. The existence of an ipsilateral ascending limb of the brachium conjunctivum remains controversial. Responses evoked ipsilaterally from stimulation of the dentate and interposed nuclei probably are mediated by the bilateral projections of the midline thalamic nuclei. MC = motor cortex; VL = ventrolateral nucleus of thalamus; VA = ventral anterior nucleus of thalamus.

dentate nuclei to nuclei in the thalamus and rostral brainstem[3, 7, 60] are direct, not involving ascending projections from the red nucleus.

The contralateral dentatothalamic and interpositothalamic projections terminate in several specific thalamic nuclei, including the ventral posterolateral (VPL), ventrolateral (VL), ventral anterior (VA), and ventromedial (VM) nuclei (Fig. 5).[11, 12, 18, 19, 49, 95, 116, 118, 130, 131] Some projections from the interposed and dentate nuclei terminate in separate thalamic regions, but many fibers from these two nuclei converge in regions of the ventrolateral thalamic nucleus.[113] As a result, individual thalamic neurons may receive inputs from both of these cerebellar nuclei.[116, 118, 130]

The specific thalamic nuclei, particularly VA and VL, commonly are considered to be "relay nuclei" in the cerebellothalamocortical projection. There is, however, extensive integration of inputs from extracerebellar structures to these nuclei.[60] The cerebellar and lemniscal projections to the ventral nuclear complex of the thalamus do not overlap in distribution.[138] Nevertheless, the neurons receiving inputs from the cerebellar nuclei in the ventrolateral[89, 90] and ventral posterolateral nuclei[19] are activated also by auditory, visual, and somatic stimuli. Moreover, many neurons in the ventrolateral thalamic nucleus receive inputs from the brachium conjunctivum, the basal ganglia,[51] and the regions of cerebral cortex to which they project.[130]

The ventrolateral thalamic nucleus, which receives major inputs from the interposed and dentate nuclei, projects to regions of the precentral motor cortex. This projection terminates in some cortical areas which also receive fibers from the ventral posterolateral thalamic nucleus.[122, 123] Cerebellocortical projections from the interposed and dentate nuclei that are mediated by these thalamic nuclei are localized to the primary motor cortex and premotor area.[60] Stimulation of the cerebellar nuclei evokes responses in many other cerebral cortical areas, substantiating the notion that the projections from the cerebellum activate neurons in the midline thalamic nuclei.

In commenting on the overall organization of cerebrocerebellar interconnections, Evarts and Thach[60] emphasized that portions of the cerebellocerebral and cerebrocerebellar projections are not organized reciprocally. Projections from the cerebral cortex to the dentate nucleus, for example, arise chiefly in the parietal cortex. In contrast, projections from dentate nucleus to cerebral cortex are limited to the primary motor cortex and premotor area.

The properties of the cerebral cortical responses are determined by the characteristics of the thalamocortical projections by which they are mediated.[116, 117] Studies in cats have compared the cerebral cortical field potentials evoked by stimulating the interposed and dentate nuclei and the thalamus.[116] These studies show that the ventral anterior nucleus mediates responses in the parietal region of the cerebral cortex and the ventrolateral nucleus mediates responses in the pericruciate area (Fig. 5). In the cat, neurons in the ventrolateral thalamic nucleus activated by dentate stimulation project to the cerebral cortex through both the so-called deep and superficial thalamocortical pathways. By contrast, in monkeys the ventral anterior nucleus projects through the superficial and the ventrolateral nucleus projects through the deep thalamocortical pathway.[116]

The work of Rispal-Padel and colleagues[91, 113, 114] has given helpful insights into the overall organization of the cerebellothalamocortical projection. In cats the cerebral cortical responses evoked from the interposed nuclei are distributed somewhat differently from those evoked from the dentate nuclei. Responses from the interposed nuclei are found in regions related to the distal and proximal forelimb muscles, while those from the dentate nuclei are in regions related to the axial and proximal musculature of the forelimb, hindlimb, and trunk. The precise distribution of these responses depends upon the latency at which they are measured. For example, the longer latency responses evoked from the dentate nucleus are located in the forelimb region only and are not found in regions related to the axial musculature.

These studies led to the formulation of an hypothesis concerning the organization of the dentatothalamocortical projections.[113] The hypothesis stated that the spatial divergence and temporal characteristics of responses in the cerebellothalamic and the thalamocortical projections ensure that the cerebral cortical responses reflect different patterns of temporal and spatial integration in the cerebellothalamocortical projection. This integration reflects the fact that a single neuron in the ventrolateral thalamic nucleus receives inputs from many regions of the dentate and interposed nuclei and that neurons in a specific cerebral cortical region receive inputs from several converging neurons in the ventrolateral thalamic nucleus. Moreover, localized responses in the cerebral cortex result from critical patterns of convergence from several components of the cerebellothalamocortical projections.[113]

REFERENCES

1. ACHENBACH, K. E., AND GOODMAN, D. C.: *Cerebellar projections to pons, medulla and spinal cord in the albino rat.* Brain Behav. Evol. 1:43, 1968.

2. ALLEN, G. I., OSHIMA, T., AND TOYAMA, K.: *Unitary components in corticopontine activation of the cat.* Brain Res. 35:245, 1971.

3. ALLEN, G. I., AND TSUKAHARA, N.: *Cerebrocerebellar communication systems.* Physiol. Rev. 54:957, 1974.

4. ALLEN, W. F.: *Distribution of the fibers originating from the different basal cerebellar nuclei.* J. Comp. Neurol. 36:399, 1924.

5. ADERSON, M. E.: *Cerebellar and cerebral inputs to physiologically identified efferent cell groups in the red nucleus of the cat.* Brain Res. 30:49, 1971.

6. ANGAUT, P.: *The ascending projections of the nucleus interpositus posterior of the cat cerebellum.* Brain Res. 24:377, 1970.

7. ANGAUT, P.: *Bases anatomo-fonctionelles des interrelations cérébello-cérébrales.* J. Physiol. (Paris) 67:53A, 1973.

8. ANGAUT, P., AND BOWSHER, D.: *Cerebello-rubral connexions in the cat.* Nature 208:1002, 1965.

9. ANGAUT, P., AND BOWSHER, D.: *Ascending projections of the medial cerebellar (fastigial) nucleus: An experimental study in the cat.* Brain Res. 24:49, 1970.

10. ANGAUT, P., AND BRODAL, A.: *The projection of the 'vestibulocerebellum' onto the vestibular nuclei in the cat.* Arch. Ital Biol. 105:441, 1967.

11. ANGAUT, P., AND GUILBAUD, G.: *Étude chez le chat anesthésié au chloralose des projections du noyau fastigial du cervelet sur les structures diencéphaliques.* J. Physiol. (Paris) 56:273, 1964.

12. ANGAUT, P., GUILBAUD, G., AND REYMOND, M. C.: *An electrophysiological study of the cerebellar projections to the nucleus ventralis-lateralis of thalamus in the cat. I. Nuclei fastigii et interpositus.* J. Comp. Neurol. 134:9, 1968.

13. BAN, M., AND OHNO, T.: *Projection of cerebellar nuclear neurones to the inferior olive by descending collaterals of ascending fibres.* Brain Res. 133:156, 1977.

14. BANTLI, H., AND BLOEDEL, J. R.: *Monosynaptic activation of a direct reticulospinal pathway by the dentate nucleus.* Pflügers Arch. 357:237, 1975.

15. BARNES, C. D., AND POMPEIANO, O.: *Dissociation of presynaptic and postsynaptic effects produced in the lumbar cord by vestibular volleys.* Arch. Ital. Biol. 108:295, 1970.

16. BATTON, R. R., III, JAYARAMAN, A., RUGGIERO, D. ET AL.: *Fastigial efferent projections in the monkey: an autoradiographic study.* J. Comp. Neurol. 174:281, 1977.

17. BAUTISTA, N. S., AND MATZKE, H. A.: *The degeneration study of cerebellifugal fibers in monkey.* J. Hirnforsch. 8:283, 1966.

18. BAVA, A., CICIRATA, F., AND MARICCHIOLO, M.: *Cortical projections and transcomissural reactivity of neurones sampled from the thalamic relay-nucleus of the cerebello-cortical pathway (VL).* Electroenceph. Clin. Neurophysiol. 35:435, 1973.

19. BAVA, A., MANZONI, T., AND URBANO, A.: *Cerebellar influences on neuronal elements of thalamic somatosensory relay-nuclei.* Arch. Sci. Biol. (Bologna) 50:181, 1966.

20. BEITZ, A. J.: *The topographical organization of the olivo-dentate and dentato-olivary pathways in the cat.* Brain Res. 115:311, 1976.

21. BLOEDEL, J. R., AND BANTLI, H.: *A spinal action of the dentate nucleus mediated by descending systems originating in the brain stem.* Brain Res. 153:602, 1978.

22. BLOEDEL, J. R., HAMES, E. G., BANTLI, H. ET AL.: *The organization of descending projections from the brainstem activated by the output of the dentate nucleus.* Neurosci. Abstr. 4:63, 1978.

23. BRODAL, A.: *Anatomical studies of cerebellar fibre connections with special reference to prob-*

lems of functional localization, in Fox, C. A., and Snider, R. S. (eds.): *The Cerebellum.* Prog. Brain Res. 25:135, 1967.

24. BRODAL, A., DESTOMBES, J., LACERDA, A. M. ET AL.: *A cerebellar projection onto the pontine nuclei. An experimental anatomical study in the cat.* Exp. Brain Res. 16:115, 1972.

25. BRODAL, A., POMPEIANO, O., AND WALBERG, F.: *The Vestibular Nuclei and Their Connections: Anatomy and Functional Correlations.* Oliver and Boyd, Edinburgh, 1962.

26. BRODAL, A., AND SZIKLA, G.: *The termination of the brachium conjunctivum descendens in the nucleus reticularis tegmenti pontis. An experimental anatomical study in the cat.* Brain Res. 39: 337, 1972.

27. BRUGGENCATE, G. TEN, TEICHMANN, R., AND WELLER, E.: *Neuronal activity in the lateral vestibular nucleus of the cat. III. Inhibitory actions of cerebellar Purkinje cells evoked via mossy and climbing fibre afferents.* Pflügers Arch. 337:147, 1972.

28. BRUGGENCATE, G. TEN, TEICHMANN, R., AND WELLER, E.: *Neuronal activity in the lateral vestibular nucleus of the cat. IV. Postsynaptic potentials evoked by stimulation of peripheral somatic nerves.* Pflügers Arch. 360:301, 1975.

29. BRUGGENCATE, G. TEN, SCHERER, H., AND TEICHMANN, R.: *Neuronal activity in the lateral vestibular nucleus of the cat. V. Topographical distribution of inhibitory effects mediated by the spino-olivocerebellar pathway.* Pflügers Arch. 360:321, 1975.

30. CANGIANO, A., COOK, W. A., JR., AND POMPEIANO, O.: *Primary afferent depolarization in the lumbar cord evoked from the fastigial nucleus.* Arch. Ital. Biol. 107:321, 1969.

31. CANGIANO, A., COOK, W. A. JR., AND POMPEIANO, O.: *Cerebellar inhibitory control of the vestibular reflex pathways to primary afferents.* Arch. Ital. Biol. 107:341, 1969.

32. CARPENTER, D., ENGBERG, I., AND LUNDBERG, A.: *Primary afferent depolarization evoked from the brain stem and the cerebellum.* Arch. Ital. Biol. 104:73, 1966.

33. CARPENTER, M. B., BRITTIN, G. M., AND PINES, J.: *Isolated lesions of the fastigial nuclei in the cat.* J. Comp. Neurol. 109:65, 1958.

34. CARPENTER, M. B., AND NOVA, H. R.: *Descending division of the brachium conjunctivum in the cat: a cerebello-reticular system.* J. Comp. Neurol. 114:295, 1960.

35. CARPENTER, M. B., AND STEVENS, G. H.: *Structural and functional relationships between the deep cerebellar nuclei and the brachium conjunctivum in the rhesus monkey.* J. Comp. Neurol. 107:109, 1957.

36. CARREA, R. M. E., AND METTLER, F. A.: *Function of the primate brachium conjunctivum and related structures.* J. Comp. Neurol. 102:151, 1955.

37. CAUGHELL, K. A., AND FLUMERFELT, B. A.: *The organization of the cerebello-rubral projection. An experimental study in the rat.* J. Comp. Neurol. 176:295, 1977.

38. CHAN-PALAY, B.: *Cerebellar Dentate Nucleus. Organization, Cytology, and Transmitters.* Springer-Verlag, New York, 1977.

39. COHEN, D., CHAMBERS, W. W., AND SPRAGUE, J. M.: *Experimental study of the efferent projections from the cerebellar nuclei to the brainstem of the cat.* J. Comp. Neurol. 109:233, 1958.

40. COMBS, C. M., AND DENNERY, J. M.: *Cerebello-cerebral exconnections in the monkey as revealed by the evoked-potential method.* Exp. Neurol. 2:613, 1960.

41. COMBS, C. M., AND SAXON, S. V.: *Evoked potential evidence for connections from the cerebellar hemispheres to the sigmoid gyri.* Exp. Neurol. 1:583, 1959.

42. COOK, W. A., JR., CANGIANO, A., AND POMPEIANO, O.: *Vestibular influences on primary afferents in the spinal cord.* Pflügers Arch. 299:334, 1968.

43. COOK, W. A., JR. CANGIANO, A., AND POMPEIANO, O.: *Controllo cerebellare sulla trasmissione di impulsi spinali lungo le fibre afferenti muscolari di gruppo I.* Boll. Soc. Ital. Biol. Sper. 44:20, 1968.

44. COOK, W. A., JR., CANGIANO, A., AND POMPEIANO, O.: *Dorsal root potentials in the lumbar cord evoked from the vestibular system.* Arch. Ital. Biol. 107:275, 1969.

45. COOK, W. A., JR., CANGIANO, A. AND POMPEIANO, O.: *Vestibular control of transmission in primary afferents to the lumbar spinal cord.* Arch. Ital. Biol. 107:296, 1969.

46. COURVILLE, J.: *Somatotopical organization of the projection from the nucleus interpositus anterior of the cerebellum to the red nucleus. An experimental study in the cat with silver impregnation methods.* Exp. Brain Res. 2:191, 1966.

47. COURVILLE, J.: *Connections of the red nucleus with the cerebellum and certain caudal brain stem structures. A review with functional considerations.* Rev. Canad. Biol. 27:127, 1968.

48. COURVILLE, J., AND OTABE, S.: *The rubro-olivary projection in the macaque: An experimental study with silver impregnation methods.* J. Comp. Neurol. 158:479, 1974.

49. CROSBY, E. C., SCHNEIDER, R. C., DEJONGE, B. R. ET AL.: *The alterations of tonus and movements through the interplay between the cerebral hemispheres and the cerebellum.* J. Comp. Neurol. 127:1, 1966.

50. CURTIS, D. R., DUGGAN, A. W., AND FELIX, D.: *GABA and inhibition of Deiters' neurones.* Brain Res. 23:117, 1970.

51. DESIRAJU, T., AND PURPURA, D. P.: *Synaptic convergence of cerebellar and lenticular projections to thalamus.* Brain Res. 15:544, 1969.

52. DOW, R. S.: *The fiber connections of the posterior parts of the cerebellum in the rat and cat.* J. Comp. Neurol. 63:527, 1936.

53. DOW, R. S.: *Efferent connections of the flocculo-nodular lobe in Macaca mulatta.* J. Comp. Neurol. 68:297, 1938.

54. EAGER, R. P.: *Cortical association pathways in the cerebellum of the cat.* J. Comp. Neurol. 121:381, 1963.

55. EAGER, R. P.: *Efferent cortico-nuclear pathways in the cerebellum of the cat.* J. Comp. Neurol. 120:81, 1963.

56. EBBESSON, S. O. E., AND CAMPBELL, C. B. G.: *On the organization of cerebellar efferent pathways in the nurse shark (Ginglymostoma cirratum).* J. Comp. Neurol. 152:233, 1973.

57. ECCLES, J. C., NICOLL, R. A. SCHWARZ, D. W. F. ET AL.: *Cerebello-spinal pathway via the fastigial nucleus and the medial reticular nucleus.* Brain Res. 66:525, 1974.

58. ECCLES, J. C., NICOLL, R. A., SCHWARZ, D. W. F. ET AL.: *Reticulo-spinal neurons with and without monosynaptic inputs from cerebellar nuclei.* J. Neurophysiol. 38:513, 1975.

59. EDWARDS, S. B.: *The ascending and descending projections of the red nucleus in the cat: An experimental study using an autoradiographic tracing method.* Brain Res. 48:45, 1972.

60. EVARTS, E. V., AND THACH, W. T., JR.: *Motor mechanisms of the CNS: Cerebrocerebellar interrelations.* Ann. Rev. Physiol. 31:451, 1969.

61. FANARDJIAN, V. V., AND DONHOFFER, H.: *An electrophysiological study of cerebello-hippocampal relationships in the unrestrained cat.* Acta Physiol. Acad. Sci. Hung. 24:321, 1964.

62. FAULL, R. L. M.: *The cerebello-fugal projections in the brachium conjunctivum of the rat. II. The ipsilateral and contralateral descending pathways.* J. Comp. Neurol. 178:519, 1978.

63. FAULL, R. L. M., AND CARMAN, J. B.: *The cerebello-fugal projections in the brachium conjunctivum of the rat. I. The contralateral ascending pathway.* J. Comp. Neurol. 178:495, 1978.

64. FLOOD, S., AND JANSEN, J.: *On the cerebellar nuclei in the cat.* Acta Anat. 46:52, 1961.

65. FLOOD, S., AND JANSEN, J.: *The efferent fibres of the cerebellar nuclei and their distribution on the cerebellar peduncles of the cat.* Acta Anat. 63:137, 1966.

66. FLUMERFELT, B. A., AND CAUGHELL, K. A.: *A horseradish peroxidase study of the cerebello-rubral pathway in the rat.* Exp. Neurol. 58:95, 1978.

67. FLUMERFELT, B. A., OTABE, S., AND COURVILLE, J.: *Distinct projections to the red nucleus from the dentate and interposed nuclei in the monkey.* Brain Res. 50:408, 1973.

68. FUKUSHIMA, K., PETERSON, B. W., UCHINO, Y. ET AL.: *Direct fastigiospinal fibers in the cat.* Brain Res. 126:538, 1977.

69. GACEK, R. R.: *A cerebellocochlear nucleus pathway in the cat.* Exp. Neurol. 41:101, 1973.

70. GOODMAN, D. C., HALLETT, R. E., AND WELCH, R. B.: *Patterns of localization in the cerebellar cortico-nuclear projections of the albino rat.* J. Comp. Neurol. 121:51, 1963.

71. GRAYBIEL, A. M., NAUTA, H. J. W., LASEK, R. J. ET AL.: *A cerebello-olivary pathway in the cat: An experimental study using autoradiographic tracing techniques.* Brain Res. 58:205, 1973.

72. HARPER, J. W., AND HEATH, R. G.: *Ascending projections of the cerebellar fastigial nuclei: Connections to the ectosylvian gyrus.* Exp. Neurol. 42:241, 1974.

73. HOPKINS, D. A., AND LAWRENCE, D. G.: *On the absence of a rubrothalamic projection in the monkey with observations on some ascending mesencephalic projections.* J. Comp. Neurol. 161:269, 1975.

74. ITO, M., OBATA, K., AND OCHI, R.: *The origin of cerebellar-induced inhibition of Deiters' neurones. II. Temporal correlation between the transsynaptic activation of Purkinje cells and the inhibition of Deiters' neurones.* Exp. Brain Res. 2:350, 1966.

75. ITO, M., UDO, M., MANO, N. ET AL.: *Synaptic action of fastigiobulbar impulses upon neurones in the medullary reticular formation and vestibular nuclei.* Exp. Brain Res. 11:29, 1970.

76. ITO, M., AND YOSHIDA, M.: *The cerebellar-evoked monosynaptic inhibition of Deiters' neurones.* Experientia 20:515, 1964.

77. JANSEN, J.: *On the efferent connections of the cerebellum,* in Kappers, J. A. (ed.): *Progress in Neurobiology,* Vol. 1. Elsevier, Amsterdam, 1956, pp. 232–239.

78. JANSEN, J., AND BRODAL, A.: *Experimental studies on the intrinsic fibers of the cerebellum. II. The cortico-nuclear projection.* J. Comp. Neurol. 73:267, 1940.

79. JANSEN, J., AND BRODAL, A.: *Experimental studies on the intrinsic fibers of the cerebellum. The cortico nuclear projection in the rabbit and the monkey (Macaca rhesus).* Norske Vid. Akad. Oslo (Avh) I. Mat. Naturv. K., 3:1, 1942.

80. KING, J. S., DOM, R. M., CONNER, J. B. ET AL.: *An experimental light and electron microscopic study of cerebellorubral projections in the opposum, Didelphis marsupialis virginiana.* Brain Res. 52:61, 1973.

81. KITANO, K., ISHIDA, Y., ISHIKAWA, T. ET AL.: *Responses of extralemniscal thalamic neurones to stimulation of the fastigial nucleus and influences of the cerebral cortex in the cat.* Brain Res. 106:172, 1976.

82. LAPRESLE, J., AND HAMIDA, M. B.: *The dentato-olivary pathway. Somatotopic relationship between the dentate nucleus and the contralateral inferior olive.* Arch. Neurol. (Chicago) 22: 135, 1970.

83. LARSELL, O., AND JANSEN, J.: *The Comparative Anatomy and Histology of the Cerebellum: The Human Cerebellum, Cerebellar Connections, and Cerebellar Cortex.* University of Minnesota Press, Minneapolis, 1972.

84. LI, C. L., AND TEW, J. M., JR.: *The effect of cerebellar stimulation on neuronal activity in the motor cortex.* Exp. Neurol. 14:317, 1966.

85. MARTIN, G. F., AND HENKEL, C. K.: *Cerebello-olivary fibers: An analysis of their origin, course and distribution using horseradish peroxidase, autoradiographic and degeneration techniques.* Neurosci. Abstr. 1:208, 1975.

86. MARTIN, G. F., HENKEL, C. K., AND KING, J. S.: *Cerebello-olivary fibers: their origin course and distribution in the North American opossum.* Exp. Brain Res. 24:219, 1976.

87. MASSION, J.: *The mammalian red nucleus.* Physiol. Rev. 47:383, 1967.

88. MASSION, J., AND ALBE-FESSARD, D.: *Dualité des voies sensorielles afférentes controlant l'activité du noyau rouge.* Electroenceph. Clin. Neurophysiol. 15:435–454, 1963.

89. MASSION, J., ANGAUT, P., AND ALBE-FESSARD, D.: *Activités évoquées chez le chat dans la région du nucleus ventralis lateralis par diverses stimulations sensorielles. I. Étude macrophysiologique.* Electroenceph. Clin. Neurophysiol. 19:433, 1965.

90. MASSION, J., ANGAUT, P., AND ALBE-FESSARD, D.: *Activités évoquées chez le chat dans la région du nucleus ventralis lateralis par diverses stimulations sensorielles. II. Étude microphysiologique.* Electroenceph. Clin. Neurophysiol. 19:452, 1965.

91. MASSION, J., AND RISPAL-PADEL, L.: *Spatial organization of the cerebello-thalamo-cortical pathway.* Brain Res. 40:61, 1972.

92. MCMASTERS, R. E., AND RUSSELL, G. V.: *Efferent pathways from the deep cerebellar nuclei of the cat.* J. Comp. Neurol. 110:205, 1958.

93. MCMULLEN, T., AND BLOEDEL, J. R.: *Effects of bulbospinal systems activated from the dentate nucleus on the stretch reflex.* Neurosci. Abstr. 5:104, 1979.

94. MEHLER, W. R.: *Double descending pathways originating from the superior cerebellar peduncle. An example of neural species differences.* Anat. Rec. 157:374, 1967.

95. MEHLER, W. R., VERNIER, V. G., AND NAUTA, W. J. H.: *Efferent projections from dentate and interpositus nuclei in primates.* Anat. Rec. 130:430, 1958.

96. METTLER, F. A., ORIOLI, F. L., GRUNDFEST, H. ET AL.: *The descending limb of the brachium conjunctivum.* Trans. Am. Neurol. Assoc. 79:79, 1954.

97. MILLER, R. A., AND STROMINGER, N. L.: *Efferent connections of the red nucleus in the brainstem and spinal cord of the rhesus monkey.* J. Comp. Neurol. 152:327, 1973.

136

98. MILLER, R. A., AND STROMINGER, N. L.: *An experimental study of the efferent connections of the superior cerebellar peduncle in the rhesus monkey.* Brain Res. 133:237, 1977.

99. MURAKAMI, F., TSUKAHARA, N., AND FUJITO, Y.: *Properties of the synaptic transmission of the newly formed cortico-rubral synapses after lesion of the nucleus interpositus of the cerebellum.* Exp. Brain Res. 30:245, 1977.

100. MURAKAMI, F., TSUKAHARA, N., AND FUJITO, Y.: *Analysis of unitary EPSPs mediated by the newly formed cortico-rubral synapses after lesion of the nucleus interpositus of the cerebellum.* Exp. Brain Res. 30:233, 1977.

101. NIIMI, K., FUJIWARA, N., TAKIMOTO, T. ET AL.: *The course and termination of the ascending fibers of the brachium conjunctivum in the cat as studied by the Nauta method.* Tokushima J. Exp. Med. 8:269, 1962.

102. OBATA, K., TAKEDA, K., AND SHINOZAKI, H.: *Further study on pharamacological properties of the cerebellar-induced inhibition of Deiters' neurones.* Exp. Brain Res. 11:327, 1970.

103. ORIOLI, F. L.: *Descending limb of brachium conjunctivum in cat. An electrophysiological study.* J. Neurophysiol. 24:583, 1961.

104. ORIOLI, F. L., AND METTLER, F. A.: *Descending limb of the brachium conjunctivum in Macaca mulatta.* J. Comp. Neurol. 106:339, 1956.

105. POIRIER, L. J., AND BOUVIER, G.: *The red nucleus and its efferent nervous pathways in the monkey.* J. Comp. Neurol. 128:223, 1966.

106. POMPEIANO, O.: *Cerebellar control of the vestibular pathways to spinal motoneurons and primary afferents.* Prog. Brain Res. 37:391, 1972.

107. POMPEIANO, O, AND BRODAL, A.: *Experimental demonstration of a somatotopical origin of rubrospinal fibers in the cat.* J. Comp. Neurol. 108:225, 1957.

108. POMPEIANO, O., AND BRODAL, A.: *The origin of vestibulospinal fibres in the cat. An experimental-anatomical study, with comments on the descending medial longitudinal fasciculus.* Arch. Ital. Biol. 95:166, 1957.

109. RAMON Y CAJAL, S.: *Histologie du système nerveux de l'homme et des vertébrés,* Vol. I. Maloine, Paris, 1909.

110. RAND, R. W.: *An anatomical and experimental study of the cerebellar nuclei and their efferent pathways in the monkey.* J. Comp. Neurol. 101:167, 1954.

111. RASMUSSEN, A. T.: *Origin and course of the fasciculus uncinatus (Russell) in the cat, with observations on other fiber tracts arising from the cerebellar nuclei.* J. Comp. Neurol. 57:165, 1933.

112. RENAUD, L. P., AND COURVILLE, J.: *Projections of nuclei interpositus anterior and lateralis to the red nucleus and thalamus in the cat.* Anat. Rec. 163:249, 1969.

113. RISPAL-PADEL, L., AND GRANGETTO, A.: *The cerebello-thalamo-cortical pathway. Topographical investigation at the unitary level in the cat.* Exp. Brain Res. 28:101, 1977.

114. RISPAL-PADEL, L., AND LATREILLE, J.: *The organization of projections from the cerebellar nuclei to the contralateral motor cortex in the cat.* Exp. Brain Res. 19:36, 1974.

115. SACHS, E., FINCHER, E. F., JR.: *Anatomical and physiological observations on lesions in the cerebellar nuclei in Macacus rhesus. Preliminary report.* Brain 50:350, 1927.

116. SASAKI, K., KAWAGUCHI, S., MATSUDA, Y. ET AL.: *Electrophysiological studies on cerebello-cerebral projections in the cat.* Exp. Brain Res. 16:75, 1972.

117. SASAKI, K., KAWAGUCHI, S., OKA, H. ET AL.: *Electrophysiological studies on the cerebellocerebral projections in monkeys.* Exp. Brain Res. 24:495, 1976.

118. SASAKI, K., MATSUDA, Y., KAWAGUCHI, S. ET AL.: *On the cerebello-thalamo-cerebral pathway for the parietal cortex.* Exp. Brain Res. 16:89, 1972.

119. SCHMIDT, R. F.: *Control of the access of afferent activity to somatosensory pathways, in Iggo, A. (ed.): Handbook of Sensory Physiology,* Vol II. Springer-Verlag, New York, 1973, pp. 151–206.

120. SHAPOVALOV, A. I., KARAMJIAN, O. A., TAMAROVA, Z. A., ET AL.: *Cerebello-rubrospinal effects on hindlimb motoneurons in the monkey.* Brain Res. 47:49, 1972.

121. SNIDER, R. S.: *Further evidence for a cerebellar influence on the "reticular activating" system.* Anat. Rec. 124:441, 1956.

122. STRICK, P. L.: *Activity of ventrolateral thalamic neurons during arm movements.* J. Neurophysiol. 39:1032, 1976.

137

123. STRICK, P. L.: *Anatomical analysis of ventrolateral thalamic input to primate motor cortex.* J. Neurophysiol. 39:1020, 1976.

124. THOMAS, A.: *Le faisceau cérébelleaux descendant.* CR Soc. Biol. 49:36, 1897.

125. THOMAS, D. M., KAUFMAN, R. P., SPRAGUE, J. M. ET AL.: *Experimental studies of the vermal cerebellar projections in the brain stem of the cat (fastigiobulbar tracts).* J. Anat. (London) 90: 371, 1956.

126. TOLBERT, D. L., BANTLI, H., AND BLOEDEL, J. R.: *Organizational features of the cat and monkey cerebellar nucleocortical projection.* J. Comp. Neurol. 182:39, 1978.

127. TOLBERT, D. L., BANTLI, H., AND BLOEDEL, J. R.: *Multiple branching of cerebellar efferent projections in cats.* Exp. Brain Res. 31:305, 1978.

128. TOLBERT, D. L., MASSOPUST, L. C., MURPHY, M. G. ET AL.: *The anatomical organization of the cerebello-olivary projection in the cat.* J. Comp. Neurol. 170:525, 1976.

129. TSUKAHARA, N., AND FUJITO, Y.: *Physiological evidence of formation of new synapses from cerebrum in the red nucleus neurons following crossunion of forelimb nerves.* Brain Res. 106: 184, 1976.

130. UNO, M., YOSHIDA, M., AND HIROTA, I.: *The mode of cerebello-thalamic relay transmission investigated with intracellular recording from cells of the ventrolateral nucleus of the cat's thalamus.* Exp. Brain Res. 10:121, 1970.

131. VAN BUREN, J. M., AND BORKE, R. C.: *Re-evaluation of the "nucleus ventralis lateralis" and its cerebellar connections. A study in man and chimpanzee.* Int. J. Neurol. 8:155, 1971.

132. VOOGD, J.: *The Cerebellum of the Cat.* F. A. Davis, Philadelphia, 1964.

133. WALBERG, F.: *Descending connections to the inferior olive. An experimental study in the cat.* J. Comp. Neurol. 104:77, 1956.

134. WALBERG, F.: *Cerebellovestibular relations: anatomy.* Prog. Brain Res. 37:361, 1972.

135. WALBERG, F., AND JANSEN, J.: *Cerebellar cortico-vestibular fibers in the cat.* Exp. Neurol. 3:32, 1961.

136. WALBERG, F., AND POMPEIANO, O.: *Fastigiofugal fibers to the lateral reticular nucleus: An experimental study in the cat.* Exp. Neurol. 2:40, 1960.

137. WALBERG, F., POMPEIANO, O., BRODAL, A. ET AL.: *The fastigiovestibular projection in the cat. An experimental study with silver impregnation methods.* J. Comp. Neurol. 118:49, 1962.

138. WALSH, T. M., AND EBNER, F. F.: *Distribution of cerebellar and somatic lemniscal projections in the ventral nuclear complex of the Virginia opossum.* J. Comp. Neurol. 147:427, 1973.

139. WHITESIDE, J. A., AND SNIDER, R. S.: *Relation of cerebellum to upper brain stem.* J. Neurophysiol. 16:397, 1953.

CHAPTER 7

Postural Regulation in Animals

Our understanding of the functions of the cerebellum in the control of posture stems from a series of studies that serves as the very foundation of cerebellar physiology. Dow and Moruzzi have reviewed and discussed these studies in an historic volume.[35] Their perspective provides a valuable basis for understanding the effects of cerebellar ablation and stimulation on posture and movement. This chapter contains a synthesis of the observations and conclusions from the older studies together with recent observations to provide an updated overview of this subject.

CEREBELLAR STIMULATION AND ABLATION IN SUBPRIMATES

Acute Effects of Cerebellar Ablation

Midline Ablation and Complete Cerebellectomy

Since the early studies of Luciani,[61, 62] the effects of total cerebellar ablation have been classified into periods of unstabilized and stabilized deficiency. These periods indicate the phases of acute and chronic neurologic deficits, respectively. In the acute phase immediately after complete cerebellar ablation in the cat or dog, the animal develops a marked increase in extensor tone of all four extremities together with opisthotonos (Fig. 1). The anatomic structures responsible for these deficits were established by a series of studies beginning with the finding that ablation of the anterior lobe alone can duplicate the effects of total cerebellar ablation.[14, 21, 22, 102] Similar effects occurred in cats after ligation of both carotid arteries and the basilar artery.[86-89] This procedure, termed anemic decerebration, results in ischemic injury of the cerebrum and the anterior lobe of the cerebellum. The result is equivalent to the effects of transecting the brainstem at the intercollicular level and ablating the cerebellar anterior lobe. Other portions of the cerebellar vermis are partially responsible for these effects.[102] Similar but less marked deficits result from ablating the posterior lobe, with the anterior lobe remaining intact. In addition, completely ablating the fastigial nucleus causes an extensor hypertonus similar to that following ablation of the anterior lobe.[6, 57] These studies indicate that the manifestations of unstabilized deficiency result chiefly from damage to midline cerebellar structures.

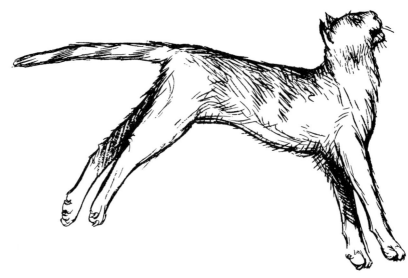

Figure 1. The acute effects of ligating both carotid arteries and the basilar artery in the cat. This procedure results in ischemic injury to the cerebrum and the anterior lobe of the cerebellum. The results are similar to those following complete surgical ablation of the cerebellum; the animal shows marked opisthotonos and extensor rigidity of the limbs. (From Pollock and Davis,[87] with permission.)

Several studies have elucidated the pathways descending into the spinal cord that mediate the rigidity following cerebellar ablation. The vestibulospinal projections were implicated by demonstrating that destruction of the vestibular labyrinths or section of the eighth cranial nerve decreases the hypertonus and opisthotonos resulting from ablation of the anterior lobe or anemic decerebration (Fig. 2).[3-5, 87-89, 107, 108] Some extensor hypertonus still can occur, however, after cerebellar ablation or ablation of the midline nuclei in decerebrate animals with bilaterally sectioned eighth nerves (Fig. 2).[5] This observation has been taken to indicate that pathways in addition to the vestibulospinal projection, most likely the reticulospinal pathways, are involved in these deficits. These studies demonstrate that the acute effects of cerebellar ablation in the cat and dog result chiefly from interrupting the interactions between the midline cerebellar region, particularly the anterior lobe, and the descending vestibulospinal and reticulospinal projections.[35]

The tonic actions of the output projections from the cerebellar cortex and the fastigial nuclei were investigated in studies employing selective ablation and stimulation of these structures. The ipsilateral extensor hypertonus resulting from ablation of the vermis of the anterior lobe unilaterally can be reversed by a lesion of the corresponding fastigial nucleus (Fig 3).[77, 81, 105, 109] This finding indicates that the output of the cerebellar cortex has different actions than the output of the fastigial nucleus. Subsequent studies have shown this conclusion to be essentially correct, however, ablations of various portions of the fastigial nuclei have different effects on posture.[6, 27, 78, 79, 81] Ablating the caudal portion of the fastigial nucleus results in hypotonia of the extensor muscles in the contralateral limbs.[6, 27, 78, 79, 81] Consistent with this observation, stimulating the caudal portion of the fastigial nucleus results in hypertonia of the same extremities.[78, 79] These studies indicate that projections from the caudal fastigial nucleus have a tonic ex-

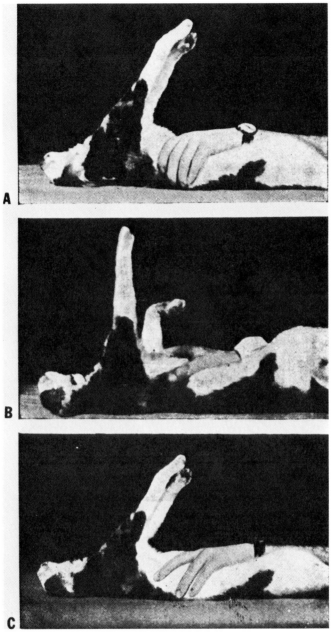

Figure 2. The effects of sectioning the eighth nerve on the rigidity and opisthotonos resulting from complete destruction of the fastigial nucleus, a lesion interrupting all of the output from the anterior lobe. A, the cat was decerebrated at the intercollicular level and had a bilateral dorsal rhizotomy from C_5 to T_2, transection of the spinal cord at T_{12}, and bilateral destruction of the roof nuclei. The animal shows marked extensor rigidity and opisthotonos. B, Section of the left eighth nerve resulted in a decrease of rigidity in the left forelimb. C, Following section of the right eighth nerve, rigidity was restored bilaterally, but the opisthotonos disappeared. The rigidity results in part from the Schiff-Sherrington release phenomenon produced by the cord section at T_{12}. (From Batini et al.,[5] with permission.)

141

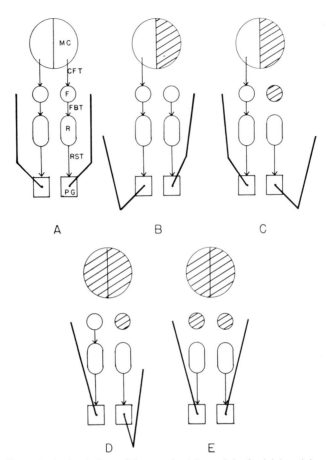

Figure 3. The effects of selective lesions of the anterior lobe and the fastigial nuclei on the postures of the forelimbs in cats. These diagrams illustrate the predominant effects responsible for changes in the tonic position of the forelimbs following ablations of the anterior lobe and fastigial nuclei. A, The structures involved. B, Ablation of the ipsilateral anterior lobe results in marked extension of the ipsilateral extremity with contralateral flexion. C, Following ablation of the fastigial nucleus, the previous postural asymmetry is reversed. D, Ablation of the entire anterior lobe of the cerebellum further accentuates the posture. E, Following ablation of the remaining fastigial nucleus, marked extensor hypertonia exists in both extremities similar to that seen following complete removal of the cerebellum. MC = anterior lobe; CFT = corticofastigial tract; F = fastigial nucleus; FBT = fastigiobulbar tract; R = reticular nucleus; RST = reticulospinal tract; PG = pectoral girdle and brachial spinal cord. (From Sprague and Chambers,[105] with permission.)

citatory effect on motoneurons innervating the contralateral extensor muscles.

The output of the caudal fastigial nucleus is organized somatotopically. Stimulating its rostral and caudal portions evokes hypertonia limited to the contralateral forelimb and contralateral hindlimb, respectively.[93] Topographically organized pathways extend from each of these regions in the caudal fastigial nucleus through the crossed fastigiovestibular projection and into the regions of the lateral vestibular (Deiters') nucleus[95] that project to forelimb and hindlimb segments of the spinal cord. Thus, the anatomic connections between the fastigial nucleus and Dei-

142

ters' nucleus account for the selective effects of stimulating or ablating the two components of the posterior fastigiovestibulospinal projections.

The results of ablating the rostral portion of the fastigial nucleus are more difficult to interpret based upon current knowledge of cerebellar efferent projections. Lesions of the rostral or rostrolateral fastigial nucleus cause hypertonia of the extensor muscles in the ipsilateral limbs,[80] while lesions of the rostromedial part of this nucleus cause hypotonia of the same muscles. Understanding the basis for these postural changes requires a review of additional neurophysiologic and neuroanatomic characteristics of the cerebellar vermis and fastigial nuclei.

Stimulating the cerebellar anterior lobe strongly affects extensor tone in cats decerebrated surgically at the midcollicular level.[17, 32, 60] The effects of this procedure depend upon stimulus frequency. High frequency stimulation decreases the extensor rigidity of the decerebrate animal and low frequency stimulation (2 to 20 Hz) increases the extensor rigidity.[69-76] It is important to appreciate that, even in preparations in which the vestibular nerves are cut, both ablating and stimulating the cerebellar anterior lobe at low frequency cause an increase of extensor rigidity.[114] The fact that both of these procedures cause hypertonia serves as the basis of the fundamental concept that the inhibitory action of the midline portion of the cerebellum on the spinal cord is mediated indirectly by the inhibition of excitatory bulbospinal pathways.[59, 111, 114]

The advent of single unit recording techniques made it possible to examine the mechanisms underlying the effects of cerebellar output on the excitability of spinal motoneurons. Ablation of the anterior lobe results in a 10 to 15 millivolt depolarization of alpha motoneurons innervating extensor muscles.[38] In contrast, stimulation of the anterior lobe causes hyperpolarization of these neurons even when their membrane potentials exceed that of the reversal potential for the Ia IPSPs (Fig. 4).[59, 111] This finding shows that the decreased excitability produced by stimulating the cerebellar surface results from decreasing an excitatory input to the alpha motoneurons rather than activating a direct inhibitory input to these cells.[59, 111] Similarly, cerebellar rebound, the increased tone observed immediately after discontinuation of cerebellar stimulation, results from a prolonged depolarization of alpha motoneurons which substantially increases their excitability. The effects of cerebellar stimulation are mediated by both vestibulospinal and reticulospinal pathways.[59]

The output of the cerebellar cortex has different synaptic actions than the output of the cerebellar nuclei. One of the first indications of this fact came from the finding that ablation of the cerebellar cortex has effects on postural tone opposite to those resulting from ablation of the fastigial nuclei.[77, 79, 105, 109] As mentioned earlier, the extensor hypertonus induced by ablating the vermis of the ipsilateral anterior lobe can be reversed by ablating the corresponding fastigial nucleus. It was not until the synaptic effects of cerebellar neurons were examined electrophysiologically, however, that the inhibitory actions of Purkinje cells[52-54] and the excitatory actions of the cerebellar nuclear neurons[119, 120] were understood fully. Once this was established, many of the effects of stimulating or ablating regions of the cerebellar cortex and nuclei could be explained.

The consequences of high-frequency stimulation and ablation of the anterior lobe result from the effects of these procedures on the inhibitory output of the Purkinje cells on the fastigial and vestibular nuclei. Similarly, the effects of stimulating or ablating the caudal part of the fastigial nucleus can be attributed to

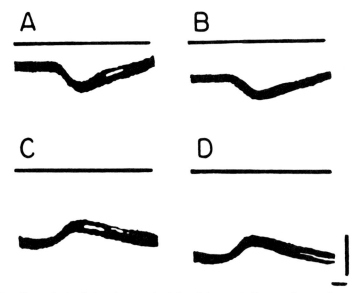

Figure 4. The effects of stimulating the anterior lobe of the cerebellum on the membrane potential of extensor alpha motoneurons. The records in A through D were obtained by recording intracellularly from a single motoneuron. The lower trace in each record is a DC recording indicating both the resting potential of the neuron and the amplitude and polarity of the response evoked by stimulating Ia afferents from the antagonistic muscle. The upper trace in each record is a reference permitting visualization of changes in DC potential from cerebellar stimulation. A and C: Control responses to stimulating the Ia afferents from the antagonistic muscle at two different membrane potentials. The membrane potential in A is depolarized from the normal resting potential and that in C is hyperpolarized to a voltage exceeding the reversal potential for the Ia IPSP. In the condition shown in C, stimulating the Ia afferents evokes depolarization. B and D: Stimulating the anterior lobe of the cerebellum evokes hyperpolarization of the motoneuron independent of whether the voltage of its membrane is above or below the reversal potential for the IPSP at the time the cerebellar stimulus is applied. These findings demonstrate that the hyperpolarization from stimulation of the anterior lobe of the cerebellum does not result from the activation of a direct inhibitory input to these neurons. Rather, the hyperpolarization results from the decreased action of an excitatory input to the motoneuron. (From Terzuolo,[111] with permission.)

effects on the excitatory action of the crossed fastigiobulbar pathway. These findings, however, do not explain the differential effects of lesions in the rostrolateral and rostromedial fastigial nucleus or the effects of stimulating the anterior lobe at high and low frequencies.

The opposite effects of rostrolateral and rostromedial fastigial nuclear lesions can be understood with additional data from studies on the combined results of ablating the fastigial nucleus and stimulating the vermis of the anterior lobe. The ipsilateral extensor hypertonus following a lesion of the rostrolateral fastigial nucleus is increased further by stimulating the cerebellar anterior lobe at the same high frequency which suppresses decerebrate rigidity in the absence of a fastigial lesion.[75] Thus, a lesion of the rostrolateral fastigial nucleus can reverse the effects of stimulating the cerebellar anterior lobe at high frequencies. Furthermore, the increase in extensor tone produced by this stimulus is abolished by destroying the rostromedial fastigial nucleus, a lesion resulting in hypotonia of the extensor muscles in the ipsilateral limb.[7, 8] These findings indicate that the selective effects of ablating the rostromedial and rostrolateral parts of the fastigial nucleus result from

144

interrupting two different projections. Lesions of the rostrolateral fastigial nucleus interrupt a major portion of the corticovestibular projection that passes through this region. These fibers directly inhibit bulbospinal neurons, particularly those originating in the vestibular nuclei. Consequently, stimulation of the cerebellar anterior lobe after ablation of the rostrolateral fastigial nucleus cannot activate the direct inhibitory input to the vestibular nuclei from the cerebellar cortex. Lesions of the rostromedial fastigial nucleus probably interrupt only the fastigiobulbar projection, an excitatory pathway to the brainstem.

Other effects of stimulating the anterior lobe of the cerebellum in the decerebrate cat, including the different effects of stimulation at high and low frequencies, depend upon several factors. Undoubtedly, stimulating the cerebellar surface activates many different neuronal elements. A specific study of this issue revealed that, in addition to activating Purkinje cells, surface stimulation can activate mossy fibers and climbing fibers.[2] Moreover, the intracellular studies of Ito and his colleagues[51-53] demonstrated that stimulating the surface of the anterior lobe can evoke short latency excitatory postsynaptic potentials in neurons located in Deiters' nucleus. Thus, surface stimulation actually can activate vestibulospinal projections. Surface stimulation also can activate neurons in the deep cerebellar nuclei through antidromic activation of both nucleocortical fibers and cerebellar afferent fibers.[116-118] Because many neurons in the cerebellar nuclei project to extracerebellar structures, cerebellar surface stimulation also can activate these efferent projections.[118] These findings demonstrate the complexity of neuronal interactions that can result from stimulating the cerebellar surface. Undoubtedly the effects of the stimulus on cerebellar output depend strongly upon the rate and intensity of stimulation. These factors probably account for the diversity of results in the literature. Stimulating the cerebellar anterior lobe, for example, can increase or decrease neuronal activity in Deiters' nucleus.[33, 96-99] In addition, stimulating the same cerebellar region can inhibit[10, 68] or excite some bulboreticular neurons.[9, 103]

The complex neuronal effects of stimulating the cerebellar surface undoubtedly account for several observations that seem otherwise inconsistent with the known inhibitory actions of Purkinje cells and the excitatory actions of neurons projecting from cerebellar nuclei. For example, stimulating or ablating portions of the posterior lobe vermis produces effects that are similar rather than opposite to the effects of stimulating or ablating the posterior portion of the fastigial nucleus. Ablating either the cerebellar cortex or the caudal portion of the fastigial nucleus leads to hypotonia in the extensor muscles of the contralateral limbs. In contrast, stimulating both these regions increases the extensor tone in limbs contralateral to the stimulus.[14, 26, 46, 78, 79, 106] In another example, ablating the pyramis and uvula decreases postural tone in the contralateral extensor muscles, an effect similar to that resulting from lesions in the caudal fastigial nucleus.[55, 56] The similarity in the effects of stimulating the posterior lobe vermis and the posterior portion of the fastigial nucleus may be due to the activation of efferent fastigial neurons by stimulating the nucleocortical fibers.[116-118] The similarity in the effects of ablating these two regions of the midline cerebellum, however, cannot be explained on this basis. Additional studies will be required to resolve this point.

Several studies have addressed the spinal mechanisms by which total cerebellar ablation or ablation of the anterior lobe causes an increase of extensor tone. A tonic increase in the excitability of the myotatic reflex resulting from the tonic activation of gamma motoneurons cannot account for this deficit, because hypertonia of the extensor muscles in the forelimb can occur in animals when this reflex arc is interrupted by chronic deafferentation of the forelimb.[110, 112, 113] Extensor rigidity also can be produced in deafferented preparations by anemically decerebrating the animal, a procedure that results in ablation of the cerebellar anterior lobe.[90] Thus, extensor rigidity following complete cerebellar ablation or ablation of the anterior lobe stems from an increase in the excitatory action of descending pathways directly on spinal alpha motoneurons rather than on gamma motoneurons (fusimotor neurons).

Extensor rigidity in the decerebellate animal results from an increase in alpha motoneuron activity which does not depend upon fusimotor activity. Consistent with this view are several studies showing that cerebellar ablation results in a decrease rather than an increase in the tonic discharge of fusimotor neurons and an associated decrease in the sensitivity of the stretch reflex.[40-42, 44, 67] The decrease in the sensitivity of the stretch reflex following cerebellar ablation is apparent in the dynamic responses of motoneurons to sinusoidal muscle stretch.[47, 48] A reduction in gain of this reflex is associated temporally with the animals' inability to stand or walk. The animals' recovery of function with time occurs in parallel with a progressive restoration of the reflex gain and a normal phase lead of the response to changes in muscle length. In addition, stimulation of the anterior lobe at frequencies low enough to cause increased extensor rigidity in decerebrate preparations increases the excitability of the monosynaptic reflex.[20] The monosynaptic reflexes in these preparations were evoked electrically by peripheral nerve stimulation and thus reflect only changes in the excitability of alpha motoneurons and not in the sensitivity of muscle spindle receptors.

Despite the marked changes that have been found in motoneuron excitability, cerebellar ablation does not affect equally all populations of motoneurons. In cats, cerebellar ablation affects selectively populations of neurons responding in a characteristic way to repetitive activation of peripheral afferent fibers.[43] In addition, cerebellar ablation affects the excitability of only certain naturally evoked reflexes.[30] Specifically, the responses of motoneurons to neck extension and to manipulation of distal joints are accentuated.[30]

Although changes in excitability of spinal reflexes do not contribute to the extensor hypertonus following bilateral anterior lobe lesions or total cerebellar ablation, these changes account for some of the effects of unilateral lesions. The ipsilateral extensor hypertonus following unilateral fastigial ablation occurs together with contralateral extensor hypotonus. These postures change dramatically after deafferentation of the ipsilateral forelimb by sectioning the dorsal roots from segments C_5 to T_2.[81] The ipsilateral forelimb becomes flaccid while the contralateral limb becomes hypertonic. These observations show that reflexes tonically active in the hypertonic extremity are responsible for the hypotonus in the opposite extremity.

Ablation and Stimulation of the Intermediate Zone

The initial investigations into the functions of the intermediate zone concerned the postural effects of stimulating and ablating this region.[108] In the decerebrate cat, stimulation of the intermediate zone of the cerebellar cortex results in flexion of the ipsilateral limbs.[108] This postural change does not result from stimulation of neuronal elements in the midline sagittal zone because ablation of the anterior lobe[108] or bilateral ablation of the fastigial nucleus does not affect the response to stimulation.[91, 105] In contrast, the effect of stimulating the paravermal cortex is eliminated by lesions of the interposed nuclei.[26] Thus, the output of the intermediate zone is separate from that of the midline zone.

Ablating the paravermal region of the cerebellar cortex results in marked flexion of the ipsilateral extremities.[125, 126] The effects of stimulating this region, however, depend upon the mediolateral location of the stimulating electrode. Stimulating the medial portion of the intermediate zone evokes flexion of the ipsilateral forelimb and stimulating the lateral region evokes extension of the ipsilateral hindlimb.[91] Both of these postural changes persist after fastigial ablation.[91] The red nucleus mediates the postural effects of stimulating the medial part of the intermediate zone because the postural changes are lost after postcollicular decerebration, midline sagittal section of the mesencephalon, or destruction of the posterior red nucleus.[91] The anterior part of the interposed nuclei is also essential for the postural response to stimulating the medial portion of the intermediate zone, as shown by the fact that ablation of this structure abolishes the response. The postural effects of stimulating the lateral region of the intermediate zone are not modified by postcollicular decerebration, indicating that these effects do not involve the red nucleus. These postural changes may be mediated by the descending limb of the brachium conjunctivum, but this has not been investigated.

Stimulating the interposed nuclei induces postural changes similar to those resulting from stimulating the paravermal cortex. The usual result is flexion of the ipsilateral extremities.[35, 94] The output projections responsible for these postural changes are organized somatotopically to some extent, because stimulation in specific regions within the anterior interposed nucleus causes selective flexion of either the forelimb or the hindlimb.[92] The red nucleus mediates these postural changes, as shown by the fact that the ipsilateral flexion resulting from stimulating the anterior interposed nucleus disappears after ablation of the red nucleus or low decerebration.[91] These findings reflect the excitatory action of neurons in the anterior interposed nuclei on rubrospinal neurons in the contralateral red nucleus.[66, 120]

The red nucleus also mediates the postural changes induced by stimulating the paramedian lobule and the posterior interposed nucleus.[63-65] Stimulating the paramedian lobule causes hypertonus of the ipsilateral extensor muscles. In contrast, stimulating the posterior interposed nucleus results in hypertonus of the ipsilateral flexor muscles. These postural changes disappear after ablation of the red nucleus. These studies indicate that the intermediate zone affects the excitability of spinal neurons primarily through the cerebellorubrospinal projection. Most of the postural changes resulting from stimulating and ablating the intermediate cortical zone and the interposed nuclei can be explained on this basis. The output of the interposed nuclei mediated by the descending limb of the brachium conjunctivum also may modify neural activity in the spinal cord, but this has not been established.

Chronic Effects of Cerebellar Ablation

Following the interval of unstabilized deficiency from cerebellar ablation in the cat and dog, the animal undergoes a progressive recovery from the disabling extensor hypertonus and opisthotonos. Luciani[61, 62] referred to this as the period of stabilized deficiency. In describing this period, Rademaker[100] established five categories of postural changes. First, he observed that the *Stützreaktion* (the supporting reaction) is exaggerated in the chronically decerebellate dog. He also observed that the deep tendon reflexes are hyperactive. Second, he found that the *Stütztonusstarke* (strength of supporting tonus) is reduced somewhat during recovery from cerebellectomy. Third, he found that the *Schunkelreaktion* (swaying reaction), the animals' ability to change body position properly in response to the movement of an extremity, is exaggerated and poorly controlled. Last, he found two other reactions to changes in body position, the *Stemmbeinreaktion* (bracing reaction) and *Hinkebeinreaktion* (hopping reaction), also are controlled poorly in the decerebellate dog. The former is slightly decreased while the latter is somewhat exaggerated.

The basis of the gradual disappearance of extensor hypertonus is not completely clear. One possibility involves the interactions responsible for mediating Schiff-Sherrington inhibition. This is the inhibition exerted on brainstem neurons by spinobulbar fibers from the lumbar spinal cord. It has been proposed that, in the chronically decerebellate animal, these fibers suppress the excitability of vestibulospinal neurons which have a tonic excitatory action on extensor motoneurons.[5, 35] This notion is supported by the observation that the rigidity produced by decerebration in the chronically decerebellate cat disappears after deafferentation of the limbs, indicating that compensation for the hypertonia produced by cerebellectomy has occurred. In this preparation, subsequent postbrachial transection of the spinal cord results in a return of forelimb extensor rigidity. This is an alpha rigidity, the type of hypertonus observed in deafferented preparations after acute removal of the cerebellum. These observations indicate that projections ascending from the lumbar region of the spinal cord exert a progressively greater inhibitory action on vestibulospinal neurons during the disappearance of extensor hypertonus in the chronically decerebellate animal. During this same period, the sensitivity of muscle spindle afferents, which is exaggerated in flexor muscles, returns to a normal range.[47, 48, 122] The depressed sensitivity of the stretch reflex in extensor muscles also returns to more normal values[45, 47] This change in reflexes occurs in parallel with a progressive recovery of the ability to stand and walk.

The rate of recovery from cerebellar ablation is species dependent.[35, 83, 124] Although the acute deficit after cerebellar ablation is most marked in quadripeds which have evolved most recently, the rate of recovery is also faster in these species.[124] The capability of recovery may be related to the greater cerebration in higher mammals.

CEREBELLAR ABLATION IN PRIMATES

Complete Cerebellectomy

The clinical manifestations of cerebellar ablation in primates cannot be divided clearly into acute and chronic phases. The disorders occurring acutely undergo a progressive improvement instead of a marked change in basic characteristics. The abnormalities can be classified into four categories:[11, 123] tremor, hypotonia, ataxia, and nystagmus. Both kinetic and static tremors occur. Kinetic tremor refers to the oscillatory movements observed during the execution of an active movement. Static tremor indicates the oscillatory movements which occur during a maintained posture. Hypotonia is a decreased resistance to passive manipulation of the limbs. Ataxia includes both postural instability and disorders of movement such as errors of range (dysmetria), inadequate performance of skilled limb movements (dyssynergia), and errors of rate.

148

The deficits immediately after cerebellar ablation in monkeys differ from those in subprimates.[1, 61, 82, 85, 100] Rather than a marked extensor rigidity, hypotonia occurs and is particularly marked in the extensor and truncal muscles. Similar disorders occur after ablations restricted to the anterior lobe.[24, 36] Decerebellate monkeys initially cannot maintain the postural support of the trunk and extremities necessary for standing and walking. Attempted movements or postural fixation result in a marked truncal tremor and ataxic movements of the limbs. Reactive movements are ataxic and may be accompanied by marked tremor, both static and kinetic. The tonic labyrinthine reflexes are unresponsive for as long as three months after the procedure,[31] and the proprioceptive reflexes are severely depressed.[24, 31] Postures of persistent flexion of the limbs (flexion dystonia) occur during the first few months.[31] The grasp reflex remains present throughout the postoperative period, but the magnet reaction with consequent extension of the lower extremities cannot be evoked immediately after complete cerebellar ablation. This reflex, consisting of limb extension in response to a light cutaneous contact with the digits of that limb, reappears approximately one week postoperatively. The positive supporting reaction, however, is depressed severely for four to six weeks. Its return occurs in parallel with the reappearance of the animal's ability to maintain adequate truncal support.[31] Spontaneous attempts at locomotion usually do not appear for as long as 4 to 6 months after the ablation. Nystagmus often persists for as long as 1½ to 2 months after cerebellar ablation. Hypotonia also persists, though decreasing somewhat with time. This deficit is most marked among higher primates such as the chimpanzee and baboon.[24, 37]

Dyssynergia and dysmetria become particularly apparent in the decerebellate monkey as the animal recovers and begins to move frequently, particularly when movement involves more than a single joint.[24, 82] As early as the experiments of Munk,[82] it was appreciated that movements requiring only the use of the distalmost extremities can be performed quite normally after cerebellar ablation. When these movements are associated with changes in posture or movement of the proximal muscles, however, a clearly dysmetric, dyssynergic pattern of movement occurs.

The degree to which primates can recover from total cerebellectomy still is not resolved completely. Hypotonia and marked ataxia persist for several months,[1, 82, 100] though these abnormalities continue to decrease. Although completely normal motor behavior does not reappear, the deficits remaining after periods greater than one year are minimal and may only be observable in certain experimental paradigms.[124]

Partial Ablation

Lesions of the Cerebellar Cortex

Removing large regions of the cerebellar cortex, particularly within the neocerebellum, generally results in neurologic disturbances similar to those following complete cerebellar ablation. Less severe deficits appear with restricted ablations, however, and the animal appears better able to compensate.[13, 24] Complete recovery can occur after restricted lesions of the cerebellar cortex.[13]

Errors of rate and force during active limb movements are the most apparent abnormalities after limited cerebellar cortical ablations, though hypotonia also occurs.[13] The occurrence of tremor following these lesions is controversial. When it occurs, tremor persists for only a few days.[13, 24] It has been concluded that tremor following cerebellar lesions requires destruction of at least a portion of the cerebellar nuclei.

In more restricted cerebellar cortical lesions, ablation of the anterior lobe vermis causes a mild dysmetria and lesions of the posterior lobe vermis cause ataxia.[24, 85] Truncal ataxia is associated most commonly with lesions of the uvula, nodulus, and the fastigial nucleus. In contrast, dysmetria most commonly results from combined lesions of the anterior and posterior lobes.[85] Only minimal deficits appear after partial ablations of the cerebellar hemispheres.[85]

Cerebellar lesions that include the fastigial nucleus and parts of the vermal cortex result in truncal ataxia.[12, 85] Tremor is notably absent in these animals[12] as long as the interposed and dentate nuclei remain intact. In addition, the ataxia resulting from fastigial lesions chiefly affects the trunk and does not affect greatly the movements of the distal extremities.

Lesions of the Dentate, Emboliform, and Globose Nuclei

Transection of the superior cerebellar peduncle has been used to study the effects of interrupting the output projections of the interposed and dentate nuclei. Complete section of the superior cerebellar peduncle in the monkey results in hypotonia, ataxia, and tremor, deficits that occur also after complete cerebellectomy.[25, 123] These deficits persist longer after bilateral than after unilateral pedunculotomy. Carrea and Mettler studied the effects of sectioning selectively the ascending and descending limbs of the brachium conjunctivum.[24, 25] They concluded that ataxia results from interrupting fibers in the descending limb and tremor results from interrupting the crossed ascending limb.

The most precise descriptions of the deficits resulting from ablation of the dentate or interposed nuclei in primates have come from studies of the kinematic variables describing various movements. Interference with the function of the dentate nucleus by cooling this structure causes marked errors in the rate and range of self-paced controlled movements in the monkey.[16, 17] With the onset of cooling, the movements become dysmetric, showing undershooting and overshooting of the target. As cooling continues during an individual session, the errors of range decrease considerably. The data indicate that the monkey develops a strategy that improves the accuracy of the movement. This is done principally by executing the movement more slowly. Errors in the rate of the movement are particularly marked and do not improve with practice. There is an increase in both peak acceleration and deceleration and in peak velocity.[17]

Abnormalities of rapidly alternating movements have long been known to occur after cerebellar lesions in humans and animals.[49, 50] Selectively cooling the dentate nucleus also causes this deficit.[28, 29, 50] During alternating movements there is a delay in the initiation of EMG activity in the antagonistic muscle, thus delaying the initiation of the return movement and decreasing the frequency with which alternating movements can be performed (Fig. 5).[28, 29] Dentate lesions also affect ballistic movements in human and nonhuman primates.[104, 115] The alternating pattern of activity in agonist and antagonist muscles observed normally during ballistic movements is disorganized. In addition, there is a delay in the onset of activity in the antagonist muscle which is necessary to stop the ballistic movement, and there is also a considerable amount of cocontraction.

There are few studies of the effects of selective lesions of the interposed nuclei.

150

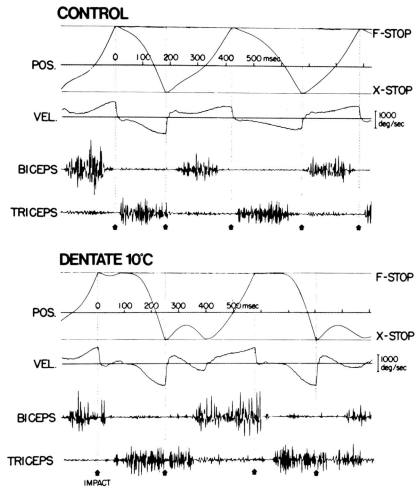

Figure 5. The effects of cooling the dentate nucleus on the performance of alternating movements in monkeys. A monkey was trained to alternate the positions of a lever between two stops designated the F stop and the X stop. Recordings were taken of the position (POS) of the lever, the velocity (VEL) of the movement, and EMG activity in the biceps and triceps muscles. Cooling the dentate nucleus to 10° C caused marked disorganization of the movements. The movements became less precise and the rate of the alternating movements was decreased. The abnormalities were associated with a prolongation of activity in the biceps and triceps muscles after the limb reached its target in flexion or extension, respectively. (From Conrad and Brooks,[28] with permission.)

When these nuclei are inactivated by cooling during a self-paced alternating movement, no increase in peak acceleration or velocity occurs.[121] Instead, the alternating movement slows and movement velocity decreases. These findings contrast markedly with those resulting from cooling of the dentate nucleus.

Neuroanatomic Basis of the Deficits Following Cerebellar Ablation

In the studies of Brooks and his colleagues,[28, 29, 50] the marked increase in peak acceleration and velocity of a limb during alternating movements was due princi-

151

pally to interrupting the output of the dentate nuclei. Cooling the interposed nuclei did not duplicate these findings. As described in Chapter 8, the hypotonia following cerebellar ablation also can be ascribed in large measure to interrupting the output projections of the dentate nucleus. Further studies will be needed to determine the relative importance of these nuclei in the other deficits following cerebellar lesions.

The descending pathways mediating the movement disorders following cerebellar ablation have not been established with certainty. The corticospinal tract has been implicated because sectioning the dorsolateral fasciculus of the decerebellate animal abolishes cerebellar dyskinesia.[23] The paresis resulting from the lesion in the dorsolateral fasciculus may be so severe, however, that the motor deficit from the cerebellar lesion cannot appear. This notion is consistent with studies showing that dyskinesia and tremor after cerebellar ablation actually can be increased by sectioning the pyramidal tract.[45] Thus, cerebellar dyskinesia depends upon the function of extrapyramidal projections, or, more likely, upon both pyramidal and extrapyramidal pathways. Cerebellar dyskinesia does not depend upon the myotatic reflex, because ataxic limb movements occur in the deafferented limbs of animals with cerebellar lesions.[39, 58] Nevertheless, peripheral inputs and spinal reflexes can modify abnormalities of ballistic limb movements following dentate lesions.[104, 115]

Interrupting certain afferent projections to the cerebellum leads to motor abnormalities comparable to those observed following ablation of the cerebellum. Lesions of the olivocerebellar pathway, for example, yield deficits similar to those following ablation of the lateral cerebellar nuclei.[104] In addition, lesions of the brachium pontis duplicate many of the neurologic deficits resulting from ablation of this cerebellar region.[34] The actions of the pontocerebellar fibers can affect the excitability of the cerebellar output projections, as shown by the fact that stimulating the brachium pontis evokes contractions of individual flexor and extensor muscles.[84]

CEREBELLAR ABLATION IN PRIMATES AND SUBPRIMATES

The differences in the effects of cerebellar ablations between primates and subprimates result from at least two factors: 1) the difference in the output projections from the vermis of the anterior lobe and 2) the predominance of projections from the cerebellar hemispheres in primates. The most striking difference in the deficits in primates and subprimates relates to the neurologic disorder following ablation of the cerebellar anterior lobe. In subprimates the disorder duplicates the acute effects of total cerebellectomy, including the marked opisthotonos and extensor rigidity. In primates the disorder consists only of a mild ataxia. This striking difference results from the fact that the subprimate cerebellum contains a large direct projection between the cerebellar anterior lobe and the vestibular nuclei, the corticovestibular projection. The marked hypertonus in subprimates results from interrupting the tonic inhibitory action of this projection on the neurons of origin of the vestibulospinal and reticulospinal tracts. A comparably developed projection from the cerebellar cortex to the vestibular nuclei has not been found in primates.

The output projections of the cerebellar hemispheres in primates are developed more fully than in subprimates and provide a much greater proportion of the total cerebellar output. Thus total cerebellar ablation in primates interrupts predominantly the output pathways from the lateral cerebellum. As a consequence, complete ablation in primates produces deficits which are comparable to the effects of ablations restricted to the cerebellar hemispheres in subprimates.[13]

REFERENCES

1. ARING, C. D., AND FULTON, J. F.: *Relation of the cerebrum to the cerebellum. II. Cerebellar tremor in the monkey and its absence after removal of the principal excitable areas of the cerebral cortex (area 4 and 6a, upper part). III. Accentuation of cerebellar tremor following lesions of the premotor area (area 6a, upper part).* Arch. Neurol. Psychiat. 35:439, 466, 1936.

2. BANTLI, H., BLOEDEL, J. R., AND TOLBERT, D. L.: *Activation of neurons in the cerebellar nuclei and ascending reticular formation by stimulation of the cerebellar surface.* J. Neurosurg. 45:539, 1976.

3. BATINI, C., MORUZZI, G., AND POMPEIANO, O.: *Origine e meccanismi di compensazione dei fenomeni dinamici di Luciani.* R. C. Accad. Lincei. 21:474, 1956.

4. BATINI, C., MORUZZI, G., AND POMPEIANO, O.: *Componenti labirintiche ed estralabirintiche nelle manifestazioni spastiche del gatto decerebrato e decerebellato.* R. C. Accad. Lincei. 21:328, 1956.

5. BATINI, C., MORUZZI, G., AND POMPEIANO, O.: *Cerebellar release phenomena.* Arch. Ital. Biol. 95:71, 1957.

6. BATINI, C., AND POMPEIANO, O.: *Chronic fastigial lesions and their compensation in the cat.* Arch. Ital. Biol. 95:147, 1957.

7. BATINI, C., AND POMPEIANO, O.: *Opposi effetti esercitati sulla rigidità da decerebrazione dalle porzioni rostro-mediali e rostro-laterali del nucleo del tetto.* Bull. Soc. Ital. Biol. Sper. 32:1452, 1956.

8. BATINI, C., AND POMPEIANO, O.: *Effects of rostro-medial and rostro-lateral fastigial lesions on decerebrate rigidity.* Arch. Ital. Biol. 96:315, 1958.

9. BAUMGARTEN, R., VON, AND MOLLICA, A.: *Der Einfluss sensibler Reizung auf die Entladungsfrequenz kleinhirnabhängiger Reticulariszellen.* Arch. Ges. Physiol. 259:79, 1954.

10. BAUMGARTEN, R., VON, MOLLICA, A., AND MORUZZI, G.: *Modulierung der Entladungsfrequenz einzelner Zellen der Substantia reticularis durch corticofugale and cerebelläre Impulse.* Pflügers Arch. 259:56, 1954.

11. BOTTERELL, E. H., AND FULTON, J. F.: *Functional localization in the cerebellum of primates. I. Unilateral section of the peduncles.* J. Comp. Neurol. 69:31, 1938.

12. BOTTERELL, E. H., AND FULTON, J. F.: *Functional localization in the cerebellum of primates. II. Lesions of the midline structures (vermis) and deep nuclei* J. Comp. Neurol. 69:47, 1938.

13. BOTTERELL, E. H., AND FULTON, J. F.: *Functional localization in the cerebellum of primates. III. Lesions of hemispheres (neocerebellum).* J. Comp. Neurol. 69:63, 1938.

14. BREMER, F.: *Contribution à l'étude de la physiologie du cervelet: La fonction inhibitrice du paléo-cerebellum.* Arch. Internat. Physiol. 19:189, 1922.

15. BREMER, F.: *Le cervelet,* in Roger, G. H., and Binet, L. (eds.): *Traité de physiologie normale et pathologique.* Masson, Paris, 1935, Vol. 10, Part 1, pp. 39–134.

16. BROOKS, V. B., ADRIEN, J., AND DYKES, R. W.: *Task-related discharge of neurons in motor cortex and effects of dentate cooling.* Brain Res. 40:85, 1972.

17. BROOKS, V. B., KOZLOVSKAYA, I. B., ATKIN, A. ET AL.: *Effects of cooling dentate nucleus on tracking-task performance in monkeys.* J. Neurophysiol. 36:974, 1973.

18. BÜRGI, S.: *Reizung und Ausschaltung des Brachium conjunctivum. I. Experimenteller Teil.* Helv. Physiol. Pharmacol. Acta 1:359, 1943.

19. BÜRGI, S.: *Reizung und Ausschaltung des Brachium conjunctivum. II. Bindearme and Kleinhirnfunktion.* Helv. Physiol. Pharmacol. Acta 1:467, 1943.

20. CALMA, I., AND KIDD, G. L.: *The action of the anterior lobe of the cerebellum on alpha motoneurones.* J. Physiol. 149:626, 1959.

21. CAMIS, M.: *Nuove osservasioni sui movimenti deambulatori: L'azione delle basse temperature sul cervelletto.* Boll. Soc. Med. Parma 15:54, 1922.

22. CAMIS, M.: *Recherches sur le mécanisme central des mouvements de deambulation.* Arch. Internat. Physiol. 20:340, 1923.

23. CARPENTER, M. B., AND CORRELL, J. W.: *Spinal pathways mediating cerebellar dyskinesia in Rhesus monkey.* J. Neurophysiol. 24:534, 1961.

24. CARREA, R. M. E., AND METTLER, F. A.: *Physiologic consequences following extensive removals of the cerebellar cortex and deep cerebellar nuclei and effect of secondary cerebral ablations in the primate.* J. Comp. Neurol. 87:169, 1947.

25. CARREA, R. M. E., AND METTLER, F. A.: *Function of the primate brachium conjunctivum and related structures.* J. Comp. Neurol. 102:151, 1955.

26. CHAMBERS, W. W., AND SPRAGUE, J. M.: *Functional localization in the cerebellum. I. Organization in longitudinal cortico-nuclear zones and their contribution to the control of posture, both extrapyramidal and pyramidal.* J. Comp. Neurol. 103:105, 1955.

27. COHEN, D., CHAMBERS, W. W., AND SPRAGUE, J. M.: *Experimental study of the efferent projections from the cerebellar nuclei to the brainstem of the cat.* J. Comp. Neurol. 109:233, 1958.

28. CONRAD, B., AND BROOKS, V. B.: *Effects of dentate cooling on rapid alternating arm movements.* J. Neurophysiol. 37:792, 1974.

29. CONRAD, B., AND BROOKS, V. B.: *Cerebellar movement disorders in monkeys: comparison of rapidly alternating and slower target movements during cooling of the dentate nucleus.* J. Neurol. 209:165, 1975.

30. COPACK, P. B., LIEBERMAN, J. S., AND GILMAN, S.: *Alpha motoneuron responses to natural stimuli in decerebellate cats.* Brain Res. 95:75, 1975.

31. DENNY-BROWN, D.: *The Cerebral Control of Movement.* Charles C Thomas, Springfield, Ill., 1966.

32. DENNY-BROWN, D., ECCLES, J. C., AND LIDDELL, E. G. T.: *Observations on electrical stimulation of the cerebellar cortex.* Proc. Roy. Soc. London SB 104:518, 1929.

33. DeVITO, R. V., BRUSA, A., AND ARDUINI, A.: *Cerebellar and vestibular influences on Deitersian units.* J. Neurophysiol. 19:241, 1956.

34. DIMANCESCU, M. D., AND SCHWARTZMAN, R. J.: *Cerebello-pontine influence on the motor system: A functional and anatomical study following section of the brachium pontis in trained macaque monkeys.* Trans. Am. Neurol. Assoc. 98:33, 1973.

35. DOW, R. S., AND MORUZZI, G.: *The Physiology and Pathology of the Cerebellum.* University of Minnesota Press, Minneapolis, 1958.

36. FULTON, J. F., AND CONNOR, G.: *The physiological basis of three major cerebellar syndromes.* Trans. Am. Neurol. Assoc. 65:53, 1939.

37. FULTON, J. F., AND DOW, R. S.: *The cerebellum: A summary of functional localization.* Yale J. Biol. Med. 10:89, 1937.

38. GIDLÖF, A.: *Intracellular aspects of 'release' phenomena in α-extensor motoneurones of the cat.* Acta Physiol. Scand. 68 (Suppl.) 277:58, 1968.

39. GILMAN, S., CARR, D., AND HOLLENBERG, J.: *Kinematic effects of deafferentation and cerebellar ablation.* Brain 99:311, 1976.

40. GILMAN, S., AND EBEL, H. C.: *Fusimotor neuron responses to natural stimuli as a function of prestimulus fusimotor activity in decerebellate cats.* Brain Res. 21:367, 1970.

41. GILMAN, S., AND McDONALD, W. I.: *Cerebellar facilitation of muscle spindle activity.* J. Neurophysiol. 30:1494, 1967.

42. GILMAN, S., AND McDONALD, W. I.: *Relation of afferent fiber conduction velocity to reactivity of muscle spindle receptors after cerebellectomy.* J. Neurophysiol. 30:1513, 1967.

43. GRANIT, R., HENATSCH, H. D., AND STEG, G.: *Tonic and phasic ventral horn cells differentiated by post-tetanic potentiation in cat extensors.* Acta Physiol. Scand. 37:114, 1956.

44. GRANIT, R., HOLMGREN, B., AND MERTON, P. A.: *The two routes for excitation of muscle and their subservience to the cerebellum.* J. Physiol. 130:213, 1955.

45. GROWDON, J. H., CHAMBERS, H. W., AND LIU, C. N.: *An experimental study of cerebellar dyskinesia in the rhesus monkey.* Brain 90:603, 1967.

46. HAMPSON, J. L., HARRISON, C. R., AND WOOLSEY, C. M.: *Cerebro-cerebellar projections and*

154

the somatotopic localization of motor function in the cerebellum. Res. Publ. Assoc. Nervous Mental Dis. 30:299, 1952.

47. HIGGINS, D. C., AND GLASER, G. H.: *Stretch responses during chronic cerebellar ablation. A study of reflex instability.* J. Neurophysiol. 27:49, 1964.

48. HIGGINS, D. C., AND GLASER, G. H.: *Recovery of motor stability after cerebellectomy.* Neurol. 15:794, 1965.

49. HOLMES, G.: *The Croonian Lectures on the clinical symptoms of cerebellar disease and their interpretation. Lecture IV.* Lancet 2:111, 1922.

50. HORVATH, F. E., ATKIN, A., KOZLOVSKAYA, I. ET AL.: *Effects of cooling the dentate nucleus on alternating bar-pressing performance in monkey.* Intl. J. Neurol. 7:252, 1970.

51. ITO, M., KAWAI, N., AND UDO, M.: *The origin of cerebellar-induced inhibition of Deiters' neurones. III. Localization of the inhibitory zone.* Exp. Brain Res. 4:310, 1968.

52. ITO, M., AND YOSHIDA, M.: *The cerebellar-evoked monosynaptic inhibition of Deiters' neurones.* Experientia 20:515, 1964.

53. ITO, M., AND YOSHIDA, M.: *The origin of cerebellar-induced inhibition of Deiters' neurones. I. Monosynaptic initiation of the inhibitory postsynaptic potentials.* Exp. Brain Res. 2:330, 1966.

54. ITO, M., YOSHIDA, M., AND OBATA, K.: *Monosynaptic inhibition of the intracellular nuclei induced from the cerebellar cortex.* Experientia 20:575, 1964.

55. JANSEN, J., AND BRODAL, A.: *Experimental studies on the intrinsic fibers of the cerebellum. II. The cortico-nuclear projection.* J. Comp. Neurol. 73:267, 1940.

56. JANSEN, J., AND BRODAL, A.: *Experimental studies on the intrinsic fibers of the cerebellum. The cortico-nuclear projection in the rabbit and the monkey (Macacus rhesus).* Oslo (Avh): Norske Vid-Akad, I. Mat. Naturv. K. 3:1, 1942.

57. LINDSLEY, D. B., SCHREINER, L. H., AND MAGOUN, H. W.: *An electromyographic study of spasticity.* J. Neurophysiol. 12:197, 1949.

58. LIU, C. N., AND CHAMBERS, W. W.: *A study of cerebellar dyskinesia in the bilaterally deafferented forelimbs of the monkey (Macaca mulatta and Macaca speciosa).* Acta Neurobiol. Exp. 31: 263, 1971.

59. LLINÁS, R.: *Mechanisms of supraspinal actions upon spinal cord activities. Differences between reticular and cerebellar inhibitory actions upon alpha extensor motoneurons.* J. Neurophysiol. 27:1117, 1964.

60. LOWENTHAL, M., AND HORSLEY, V.: *On the relations between the cerebellar and other centers (namely cerebral and spinal) with special reference to the action of antagonistic muscles.* Proc. Roy. Soc. London 61:20, 1897.

61. LUCIANI, L.: *Il cervelletto: Nuovi studi di fisiologia normale e pathologica.* LeMonnier, Florence, 1891.

62. LUCIANI, L.: *Muscular and nervous system,* in *Human Physiology, Vol. 3.* Macmillan, London, 1911–1917.

63. MAFFEI, L., AND POMPEIANO, O.: *Analisi delle risposte posturali alla stimolazione del lobulo paramediano e dei suoi "relays" nucleocerebellari nel gatto decerebrato.* Boll. Soc. Ital. Biol. Sper. 37:918, 1961.

64. MAFFEI, L., AND POMPEIANO, O.: *Inversione degli effetti die stimolazione del lobulo paramediano prodotta dall distruzione parziale del nucleo interposito.* Boll. Soc. Ital. Biol. Sper. 37:921, 1961.

65. MAFFEI, L., AND POMPEIANO, O.: *Cerebellar control of flexor motoneurons. An analysis of the postural responses to stimulation of the paramedian lobule in the decerebrate cat.* Arch. Ital. Biol. 100:476, 1962.

66. MASSION, J.: *The mammalian red nucleus.* Physiol. Rev. 47:383, 1967.

67. MCLEOD, J. G., AND VAN DER MEULEN, J. P.: *Effect of cerebellar ablation on the H reflex in the cat.* Arch. Neurol. 16:421, 1967.

68. MOLLICA, A., MORUZZI, G., AND NAQUET, R.: *Décharges réticulaires induites par la pólarisation du cervelet: Leurs rapports avec le tonus postural et la réaction d'éveil.* Electroencephal. Clin. Neurophysiol. 5:571, 1953.

69. MORUZZI, G.: *Ricerche sperimentali e una nuova ipotesi sulla natura del rimbalzo cerebellare.* Boll. Soc. Ital. Biol. Sper. 24:397, 1948.

70. MORUZZI, G.: *Nuove ricerche sugli effetti paleocerebellari aumentatori del tono.* Boll. Soc. Ital. Biol. Sper. 24:753, 1948.

71. MORUZZI, G.: *L'irradiazióne degli effetti paleocerebellari inibitori del tono.* Boll. Soc. Ita!. Biol. Sper. 24:755, 1948.

72. MORUZZI, G.: *Le vie efferenti per l'inibizione paleocerebellare del tono.* Boll. Soc. Ital. Biol. Sper. 24:756, 1948.

73. MORUZZI, G.: *Nuove osservazioni intorno agli effetti della stimolazione del cervelletto sul sistema nervoso autonomo.* Boll. Soc. Ital. Biol. Sper. 24:752, 1948.

74. MORUZZI, G.: *L'action du paléocervelet sur le tonus postural.* J. Physiol. Paris 41:371, 1949.

75. MORUZZI, G.: *Problems in Cerebellar Physiology.* Charles C Thomas, Springfield, Ill., 1950.

76. MORUZZI, G.: *Effects at different frequencies of cerebellar stimulation upon postural tonus and myotatic reflexes.* Electroencephal. Clin. Neurophysiol. 2:463, 1950.

77. MORUZZI, G., AND POMPEIANO, O.: *Influenze cerebellari crociate sul tono posturale.* R. C. Accad. Lincei 18:420, 1955.

78. MORUZZI, G., AND POMPEIANO, O.: *Crossed fastigial atonia.* Experientia (Basel) 12:35, 1956.

79. MORUZZI, G., AND POMPEIANO, O.: *Crossed fastigial influence on decerebrate rigidity.* J. Comp. Neurol. 106:371, 1956.

80. MORUZZI, G., AND POMPEIANO, O.: *Inhibitory mechanisms underlying the collapse of decerebrate rigidity after unilateral fastigial lesions.* J. Comp. Neurol. 107:1, 1957.

81. MORUZZI, G., AND POMPEIANO, O.: *Effects of vermal stimulation after fastigial lesions.* Arch. Ital. Biol. 95:31, 1957.

82. MUNK, H.: *Über die Funktionen des Kleinhirns.* Akad. Wissensch. 1906, pp. 443–480; 1907, pp. 16–32; 1908, pp. 294–396.

83. MURPHY, M. G., AND O'LEARY, J. L.: *Hanging and climbing functions in raccoon and sloth after total cerebellectomy.* Arch. Neurol. 28:111, 1973.

84. PERCIAVALLE, V., SANTANGELO, F., SAPIENZA, S. ET AL.: *Motor effects produced by microstimulation of brachium pontis in the cat.* Brain Res. 126:557, 1977.

85. POIRIER, L. J., LAFLEUR, J., DELEAN, J. ET́AL.: *Physiopathology of the cerebellum in the monkey. Part 2. Motor disturbances associated with partial and complete destruction of cerebellar structures.* J. Neurol. Sci. 22:491, 1974.

86. POLLOCK, L. J., AND DAVIS, L.: *Studies in decerebration. I. A method of decerebration.* Arch. Neurol. Psychiat. 10:391, 1923.

87. POLLOCK, L. J., AND DAVIS, L.: *The influence of the cerebellum upon the reflex activities of the decerebrate animal.* Brain 50:277, 1927.

88. POLLOCK, L. J., AND DAVIS, L.: *Studies in decerebration. V. The tonic activities of a decerebrate animal exclusive of the neck and labyrinthine reflexes.* Am. J. Physiol. 92:625, 1930.

89. POLLOCK, L. J., AND DAVIS, L.: *The reflex activities of a decerebrate animal.* J. Comp. Neurol. 50:377, 1930.

90. POLLOCK, L. J., AND DAVIS, L.: *Studies in decerebration. VI. The effect of deafferentation upon decerebrate rigidity.* Am. J. Physiol. 98:47, 1931.

91. POMPEIANO, O.: *Responses to electrical stimulation of the intermediate part of the cerebellar anterior lobe in the decerebrate cat.* Arch. Ital. Biol. 96:330, 1958.

92. POMPEIANO, O.: *Organizzazione somatotopica delle risposte flessorie alla stimolazione elettrica del nucleo interposito nel gatto decerebrato.* Arch. Sci. Biol. 43:163, 1959.

93. POMPEIANO, O.: *Somatotopic organization of the postural responses to stimulation and destruction of the caudal part of the fastigial nucleus.* Arch. Ital. Biol. 100:259, 1962.

94. POMPEIANO, O.: *Functional organization of the cerebellar projections to the spinal cord,* in Fox, C. A., and Snyder, R. S. (eds.): *The Cerebellum.* Prog. Brain Res. 25:282, 1967.

95. POMPEIANO, O.: *Cerebellar control of the vestibular pathways to spinal motoneurons and primary afferents.* Prog. Brain Res. 37:391, 1972.

96. POMPEIANO, O., AND COTTI, E.: *Risposte di unita deitersiane alla stimolazione galvanica localizzata della corteccia cerebellare vermiana del "lobus anterior."* Boll. Soc. Ital. Biol. Sper. 35: 383, 1959.

97. POMPEIANO, O., AND COTTI, E.: *Localizzazione topografica delle risposte deitersiane alla po-*

larizzazione della corteccia cerebellare vermiana del "lobus anterior." Boll. Soc. Ital. Biol. Sper. 35:385, 1959.

98. POMPEIANO, O., AND COTTI, E.: *Analisi microelettrodica delle proiezioni cerebellodeitersiane.* Arch. Sci. Biol. 43:57, 1959.

99. POMPEIANO, O., AND COTTI, E.: *Effetti della stimolazione corticocerebellare sull' attivitá di singole unitá deitersiane provocata da stimolazione libirintiche.* Boll. Soc. Ital. Biol. Sper. 36: 303, 1960.

100. RADEMAKER, G. G. J.: *Das Stehen: Statische Reaktionen, Gleichgewichtsreaktionen und Muskeltonus unter besonderer Berücksichtigung ihres Verhaltens bei kleinhirnlosen Tieren.* Springer, Berlin, 1931.

101. RANISH, N. A., AND SOECHTING, J. F.: *Studies on the control of some simple motor tasks. Effects of thalamic and red nuclei lesions.* Brain Res. 102:339, 1976.

102. ROTHMANN, M.: *Die Funktion des Mittellappens des Kleinhirns.* Monatsschr. Psychiat. Neurol. 34:389, 1913.

103. SCHEIBEL, M., SCHEIBEL, A., MOLLICA, A. ET AL.: *Convergence and interaction of afferent impulses on single units of reticular formation.* J. Neurophysiol. 18:309, 1955.

104. SOECHTING, J. F., RANISH, N. A., PALMINTERI, R. ET AL.: *Changes in a motor pattern following cerebellar and olivary lesions in the squirrel monkey.* Brain Res. 105:21, 1976.

105. SPRAGUE, J. M., AND CHAMBERS, W. W.: *Regulation of posture in intact and decerebrate cat. I. Cerebellum, reticular formation, vestibular nuclei.* J. Neurophysiol. 16:451, 1953.

106. SPRAGUE, J. M., AND CHAMBERS, W. W.: *Control of posture by reticular formation and cerebellum in the intact, anesthetized and unanesthetized and in the decerebrated cat.* Am. J. Physiol. 176:52, 1954.

107. STELLA, G.: *Sul meccanismo della rigidita da decerebrazione in arti deafferentati.* Atti Soc. Med. Chir. (Padua) 23:5, 1944.

108. STELLA, G.: *Influenza del cervelletto sulla rigidita da decerebrazione.* Atti Soc. Med. Chir. (Padua) 23:17, 1944.

109. STELLA, G., ZATTI, P., AND SPERTI, L.: *Decerebrate rigidity in forelegs after deafferentation and spinal transection in dogs with chronic lesions in different parts of the cerebellum.* Am. J. Physiol. 181:230, 1955.

110. TERZIAN, H., AND TERZUOLO, C.: *Le componenti automatiche e riflesse del tono posturale.* Arch. Fisiol. 54:37, 1954.

111. TERZUOLO, C. A.: *Cerebellar inhibitory and excitatory actions upon spinal extensor motoneurons.* Arch. Ital. Biol. 97:316, 1959.

112. TERZUOLO, C. A., AND TERZIAN, H.: *Sul meccanismo della rigiditá da decerebrazione in arti anteriori cronicamente deafferentati.* Boll. Soc. Ital. Biol. Sper. 27:1317, 1951.

113. TERZUOLO, C. A., AND TERZIAN, H.: *Riflessi di magnus e tono posturale in arti sottoposti a deafferentazione acuta o cronica.* Boll. Soc. Ital. Biol. Sper. 27:1319, 1951.

114. TERZUOLO, C. A., AND TERZIAN, H.: *Cerebellar increase of postural tonus after deafferentation and labyrinthectomy.* J. Neurophysiol. 16:551, 1953.

115. TERZUOLO, C. A., AND VIVIANI, P.: *Parameters of motion and EMG activities during some simple motor task in normal subjects and cerebellar patients,* in Cooper, I. S., Riklan, M., and Snider, R. S. (eds.): *The Cerebellum, Epilepsy and Behavior.* Plenum Press, New York, 1974, pp. 173–215.

116. TOLBERT, D. L., BANTLI, H., AND BLOEDEL, J. R.: *Anatomical and physiological evidence for a cerebellar nucleocortical projection in the cat.* Neurosci. 1:205, 1976.

117. TOLBERT, D. L., BANTLI, H., AND BLOEDEL, J. R.: *The intracerebellar nucleocortical projection in a primate.* Exp. Brain Res. 30:425, 1977.

118. TOLBERT, D. L., BANTLI, H., AND BLOEDEL, J. R.: *Multiple branching of cerebellar efferent projections in cats.* Exp. Brain Res. 31:305, 1978.

119. TOYAMA, K., TSUKAHARA, N., KOSAKA, K. ET AL.: *Synaptic excitation of red nucleus neurones by fibres from interpositus nucleus.* Exp. Brain Res. 11:187, 1970.

120. TSUKAHARA, N., TOYAMA, K., AND KOSAKA, K.: *Electrical activity of the red nucleus neurons investigated with intracellular microelectrodes.* Exp. Brain Res. 4:18, 1967.

121. UNO, M., KOZLOVSKAYA, I. B., AND BROOKS, V. B.: *Effects of cooling interposed nuclei on tracking-task performance in monkeys.* J. Neurophysiol. 36:996, 1973.

157

122. VAN DER MEULEN, J. P., AND GILMAN, S.: *Recovery of muscle spindle activity in cats after cerebellar ablation.* J. Neurophysiol. 28:943, 1965.

123. WALKER, A. E., AND BOTTERELL, E. H.: *The syndrome of the superior cerebellar peduncle in the monkey.* Brain 60:329, 1937.

124. WIRTH, F. P., AND O'LEARY, J. L.: *Locomotor behavior of decerebellated arboreal mammals — monkey and raccoon.* J. Comp. Neurol. 157:53, 1974.

125. YU, J.: *The pathway mediating ipsilateral limb hyperflexion after cerebellar paravermal cortical ablation or cooling in cats.* Exp. Neurol. 36:549, 1972.

126. YU, J., TARNECKI, R., CHAMBERS, W. W. ET AL.: *Mechanisms mediating ipsilateral limb hyperflexion after cerebellar paravermal cortical ablation or cooling.* Exp. Neurol. 38:144, 1973.

CHAPTER 8

Cerebellar Hypotonia and Tremor

CEREBELLAR HYPOTONIA

Structures Involved

Relation of the Cerebellum to the Cerebral Hemispheres

Gordon Holmes[72] in his Croonian lectures of 1922 discussed the physiologic significance of the symptoms and signs that result from injury of the cerebellum. He devoted his first lecture to hypotonia, the disturbance of muscle tone produced by destructive cerebellar lesions in the human. His definition of muscle tone was " . . . that slight constant tension characteristic of healthy muscle, owing to which the limbs when handled or moved passively offer a definite resistance to displacement." He concluded that lesions of the cerebellum consistently decrease the resistance to passive stretch of the limb muscles. He stated that a series of other symptoms and signs can be attributed directly to cerebellar hypotonia: abnormal attitudes, excessive associated movements, pendular deep tendon reflexes, static tremor, and the rebound phenomenon. He also concluded that hypotonia contributes to the "clonic and discontinuous character of movements met with in cerebellar disease, and to the asthenia and hypermetria that follow cerebellar injury."

Holmes concluded that hypotonia is one of the fundamental disturbances in posture and movement resulting from cerebellar disease. His view was compatible with the conclusions of Luciani[94] who studied the effects of cerebellar lesions in animals a couple of decades earlier. From his studies on the effects of extensive cerebellar ablation in the dog and monkey, Luciani concluded that "atonia," as evidenced by a decrease in the supporting reaction of the limb extensor muscles, was one of the cardinal symptoms of cerebellar deficiency in experimental animals. Subsequent studies have shown that the hypotonia of Holmes and the atonia of Luciani are analogous disturbances, representing disorders of the proprioceptive control of posture. The disturbances present differently because of differences in the nervous systems of the species studied.

In synthesizing the results of cerebellar ablations in primates and subprimates, Bremer[19] pointed out that various regions of the cerebellum have different functions in the governance of posture and movement. He concluded that the lateral regions of the cerebellum, the neocerebellum, interact chiefly with the cerebral cortex in regulating posture and movement. In contrast, the midline cerebellum (the paleocerebellum) interacts with ascending and descending spinal pathways in regulating equilibrium and truncal coordination. Bremer also concluded that the output of the lateral regions of the cerebellum has a facilitatory action on cerebral cortical neurons.

Many early studies support Bremer's view. In a major discovery, Rossi[101] demonstrated that stimulation of the lateral cerebellum reduced the stimulus intensity needed to evoke movements by stimulating the cerebral cortex. Although similar observations had been made previously,[93] Rossi clearly described the importance of the lateral region of the cerebellum for movements evoked from the cerebral cortex. In expanding on the early experiments of Russell[103] and Luciani,[94, 95] Rossi[102] found that cerebellar ablation increases the threshold for activating movements by cerebral cortical stimulation in cats. This finding was confirmed in other species.[43] Recent electrophysiologic studies, reviewed in Chapter 7, support the view of these early investigators that the dentate and interposed output projections exert excitatory actions on cerebral cortical neurons.

The output of the neocerebellum can increase the excitability of alpha motoneurons in the spinal cord. This finding is consistent with the observation that hypotonia is a dominant abnormality after cerebellar ablation in primates, the animals in which the cerebellar hemispheres have become the largest portion of the cerebellum. Hypotonia is particularly apparent after cerebellar ablation in the monkey and baboon[15, 17] and is even more remarkable in the chimpanzee.[52] Interrupting the output from the dentate nucleus is most essential to the production of hypotonia. Consequently, hypotonia does not result from lesions restricted to the fastigial, globose, or emboliform nuclei.[30]

Segmental Reflexes Responsible for Postural Tone

Abnormalities of the control systems in the spinal cord that regulate the sensitivity of the muscle spindle receptors are responsible for the hypotonia resulting from cerebellar ablation.[54] The intrafusal fibers of mammalian striated muscle contain specialized types of muscle fibers and nerve endings. There are two types of receptors within the muscle spindle, nuclear bag and nuclear chain.[9, 18, 50, 108, 114] Two types of nuclear bag receptors have been identified and currently are termed bag_1 and bag_2 fibers.[7] These fibers differ with respect to length, diameter, histochemical profile, and ultrastructure, with the bag_2 fiber showing characteristics intermediate between bag_1 and chain fibers.[11] Primary afferent nerve fibers from spindles arise from spiral endings in the equatorial region of bag_1, bag_2, and chain fibers and form the large diameter (12 to 20 micron) group Ia afferents.[6, 9, 18, 35] Secondary afferent nerve fibers arise chiefly from nuclear chain muscle fibers, though many also originate on bag_1 and bag_2 fibers.[6, 12, 18] The secondary afferents, located on the myotube or polar regions of the muscle fiber, form the small diameter (4 to 12 micron) group II nerve fibers. In the absence of motor innervation, there are striking differences in the responses of primary and secondary afferent endings to muscle stretch.[13, 33, 34, 71] Changes in the impulse activity of primary afferents generally reflect changes in the rate of muscle stretch, whereas the activity of secondary afferents reflects principally the length of the muscle when ramp and hold stimuli are employed.[97]

The motor fibers innervating muscle spindles terminate either as endplates or as diffuse (trail) endings.[10, 18] Both types of endings are terminations of gamma efferent fibers called "gamma plates" (γ_1 endings of Boyd) or "gamma trails" (γ_2), respectively.[66] The motor fibers innervating the muscle spindles have been termed "fusimotor" fibers, a term coined by Hunt and Paintal[75] to signify intrafusal innervation regardless of their diameter.

The output of the fusimotor neurons alters the sensitivity of the muscle spindle receptors. Two types of fusimotor fibers, dynamic and static, have been identified by examining the effects of stimulating individual fibers on the responses of spindle endings during phasic or tonic extension of muscle.[96] Both types of fusimotor fiber affect the responses of primary afferents.[73, 74] Dynamic fusimotor fibers enhance the responses of the spindle primary endings during phasic stretch of muscle, but have little effect when muscle length remains constant. Static fusimotor fibers increase the firing rate of spindle primary endings when the muscle is kept at a fixed length but fail to increase the response to phasic extension of the muscle.[14, 22, 77, 96, 97] The major effect of both static and dynamic fusimotor action upon primary afferents is to regulate the sensitivity of the primary ending to stretching for all amplitudes of movement.[73, 74] The responses of muscle spindle secondary endings to ramp and hold stimuli are affected by static fusimotor fibers but not by dynamic fusimotor fibers, except for the few secondary endings that show some sensitivity to the rate of change of muscle length (dynamic sensitivity).[2, 3, 37, 38] Fusimotor stimulation actually decreases the responses of secondary afferents to sinusoidal muscle extension at low frequency.[39] Dynamic fusimotor fibers terminate principally in the "gamma plate" endings.[11] Dynamic effects result chiefly from activation of the bag$_1$ intrafusal muscle fiber.[5, 11, 51] Static fusimotor fibers terminate mostly in the "gamma trail" endings.[11] Static fusimotor effects result chiefly from activation of the bag$_2$ and chain intrafusal fibers.[5, 11, 51]

Effects of Muscle Spindle Receptors on the Excitability of Alpha Motoneurons

The activation of primary endings by muscle stretch excites monosynaptically the motoneurons innervating the muscle from which these afferents originate as well as some synergistic muscles.[45, 85, 92] Motoneurons innervating antagonistic muscles are inhibited via a disynaptic arc.[20, 49] A large proportion of spindle primary afferents in a hindlimb extensor muscle of the intact, lightly anesthetized cat[61] or monkey[54] discharges even in the absence of applied stretch (i.e., with muscle at its shortest natural length). In part, this is the consequence of the tonic action of fusimotor neurons[78] on the sensitivity of the muscle spindle receptors.[69]

Activation of muscle spindle secondary endings has been thought to excite polysynaptically the motoneurons innervating flexor muscles and inhibit those innervating extensor muscles, regardless of the muscle of origin of the secondary endings.[21, 83, 92] Recent evidence, however, indicates that some muscle spindle secondary afferents have monosynaptic connections with motoneurons similar to those of muscle spindle primary afferents.[105, 108] Golgi tendon organs, which have no direct efferent control from the central nervous system, are more sensitive to muscle twitch than to passive muscle extension. Centrally, activation of Golgi tendon organs inhibits motoneurons innervating the muscle from which they originate as well as the motoneurons of synergistic muscles.[46, 47, 66, 85]

Pathophysiology of Cerebellar Hypotonia

The first clue to the physiologic mechanism underlying cerebellar hypotonia came from studies of the effects of cerebellar ablation on the responses of muscle spindle afferents in the decerebrate cat.[68] Interrupting the output of the cerebellar anterior lobe by cooling or ablation decreases the responses of spindle afferents to maintained extension of the soleus muscle. Acute cerebellar ablation decreases the responses of spindle afferents to stretch of both flexor and extensor limb muscles.[110] In recently decerebellate cats, the responses to static extension of muscle spindle afferents in the medial gastrocnemius muscle are more depressed than the responses to other forms of natural stimuli.[61, 62] In chronically decerebellate cats, the spindle responses to stretch improve as the proprioceptive positive supporting reaction recovers, that is, as signs of Luciani's atonia diminish.[110] These studies, corroborated by recordings from fusimotor neurons,[53] demonstrate that cerebellar ablation results in decreased fusimotor activity which, in turn, decreases the responses of muscle spindle afferents.

Although the positive supporting reaction is abnormal in the decerebellate cat and fusimotor activity is decreased, hypotonia is not apparent. Instead, there is an enhancement of the resistance to passive manipulation of the limbs resulting from a marked increase in the excitability of alpha motoneurons. Accordingly, it is necessary to use a primate species to elucidate the mechanisms underlying cerebellar hypotonia.[54]

The most remarkable abnormality after complete cerebellar ablation in the macaque monkey is a severe disturbance of stance and gait. For the first several weeks after operation, the animal cannot stand or walk. Usually the animal lies prone on the floor with the head erect and all limbs closely flexed under the body. Any active movement of the trunk or limbs initiates a coarse, rhythmical tremor of the trunk and head. Movement is performed by ataxic movements of the limbs which are kept widely abducted. The abdomen drags along the floor except during brief running movements. If stood erect on all four limbs, the animal immediately collapses to the floor when passive support is discontinued. Passive manipulation of the limbs reveals a soft, plastic resistance in the flexor muscles, particularly at proximal joints, but clearly diminished resistance (hypotonia) occurs in the extensor muscles. The deep tendon reflexes of the ankles, knees, and wrists are slow and pendular. If the animal is suspended in air in the upright or prone position from the trunk or pelvis, the limbs remain flexed close to the body. In the second week after operation, with the animal held from the trunk suspended in air, a light contact with the plantar surface of the distal pads of the toes or fingers leads to a gradual extension of the limb. This response has been termed the magnet reaction.[100] Despite the sustained extension of the limb during the magnet reaction, however, the limb fails to sustain the weight of the body and, if stood on the extended limb, the animal collapses to the floor.

In time, usually by 6 to 8 weeks postoperatively, the supporting reactions of the limbs recover partially so that progressively the animal is able to sustain an upright posture, particularly when the side of the body remains in contact with a wall. Eventually the animal begins to walk in the erect position on all four limbs, developing a coarse tremor of trunk and limbs. As the proprioceptive positive supporting reactions of the limbs increase in intensity, the hypotonia of the limb extensor muscles progressively decreases. Correspondingly, the tendon reflexes become less pendular.

In the second month of the recovery process, denervation of the foot or hand by sectioning all nerves at the ankle or wrist abolishes the magnet reaction completely.[41, 42] If a single cutaneous nerve in the hand or foot is preserved, contact with the innervated area of skin still can evoke the magnet reaction. Interactions between the magnet and the positive supporting reactions can be studied in the chronically decerebellate monkey by sectioning the dorsal roots L3, 4 and 5. This procedure deafferents the quadriceps muscle but leaves intact the cutaneous innervation of the foot. The result is a depression of both the positive supporting and the magnet reactions for several weeks, preserving only sustained postures of flexion at the knees. Eventually, however, a strong magnet reaction reappears. Although sustained extension of the leg can be evoked, the amount of weight the knee can support is completely inadequate for maintaining the animal's body in the upright position.

The prolonged initial loss of positive supporting reactions after cerebellectomy results from a decrease of the responses to stretch of spindle afferents in limb muscles, particularly the antigravity extensor muscles.[42] This disorder is superimposed upon a series of preserved tactile reactions of opposite type: a magnet reaction that can evoke limb extension and a more dominant truncal contactual reaction that produces the predominant postures of limb flexion. In time, compensatory processes restore the spindle responses partially, so that the proprioceptive positive supporting reactions reappear and the hypotonia diminishes. The observation that a partially compensated positive supporting reaction in the hindlimb is depressed severely by deafferentiation of the knee musculature emphasizes the importance of the input to alpha motoneurons from muscle spindles in evoking the supporting reactions.

Study of the effects of hemicerebellar ablation in the monkey permits a quantitative comparison between the positive supporting responses and the resistance to

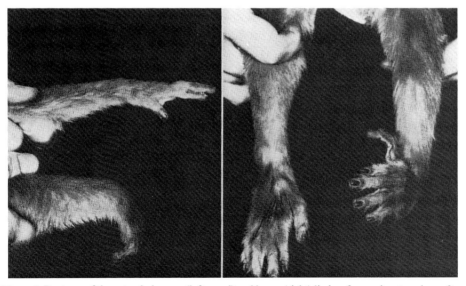

Figure 1. Postures of the extended upper (left panel) and lower (right) limbs of a monkey two days after right hemicerebellectomy, showing flexion of the right wrist and plantar flexion with pronation of the right ankle under the influence of gravity. (From Gilman,[54] with permission.)

163

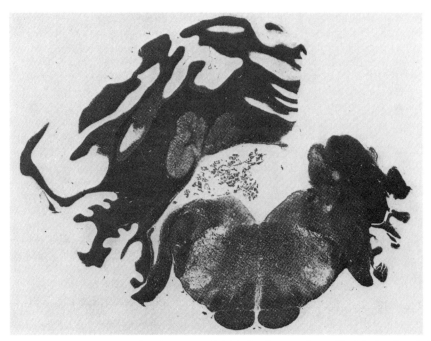

Figure 2. Histologic section showing the extent of the lesion in a monkey with right hemicerebellectomy of 99 days duration. Luxol fast blue stain. Other records from this animal appear in Figures 1 and 3. (From Gilman,[54] with permission.)

passive manipulation of the limbs on the two sides of the body.[54] In the animal with a hemicerebellar ablation of 1 to 2 days duration (Figs. 1 and 2), passive manipulation of the limbs reveals diminished resistance in the extensor muscles of the limbs on the side of the ablation. When the limbs are held extended in the horizontal position, the wrist and ankle flex under the influence of gravity more on the side of the ablation than on the opposite side (Fig. 1). The positive supporting reactions of the limbs are decreased to 20 percent of those on the opposite side in the first postoperative week, 50 percent in the fifth, and 75 percent in the eighth. The depressed excitability of stretch reflexes in the affected limbs can be measured with electromyographic recordings. These reveal that a greater degree of extension is required to initiate EMG activity on the side of the ablation compared

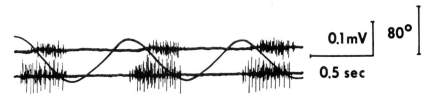

Figure 3. Electromyogram recorded from the right (upper trace) and left (lower) quadriceps muscles of a monkey two days after right hemicerebellar ablation. The middle trace records the rate, extent, and direction of passive movements of the lower limbs at the knees, downward deflection signifying flexion. Voltage and time calibration apply to both EMG tracings. Angular movement calibration applies to the middle trace indicating the extent of movement at the knees. Note that a greater degree of flexion is required to evoke EMG responses on the right than on the left. (From Gilman,[54] with permission.)

164

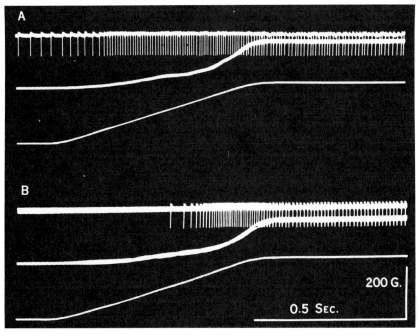

Figure 4. A, Control monkey lightly anesthetized with pentobarbital. Response to 24 mm/sec dynamic extension of a medial gastrocnemius muscle spindle afferent (conduction velocity 94.1 meters per second) recorded from a filament of S_1 dorsal root (upper trace). Gastrocnemius muscle extended 16 mm beyond starting length. Muscle tension and length shown in middle and lower traces, respectively. B, Five day decerebellate monkey lightly anesthetized with pentobarbital. Stretch response of a medial gastrocnemius muscle spindle primary afferent (conduction velocity 95.6 meters per second). Site and conditions of recording, rate and extent of muscle stretch as in A. Occurring at minimum length in the control animal, the afferent discharge increases soon after the stretch begins. In the decerebellate animal, discharge begins only after considerable (about 8.5 mm) stretch has been applied. (From Gilman,[54] with permission.)

with the opposite side (Fig. 3).[54] This abnormality lessens in a time course similar to that of the recovery of the positive supporting response. Both of these responses depend upon the integrity of the segmental stretch reflex. Thus their initial depression and their parallel recovery suggest that both result from a common abnormality, possibly a depression of spindle afferent responses, as had been suggested earlier.[42, 110]

Direct recordings of the responses of spindle afferents to extension of the gastrocnemius muscle in monkeys confirm that these responses are decreased after recent cerebellectomy (Figs. 4 and 5A).[54] Only the responses of spindle primaries are affected; the responses of spindle secondary afferents are essentially unchanged. The responses of muscle spindle primary afferents to various rates of muscle extension are similar to the reflex responses of motor units in electromyographic recordings to comparable stimuli. The conclusion is that the abnormal responses of spindle afferents are directly and possibly causally related to the abnormal responses recorded electromyographically and observed clinically. Thus, depressed sensitivity of the muscle spindles underlies the clinical hypotonia so characteristic of acute cerebellar lesions in higher apes and man.[52, 72]

Cerebellectomy affects chiefly the spindle primary afferents in the upper range

165

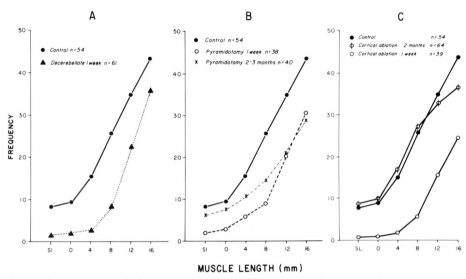

Figure 5. Graphs of mean discharge frequencies of medial gastrocnemius muscle spindle primary afferents (ordinate) as a function of muscle length (abscissa) in monkeys. A, Responses of control animals compared with those of animals decerebellate for 5 to 6 days. B, Responses of control animals compared with those of animals with bilateral medullary pyramidotomy of 4 to 7 days and of 2 to 3 months duration. C, Responses of control animals compared with those of animals with ablation of cortical areas 4 and 6 in the cerebral hemisphere opposite the side of recording one week and two months after operation. (A from Gilman,[54] B from Gilman et al.,[60] C from Gilman et al.,[58] with permission.)

of axonal conduction velocities,[61, 62] depressing either their responses to maintained stimuli or to changes in muscle length.[54] In addition, cerebellectomy decreases the initial increase of muscle tension induced by sinusoidal stretching of the ankle extensor muscles in decerebrate cats.[63] This latter effect can also be achieved without cerebellectomy by blocking fusimotor fibers with a local anesthetic agent.[64] The results indicate that cerebellar ablation leads to hypotonia and a reduction of the proprioceptive positive supporting reaction by decreasing the resting discharge of both static and dynamic fusimotor fibers, thus impairing the corresponding responses of the spindle primary afferents in extensor muscles. Indeed, direct recordings from fusimotor fibers in dissected peripheral nerves of cats have shown a decrease of resting discharge after cerebellectomy.[53] The depressed fusimotor units still respond to natural vestibular, cutaneous, or proprioceptive stimuli. These findings may be related to the abnormalities of coordinated movement of the decerebellate animal, but direct evidence for this assumption is lacking.

Central Pathways Involved in Hypotonia

A Cerebello-thalamo-corticospinal Circuit

Bremer[19] concluded that the paleocerebellum, through bulbospinal relays, tonically inhibits spinal neurons affecting extensor muscles involved in postural mechanisms, whereas the neocerebellum facilitates these neurons tonically by way of the cerebral cortex. In support of this hypothesis, Dow and Moruzzi[44] cited the similarity in the hypotonia resulting from cerebellar lesions[16, 17] and from medullary pyramidotomy in primates.[109] An excitatory projection from the neocerebellum to the cerebral cortex originates in the lateral cerebellar nuclei, the dentate and interposed nuclei. This projection involves neurons in the ventrolateral nucleus of the thalamus and the precentral motor cortex.

The notion that the interruption of a pathway extending from the cerebellum to the thalamus is important for the production of hypotonia is based on studies examining the effects of interrupting the projections from the lateral cerebellar nuclei to the ventrolateral nucleus. Sectioning the superior cerebellar peduncles reduces the responses to extension of gastrocnemius muscle spindle primary afferents.[61] Interrupting the function of the ventrolateral nucleus with a cryogenic technique also depresses the responses of muscle spindle afferents.[57, 89] Moreover, the decrease of muscle spindle responses resulting from these two procedures is virtually identical. Thus, the ventrolateral nucleus mediates a tonic facilitatory action of the neocerebellum on segmental fusimotor neurons, probably by means of a pathway involving the cerebral cortex. Depression of fusimotor activity from lesions of the ventrolateral nucleus is an important mechanism underlying the beneficial effects of ventrolateral nuclear lesions in humans with limb hypertonia from disorders such as Parkinson disease.

Precentral Cortex

The major projection of the ventrolateral nucleus terminates in the precentral cortex in subhuman primates and man. Ablation of this cortical region by the unilateral removal of areas 4 and 6 of Brodmann (Fig. 6) results initially in a contralateral hypotonic hemiplegia followed in 3 to 4 weeks by a hypertonic hemiplegia.[41, 58] The hypotonic hemiplegia is characterized by diminished resistance to passive manipulation at all joints of the affected opposite limbs, diminished to absent deep tendon reflexes, and absence of the oriented grasping, avoiding, and traction responses. Electromyographic recordings from hindlimb extensor muscles reveal a raised threshold for muscle discharge in response to passive dorsiflexion of the ankles on the paretic side relative to the control side.[58]

Developing hypertonia generally becomes apparent in the third week when a slight resistance to passive manipulation of the hemiparetic limbs becomes detectable and then increases progressively in intensity. By the fourth week a definite heightening of resistance to dorsiflexion of the ankle and wrist appears, and the deep tendon reflexes of the hemiparetic limbs become hyperactive and abnormally spreading. During the subsequent month, increasing plastic resistance to passive manipulation involves the shoulder, wrist, and ankle, little or no increase of resistance appears at the knee, and the resistance at the elbow usually is variable. Correspondingly, EMG recordings reveal a lowered threshold for the onset of responses to passive stretch in the extensor muscles of the hemiparetic hindlimb.

The mechanisms underlying the postural changes from cerebral cortical lesions were studied by examining the responses of muscle spindle afferents to extension of the gastrocnemius muscle in the hemiplegic hindlimb of the monkey following ablation of areas 4 and 6.[58] The responses of the spindle afferents are severely depressed during the first postoperative week (see Fig. 5C). During the second week they recover considerably but remain somewhat depressed. The initial hypotonic hemiplegia results from a depression of the responses of both alpha motoneurons and fusimotor neurons. The depression of these responses stems from the

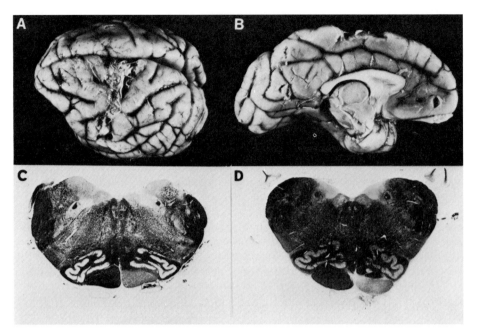

Figure 6. Photographs of the external surface laterally (A) and medially (B) of the brain of a monkey 57 days after operation showing the extent of the ablation of areas 4 and 6 in the left precentral cortex. Note the sparing of the postcentral cortex in A and of the cortex about the cingulate sulcus in B. C, Photomicrograph through the medulla of the brain illustrated in A and B showing degeneration of pyramidal tract fibers on the left side. Mahon stain. D, Photomicrograph through the medulla of an animal 8 months after unilateral section of the medullary pyramid showing the extent of degeneration of the pyramid caudal to the lesion. Luxol fast blue stain. (A, B and C from Gilman et al.,[58] D from Gilman and Marco,[59] with permission.)

withdrawal of excitatory influences mediated by pyramidal and extrapyramidal corticospinal projections originating in the ablated cortical regions.

During the phase of hypertonic hemiparesis the spindle afferent responses become essentially equal to those of control animals, showing no enhancement that corresponds to the marked clinical hypertonia.[58] Thus the hypertonic hemiplegia observed clinically results from an increase in the excitability of alpha motoneurons that is not entirely reflex in origin. No evidence has been adduced indicating that the excitability of fusimotor neurons is increased, because spindle afferent responses are normal during this period. The recovery of fusimotor activity to normal levels results from a combination of the depressant effects of interrupting the corticospinal projections and the excitatory effects of interrupting the extrapyramidal projections. The mechanisms underlying these changes have not been determined.

Pyramidal Tract

The nature of the motor defects resulting from lesions of the pyramidal tract in man and animals has become a controversial issue. According to early neurologic concepts, chronic pyramidal tract lesions produce a hypertonic (spastic) paresis. The initial animal experiments bearing on this issue, however, revealed that an

168

enduring hypotonic paresis of the limbs results from section of the medullary pyramidal tracts in the monkey.[109] In this study, Tower characterized the disorder as a decreased resistance to passive manipulation at all joints in the affected limbs, defects in the initiation and execution of active movements, and loss of discrete digital movements. Subsequent observations have given conflicting evidence about the uniformity of hypotonia in all skeletal muscles, the duration of hypotonia in the chronic preparation, and the occurrence of increased resistance to passive manipulation of the limbs after pyramidotomy.[41, 64, 70, 90, 112]

Shortly after Tower's report, Wagley[112] found that unilateral medullary pyramidotomy in monkeys resulted in decreased resistance to passive manipulation of the contralateral limbs at all joints except the hip in which "hypertonic" adductor muscles were found. In a single monkey with unilateral medullary pyramidotomy, Liu and Chambers[90] found motor disorders similar to those described by Tower.[109] In a larger series with unilateral and bilateral lesions, Growdon and colleagues[70] reported an initial decrease of the resistance to passive manipulation of the appropriate limbs at all joints, but in the chronic animal he observed an increase of resistance in the forelimb flexors, hip adductors, ankle extensors, and foot invertors. Denny-Brown[40, 41] also found evidence of hypertonia after unilateral medullary pyramidotomy in the monkey, consisting of a slight increase of stretch reflexes in the contralateral limbs during the second postoperative week. With lesions incompletely transecting the pyramidal tract, slight spasticity was observed in flexor and extensor muscles of the affected limbs. Clonus of the tendon reflexes in fingers and toes, Hoffman responses, and very brisk, repetitive biceps and quadriceps tendon reflexes also were found. Contrary to these observations, Goldberger[64] found no evidence of increased myotatic reflexes after unilateral medullary pyramidotomy in the monkey. Conflicting evidence has accumulated also about the degree of limb paresis resulting from pyramidotomy. Tower[109] found a severe paresis, but Lawrence and Kuypers[88] reported a considerably less severe paresis and emphasized the degree of preservation of limb function.

Conflicting results have emerged also from study of the effects of interrupting corticospinal fibers at the level of the cerebral peduncle in monkeys. Cannon, Magoun and Windle[29] found a hypotonic paresis with hyperactive deep tendon reflexes in the contralateral limbs. Bucy, Ladpli, and Ehrlich[23] also found an enduring hypotonic paresis, but no increase in tendon reflexes. In contrast, Walker and Richter[113] found that an initial hypotonic paresis with depressed tendon reflexes evolved into a hypertonic paresis with heightened deep tendon reflexes.

Recent studies have confirmed Tower's initial finding of a hypotonic paresis after medullary pyramidotomy (Fig. 7).[59, 60, 104] The major clinical defects in the chronic animal after bilateral pyramidotomy include: loss of contactual orienting responses of the hands and feet (tactile placing, grasping, and avoiding); defective use of the fingers and toes for finely coordinated movement; hypotonia (decreased resistance to passive manipulation) of the limbs without hyperreflexia; and various transient disorders of posture and limb placement. Electromyographic examination reveals a depression of the responses to stretch of hindlimb extensor muscles in the immediate postoperative period, an effect that regresses partially with time. The decrease of responses is similar to that described in monkeys with cerebellar ablation,[54] consisting of a raised threshold for the responses to muscle stretch. Thus no clinical or EMG evidence of heightened myotatic reflexes could be found after pyramidotomy.

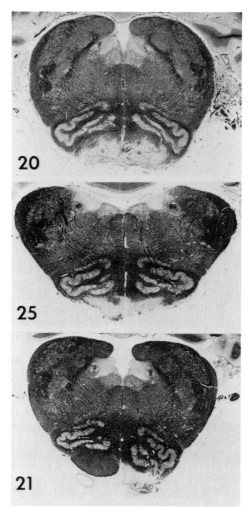

Figure 7. Photomicrographs of lesions in animals with bilateral pyramid section of one week (animal #20) and 6 months (animal #25) duration; unilateral pyramid section of 8 months duration (animal #21). Sections stained with Luxol fast blue. (From Gilman and Marco,[59] with permission.)

Shortly after pyramidotomy in monkeys, the responses to passive extension of the spindle primaries in the gastrocnemius muscle are decreased significantly (see Fig. 5B).[60] These responses are not significantly different from those of decerebellate monkeys.[54] Moreover, the spindle afferent responses of the pyramid-sectioned animal are unchanged by acute ablation of the neocerebellar cortex and dentate nuclei but are decreased significantly by subsequent denervation of the muscle spindles by ventral root section. Because neocerebellar ablation produces no further decrement in the sensitivity of muscle spindles despite the presence of a tonic level of background activity in the fusimotor efferent system, it is concluded that the pyramidotomy interrupts a central pathway involving the cerebellum. In monkeys with chronic bilateral pyramidotomy, the spindle afferent responses are greater than those observed acutely after pyramidotomy, but less than those of

170

the controls (see Fig. 5). Thus, the central nervous system compensatory process can partially restore the defect from pyramidotomy, but the persistent depression of fusimotor activity results in a continuing decrease of the responses of muscle spindle primaries. This, in turn, contributes to the chronic hypotonia of the animal.

Extrapyramidal Pathways

Efferent pathways from the lateral segments of the cerebellum can influence spinal activity without involving the thalamus or cerebral cortex. Stimulation of the dentate nucleus in monkeys increases the excitability of alpha motoneurons through pathways that do not include the primary sensorimotor cortex or premotor cortex.[8] The pathways influence the excitability of some proprioceptive reflexes and also depolarize many alpha motoneurons. Because these studies were conducted in preparations with the dorsal roots sectioned, the findings indicate that the output projections from the lateral cerebellum can increase the excitability of alpha motoneurons by mechanisms that do not involve the myotatic reflex.

CEREBELLAR TREMOR

Lesions of the lateral cerebellar nuclei induce a tremor most marked during limb movements projected into space.[44, 99] Carrea and Mettler[30, 31] categorized the tremors following cerebellar ablation in primates into ataxic or intention types and three varieties observed during postural fixation: postural, propraxic, and epipraxic. Ataxic or intention tremors are the oscillations of the extremity which occur during movements. In current terminology, both of these types should be labeled "kinetic tremors." The term "intention tremor" should be avoided because of frequent misinterpretations of its meaning.

Postural tremor consists of the oscillatory movement of an extremity while an animal maintains a specific posture. Propraxic and epipraxic tremors occur just before and just after a movement, respectively. A third type of tremor, simple tremor, was described in early studies[30] in the absence of any movement or postural fixation. Carrea and Mettler[30, 31] pointed out that these various types of tremor can appear simultaneously and often have the same frequency (3 to 4 Hz). Consequently, the tremors may represent variations of the same pathophysiologic process.

Carrea and Mettler[31] maintained that cerebellar tremor should not be regarded merely as the consequence of severe ataxia. In supporting this view, they showed that interrupting different parts of the brachium conjunctivum differentially affected cerebellar ataxia and cerebellar tremor. Lesions of the ventral portion of the crossed ascending limb of the brachium conjunctivum produced a tremor, while lesions interrupting the descending limb resulted in ataxia.

Cerebellar postural tremor and the "resting" tremor accompanying basal ganglia disorders may be related pathophysiologically.[65] Administering L-dopa relieves the tremor resulting from lesions in the basal ganglia and the postural tremor following cerebellar ablations,[65] however, L-dopa does not affect the kinetic tremor resulting from cerebellar lesions. These findings indicate that different mechanisms may underlie cerebellar kinetic tremor and the postural tremors following either cerebellar or basal ganglia lesions.

171

Animal 1 CO   Animal 1 DA 15 days   Animal 3 DB 14 days   Animal 1 DA 38 days DB 10 days

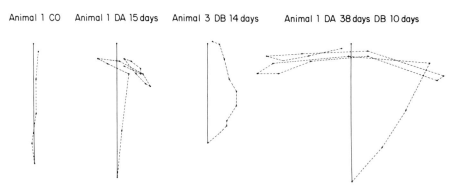

Figure 8. Kinematic records of trajectory and velocity of movements made by monkeys reaching for food. The reaching movement was along a horizontal table top and was filmed by a movie camera pointing vertically downward. The location of the reaching hand was represented by the mid-point between the first and second metacarpophalangeal joints. Dots mark positions of this point at intervals of approximately 63 millisec. They are interconnected by dotted lines. The average distance of the food target was 15 cm; its direction was varied randomly between five positions. CO = unoperated control; DA = deafferented; DB = decerebellate; DADB = deafferented and later decerebellate. (From Gilman et al.,[55] with permission.)

A rubro-olivo-cerebello-rubral circuit is implicated in experimentally induced postural tremors in the monkey.[86, 87] Lesions interrupting this circuit predispose a monkey to acquire a tremor if there is a decrease in the concentration of monoamines in the central nervous system or if central lesions interrupt the monoaminergic pathways. On the basis of this conception, interrupting the rubrocerebellar circuits by lesions of the cerebellar nuclei could result in a tremor, particularly if there are associated lesions in other central nuclei.

Recent studies have given further insights into the mechanisms underlying cerebellar tremor. Cooling the dentate nucleus in monkeys markedly decreases the damping of oscillations produced by stimulation of the brachium conjunctivum or interposed nucleus during self-paced, goal-directed movements.[4] The oscillatory movements accentuated by dentate cooling have a power spectrum with peaks at the same frequencies (3 to 5 Hz) as the kinetic tremor in these animals.[32] These oscillations cannot be ascribed solely to oscillations in segmental reflexes, because the deficit occurs in animals in which the dorsal roots have been cut (Fig. 8).[55, 90, 98]

Although the spinal reflexes do not need to be intact for tremor to appear, they contribute to specific features of the tremor.[4, 32, 98, 111] When monkeys are trained to resist imposed perturbations during fast flexion and extension movements, cooling of the dentate nucleus leads to a tremor with a frequency of 3 to 5 Hz. The frequency of this tremor can be increased by increasing the torque or spring stiffness of the imposed load. Moreover, changes in limb position can vary the frequency of the tremor, with a higher frequency observed in flexion than in extension. It was proposed that this deficit does not result from a change in gain of these reflexes, but rather from a change in the temporal relationship (phase) of the reflexes to time-variant peripheral inputs.[111]

In summary, the tremor produced by interrupting the output of the dentate nucleus does not depend upon the myotatic reflex. The characteristics of the oscillations can be modified, however, by alterations in segmental reflexes from pe-

172

ripheral stimuli. The kinetic tremors may result from loss of the mechanisms required for the proper damping of oscillations produced during the performance of goal-directed movements.

REFERENCES

1. ALNAES, E.: *Static and dynamic properties of Golgi tendon organs in the anterior tibial and soleus muscles of the cat.* Acta Physiol. Scand. 70:176, 1967.

2. APPELBERG, B., BESSOU, P., AND LAPORTE, Y.: *Effects of dynamic and static fusimotor gamma fibres on the responses of primary and secondary endings belonging to the same spindle.* J. Physiol. (Lond.) 177:29P, 1965.

3. APPELBERG, B., BESSOU, P., AND LAPORTE, Y.: *Action of static and dynamic fusimotor fibres on secondary endings of cat's spindles.* J. Physiol. (Lond.) 185:160, 1966.

4. ATKIN, A., AND KOSLOVSKAYA, I. B.: *Effects of cooling cerebellar nuclei on evoked forearm oscillations.* Exp. Neurol. 50:766, 1976.

5. BANKS, R. W., BARKER, D., BESSOU, P. ET AL.: *Histological analysis of cat muscle spindles following direct observation of the effects of stimulating dynamic and static motor axons.* J. Physiol. 283:605, 1978.

6. BANKS, R. W., BARKER, D., AND STACEY, M. J.: *Sensory innervation of cat hind-limb muscle spindles.* J. Physiol. 293:40P, 1979.

7. BANKS, R. W., HARKER, D. W., AND STACEY, M. J.: *A study of mammalian intrafusal muscle fibres using a combined histochemical and ultrastructural technique.* J. Anat. 123:783, 1977.

8. BANTLI, H., AND BLOEDEL, J. R.: *Characteristics of the output of the dentate nucleus to spinal neurons via pathways which do not involve the primary sensorimotor cortex.* Exp. Brain Res. 25:199, 1976.

9. BARKER, D.: *The structure and distribution of muscle receptors,* in Barker, D. (ed.): *Symposium on Muscle Receptors.* Hong Kong University Press, Hong Kong, 1962, pp. 227–240.

10. BARKER, D., AND COPE, M.: *The innervation of individual intrafusal muscle fibres,* in Barker, D. (ed.): *Symposium on Muscle Receptors.* Hong Kong University Press, Hong Kong, 1962, pp. 263–249.

11. BARKER, D., EMONET-DENAND, F., HARKER, D. W. ET AL.: *Distribution of fusimotor axons to intrafusal muscle fibres in cat tenuissimus spindles as determined by the glycogen-depletion method.* J. Physiol. 261:49, 1976.

12. BARKER, D., AND IP, M. C.: *A study of single and tandem types of muscle-spindle in the cat.* Proc. R. Soc. Biol. 154:377, 1961.

13. BESSOU, P., AND LAPORTE, Y.: *Responses from primary and secondary endings of the same neuromuscular spindle of the tenuissimus muscle of the cat,* in Barker, D. (ed.): *Symposium on Muscle Receptors.* Hong Kong University Press, Hong Kong, 1962, pp. 105–119.

14. BESSOU, P., AND LAPORTE, Y.: *Observations on static fusimotor fibers,* in Granit, R. (ed.): *Nobel Symposium I, Muscular Afferents and Motor Control.* Almqvist and Wiksell, Stockholm, 1966, pp. 81–89.

15. BOTTERELL, E. H., AND FULTON, J. F.: *Relations of the cerebrum to the cerebellum. IV. Functions of the paleo and neocerebellum in chimpanzees and monkeys.* Trans. Am. Neurol. Assoc. 62:172, 1936.

16. BOTTERELL, E. H., AND FULTON, J. F.: *Functional localization in the cerebellum of primates. I. Unilateral section of the peduncles.* J. Comp. Neurol. 69:31, 1938.

17. BOTTERELL, E. H., AND FULTON, J. F.: *Functional localization in the cerebellum of primates. III. Lesions of hemispheres (neocerebellum).* J. Comp. Neurol. 69:63, 1938.

18. BOYD, I. A.: *The structure and innervation of the nuclear bag muscle fibre system and the nuclear chain muscle fibre system in mammalian muscle spindles.* Phil. Trans. Roy. Soc. B. 245:81, 1962.

19. BREMER, F.: *Le cervelet,* In Roger, G. H., and Binet, L. (eds.): *Traité de physiologie normale et pathologique.* Masson, Paris, vol. 10, pt. 1, 1935, pp. 39–134.

20. BROCK, L. G., COOMBS, J. S., AND ECCLES, J. C.: *The recording of potentials from motoneurones with an intracellular electrode.* J. Physiol. (Lond.) 117:431, 1952.

21. BROCK, L. G., ECCLES, J. C., AND RALL, W.: *Experimental investigations on the afferent fibres in muscle nerves.* Proc. R. Soc. B. 138:453, 1951.

22. BROWN, M. C., AND MATTHEWS, P. B. C.: *On the subdivision of the efferent fibres to muscle spindles into static and dynamic fusimotor fibres,* in Andrew, B. L. (ed.): *Control and Innervation of Skeletal Muscle.* Thompson, Dundee, 1966, pp. 18–31.

23. BUCY, P. C., LADPLI, R., AND EHRLICH, A.: *Destruction of the pyramidal tract in the monkey.* J. Neurosurg. 25:1, 1966.

24. BURKE, R. E.: *Motor unit types of cat triceps surae muscle.* J. Physiol. (Lond.) 193:141, 1967.

25. BURKE, R. E.: *Composite nature of the monosynaptic excitatory postsynaptic potential.* J. Neurophysiol. 30:1114, 1967.

26. BURKE, R. E.: *Group Ia synaptic input to fast and slow twitch motor units of cat triceps surae.* J. Physiol. (Lond.) 196:605, 1968.

27. BURKE, R. E.: *Firing patterns of gastrocnemius motor units in the decerebrate cat.* J. Physiol. (Lond.) 196:631, 1968.

28. BURKE, R. E., LEVINE, D. N., ZAJAC, F. E., III. ET AL.: *Mammalian motor units: physiological-histochemical correlation in three types in cat gastrocnemius.* Science 174:709, 1971.

29. CANNON, W., MAGOUN, H. W., AND WINDLE, W. F.: *Paralysis with hypotonicity and hyperreflexia subsequent to section of the basis pedunculi in monkeys.* J. Neurophysiol. 7:425, 1944.

30. CARREA, R. M. E., AND METTLER, F. A.: *Physiologic consequences following extensive removal of the cerebellar cortex and deep cerebellar nuclei and effect of secondary cerebral ablations in the primate.* J. Comp. Neurol. 87:169, 1947.

31. CARREA, R. M. E., AND METTLER, F. A.: *Function of the primate brachium conjunctivum and related structures.* J. Comp. Neurol. 102:151, 1955.

32. COOKE, J. D., AND THOMAS, J. S.: *Forearm oscillation during cooling of the dentate nucleus in the monkey.* Can. J. Physiol. Pharmacol. 54:430, 1976.

33. COOPER, S.: *The secondary endings of muscle spindles.* J. Physiol. (Lond.) 149:27P:, 1959.

34. COOPER, S.: *The responses of the primary and secondary endings of muscle spindles with intact motor innervation during applied stretch.* Quart. J. Exp. Physiol. 46:389, 1961.

35. COOPER, S., AND DANIEL, P. M.: *Muscle spindles in man: their morphology in the lumbrical and the deep muscles of the neck.* Brain 86:563, 1963.

36. CROSBY, E. C., SCHNEIDER, R. C., DEJONGE, B. R. ET AL.: *The alterations of tonus and movements through the interplay between the cerebral hemispheres and the cerebellum.* J. Comp. Neurol. 127:(Suppl. 1, Part II) 1, 1966.

37. CROWE, A., AND MATTHEWS, P. B. C.: *The effects of stimulation of static and dynamic fusimotor fibres on the response to stretching of the primary endings of muscle spindles.* J. Physiol. (Lond.) 174:109, 1964.

38. CROWE, A., AND MATTHEWS, P. B. C.: *Further studies of static and dynamic fusimotor fibres.* J. Physiol. (Lond.) 174:132, 1964.

39. CUSSONS, P. D., HULLIGER, M., AND MATTHEWS, P. B. C.: *Effects of fusimotor stimulation on the response of the secondary ending of the muscle spindle to sinusoidal stretching.* J. Physiol. 270:835, 1977.

40. DENNY-BROWN, D.: *The extrapyramidal system and postural mechanisms.* Clin. Pharmacol. Ther. 5:812, 1964.

41. DENNY-BROWN, D.: *The cerebral control of movement.* Liverpool University Press, Liverpool, 1966.

42. DENNY-BROWN, D., AND GILMAN, S.: *Depression of gamma innervation by cerebellectomy.* Trans. Am. Neurol. Assoc. 90:96, 1965.

43. DIGIORGIO, A. M.: *Persistenza di effetti cerebellari nella corteccia cerebrale.* Boll. Soc. Ital. Biol. Sper. 17:101, 1942.

44. DOW, R. S., AND MORUZZI, G.: *The Physiology and Pathology of the Cerebellum.* University of Minnesota Press, Minneapolis, 1958.

45. ECCLES, J. C., ECCLES, R. M., AND LUNDBERG, A.: *The convergence of monosynaptic excitatory afferents on to many different species of alpha motoneurones.* J. Physiol. (Lond.) 137:22, 1957.

46. ECCLES, J. C., ECCLES, R. M., AND LUNDBERG, A.: *Synaptic actions on motoneurones in relation to the two components of the group I muscle afferent volley.* J. Physiol. (Lond.) 136:527, 1957.

47. ECCLES, J. C., ECCLES, R. M., AND LUNDBERG, A.: *Synaptic actions on motoneurones caused by impulses in Golgi tendon organ afferents.* J. Physiol. (Lond.) 138:227, 1957.

48. ECCLES, J. C., ECCLES, R. M., AND LUNDBERG, A.: *The action potentials of the alpha motoneurones supplying fast and slow muscles.* J. Physiol. (Lond.) 142:275, 1958.

49. ECCLES, J. C., FATT, P., AND LANDGREN, S.: *The central pathway for the direct inhibitory action of impulses in the largest afferent nerve fibres to muscle.* J. Neurophysiol. 19:75, 1956.

50. ELDRED, E., BRIDGMAN, C. F., SWETT, J. E. ET AL.: *Quantitative comparisons of muscle receptors of the cat's medial gastrocnemius, soleus, and extensor digitorum brevis muscles,* in Barker, D. (ed.): *Symposium on Muscle Receptors.* Hong Kong University Press, Hong Kong, 1962, pp. 207–213.

51. EMONET-DÉNAND, F., LAPORTE, Y., MATTHEWS, P. B. C. ET AL.: *On the subdivision of static and dynamic fusimotor actions on the primary ending of the cat muscle spindle.* J. Physiol. 268: 827, 1977.

52. FULTON, J. F., AND DOW, R. S.: *The cerebellum: A summary of functional localization.* Yale J. Biol. Med. 10:89, 1937.

53. GILMAN, S.: *Fusimotor fiber responses in the decerebellate cat.* Brain Res. 14:218, 1969.

54. GILMAN, S.: *The mechanism of cerebellar hypotonia. An experimental study in the monkey.* Brain 92:621, 1969.

55. GILMAN, S., CARR, D., AND HOLLENBERG, J.: *Kinematic effects of deafferentation and cerebellar ablation.* Brain 99:311, 1976.

56. GILMAN, S., AND EBEL, H. C.: *Fusimotor neuron responses to natural stimuli as a function of prestimulus fusimotor activity in decerebellate cats.* Brain Res. 21:367, 1970.

57. GILMAN, S., LIEBERMAN, J. S., AND COPACK, P.: *A thalamic mechanism of postural control.* Int. J. Neurol. 8:260, 1971.

58. GILMAN, S., LIEBERMAN, J. S., AND MARCO, L. A.: *Spinal mechanisms underlying the effects of unilateral ablation of areas 4 and 6 in monkeys.* Brain 97:49, 1974.

59. GILMAN, S., AND MARCO, L. A.: *Effects of medullary pyramidotomy in the monkey. I. Clinical and electromyographic abnormalities.* Brain 94:495, 1971.

60. GILMAN, S., MARCO, L. A., AND EBEL, H. C.: *Effects of medullary pyramidotomy in the monkey II. Abnormalities of spindle afferent responses.* Brain 94:515, 1971.

61. GILMAN, S., AND MCDONALD, W. I.: *Cerebellar facilitation of muscle spindle activity.* J. Neurophysiol. 30:1494, 1967.

62. GILMAN, S., AND MCDONALD, W. I.: *Relation of afferent fiber conduction velocity to reactivity of muscle spindle receptors after cerebellectomy.* J. Neurophysiol. 30:1513, 1967.

63. GLASER, G. H., AND HIGGINS, D. C.: *Motor stability, stretch responses and the cerebellum,* in Granit, R. (ed.): *Nobel Symposium I: Muscular Afferents and Motor Control.* Almqvist and Wiksell, Stockholm, 1966, pp. 121–138.

64. GOLDBERGER, M. E.: *The extrapyramidal systems of the spinal cord II. Results of combined pyramidal and extrapyramidal lesions in the macaque.* J. Comp. Neurol. 135:1, 1969.

65. GOLDBERGER, M. E., AND GROWDEN, J. H.: *Tremor at rest following cerebellar lesions in monkeys: effect of L-dopa administration.* Brain Res. 27:183, 1971.

66. GRANIT, R.: *The Basis of Motor Control.* Academic Press, London, 1970.

67. GRANIT, R., HENATSCH, H. D., AND STEG, G.: *Tonic and phasic ventral horn cells differentiated by post-tetanic potentiation in cat extensors.* Acta Physiol. Scand. 37:114, 1956.

68. GRANIT, R., HOLMGREN, B., AND MERTON, P. A.: *The two routes for excitation of muscle and their subservience to the cerebellum.* J. Physiol. (Lond.) 130:213, 1955.

69. GRANIT, R., KELLERTH, J. O., AND SZUMSKI, A. J.: *Intracellular recording from extensor motoneurons activated across the gamma loop.* J. Neurophysiol. 29:530, 1966.

70. GROWDON, J. H., CHAMBERS, W. W., AND LIU, C. N.: *An experimental study of cerebellar dyskinesia in the rhesus monkey.* Brain 90:603, 1967.

71. HARVEY, R. J., AND MATTHEWS, P. B. C.: *The response of de-efferented muscle spindle endings in the cat's soleus to slow extension of the muscle.* J. Physiol. (Lond.) 157:370, 1961.

72. HOLMES, G.: *The clinical symptoms of cerebellar diseases and their interpretation.* Lancet 1: 1177, and 2:59, 1922.

73. HULLINGER, M., MATTHEWS, P. B. C., AND NOTH, J.: *Static and dynamic fusimotor action on*

the response of IA fibres to low frequency sinusoidal stretching of widely ranging amplitude. J. Physiol. 267:811, 1977.

74. HULLINGER, M., MATTHEWS, P. B. C., AND NOTH, J.: *Effects of combining static and dynamic fusimotor stimulation on the response of the muscle spindle primary ending to sinusoidal stretching.* J. Physiol. 267:839, 1977.

75. HUNT, C. C., AND PAINTAL, A. S.: *Spinal reflex regulation of fusimotor neurones.* J. Physiol. (Lond.) 143:195, 1958.

76. JANSEN, J. K. S., AND RUDJORD, T.: *On the silent period and Golgi tendon organs of the soleus muscle of the cat.* Acta Physiol. Scand. 62:364, 1964.

77. JANSEN, J. K. S.: *On fusimotor reflex activity,* in Granit, R. (ed.): *Nobel Symposium I, Muscular Afferents and Motor Control.* Almqvist and Wiksell, Stockholm, 1966, pp. 91–105.

78. KEMM, R. E., AND WESTBURY, D. R.: *Some properties of spinal γ-motoneurones in the cat, determined by micro-electrode recording.* J. Physiol. 282:59, 1978.

79. KERNELL, D.: *High-frequency repetitive firing in cat lumbosacral motoneurones stimulated by long-lasting injected currents.* Acta Physiol. Scand. 65:74, 1965.

80. KERNELL, D.: *The limits of firing frequency in cat lumbosacral motoneurones possessing different time course of afterhyperpolarization.* Acta Physiol. Scand. 65:87, 1965.

81. KERNELL, D.: *Input resistance, electrical excitability, and size of ventral horn cells in the cat spinal cord.* Science 152:1637, 1966.

82. KIRKWOOD, P. A., AND SEARS, T. A.: *Monosynaptic excitation of motoneurones from secondary endings of muscle spindles.* Nature 252:243, 1974.

83. KUNO, M.: *Excitability following antidromic activation in spinal motoneurones supplying red muscles.* J. Physiol. (Lond.) 149:374, 1959.

84. LAPORTE, Y., AND BESSOU, P.: *Modifications d'excitabilité de motoneurones homonymes provoqués par l'activation physiologique de fibres afférentes d'origine musculaire du groupe II.* J. Physiol. (Paris) 51:897, 1959.

85. LAPORTE, Y., AND LLOYD, D. P. C.: *Nature and significance of the reflex connections established by large afferent fibers of muscular origin.* Am. J. Physiol. 169:609, 1952.

86. LAROCHELLE, L., BEDARD, P., BOUCHER, R. ET AL.: *The rubro-olivo-cerebello-rubral loop and postural tremor in the monkey.* J. Neurol. Sci. 11:53, 1970.

87. LAROCHELLE, L., BEDARD, P., POIRIER, L. J. ET AL.: *Correlative neuroanatomical and neuropharmacological study of tremor and catatonia in the monkey.* Neuropharmacol. 10:273, 1971.

88. LAWRENCE, D. G., AND KUYPERS, H. G. J. M.: *The functional organization of the motor system in the monkey I. The effects of bilateral pyramidal lesions.* Brain 91:1, 1968.

89. LIEBERMAN, J. S., COPACK, P. B., AND GILMAN, S.: *Fusimotor effects of cryogenic lesions in ventrolateral nucleus and pulvinar.* Arch. Neurol. 30:375, 1974.

90. LIU, C. N., AND CHAMBERS, W. W.: *An experimental study of the corticospinal system in the monkey (Macaca mulatta).* J. Comp. Neurol. 123:257, 1964.

91. LIU, C. N., AND CHAMBERS, W. W.: *A study of cerebellar dyskinesia in the bilaterally deafferented forelimbs of the monkey (Macaca mulatta and Macaca speciosa).* Acta Neurobiol. Exp. 31:263, 1971.

92. LLOYD, D. P. C.: *Facilitation and inhibition of spinal motoneurons.* J. Neurophysiol. 9:421, 1946.

93. LÖWENTHAL, M., AND HORSLEY, V.: *On the relations between the cerebellar and other centers (namely cerebral and spinal) with special reference to the action of antagonistic muscles.* Proc. Roy. Soc. Lond. 61:20, 1897.

94. LUCIANI, L.: *Il cervelletto: Nuovi studi di fisiologia normale e patologica.* Le Monnier, Florence, 1891.

95. LUCIANI, L.: *De l'influence qu'exercent les mutilations cérébelleuses sur l'excitabilité de l'écorce cérébrale et sur les réflexes spinaux.* Arch. Ital. Biol. 21:190, 1894.

96. MATTHEWS, P. B. C.: *The differentation of two types of fusimotor fibres by their effects on the dynamic response of muscle spindle primary endings.* Quart. J. Exp. Physiol. 47:324, 1962.

97. MATTHEWS, P. B. C.: *Mammalian muscle receptors and their central actions.* Williams and Wilkins, Baltimore, 1972.

98. MURPHY, J. T., KWAN, H. C., MACKAY, W. A., ET AL.: *Physiological basis of cerebellar dysmetria.* J. Neurol. Sci. 2:279, 1975.

 99. OHYE, C., BOUCHARD, R., LAROCHELLE, L. ET AL.: *Effect of dorsal rhizotomy on postural tremor in the monkey.* Exp. Brain Res. 10:140, 1970.

100. RADEMAKER, G. G. J.: *Das Stehen.* J. Springer, Berlin, 1931.

101. ROSSI, G.: *Ricerche sulla eccitabilità della corteccia cerebrale in cani sottoposti ad emiestirpazione cerebellare.* Arch. Fisiol. 10:257, 1912.

102. ROSSI, G.: *Sugli effetti conseguenti alla stimolazione contemporanea della corteccia cerebrale e di quella cerebellare.* Arch. Fisiol. 10:389, 1912.

103. RUSSELL, J. S. R.: *Experimental researches into the functions of the cerebellum.* Philos. Tr. Roy. Soc. Lond. 185:819, 1894.

104. SCHWARTZMAN, R. J.: *A behavioral analysis of complete unilateral section of the pyramidal tract at the medullary level in Macaca mulatta.* Ann. Neurol. 4:234, 1978.

105. STAUFFER, E. K., WATT, D. G. D., TAYLOR, A. ET AL.: *Analysis of muscle receptor connections by spike-trigger averaging. 2. Spindle group II afferents.* J. Neurophysiol. 39:1393, 1976.

106. STEG, G.: *The function of muscle spindles in spasticity and rigidity.* Acta Neurol. Scand. 39:53, 1962.

107. STEG, G.: *Efferent muscle innervation and rigidity.* Acta Physiol. Scand. 61: (Suppl. 225) 1, 1964.

108. SWETT, J. E., AND ELDRED, E.: *Comparisons in structure of stretch receptors in medial gastrocnemius and soleus muscles of the cat.* Anat. Rec. 137:461, 1960.

109. TOWER, S. S.: *Pyramidal lesion in the monkey.* Brain 63:36, 1940.

110. VAN DER MEULEN, J. P., AND GILMAN, S.: *Recovery of muscle spindle activity in cats after cerebellar ablation.* J. Neurophysiol. 28:943, 1965.

111. VILLIS, T., AND HORE, J.: *Effects of changes in mechanical state of limb on cerebellar intention tremor.* J. Neurophysiol. 40:1214, 1977.

112. WAGLEY, P. F.: *A study of spasticity and paralysis.* Bull. Johns Hopkins Hosp. 77:218, 1945.

113. WALKER, A. E., AND RICHTER, H.: *Section of the cerebral peduncle in the monkey.* Arch. Neurol. 14:231, 1966.

114. WALKER, L. B., JR.: *Diameter spectrum of intrafusal muscle fibers in muscle spindles of the dog.* Anat. Rec. 130:385, 1958.

CHAPTER 9

Cerebellar Regulation of Movement

As described in the preceding chapters, the cerebellum participates in many aspects of motor control. It is a component of various open and closed loop systems responsible for coordinating the movements of several extremities as well as the eyes, head, and neck. Each of the three major cerebellar zones appears to function differently as a component of these systems. Nevertheless, many aspects of motor function require the coordinated action of all three zones simultaneously.

THE MIDLINE ZONE OF THE CEREBELLUM

The components of the midline zone of the cerebellum, the cerebellar vermis and the fastigial nucleus, may be viewed as a closed loop control system that regulates the segmental reflexes important in postural fixation or truncal movement.[14, 15] Many of the initial ablation studies demonstrate the importance of these midline cerebellar structures in postural control. These studies show that the tonic action of the vermal cerebellar cortex and fastigial nucleus can affect the excitability of neurons in the vestibulospinal and reticulospinal projections, and that these projections regulate the tonic activity of alpha and gamma motoneurons in the spinal cord. The specific mechanisms responsible for the action of the midline zone of the cerebellum in postural control are not yet known.

The midline region of the cerebellum participates not only in postural control, but also in many dynamic features of motor behavior. These features include phasic eye and head movements and the movements of the trunk and extremities required to maintain equilibrium during complex motor tasks. The influence of the midline zone upon dynamic movements has been underemphasized in the past because of the tonic nature of the deficits resulting from ablation of the midline region of the cerebellum in subprimates. The ascending projections of the fastigial nucleus may regulate some aspects of phasic movements, but the extent of this is presently unknown. It is possible that neural activity projecting from the fastigial nucleus to the thalamus and cerebral cortex interacts with activity in the ascending projections from the lateral regions of the cerebellum during goal directed movements of the extremities.

The midline zone of the cerebellum participates in the control of eye movements by regulating the vestibulo-ocular reflex. Regulation of this reflex occurs through interactions between the flocculonodular lobe and the vestibular nuclei.

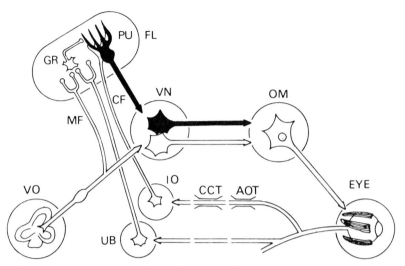

Figure 1. The control system proposed by Ito for the modification of the vestibulo-ocular reflex by the flocculus. In this system the flocculus acts as a component of an open loop control system for stabilizing retinal images during movements of the head and eyes. The climbing fiber input can modify the responses of Purkinje cells to mossy fiber inputs in order to optimize the characteristics of the control system. VO = vestibular receptor; MF = mossy fiber; GR = granule cell; PU = Purkinje cell; CF = climbing fiber; FL = flocculus; VN = vestibular nuclei; OM = oculomotor nucleus; UB = unknown brainstem nucleus; IO = inferior olive; CCT = central tegmental tract; AOT = accessory optic tract. (From Ito,[15] with permission.)

The Purkinje cells in the flocculonodular lobe suppress the vestibulo-ocular reflex during head movement when visual fixation requires that the eyes remain immobile.[17, 18] Mossy fibers activated by vestibular stimuli, and presumably by eye movement, modulate the Purkinje cell activity required to modify the vestibulo-ocular reflex. Thus, the modulation of Purkinje cell activity equals the vector sum of the head movements and eye movements occurring simultaneously.[17, 18] The result is a change in gain of the vestibulo-ocular reflex consistent with the behavioral requirements.[23] A change in gain of this reflex also underlies the alterations in reflexly evoked eye movements which occur when visual prisms are used to change the movement of the environment relative to the movement of the head.

Ito[15] proposed that the flocculus is a component of an open loop control system that requires the action of climbing fiber inputs to modify the effects of vestibular afferents on eye movements (Fig. 1). This control system is thought to minimize the slippage of a visual image on the retina during movements of both the eyes and the head. The climbing fiber input activated by moving visual stimuli is thought to be responsible for the long term modification in the action of the mossy fiber–parallel fiber projection to Purkinje cells, a modification resulting in progressive changes in gain of the vestibulo-ocular reflex.

THE INTERMEDIATE ZONE OF THE CEREBELLUM

The intermediate zone of the cerebellum, like the midline zone, receives inputs from the spinal cord. The connections of the intermediate zone with forebrain structures, however, are more extensive than those of the midline zone. Much of our knowledge concerning the participation of the intermediate zone in the control of movements stems from the ablation studies reviewed in Chapter 7 and investigations in which single units in the intermediate region of the cerebellar cortex and interposed nuclei are recorded during specific motor tasks in the awake animal.

Many neurons in the interposed nuclei show changes in discharge rate during both phasic movements and maintained positions of an extremity,[28-31] suggesting that the intermediate zone participates in the regulation of both types of movement. The intermediate zone interconnects with the spinal cord and the cerebral cortex, and thus the modulation of activity in the interposed nuclei can occur through several mechanisms. These include the actions of ascending nervous system pathways activated during a movement, the effects of descending pathways that initiate or direct the movement, or the combined results of activating both ascending and descending projections. Attempts have been made to differentiate these possibilities by examining the relationships of activity in the interposed nuclei to the features of a goal directed movement. Burton and Onoda found that neurons in the interposed nuclei of the cat discharge in proportion to the velocity of a ballistic movement performed with an upper extremity.[7] The findings indicate that the output of the interposed nuclei can be modified by inputs responding to rate sensitive receptors in muscles affected by the movement. Indirect evidence from the study suggests that the output of the interposed nucleus is involved also in the activation of motoneurons responsible for producing the movement. Other studies have shown that neurons in the interposed nuclei respond well before the initiation of a movement and thus may be activated by the actions of descending pathways.[30] Purkinje cells in the intermediate zone of the cerebellar cortex respond proportionally to the velocity of a movement or muscle stretch.[20, 31] Based on this finding, a hypothesis was formulated stating that some neurons of the interposed nuclei provide the substrate for a feedback system which senses the velocity of an executed movement and alters the output of the cerebral cortex based on information concerning velocity.[20] According to this view, the intermediate cerebellar zone serves as a component of a position control system that regulates movements of the extremities.

THE LATERAL ZONE OF THE CEREBELLUM

Concepts regarding the function of the lateral cerebellar zone have evolved considerably in recent years. The function of the dentate nucleus appears to be distinct from that of the interposed nuclei, because certain motor deficits appear only when the output projections of the dentate nucleus are interrupted. The notion of different functions for the dentate and interposed nuclei was not supported by initial studies of the relationship between the responses of dentate neurons and the time course of goal directed movements of the extremities.[30] The discharge rate of some dentate neurons was found to change during maintained positions as well as during phasic movements, similar to the responses of neurons in the interposed nuclei.[30] However, other neurons in the dentate nucleus responded somewhat earlier than those in the interposed nuclei relative to the onset of the movement. Elucidation of the difference in behavior of dentate and interposed neurons comes from studies of complex movements.

The discharge of dentate neurons can be related to very complex features of movement. In a study of the behavior of dentate neurons during a visually guided task, a monkey was required to push a sequence of illuminated buttons.[13, 22] During the task the discharge of dentate neurons was not correlated with any particular feature or phase of the movement. Rather, the firing rate often increased with a time course extending over a large portion of the task. The activity of other cells was modulated slightly during the course of the movement, but again not in relation to any specific feature of the movement. This type of response has not been observed in the interposed nuclei.

Other differences between the discharge of neurons in the interposed and dentate nuclei emerged from investigations using a different type of paradigm. One study was designed to differentiate between neurons responding in association with the initiation of a movement and those responding to peripheral stimuli activated during the execution of a movement.[26] Monkeys were conditioned either to push or to pull a lever upon receiving an appropriate visual command. A force then was applied to the manipulandum in a direction which was either the same or opposite that of the requested movement. The discharge of many interposed neurons was correlated principally with the direction of the imposed displacement rather than the direction of the initial movement. In contrast, the discharge of neurons in the dentate nucleus was correlated chiefly with the direction of the initial movement rather than the imposed displacement. These findings demonstrate that neurons in the interposed nuclei respond chiefly to peripheral inputs activated during the movement, while neurons in the dentate nucleus respond to characteristics of the initial movement which the monkey "intended" to perform.

Additional evidence for differences in the behavior of neurons in the interposed and dentate nuclei came from studies of neuronal activity during an 8-step motor task.[33] Neural activity in the motor cortex was recorded also. The actual discharge of the cerebellar neurons was compared with hypothetical responses based upon the assumption that the discharge pattern would be correlated with: 1) joint position; 2) load; or 3) direction of the next intended movement in sequence (Fig. 2). Neurons in both the dentate and interposed nuclei responded to changes in joint position and load. However, the latency of the neuronal responses to passive perturbation of the wrist was appreciably shorter m the interposed nuclei than in the dentate nucleus or motor cortex. The neurons in the interposed and dentate nuclei showed another striking difference in their responses. The discharge of several dentate neurons was correlated with the direction of the next intended movement. This characteristic was observed also among cerebral cortical cells, but not among neurons in the interposed nuclei. These observations led to the conclusion that only neurons in the dentate nucleus and motor cortex discharge in association with conditions underlying the planned sequence of a movement. In contrast, neurons in the interposed nuclei respond in relation to characteristics of the movement itself or to sensory inputs activated during the execution of the movement.

Interactions between the dentate nucleus and the cerebral cortex are important in goal directed movements. Inactivating the dentate nucleus by local cooling disrupts the relationship between the discharge of neurons in the cerebral cortex and the kinematic variables of a limb movement, particularly velocity.[6] In addition, cooling the dentate nucleus results in an oscillation of neuronal discharge in the cerebral cortex which is correlated with the oscillation of the extremity during movement.[19] Cooling the dentate nucleus also affects the responses of neurons in the precentral cortex to torque stimuli applied to the arm.

Other findings have implicated the dentatothalamocortical pathway in the initiation of movement.[10, 32, 33] Many neurons in the dentate nucleus discharge either about the same time or somewhat in advance of the discharge of cells in the primary motor cortex during goal directed movements.[32, 33] According to Deecke

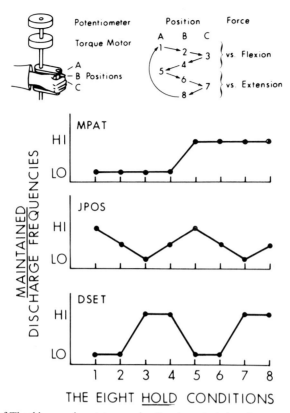

Figure 2. Diagram of Thach's experiment to examine the characteristics of neuronal discharge in cerebellar nuclei and motor cortex during different motor tasks. The monkey was trained to move the lever through three positions, A (in flexion at the wrist), B (in neutral), and C (in extension). The monkey moved the manipulandum through the sequence of movements numbered 1 through 8 and then returned it to position 1. During movements 1 through 4, a 1 lb torque load was applied directed against flexion. During movements 5 through 8 the same torque load was directed against extension. The monkey was trained to hold the manipulandum for 2 to 5 sec in the eight positions during the task and received a reward for remaining in each numbered position. The graphs indicate the anticipated changes in maintained discharge frequencies of a hypothetical nuclear neuron during the sequence of movements. The differences between each graph reflect changes in impulse activity expected if the cell were participating in one of three different functional interactions. MPAT indicates the hypothetical discharge of a neuron firing in relation to the pattern of muscular activity required for the task. Plot JPOS indicates the hypothetical changes in discharge due to joint position. Plot DSET indicates the expected changes if the impulse activity were related to the direction of the next intended light triggered movement. (From Thach,[33] with permission.)

and coworkers,[10] the actual initiation of a goal directed movement may occur within the association cortex. The output of the association cortex is thought to initiate a sequence of neuronal activity involving the dentate nucleus, the primary motor cortex, and descending corticofugal pathways.[32, 33] In this scheme the dentate nucleus participates in the neuronal interactions responsible for initiating preplanned motor behavior, but it is not considered to be the nucleus in which the pertinent sequence of neuronal interactions is initiated. Descending pathways also may affect activity in the interposed nuclei; however, interactions in these nuclei are not thought to be involved in the initiation of motor behavior.[33]

The dentate nucleus almost certainly affects motor behavior through pathways in addition to the dentatothalamocortical projection. There is ample evidence that the output of the dentate nucleus can alter the excitability of neurons in the spinal cord through pathways that do not involve the sensorimotor cortex. For example, stimulation of the dentate nucleus in decorticate monkeys alters the excitability of alpha motoneurons and the segmental actions of Ib afferent fibers.[3] In addition, the output of the dentate nucleus can activate neurons in the reticulospinal and rubrospinal projections.[2, 4, 5, 34] Moreover, stereotyped movements of the forelimb and hindlimb can be evoked by stimulation in the dentate nucleus of monkeys in which the dentatothalamocortical pathway has been interrupted.[24] Finally, lesions in the ventrolateral thalamic nucleus do not disrupt the pattern of EMG activity in agonist and antagonist muscles during a ballistic movement,[21] but lesions involving the dentate nucleus do interrupt this pattern (Figs. 3 and 4).[25] Thus, the output from the dentate nucleus can affect spinal integration by pathways other than the dentatothalamocortical projections. Indeed, there is evidence suggesting that some output projections from the lateral zone of the cerebellum are part of an automatic control system responsible for regulating patterns of muscle activity during ballistic movements.[25, 27]

In conclusion, the dentate nucleus participates in motor behavior both through dentatothalamocortical pathways and through projections involving the basal ganglia, the rubrospinal pathway, and the reticulospinal pathway. The precise role

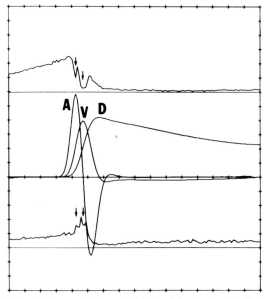

Figure 3. The relationships of biceps and triceps EMG activity during a ballistic movement in normal monkeys. The top and bottom traces show the averaged EMG responses recorded from the biceps and triceps, respectively. The data were obtained from 320 trials in five monkeys. The three superimposed traces in the middle of the graph show the calculated acceleration (A), velocity (V), and displacement (D) occurring during the ballistic movement. The two arrows in the biceps and triceps record indicate the time at which peak acceleration and velocity occurred. The arrows also help to visualize the reciprocal activity occurring in the agonist and antagonist muscles. The ordinates for each measurement are: displacement = 0.2 radians; velocity = 4 radians/sec; and acceleration = 80 radians/sec^2. The time calibration on the X axis is 50 msec/division. (From Soechting, et al.,[25] with permission.)

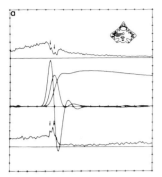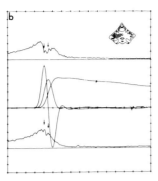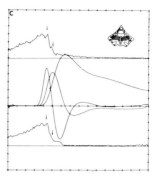

Figure 4. The effects of cerebellar lesions on biceps and triceps EMG activity during a ballistic move-ment. The organization of the data and the coordinates are identical to those described for Figure 3. The lesions of the cerebellar nuclei are shown in the insert of each graph. Graph a was obtained from an average of 146 trials and b from an average of 298 trials in monkeys with unilateral lesions. Graph c shows the effects of bilateral lesions on a ballistic movement performed with an increase in the moment of inertia (average of 130 trials). In graph a some normal features remain in the relationship between the activity of the biceps and triceps and the three parameters of movement. In b and c the presence of cocontraction and the loss of reciprocal relationships between agonist and antagonist during peak ac-celeration and velocity are evident. (From Soechting, et al.,[25] with permission.)

of the dentate nucleus remains unknown. Current evidence suggests it is involved in the initiation of movements, the execution of preplanned motor tasks, and the regulation of posture. The mechanisms underlying these functions are unknown, however, dentate efferent projections clearly affect neuronal interactions in the thalamus and cerebral cortex as well as the spinal cord.

A GENERAL PERSPECTIVE

Each of the three major cerebellar sagittal zones displays a remarkable degree of functional diversity. The lateral zone of the cerebellum, for example, is in-volved in goal directed movements of the extremities, but the anatomic connec-tions of the dentate nucleus with extraocular motor nuclei strongly suggest the lateral zone is involved also in the control of eye movements. The lateral cerebel-lar zone also may participate in the control of posture, because postural deficits clearly are apparent after dentate lesions. In addition, neurons in the dentate as well as the interposed nuclei respond during both phasic movements and tonic maintenance of posture. The output of the dentate nucleus is important in the con-trol of proximal muscles, as indicated by studies showing that dentate efferent projections affect the behavior of neurons in regions of the motor cortex related to proximal muscle groups. Similarly, the midline cerebellar zone, in addition to its involvement in postural regulation, also may participate in goal directed move-ments. The projections ascending from the fastigial nuclei to the thalamus may contribute to this function, particularly when postural fixation or associated movements of the trunk and proximal muscles are required. Consequently, it is inappropriate to consider the control of posture as restricted to the function of the cerebellar vermis, leaving the regulation of goal directed limb movements to the cerebellar hemispheres.[2, 8, 9, 11, 16]

The functions that the cerebellum performs are not necessarily engaged auto-matically by the nervous system during a specific motor task. Rather, the contribution of the cerebellum is determined by the conditions under which the task is performed. For example, the modification in gain of the vestibulo-ocular reflex resulting from the actions of the cerebellum depends upon the need for visual fixation during a head movement. The activity of neurons in the cerebellar cortex and nuclei can reflect a combination of inputs activated by stimuli of several different modalities, as a result of the marked convergence of mossy fiber projections to the cerebellum. Moreover, owing to the convergence of mossy fiber inputs from descending central nervous system pathways, cerebellar neuronal activity can respond to signals conveying the intent, initiation, time course, and magnitude of the movement. As a consequence, the cerebellar output resulting from the activation of a specific cerebellar input will vary depending upon the inputs from other sources.

Despite the extensive investigations of cerebellar anatomy and physiology, it is still not possible to define precisely how the cerebellum performs its function. Only its regulation of the gain of the vestibuloocular reflex has a sound quantitative basis. Quantitative studies of the deficits resulting from total or partial cerebellar ablation have been helpful, however, in determining the specific aspects of motor control in which the cerebellum participates. The cerebellum is intimately involved in timing the activity in agonist and antagonist muscles during the execution of preplanned ballistic movements, particularly if the movement is directed toward a restricted target. Thus, the cerebellum participates in the execution of motor tasks whose strategy must be determined before the movement is initiated. It is required for the execution of rapidly alternating repetitive movements. The cerebellum appears to be particularly important for the execution of complex smooth pursuit movements requiring the coordination of several extremities. This function may require the cerebellum to maintain the relationship between directed movements of the distal extremities and the postural fixation required for the performance of the movements. For example, the dysmetria of a learned movement following lesions of the dentate and interposed nuclei is accentuated when postural fixation of the limb is required for the movement of the distal extremities.[12] If the requirement of postural fixation is removed by passively stabilizing the extremity, the phasic movements of the distal extremities show an appreciable reduction in the amount of dysmetria. Thus, it is likely that cerebellar function is truly integrative in nature, enabling the performance of tasks which require the coordinated activation of many groups of muscles.

REFERENCES

1. ALLEN, G. I., AND TSUKAHARA, N.: *Cerebrocerebellar communication systems.* Physiol. Rev. 54:957, 1974.
2. BANTLI, H., AND BLOEDEL, J. R.: *Monosynaptic activation of a direct reticulospinal pathway by the dentate nucleus.* Pflügers Arch. 354:237, 1975.
3. BANTLI, H., AND BLOEDEL, J. R.: *Characteristics of the output from the dentate nucleus to spinal neurons via pathways which do not involve the primary sensorimotor cortex.* Exp. Brain Res. 25: 199, 1976.
4. BANTLI, H., AND BLOEDEL, J. R.: *Interactions between the dentate nucleus and the spinal cord via infratentorial nuclei.* Exp. Brain Res. (Suppl.) 1:84, 1976.
5. BLOEDEL, J. R., HAMES, E. G., BANTLI, H. ET AL.: *The organization of descending projections from the brainstem activated by the output of the dentate nucleus.* Neurosci. Abstr. 4:63, 1978.
6. BROOKS, V. B., ADRIEN, J., AND DYKES, R. W.: *Task-related discharge of neurons in motor cortex and effect of dentate cooling.* Brain Res. 40:85, 1972.

7. BURTON, J. E., AND ONODA, N.: *Interpositus neuron discharge in relation to a voluntary movement.* Brain Res. 121:167, 1977.

8. CHAMBERS, W. W., AND SPRAGUE, J. M.: *Functional localization in the cerebellum. I. Organization in longitudinal cortico-nuclear zones and their contribution to the control of posture, both extrapyramidal and pyramidal.* J. Comp. Neurol. 103:105, 1955.

9. CHAMBERS, W. W., AND SPRAGUE, J. M.: *Functional localization in the cerebellum. II. Somatotopic organization in cortex and nuclei.* Arch. Neurol. Psychiat. 74:653, 1955.

10. DEECKE, L., BECKER, W., GROZINGER, B. ET AL.: *Human brain potentials preceding voluntary limb movements.* Electroenceph. Clin. Neurophysiol. (Suppl.) 33:97, 1973.

11. ECCLES, J. C., SABAH, N. H., SCHMIDT, R. F. ET AL.: *Mode of operation of the cerebellum in the dynamic loop control of movement.* Brain Res. 40:73, 1972.

12. GOLDBERGER, M. E., AND GROWDON, J. H.: *Pattern of recovery following cerebellar deep nuclear lesions in monkeys.* Exp. Neurol. 39:307, 1973.

13. GRIMM, R. J., AND RUSHMER, D. S.: *The activity of dentate neurons during an arm movement sequence.* Brain Res. 71:309, 1974.

14. ITO, M.: *Cerebellar control of the vestibular neurones: physiology and pharmacology.* Prog. Brain Res. 37:377, 1972.

15. ITO, M.: *Learning control mechanisms by the cerebellum investigated in the flocculo-vestibulo-ocular system,* in Tower, D. B. (ed.): *The Nervous System, Vol. 1. The Basic Neurosciences.* Raven Press, New York, 1975, pp. 245–252.

16. KORNHUBER, H. H.: *Motor functions of cerebellum and basal ganglia: The cerebellocortical saccadic (ballistic) clock, the cerebello-nuclear hold regulator, and the basal ganglia ramp (voluntary speed smooth movement) generator.* Kybernetik 8:157, 1971.

17. LISBERGER, S. G., AND FUCHS, A. F.: *Role of primate flocculus during rapid behavioral modification of vestibulo-ocular reflex. I. Purkinje cell activity during visually guided horizontal smooth-pursuit eye movements and passive head rotation.* J. Neurophysiol. 41:733, 1978.

18. LISBERGER, S. G., AND FUCHS, A. F.: *Role of primate flocculus during rapid behavioral modification of vestibulo-ocular reflex. II. Mossy fiber firing patterns during horizontal head rotation and eye movement.* J. Neurophysiol. 41:764, 1978.

19. MEYER-LOHMANN, J., CONRAD, B., MATSUNAMI, K. ET AL.: *Effects of dentate cooling on precentral unit activity following torque pulse injections into elbow movements.* Brain Res. 94:237, 1975.

20. MURPHY, J. T., KWAN, H. C., MACKAY, W. A., ET AL.: *Physiological basis of cerebellar dysmetria.* Can. J. Neurol. Sci. 2:279, 1975.

21. RANISH, N. A., AND SOECHTING, J. F.: *Studies on the control of some simple motor tasks. Effects of thalamic and red nuclei lesions.* Brain Res. 102:339, 1976.

22. ROBERTSON, L. T., AND GRIMM, R. J.: *Responses of primate dentate neurons to different trajectories of the limb.* Exp. Brain Res. 23:447, 1975.

23. ROBINSON, D. A.: *Adaptive gain control of vestibulo-ocular reflex by the cerebellum.* J. Neurophysiol. 39:954, 1976.

24. SCHULTZ, W., MONTGOMERY, E. B., JR., AND MARINI, R.: *Stereotyped flexion of forelimb and hindlimb to microstimulation of dentate nucleus in cebus monkeys.* Brain Res. 107:151, 1976.

25. SOECHTING, J. F., RANISH, N. A., PALMINTERI, R., ET AL.: *Changes in a motor pattern following cerebellar and olivary lesions in the squirrel monkey.* Brain Res. 105:21, 1976.

26. STRICK, P. L.: *Cerebellar neuron response to imposed limb displacement: Dependence of short latency dentate activity on intended movement.* Neurosci. Abstr. 2:533, 1976.

27. TERZUOLO, C. A., SOECHTING, J. F., AND PALMINTERI, R.: *Studies on the control of some simple motor tasks. III. Comparison of the EMG pattern during ballistically initiated movements in man and squirrel monkey.* Brain Res. 62:242, 1973.

28. THACH, W. T.: *Discharge of Purkinje and cerebellar nuclear neurons during rapidly alternating arm movements in the monkey.* J. Neurophysiol. 31:785, 1968.

29. THACH, W. T.: *The behavior of Purkinje and cerebellar nuclear cells during two types of voluntary arm movement in the monkey,* in Fields, W. C., and Willis, W. D. (eds.): *Cerebellum in Health and Disease.* Warren H. Greene, Inc., St. Louis, 1970, pp. 217–230.

30. THACH, W. T.: *Discharge of cerebellar neurons related to two maintained postures and two prompt movements. I. Nuclear cell output.* J. Neurophysiol. 33:527, 1970.

31. THACH, W. T.: *Discharge of cerebellar neurons related to two maintained postures and two prompt movements. II. Purkinje cell output and input.* J. Neurophysiol. 33:537, 1970.

32. THACH, W. T.: *Timing of activity in cerebellar dentate nucleus and cerebral motor cortex during prompt volitional movement.* Brain Res. 88:233, 1975.

33. THACH, W. T.: *Correlation of neuron discharge with pattern and force of muscular activity, joint position and direction of intended next movement in the motor cortex and cerebellum.* J. Neurophysiol. 41:654, 1978.

34. TOLBERT, D. L., BANTLI, H., HAMES, E. G. ET AL.: *A demonstration of the dentato-reticulospinal projection in the cat.* Neuroscience (in press).

CHAPTER 10

The Symptoms and Signs of Cerebellar Disease

THE SYMPTOMS OF CEREBELLAR DISEASE

Diseases affect cerebellar function through a number of mechanisms, including direct compression or invasion of cerebellar tissue, alteration of blood supply to the cerebellum, and inflammation or edema of cerebellar structures. Cerebellar disease also causes symptoms through damage to adjacent structures such as the meninges and blood vessels in the posterior fossa and through obstruction to the flow of cerebrospinal fluid. Apart from a few exceptions, symptoms resulting directly from cerebellar injury cannot be separated clearly from symptoms due to damage of adjacent structures.[15, 16, 21, 28, 44]

The initial complaints in patients with cerebellar disease depend more on the location and rate of progression than on the pathology of the lesion. Disturbances of sudden onset, such as hemorrhages and infarctions, present with remarkably similar symptoms.[20, 34] Disturbances of gradual onset, such as certain types of neoplasms, usually cause few symptoms of cerebellar disease.[3] Other types of neoplasms, such as metastatic tumors, may produce rapidly evolving signs of both cerebellar injury and brainstem compression.[19]

Table 1 contains a list of symptoms in 162 patients with focal cerebellar lesions from recent studies by Lechtenberg and Gilman.[52, 53] The location of the lesion and type of pathology were determined by autopsy examination or surgical exploration in 90 percent of the cases and by contrast studies or CT scan in the rest. Most patients had a combination of four symptoms: headache, gait difficulty, nausea and vomiting, and dizziness. The complaint of dizziness in most patients represented a sense of light headedness and only in a few cases was described as a true vertigo. Apart from a few cases, these symptoms showed no clear correlation with the site of the pathology in the cerebellum (Tables 2, 3, and 4). Some of the symptoms, such as double vision, hearing disorder, and memory difficulty, resulted from extension of the disease beyond the confines of the cerebellum. These symptoms conform well in frequency with symptoms reported in other series of patients with cerebellar disease.[3, 19, 46, 80]

Headache

The headache resulting from cerebellar disease presents typically as a severe, dull, frontal or occipital pain, often developing early in the evolution of symptoms.

189

Table 1. Symptoms of focal cerebellar lesions in
162 patients

Symptom	Number of Patients
Headache	125
Nausea and vomiting	121
Gait difficulty	100
Dizziness	60
Double vision	27
Memory difficulty	16
Blurred vision	6
Hearing loss	6
Clumsiness	5
Altered sensation	4
Tremor	4
Limb weakness	2
Eye deviation	2
Ringing in ears	2
Head shaking	2
Head tilt	1
Difficulty swallowing	1
Illusory environmental movement	1

The pain often is limited to a small area above or behind the eye or at the base of the skull and usually does not lateralize.[42] The headache often worsens with postural changes. Lying flat for several hours may increase the pain and lead to the characteristic complaint of frontal headache, which is most severe upon awakening in the morning, subsiding as the day advances. The headache from an expanding cerebellar lesion does not show the lateralization or characteristic visual disorder seen in migraine and does not cause the autonomic phenomena associated with nocturnal cluster headaches such as conjunctival injection, unilateral lacrimation, rhinorrhea, and changes in sweating. The pain does not awaken the patient and photophobia does not accompany the pain.

The acute headache developing with cerebellar hemorrhage or infarction[36] evolves over minutes to hours and lasts hours or days depending upon how long the patient survives. The pain usually is described as more severe than any prior headache experienced by the patient. Complaints of headache persist with mild

Table 2. Headache

	Location of Lesion		
Location of Pain	Left Hemisphere	Right Hemisphere	Vermis
Frontal	15	12	6
Parietal	2	1	2
Occipital	10	8	10
Frontal and occipital (Poorly defined location 41)	6	8	4

Table 3. Diplopia

Site of Lesion	Patients Complaining
Right hemisphere	7
Left hemisphere	7
Vermis	13

analgesics or rest. Severe gait difficulty or progressive obtundation usually alerts the observer to the seriousness of this headache. With chronic lesions, such as tumors and cysts, headaches evolve over minutes, days, or weeks, and last weeks or months. Headache is the most common symptom in patients with cerebellar tumors,[3] and remitting and recurring head pain over the course of months is also common with cerebellar tumors.

The location of the lesion in the cerebellum does not affect the likelihood of developing headache; a tumor in the vermis is as likely to produce headaches as a tumor in the hemisphere (see Table 2). The frontal headache accompanying cerebellar disease reflects distortion of the meninges on the dorsal surface of the cerebellum and the tentorium; cerebellar tissue itself is insensitive and extensive damage to this structure alone does not evoke head pain. Pain fibers to the surface of the tentorium cerebelli are derived from the first division of the fifth cranial nerve.[25] Because this division of the trigeminal nerve also supplies the skin of the forehead over the eyes, the frontal headache with a posterior fossa lesion is due to referred pain.

The occipital headache occurring with cerebellar lesions results from distortion of the leptomeninges about the foramen magnum. Cervical nerve roots and perhaps some branches of the vagus nerve supply the meninges in this area. C_2 and C_3 have ascending rami that enter the posterior fossa and supply the dura on the floor of the posterior fossa.[47] Consequently, many patients complain of neck stiffness or aching as well as occipital pain.

Nausea and Vomiting

Nausea and vomiting frequently accompany headache in acute and chronic cerebellar lesions.[46, 73] As with the headaches accompanying cerebellar disease, nausea and vomiting are most severe in the morning and the nausea may subside once the patient is upright and active. Weeks of nausea remitting for months and then recurring are common also. Projectile vomiting, consisting of forceful vomiting with little or no warning,[73] occurs in some of these patients though protracted nau-

Table 4. Impaired memory

Site of Lesion	Patients Complaining
Right hemisphere	9
(Superior right hemisphere)	(5)
Left hemisphere	5
(Superior left hemisphere)	(5)
Vermis	2
(Superior vermis)	(2)

sea is more common. Vomiting may relieve temporarily both the nausea and the headache. Abdominal pain, changes in bowel patterns, and alterations in appetite are absent. With rapidly progressive cerebellar damage, nausea and vomiting may begin abruptly and terminate only as obtundation intervenes. In young children, the vomiting and resultant weight loss may so dominate the illness that an extensive abdominal evaluation may be completed before the intracranial basis for the symptom becomes apparent. The structures responsible for the nausea and vomiting accompanying cerebellar disease are unknown, but compromise of brainstem function is thought to be the significant factor.[65] Nausea and vomiting do not accompany degenerative cerebellar disease,[9, 50] lending support to the notion that no intrinsic cerebellar structure is responsible for these symptoms.

Gait Difficulty

Patients with cerebellar disease complain that they walk with a staggering gait, making it seem that they suffer from alcohol intoxication. Their difficulties include walking in a straight line directly toward a target and precise placement of their feet. They tend to lurch from side to side or to drift irresistibly to one side while trying to walk forward.[46] The patients often find that, in addition to being lifted too high, the feet are placed either too widely apart or too closely together in an irregular sequence so that successive steps are spaced irregularly.[2] Patients with cerebellar disease seldom develop the exaggerated elevation of the foot which is observed in patients with impaired position sense. The complaint of gait difficulty can be helpful in localizing the site of pathology; injury to one cerebellar hemisphere may lead the patient to deviate while walking toward the side of the lesion or to fall to that side.[46] The tendency may be substantial enough to interfere with stance as well as gait and, at its worst, the patient will complain of falling to one side on sitting. Complaints of difficulty initiating gait, changes in velocity of gait, and instability from propulsion or retropulsion are not characteristic of cerebellar disease. These symptoms often occur with basal ganglia disease and may be helpful in distinguishing basal ganglia disease from cerebellar disease.[18]

Vertigo

Patients with cerebellar disease often complain of dizziness, a symptom usually described imprecisely and with difficulty. In some patients this symptom represents vertigo, a subjective sense of rotation in space with the patient actually having the illusion of environmental or personal movement. Usually vertigo from disease of the cerebellum or brainstem consists of feelings of recurrent front-and-back or side-to-side movements of the patient or environment. In contrast, spinning sensations often stem from disease of the labyrinth. Other complaints described by patients as dizziness include feelings of instability when attempting to walk, lightheadedness, and faintness. These complaints are as common as vertigo in cerebellar disease.[46, 73] Dizziness often appears episodically[19] and may be severe enough to prevent standing or even sitting. Nausea and vomiting may appear with this symptom.

Many patients with cerebellar disease observe that dizziness may be evoked by changes in position. Turning the head to one side may elicit severe nausea and a sense of spinning. Transient nystagmus develops with the positional change and patients occasionally describe oscillopsia, or oscillations of the environment coincident with the nystagmus. Dizziness occurs in patients with a variety of cerebellar disorders including vascular lesions, neoplasms, degenerative diseases, and inflammatory processes.[46] The type of lesion and rate of progression bear no well defined relation to the development of this symptom.

Visual and Ocular Motor Disorders

A number of visual disturbances can occur in association with cerebellar diseases even though the cerebellar lesion itself usually does not cause the disturbance. Diplopia is the most common visual complaint associated with any cerebellar lesion (see Table 3).[3, 73] The diplopia may be episodic or constant and, when it lasts more than a few minutes, the patient generally recognizes the advantage of closing one eye. Dysconjugate gaze may be experienced as blurred vision by some, and these individuals may find that visual acuity improves with closing one eye. Other types of visual disorder occur less commonly. With overshoot ocular dysmetria, the patient has transient oscillations of the eyes initially upon looking toward a target. During this transient phase of gaze instability, the patient may be aware of blurred vision.[69] A patient with ocular dysmetria and a right cerebellar hemisphere tumor, for example, complained of difficulty seeing only while in motion.[17] Degenerative, neoplastic, or vascular lesions in the cerebellum may be associated with ocular motor disorders which disturb conjugate gaze or convergence. These abnormalities reflect the involvement of the cerebellum in vestibulo-ocular reflexes; maintenance of gaze on an object while the head is moving relies upon cerebellar interactions with the vestibular apparatus.

Impaired visual acuity or blindness may develop as part of degenerative,[51] metabolic, or inflammatory diseases. This may be abrupt and transient, as in the optic neuritis of multiple sclerosis,[55] or gradual and permanent, as in the pigmentary retinal degeneration of Refsum disease.[49] Some patients[53] with cerebellar neoplasms note episodic visual illusions, a complaint also reported in certain degenerative diseases.[23] These are described as a loss of perspective or a distortion of dimensions. Visual loss may be an early complaint in some familial forms of spinocerebellar degeneration.[51] In these cases the patient may be an infant who fails to respond to visual cues or a young adult with failing central, peripheral, or color vision. The "dancing" eye movements of an infant with a neuroblastoma may be the first sign of this disorder.[12] A child's commenting upon "spots" in one eye may be early indication of retinal angiomata associated with von Hippel-Lindau syndrome.[60]

Dyssynergia

A number of patients with cerebellar disease complain initially of clumsiness in performing familiar acts such as tying a knot, opening a jar, or moving small objects. Opening a lock requires increased attention to the placement and movement of the key. Few patients misconstrue this as weakness; the typical complaint is that a hand is useless even though the strength is intact. The rapidity of movements is slowed and accuracy is lost.[7, 37-39] There are no sensory changes; the limb does not feel heavy or numb and no clumsiness is apparent until the patient attempts some coordinated action.

NEUROLOGIC SYMPTOMS OCCURRING IN CONJUNCTION WITH CEREBELLAR DISEASE

Dementia

Memory impairment or transient confusion may prompt some patients with focal or widespread cerebellar disease to seek medical attention (see Table 4).[46] Obstructive hydrocephalus accounts for the altered mentation in many of these patients.[34, 73] Minor deficits in memory and attention are common complaints in patients with cerebellar degeneration,[45] but frank dementia usually can be traced to deterioration of noncerebellar structures.

Hearing Loss

Hearing loss is not by itself a symptom of cerebellar disease,[73] but may develop unilaterally or bilaterally in association with several cerebellar diseases.[1, 29, 72] A cerebellopontine angle schwannoma of the eighth cranial nerve causes slowly progressive or abrupt loss of hearing on the affected side in advance of an ipsilateral cerebellar disorder.[33] The frequent bilaterality of this lesion may produce a deceptively multifocal clinical presentation. Many of the spinocerebellar and olivo-pontocerebellar degenerations include progressive hearing loss as a symptom,[50] but the associated signs and symptoms usually clarify the diagnosis. Occlusion of the anterior inferior cerebellar artery can present with sudden unilateral deafness,[1] though usually there are enough signs of brainstem disease to indicate the diagnosis. Occlusion of the superior cerebellar artery generally does not cause deafness, but partial hearing loss may develop.[1] Less frequent causes of cerebellar disease with deafness include subpial siderosis,[72] a condition usually ascribed to recurrent subarachnoid hemorrhages with subpial accumulations of hemosiderin, and metastatic cerebellar abscess,[29] an infectious disorder resulting in compression of the eighth nerve.

THE SIGNS OF CEREBELLAR DISEASE

As pointed out in Chapter 1, the organization of the cerebellum can be viewed from several perspectives. For the clinician, at present the most helpful conceptualization is to view the cerebellum as a structure organized into a series of sagittal zones extending from medial to lateral on each side. The midline zone of the cerebellar cortex with the fastigial nuclei comprise one functional grouping, the intermediate zone with the interposed nuclei a second, and the lateral zone with the dentate nuclei a third. Although smaller divisions have been demonstrated anatomically, clinical abnormalities uniquely referable to smaller subdivisions have not been defined. Indeed, owing to the irregular and often unpredictable patterns of anatomic damage in human cerebellar disease, distinct abnormalities can be referred only to the midline and lateral zones; signs of cerebellar disease peculiar to the intermediate zone have not been identified.

In the past, distinctive cerebellar symptoms and signs have been attributed to disease of similar anatomic subdivisions, but these have included smaller segments of the cerebellum. Thus, Dow and Moruzzi[19] recommend a classification that includes: 1) the flocculonodular lobule; 2) the anterior lobe; and 3) the posterior lobe. Brown[13, 14] proposes a classification including five subdivisions based upon conceptions of the localization of function in the cerebellum. This classification includes: the basal portion (flocculonodular lobule); the midportion (simple lobule, tuber, and pyramis); the anterior portion (anterior lobe); and the right and left lateral portions (neocerebellum). The clinical signs attributed to these structures are: truncal ataxia from disease of the basal portion; disturbed speech and eye movements from involvement of the midportion; abnormalities of station and gait from damage to the anterior portion; and defects of postural fixation and skilled voluntary acts from disturbances of the lateral portion.

Recent anatomic and physiologic studies, reviewed in the earlier chapters of this monograph, have shown that cerebellar connections are organized considerably less strictly into functional zonal groups than appreciated previously. Thus, the midline cerebellar zone receives information descending from forebrain levels of the central nervous system, including the cerebral cortex, as well as from the brainstem and spinal cord. The midline zone sends projections to rostral as well as caudal regions of the nervous system. The lateral cerebellar zone also communicates with both forebrain and spinal levels of the central nervous system. In keeping with these findings, a recent study of the clinical signs resulting from focal lesions of the cerebellum revealed that the localization of clinical signs is much less precise than thought previously.[52, 53] The only localization that can be supported at this time on the basis of the available clinical studies is to distinguish between the effects of disease in the midline and lateral cerebellar zones (Table 5). In many patients, even these two cannot be distinguished with certainty; each of the signs classically attributed to midline cerebellar disease can occur with disease in the lateral zones of the cerebellum (Table 5). The most helpful signs localizing a disease process to the midline zone are the association of nystagmus with an ataxic gait without ataxia of the individual limbs. The most helpful signs localizing a disease process to the lateral zone are disorders of coordinated limb movements restricted to one side of the body, with ipsilateral hypotonia, dysdiadochokinesis, dysrhythmokinesis, nystagmus, and impaired check and excessive rebound.

Disease of the Midline Zone of the Cerebellum

The midline zone of the cerebellum consists of the anterior and posterior vermis, the flocculonodular lobe, and the fastigial nuclei. As pointed out earlier in this monograph, these regions receive many afferent projections from spinocerebellar pathways, vestibular primary afferents and nuclei, and reticulocerebellar pathways. The midline zone sends projections to brainstem structures, chiefly the vestibular and reticular nuclei, which in turn project to nuclei of the spinal cord and the extraocular muscles. Both the afferent and efferent connections of the midline cerebellar zone are involved in the balance required for ambulation, the maintenance of truncal posture, the position of the head in relation to the trunk, and the control of extraocular movements. As a consequence, the clinical signs resulting from midline cerebellar disease consist of disordered stance and gait,[57, 58] truncal titubation,[19] rotated postures of the head,[3] and disturbances of extraocular movements.[19] In the past, dysarthria has been considered a sign of midline cerebellar disease.[37, 38] However, a recent study demonstrated that dysarthria results chiefly from disease of the cerebellar hemisphere.[52, 53] Dysarthria was found to occur much more frequently from left cerebellar hemisphere disease than from vermal or right hemisphere disease.

Table 5. Effects of disease in midline and lateral cerebellar zones

Sign	Total Affected (% of those tested)	Left Hemisphere (% of those tested for group)	Right Hemisphere (% of those tested for group)	Vermis (% of those tested for group)
Gait difficulty	127 (87%)	47 (88%)	47 (94%)	33 (79%)
Dysmetria	108 (74%)	48 (87%)	36 (71%)	25 (61%)
Nystagmus (gaze evoked)				
Horizontal	85 (56%)	32 (55%)	32 (59%)	21 (51%)
Vertical	24	7	10	7
Succession deficits	77 (68%)	31 (74%)	25 (62%)	21 (68%)
Facial palsy unilateral	51	26	16	10
Kinetic tremor	50 (56%)	18 (40%)	16 (39%)	16 (44%)
Dysarthria	31 (25%)	22 (54%)	7 (15%)	2 (6%)
Impaired consciousness	38 (24%)	13 (22%)	17 (31%)	8 (19%)
Impaired memory	29 (41%)	14 (58%)	12 (40%)	3 (19%)
Past-pointing	34 (44%)	15 (60%)	12 (43%)	7 (29%)
Head tilt	23	11	8	4
VI nerve palsy	25	10	5	10
Titubation	14	6	3	5
VIII nerve deficits	9	7	1	1
Global dementia	7	4	3	0
Ocular dysmetria	4	2	0	2
V nerve deficits	3	3	0	0
Handwriting impaired	17 (33%)	9 (50%)	7 (37%)	1 (10%)
Group totals	162	59	59	44

Disorders of Stance and Gait

CHARACTERISTICS OF THE DISORDERS. Abnormalities of standing and walking are the most common clinical signs of cerebellar disease (see Table 5).[3, 19, 46] The stance usually is on a broad base with the feet several inches apart. There may be a fore-and-aft or side-to-side truncal tremor that can evolve into a severe titubation. Postural abnormalities may occur, particularly if the cerebellar disorder has existed for several years. These abnormalities consist of scoliosis, elevation or depression of a shoulder, and a pelvic tilt. These abnormalities may be so slight that the only finding is an inequality in the height of the shoulder or the hips.[73] Postural abnormalities of marked degree occur more commonly with disease of the lateral than the midline cerebellar zone. Unequal degrees of hypotonia affecting truncal musculature probably are responsible for these findings.

During walking, truncal instability may be manifested by falls to the right, left, and forward, as well as backward, in individual patients.[38] Walking is carried out with a series of steps irregularly placed, some too far forward, some not sufficiently far forward, and some too far to the left or to the right. The legs often are lifted too high during ambulation. The patient may assume transiently a posture with optimal placement of the center of gravity, but then may develop truncal instability. This instability may be decreased slightly when the patient can look about and compensate for the truncal ataxia by monitoring the degree of stability with visual cues. There is no substantial change in the inclination to fall with the eyes open or shut. The Romberg test cannot be applied to assess position sense in these patients.[38]

Gait deficits can be enhanced by various maneuvers.[18] Walking in tandem, the successive placement of the heel of one foot in line and in contact with the toe of the other foot, may disclose an inability to walk on a narrow base or a tendency to fall toward one side. Walking on the heels, on the toes, or backward serves to increase the demand on cerebellar mechanisms for balance and coordination and may bring out a subtle deficit. Walking in a circle a few feet in diameter elicits a tendency to fall or stagger when circling clockwise or counterclockwise.[73] Such techniques, of course, must be evaluated in the context of the patient's age and other disabilities. The side toward which the patient falls, swerves, drifts, or leans does not indicate with absolute certainty the side of a cerebellar lesion.[46] A vermal lesion, for example, may produce consistent falling to the left, whereas a left hemisphere lesion can lead to a gait veering consistently to the right.

THE LOCALIZING VALUE OF DISORDERED STANCE AND GAIT. Ataxia of gait with otherwise unimpaired limb coordination can occur with strictly anterosuperior vermal damage and, indeed, is a hallmark of the cerebellar disturbance resulting from nutritional and alcoholic damage to the nervous system.[57, 75] Lesions of the flocculonodular lobule also are associated with disorders of stance and gait, often in conjunction with multidirectional nystagmus and head rotation.[13, 19] Mass lesions of the midline cerebellar zone may evoke abnormalities of stance and gait, but these abnormalities can result from the combined effects of obstruction of cerebrospinal fluid flow and focal cerebellar damage. This was illustrated in a series of patients[58] with cerebellar tumors and gait disorders examined before and after cerebrospinal fluid shunting procedures. Truncal ataxia was found in patients with either vermal or hemisphere lesions, but all the cerebellar tumor patients showed an improvement of gait with cerebrospinal fluid shunting alone.

In the cases of Lechtenberg and Gilman[53] with focal cerebellar disease,

Table 6. Gait disturbance

Gait	Cerebellar Lesion					
	Left Hemisphere		Right Hemisphere		Vermis	
	Affected	% of Left	Affected	% of Right	Affected	% of Vermis
Able to walk only						
when assisted	12	23	8	16	7	17
Markedly impaired	19	55	34	68	21	50
Trace impaired	6	11	5	10	5	12
Unimpaired	6	11	3	6	9	21

87 percent of those who could be tested for gait function had disordered gait. The procedures used for localizing the lesions, consisting chiefly of surgical delineation and autopsy examination, permitted separation of the cases into three groups. These groups consisted of those in which damage involved predominantly the left hemisphere, the right hemisphere, or the vermis. The findings revealed no major difference in the incidence of gait disorders with midline as opposed to lateral hemisphere lesions (Tables 5 and 6). It is possible, of course, that these findings reflected an association of gait disorder with limb ataxia in the patients with lateral cerebellar lesions and no such association in the patients with midline cerebellar lesions. To focus on this possibility, we eliminated all cases with limb dysmetria from the sample of patients evaluated for gait function. Tabulating the incidence of gait disorders in patients without limb dysmetria (see Table 10) revealed a definite but low incidence of gait and truncal ataxia in patients with left hemisphere disease, a higher incidence with right hemisphere lesions, and an even higher incidence with midline lesions. The conclusion is that disordered stance and gait without ataxia of individual limbs can result not only from disease of the midline cerebellar zone but also from disease of the lateral zone.

Titubation

Titubation consists of a rhythmic tremor of the body or head, appearing usually as a rocking of the trunk or head forward and back, from side to side, or in a rotatory movement, occurring several times per second. The amplitude of the tremor may be fine enough to be overlooked or coarse enough to prevent sitting or standing and, as with other cerebellar tremors, disappears with complete relaxation or sleep. A fore-and-aft, side-to-side, or rotatory tremor of the head and neck without truncal movement occurs commonly in the disorder described as senile, heredofamilial or essential tremor, without evidence of cerebellar dysfunction. The tremor of the head usually is associated with a distal static tremor of the fingers and wrists. Although truncal titubation can occur from disease of the cerebellar midline zone,[19] we have found that this sign has little localizing value (see Table 5).

Rotated or Tilted Postures of the Head

Abnormal postures of the head can result from cerebellar disease and have been thought to indicate disease involving the vermis[3] or the flocculonodular lobule.[19] As conventionally used, the term "head tilt" signifies the lateral deviation of the head without rotation, so that one ear is located closer to the shoulder than the other ear. Thus, lateral deviation of the head to the right usually is described as a head tilt to the right. A rotated posture of the head indicates deviation of the occiput to one side with deviation of the chin to the opposite side.[18] Rotation of the head to the right indicates deviation of the occiput to the right. Head tilt and rotation can and often do present simultaneously with cerebellar diseases. In our patients,[53] head tilt or rotation occurred in 23 patients, but only 4 cf them had primarily midline lesions. Three of these 4 had a head tilt to the right and 1, to the left. Hemispheric lesions were associated with head tilt in 19 cases, but there was no correlation between the side of the damage and the direction of the head tilt. Eleven had head tilt ipsilateral to the side of the lesion and 8 had tilt to the contralateral side. We conclude that head tilt can be ascribed to cerebellar disease but does not have localizing significance.

Ocular Motor Abnormalities

Cerebellar diseases result in numerous and varied abnormalities of ocular motor function[46] ranging from nystagmus[18] to paresis of conjugate gaze.[27, 54] These abnormalities may be transient and asymptomatic and thus can be missed unless looked for specifically. Many of the abnormalities can be elicited on clinical examination, without specialized recording apparatus.[38] Most ocular motor abnormalities occurring with cerebellar diseases cannot be localized to specific cerebellar regions at present.

The limited localizing value of ocular motor abnormalities reflects the many regions of the cerebellum participating in the control of ocular motor functions. The flocculus is important in smooth pursuit movements, and other presently undefined areas of the cerebellum are essential in maintaining an eccentric gaze.[79] The flocculonodular lobule is important in visual-vestibular interactions. Cerebellar cortical ablation in primates[5] leads to changes in the amplitude and frequency of saccades. Some of these animals develop hypermetric saccades, and others have evident disorders of eye position on attempted fixation in the visual field ipsilateral to the cerebellar damage. This supports the view that some cerebellar hemispheric structures help maintain eccentric gaze.[79] This could be one of the functions of the fibers projecting from the cerebellar nuclei to the ocular motor nuclei.[22] The cerebellum, along with the brainstem, is involved in computing the location of targets in space, transforming spatial information into temporal information for appropriate muscle innervation, and adjusting the gain on saccadic eye movements to minimize overshoot or undershoot of a target.[5, 79] Thus, the cerebellum participates in the maintenance of lateral and vertical gaze positions, the production of smooth pursuit eye movements, and the modulation of saccadic eye movement amplitude.[30] Impaired cerebellar function causes, at least transiently, gaze-paretic nystagmus, poor following of targets without saccadic movements, abnormal optokinetic nystagmus, overshoot or undershoot ocular dysmetria, and rebound nystagmus.[17, 69, 79]

At present, the only ocular motor abnormalities known to result from midline cerebellar disease are gaze evoked nystagmus, rebound nystagmus, ocular dysmetria, and disorders of optokinetic nystagmus. Each of these abnormalities can result also from disease of other cerebellar zones.

Nystagmus

GAZE-PARETIC NYSTAGMUS. Nystagmus consists of rhythmic oscillatory movements of one or both eyes, occurring with the eyes in the primary position or with ocular deviation. Controversy has developed in recent decades over whether or not lesions restricted to the cerebellum can elicit nystagmus.[22, 24, 61, 64] Current evidence indicates that nystagmus does develop with cerebellar lesions[5, 79] and that gaze-paretic nystagmus, also termed gaze evoked nystagmus, is the most common form of nystagmus found with cerebellar disease.[6, 61] Patients with gaze-paretic nystagmus cannot maintain conjugate eye deviation away from the midposition. The drift of the eyes back to the center appears as the slow component of the nystagmus and the rapid corrective movement is seen as the fast component. The result is a series of to-and-fro jerking eye movements, occurring with conjugate ocular deviation, with a fast component in the direction of gaze and a slow component in the opposite direction. The amplitude of the fast component for gaze toward the side of a cerebellar lesion often is greater than the amplitude with gaze away from the side of the damage.[13, 54] The term "coarse" nystagmus generally refers to nystagmus with a large amplitude fast component. This nystagmus persists as long as the patient tries to look to the side or vertically. The nystagmus does not show fatigue or changes in frequency.[47] The examiner evokes nystagmus by asking the patient to follow laterally or vertically an object brought near the end points of normal gaze. The nystagmus becomes more prominent as gaze deviates in the direction of the fast component.[47] Nystagmus elicited on vertical gaze has limited localizing value (see Table 5), appearing frequently in patients with cerebellar as well as brainstem disease. Downbeat nystagmus is especially common in patients with the Arnold-Chiari malformation.

Fifty-six percent of the patients of Lechtenberg and Gilman[53] with focal cerebellar lesions had gaze evoked nystagmus (Tables 5 and 7). Fifty-one percent of patients with vermal lesions had gaze evoked nystagmus and only 12 percent of these patients had fast components of equal size on gaze to the right and left. Hemispheric lesions produced ipsilateral nystagmus in 31 percent of patients with lesions on the left and in 26 percent of those with lesions on the right. These findings indicate that nystagmus, although more frequent with vermal disease, also results from hemispheric disease.[61, 73] The findings provide no evidence supporting the notion of a midline cerebellar locus instrumental in the development of gaze evoked nystagmus.

REBOUND NYSTAGMUS. This is a disorder of ocular movements associated with disease of the midline or lateral zones of the cerebellum occurring characteristically in chronic cerebellar disease.[40, 56] Rebound nystagmus can be evoked by

Table 7. Lateral gaze evoked nystagmus

| Direction of Gaze for Maximum | Cerebellar Lesion | | | | | |
| | Left Hemisphere | | Right Hemisphere | | Vermis | |
	Affected	% of Left	Affected	% of Right	Affected	% of Vermis
Left	18	31	6	11	11	27
Right	6	10	14	26	5	12
Bilateral	8	13	12	22	5	12
Neither	26	45	22	41	20	49

having the patient deviate the eyes laterally. Nystagmus with its fast component in the direction of the gaze starts with only a few degrees of ocular movement. The amplitude and frequency of the nystagmus are the same in both eyes. As the eyes maintain eccentric gaze, the amplitude of the nystagmus decreases and the direction of the fast component reverses after about 20 sec of sustained lateral gaze. With return of the eyes to the primary position, nystagmus recurs with the fast component away from the side of the prior gaze deviation. The nystagmus with gaze directly forward also abates after several seconds unless fixation is shifted to another eccentric point. Although chronic cerebellar lesions are the typical setting in which this ocular motor dysfunction develops, it is seen also with phenytoin intoxication.[40] Rebound nystagmus generally does not result from brainstem disease and is the only type of nystagmus that can be considered specific for cerebellar disease.

OCULAR DYSMETRIA. This is a disorder of eye movements analogous to limb dysmetria which superficially may resemble nystagmus. Errors in visual fixation occur as the patient's gaze approaches a visual target and small rapid eye movements develop as the patient corrects for the inaccuracies in both the initial attempt at fixation and subsequent efforts at refixation. Both overshoot and undershoot of fixation occur so that the eyes appear to jerk back and forth because of the persistent inaccuracies in saccadic movements intended to bring the target to the fovea. These errors decrease in size progressively and, as a result, the eyes oscillate momentarily about the target.

Ocular dysmetria is most obvious on changes in fixation from an eccentric position to the primary position of gaze. The amplitude of the overshoot may be equal with gaze to either side, even when the cerebellar lesion is limited strictly to a single hemisphere.[17] Regardless of whether attempts at shifting gaze from one point to the next result in overshoot or undershoot of the target, the compensatory movements will be saccades. When ocular dysmetria is manifested by overshoot of the target, it is called saccadic overshoot dysmetria. The saccadic pattern in overshoot dysmetria has been well defined.[69] The percentage of overshoot with each attempt at refixation actually increases with smaller excursions of gaze (Fig. 1). The overshoot error is greater if a smaller arc of eye movement is required. Usually there is a maximal saccade excursion beyond which the saccades become hypometric; gaze falls short of the desired fixation point and compensatory movements must make up the difference. Although visual pursuit of an object does not normally involve saccadic eye movements, patients with overshoot dysmetria will demonstrate overshoot when following a target that stops suddenly.[17] The pursuit movement yields to compensatory saccades that correct for the overshoot error (Fig. 2). Consequently, ocular dysmetria can occur with smooth pursuit eye movements and saccadic eye movements. The underlying mechanisms in both of these situations may be "underdamping" of the eye movements caused by delays in the integration of neural activity from muscle spindles.[69]

Ocular dysmetria occurs with disease of midline[69] or lateral cerebellar structures.[70] Hereditary degenerative disorders,[6] cerebellar tumors,[3] and cerebellar infarctions can cause this disorder. An acute form of ocular dysmetria develops with rapidly progressive, widespread cerebellar disease.[70] This acute dysmetria is characterized by transiently incrementing, rather than decrementing, saccades with the usual inaccurate refixation phenomenon. These progressively enlarging saccades are called macrosaccadic oscillations.[70] Typically the oscillations disappear in complete darkness and abate spontaneously about two to three weeks af-

202

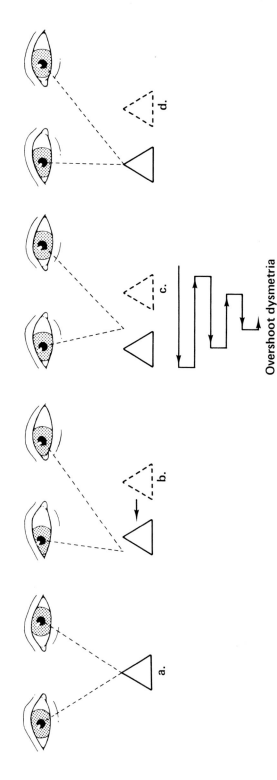

Overshoot dysmetria

Figure 1. Saccadic overshoot dysmetria. Starting with the eyes fixed on a target (a), the patient must shift his gaze when the target abruptly assumes a new position. The eyes move conjugately towards the new target position, but overshoot the actual target location (b). The saccade to compensate for the overshoot itself is larger than necessary. Consequently, the eyes seem to oscillate about the target for a fraction of a second as each successive error is corrected (c and d). The black arrows represent the direction and magnitude of successive saccadic adjustments enabling the patient to fixate accurately on the target.

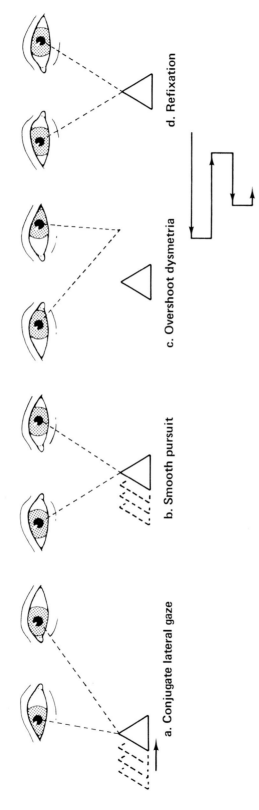

Figure 2. Overshoot dysmetria with arrested pursuit. a, The target is moving smoothly from right to left and the eyes conjugately are pursuing the target. b, The target moves into the primary position of gaze and accurate fixation is maintained. c, The target stops moving abruptly and the eyes conjugately overshoot the resting point. Arrest of eye movements lags behind arrest of the target. d, Refixation on the target is achieved with typical saccadic overshoot dysmetria. The black arrows represent the direction and magnitude of the terminal saccades required for accurate fixation on the target.

a. Conjugate lateral gaze   b. Smooth pursuit   c. Overshoot dysmetria   d. Refixation

203

ter the onset of the lesion. The occurrence of macrosaccadic oscillations in cerebellar disease provides an indication of the influence of the cerebellum on the calibration of saccade amplitude.[70]

OPTOKINETIC NYSTAGMUS. Abnormalities of optokinetic nystagmus can occur with midline cerebellar lesions. Nystagmus develops normally when an individual attempts to count the stripes on a rotating drum or moving cloth strip. The resulting eye movements, termed optokinetic nystagmus, should appear regardless of the direction in which the striped object moves, whether it be lateral or vertical, to the right or to the left. The slow component of the nystagmus is in the direction the stripes are moving. When the direction of the movement reverses, the slow component of the nystagmus reverses. As with other types of nystagmus occurring in pathologic situations, the slow and fast phases of this physiologic nystagmus should be equal in excursion and speed in both eyes. Many lesions, both infratentorial and supratentorial, can alter this nystagmus, but the pattern of the alteration usually is helpful in assessing the site of the lesion. With lesions of the medial longitudinal fasciculus, the amplitude of excursions in the two eyes is unequal. With parietal lobe disturbances, optokinetic nystagmus is asymmetric, the amplitude of the fast component being less prominent when the stripes are moved toward the side of the cerebral lesion.[10] Patients with cerebellar lesions also have disturbed optokinetic nystagmus, but the abnormality frequently is an increase in the amplitudes of the fast and slow components, particularly with chronic disease. Enhanced optokinetic nystagmus may result from decreased inhibition of the normal excursions allowed by the ocular motor apparatus.[40] The abnormality can be likened to impaired check of eye movements. Patients with more acute lesions may demonstrate inconsistent or diminished optokinetic nystagmus.[69] Tumors extending into the fourth ventricle occasionally produce an asymmetric optokinetic nystagmus with the fast component completely absent when the nystagmus is elicited in one direction.[17] Although a similar asymmetry in the nystagmus may develop with cerebellar hemisphere lesions, there is little in the pattern that indicates the side of cerebellar damage.

Disease of the Lateral (Hemispheric) Zone of the Cerebellum

For clinical purposes, the lateral cerebellar zone consists of the cerebellar hemisphere and the dentate and interposed nuclei of each side. The intermediate cerebellar zone, consisting of paravermal portions of the cerebellar cortex and the interposed nuclei, is included in the lateral zone because diseases affecting this region specifically have not been identified. The lateral cerebellar zones send projections to brainstem and thalamic structures that engage both forebrain and spinal levels of the central nervous system.

The "syndrome of the posterior lobe,"[13, 19] an older term for lateral cerebellar zone disorders, denotes a collection of signs often seen with damage to the bulk of the hemispheres and only minor or no midline cerebellar involvement. Gordon Holmes[37, 38] provided the major observations on this syndrome in patients with shrapnel injuries to the posterior fossa during World War I. The clinical signs were similar whether one hemisphere or both were damaged, although the signs were generally more severe and bilateral with damage to both hemispheres. Holmes found that an acute lesion results in decreased resistance to passive manipulation in the ipsilateral limbs. Active movement of the limbs on the affected side results in static and kinetic tremors. Movements are discontinuous and some-

204

what delayed. With unilateral lesions, movements on the affected side begin more slowly and peak force is reached more slowly than on the other side.[39] Exertion is less continuous and the involved limb appears to tire more readily. Other signs of lateral cerebellar disease include dysarthria, dysmetria, dysdiadochokinesis, excessive rebound, impaired check, kinetic and static tremors, decomposition of movements, past-pointing, and eye movement disorders.[73]

Hypotonia

Hypotonia, a decrease in the resistance to passive movement of the limbs, appears in one or several limbs at the time of cerebellar injury or in the course of cerebellar degeneration.[37] Hypotonia often abates with time, especially if the initiating lesion is not progressive. The mechanisms responsible for hypotonia are discussed in Chapter 8.

Hypotonia can be detected most easily when it follows unilateral cerebellar damage of recent onset.[73] The hypotonic limb resists passive movement considerably less than the normal limb.[18] Grasping the patient's forearm and shaking the relaxed hand at the wrist is a simple way to assess the resistance to passive manipulation. Not only will the hypotonic limb appear to have a more flail hand, but the carrying angle of the hand on the forearm will be more acute for the hypotonic arm than is normal. A normal carrying angle is about 70° between the hand and the

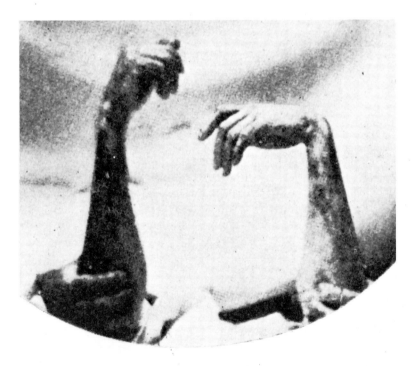

Figure 3. The forearms and hands of a patient with extensive injury of the left side of the cerebellum. This photograph was taken one week after the injury. When the forearms were held vertically, the left wrist flexed under the influence of gravity much more than the right. (From Holmes,[37] with permission.)

forearm when the forearm is held upright and the hand is allowed to fall limp at the wrist (Fig. 3). At rest the limb may assume a more flail posture than the corresponding limb[73] and on active extension of the arms forward, there appears abnormal flexion of the wrists with hyperextension at the metacarpophalangeal joints. This probably results from hypotonia that is greater in wrist extensor than flexor muscles and a similar imbalance in the finger flexors and extensors. The hypotonic limbs often show pendular deep tendon reflexes.[39] When the patellar tendon is struck, the familiar damping of tendon jerks does not occur and the lower leg swings forward and back three or more times. This sign can be demonstrated best with the patellar and triceps reflexes. The leg should hang freely over the edge of an examining table when the examiner attempts to elicit the reflex. Pendular reflexes should not be confused with the clonus resulting from corticospinal tract disease. Clonus occurs at a rate several fold faster than the rate of the pendular reflex. Moreover, sustained clonus usually requires continuous stretch of muscle. The decreased resistance to passive manipulation of the limb in cerebellar disease and increased resistance in corticospinal tract disease should leave little uncertainty over whether or not the repetitive response is clonus.

Dysarthria

In patients with cerebellar disease, speech may slow and become more labored, but comprehension remains intact and grammer does not suffer. The problem from the patient's viewpoint is the flow of speech; the facile production of words and phrases is lost. Early in the development of dysarthria, the patient is unaware of the change in the sound of his voice. Those familiar with the normal tone and rate of the patient's speech will comment that his speech is slowed, slurred, garbled, hoarse, monotonous, or shows some combination of these features. As with gait difficulties, the alterations in speech may be ascribed to alcohol intoxication by uninformed observers. The degree of dysarthria may vary greatly from day to day.

Writing may be labored in much the same way as speech. In a recent study of dysarthria from cerebellar disease,[52] patients without evident right hand tremor or dysmetria complained that the flow and form of their penmanship deteriorated in parallel with their speech. This dysgraphia with dysarthria has some similarity to the writing disorder manifest with some aphasias.[31] The patient with an expressive aphasia may have telegraphic writing associated with nonfluent telegraphic speech. The patient with dysarthria arising from a cerebellar lesion may have irregular, labored penmanship in association with slurred labored speech. There is presently no sizeable series of patients with cerebellar disease to establish whether this is a phenomenon necessarily developing with speech difficulty. Speech disorders are discussed further in Chapter 11.

Dysmetria

Dysmetria is a disturbance of the trajectory or placement of a body part during active movements (Fig. 4).[32, 43] Hypometria refers to a trajectory in which the body part falls short of its goal, and hypermetria indicates a trajectory in which the body part extends beyond its goal. To test for limb dysmetria, the physician asks the patient to use the forefinger of his outstretched arm to touch the tip of his nose with his eyes closed. Rather than alighting on the nose with one fluid movement,

206

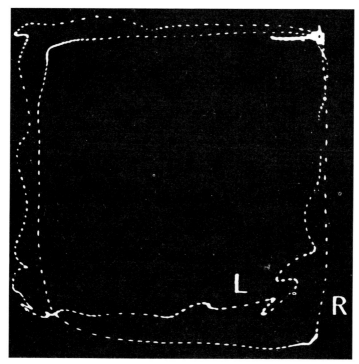

Figure 4. Records of the attempts of a patient with a lesion of the left side of the cerebellum to outline the square end of a room with the right (unaffected) and left (affected) forefingers in succession. Each flash of light represents the distance covered by the moving finger in 0.04 sec. In attempting to outline a square as slowly and accurately as possible, the patient cannot maintain a uniform rate with the affected limb. The movement consists of a series of jerks separated by considerable periods of time. The more slowly the patient attempts to perform the movement, the more irregular it becomes. There is marked dysmetria, with both hypometria and hypermetria. A marked abnormality in the rate of movement can be detected in this record. (From Holmes,[37] with permission.)

the finger takes an erratic or inaccurate approach and strikes the cheek (in a hypermetric movement) or stops before reaching the nose (in a hypometric reach). The entire movement usually contains errors in trajectory and speed.[37] Corrective movements affect the arrival at the desired point and the final elements of the movement may be short oscillations about the nose. Commonly there will be a side-to-side tremor, generated at the shoulder, as the finger approaches the nose. There are some limitations to the interpretation of the finger-to-nose test. Position sense deficits or mildly impaired strength may produce abnormalities of trajectory or placement, but these problems should be apparent on evaluation of sensory and motor function.

Often a patient with cerebellar disease can compensate somewhat with vision for dysmetric movements. With severe cerebellar dysfunction, however, visual cues cannot compensate for the errors in limb movements.[37] With both eyes open, the patient will still overshoot, undershoot, or arrest lateral to a target he is asked to touch with the finger of an outstretched arm. This form of dysmetria occasionally is termed past-pointing, but this term is at best applicable only when arm movements are hypermetric. Historically, past-pointing has referred to the inaccurate placement of a limb with movement limited to one joint. In the Barany

207

past-pointing test, the patient is asked to extend his arms in front of his body, parallel to the floor. With his eyes closed, he redirects them straight up over his head and then rapidly tries to reapproximate the initial forward position with movement only at the shoulder joints. Patients with cerebellar lesions will reposition the arms inaccurately, usually overshooting the original position or drifting laterally with one or both arms.[38]

Dysmetria can be detected in the legs by having the patient, lying supine, touch the heel of one foot to the knee of the opposite leg and run the heel down the shin. The heel must be lifted free of the shin before the patient repeats the movement, because simply running the heel up and down the shin will mask unsteadiness or a tremor in the moving leg. Errors in placement and force characterize the movements of the disabled limb which commonly deviates to the left or right while the foot moves along the shin. Tests analogous to those used for evaluating past-pointing in the upper limb involve reapproximating a leg position with movement restricted to the hip. The patient tries to touch the examiner's finger held about two feet above his great toe, moving his leg only at the hip, with his eyes open and then shut. Although dysmetria and past-pointing in the legs commonly are associated with a disorder of gait, a profound gait disorder may develop with cerebellar damage in the absence of clinically demonstrable lower limb dysmetria. Gait is a level of function vulnerable to more than just individual limb dysfunctions.

Dysdiadochokinesis and Dysrhythmokinesis

Dysdiadochokinesis is a manifestation of the decomposition of movement in cerebellar disease demonstrated by testing alternating or fine repetitive movements (Fig. 5).[37, 73] Clinical tests to elicit dysdiadochokinesis include having the patient tap one hand with the other rapidly, placing the palmar and dorsal surfaces alternatively upward. When this is performed as quickly as possible, deficits appear in the rate of alternation as well as the completeness of the sequence.[38] The hand may be supinated or pronated incompletely. The patient cannot produce regularly syncopated movements. More subtle irregularities in the rate and force of the movement may be appreciated by listening to the sound made by the hand striking a surface, alternately with the palmar and then the dorsal surface. Variations of this include having the patient rapidly open and close the fist or pantomime rapidly screwing a light bulb into an overhead socket. Apposing each finger in rapid succession against the thumb of the same hand will demonstrate finer deficits in coordination. Alternate tapping of the heel and toe on the floor will demonstrate succession deficits in the feet. Similar disturbances may appear with diseases of the basal ganglia or the corticospinal tracts, but characteristic of cerebellar disease is a disturbance in the rhythm of the activity. Dysrhythmokinesis, a disorder in the rhythm of rapidly alternating movements, can be evoked directly by asking a patient to tap out a rhythm, such as three rapid beats followed by one delayed beat. Initiation of a rhythmic sequence may be slowed with basal ganglia or corticospinal tract damage, but the rhythm typically is distorted with cerebellar lesions. Hyperreflexia, clonus, extensor plantar response, and increased resistance to passive manipulation of the limbs may be additional indications of a noncerebellar etiology for the dysdiadochokinesis.

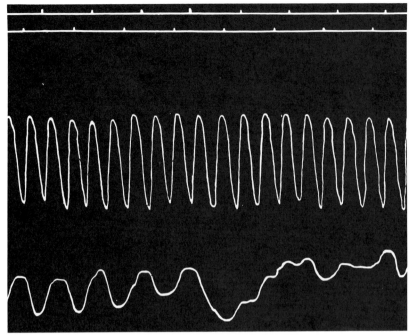

Figure 5. Tracings of rapid pronation and supination. The movements of the affected arm (below) were, for a time, regular though slower and of smaller amplitude than the movements of the unaffected arm, but grew increasingly irregular as the arm became more or less fixed in supination. (From Holmes,[37] with permission.)

Ataxia

DEFINITION. Ataxia describes comprehensively the various problems with movement resulting chiefly from the combined effects of dysmetria and decomposition of movement (Fig. 6). Decomposition of movement refers to errors in the sequence and speed of the component parts of a movement. The result is a lack of speed and skill in acts requiring the smoothly coordinated activity of several muscles.[73] Movements previously fluid and accurate become halting and imprecise.

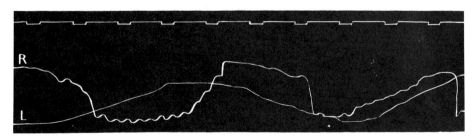

Figure 6. A patient with a right sided cerebellar lesion was requested to flex and extend each index finger at a slow and uniform rate. The separate tracings were obtained on a smoked drum during successive rotations of the drum. The jerky and tremulous character of the movements of the right finger contrast with the regular and uniform rate of those of the left. Errors in the sequence and speed of the component parts of the movement can be seen. The movements become halting and inprecise. (From Holmes,[37] with permission.)

Table 8. Limb dysmetria

Limbs Most Affected	Cerebellar Lesion					
	Left Hemisphere		Right Hemisphere		Vermis	
	Affected	% of Left	Affected	% of Right	Affected	% of Vermis
Left	37	67	6	12	6	15
Right	4	7	22	43	3	7
Both equally	7	13	8	16	16	39
Neither	7	13	15	29	16	39

The abnormalities of movement with cerebellar disease have been termed *asynergia* or *dyssynergia,* terms indicating the patient's inability to perform various components of a movement at the right time in the appropriate space.[3, 62]

THE LOCALIZING VALUE OF LIMB ATAXIA. The distribution of ataxia in the patient's limbs assists in localizing cerebellar diseases. In the series of Lechtenberg and Gilman,[53] unilateral limb dysmetria occurred uncommonly with midline cerebellar disease (Table 8), a finding consistent with the notion that lateral cerebellar disease results in this sign, as shown in prior clinical studies.[3, 46] Seventy-four percent of patients in our series had limb dysmetria, with 71 percent of those with right hemisphere disease affected, 87 percent of those with left hemisphere damage affected, and 61 percent of those with vermal lesions (see Table 5). The ipsilateral limbs were primarily affected in 67 percent of patients with left cerebellar hemisphere disease and in 43 percent of patients with right hemisphere disease. These findings give further evidence that dysmetria results chiefly from hemispheric disturbances. In addition, limb dysmetria was absent in 39 percent of the patients with vermal disease, and the majority of patients with vermal disease and dysmetria had both sides affected equally.

The distribution of dysdiadochokinesis also helps to localize the site of a cerebellar disorder (Table 9). Deficits of succession or rapid alternating movements appeared in 63 percent of our patients. Sixty-two percent of patients with right hemisphere disease were affected, 74 percent of left, and 69 percent of vermal. There was a disparity in the occurrence of this sign in the two hemisphere groups in our series. Sixty percent of patients with left hemisphere lesions had succession deficits primarily in the ipsilateral limbs, but only 27 percent of the patients with right hemisphere disease had predominantly right limb dysfunction. Although

Table 9. Succession deficits

Limbs Most Affected	Cerebellar Lesion					
	Left Hemisphere		Right Hemisphere		Vermis	
	Affected	% of Left	Affected	% of Right	Affected	% of Vermis
Left	25	60	7	18	14	45
Right	1	2	11	27	5	16
Both equally	5	12	7	18	2	6
Neither	11	26	15	37	10	32

210

Table 10. Gait in patients without limb dysmetria

| | Cerebellar Lesion | | | | | |
| | Left Hemisphere | | Right Hemisphere | | Vermis | |
Gait	Affected	% of Left	Affected	% of Right	Affected	% of Vermis
Able to walk only when assisted	0	0	2	17	2	12
Markedly impaired	0	0	6	50	7	44
Trace impaired	3	43	2	17	1	6
Unimpaired	4	57	2	17	6	38

only 2 percent of patients with left hemisphere disease had contralateral dysdiadochokinesis greater than ipsilateral dysdiadochokinesis, 18 percent of those with right hemisphere damage had primarily left limb succession deficits. Even in the group with vermal disease, 32 percent of patients had no succession deficits and 45 percent of patients had primarily left limb difficulties. As with dysmetria, ipsilateral limb dysfunction was not nearly as likely with a right hemisphere lesion as with a left hemisphere lesion. Indeed, even if the lesion was in the right hemisphere or the vermis, there was an unexpectedly high proportion of patients with left limb dysfunction.

Although the pathology in any series may occur more often in one site rather than another for no apparent reason, lesions in our series showed no evidence of disproportionate involvement of the left hemisphere.[52, 53] In addition to the autopsy material, surgical reports, and radiographic studies favoring a truly random scatter of lesions throughout the cerebellum in this series, there was evidence from the clinical findings. Kinetic tremor appeared with similar frequency in the ipsilateral limbs whether the left hemisphere or the right hemisphere was damaged. Bilateral kinetic tremors occurred most frequently in patients with vermal disease. Altered mentation and obtundation were slightly more common with right hemisphere disease than with either vermal or left hemisphere damage. In addition, severe gait dysfunction occurred in more than half of the patients without limb dysmetria when the lesion was vermal, and in none of the patients when the lesion was left hemispheric. In contrast, two-thirds of the patients with right hemisphere disease without limb dysmetria had severe gait disorders (Table 10). Our conclusions are that: 1) the patients in our series had a random distribution of lesions; 2) cerebellar hemisphere lesions result in unilateral limb dysmetria, dysdiadochokinesis, and tremor; and 3) the left and right cerebellar hemispheres show differential susceptibility to the effects of local disease processes.

Tremor

Cerebellar disease results in static and kinetic tremors. Existing terminology for these abnormalities of movement is confusing. *Intention tremor*[42, 77] is an ambiguous term because it can be used in reference to tremors on contemplating, initiating, performing, or completing a movement. *Kinetic tremor* is a more accurate term for the classic cerebellar tremor occurring with limb movement. Present terminology usually includes the term "proximal" because the tremor is generated primarily in the proximal limb musculature.

211

Static tremor can be demonstrated by asking the patient to extend the arms parallel to the floor with the hands open. Usually this position can be sustained steadily for several seconds, but then the arms develop a rhythmic oscillation generated at the shoulder. A similar tremor can be demonstrated in the lower extremities by having the patient, while supine, elevate one leg and hold the great toe of the leg adjacent to but not contacting the examiner's finger. This posture also can be held for a few seconds, but then a rhythmic oscillation develops at the hip.

The proximal kinetic tremor in cerebellar disease can be brought out by having the patient perform the finger-nose and heel-shin tests. The tremor appears when the patient initiates a movement of the limb or during the course of moving the limb. The amplitude of the oscillations increases as the limb approaches the target. The arm tremor is coarse, side-to-side, and of increasing amplitude as the arm is extended. Whether the affected limb is an arm or a leg, the tremor arises chiefly in the limb girdle. A lower limb tremor is likely to be enhanced by a maneuver requiring flexion at the knee. On attempting to touch the heel of one foot to the opposite knee, the patient develops a prominent side-to-side swinging of the knee and foot of the moving leg.

The static and kinetic tremors of cerebellar disease often need to be distinguished from the tremors of Parkinson disease, Wilson disease, essential tremor, and hyperthyroidism. Patients with parkinsonism have a distal tremor, most prominent at rest, and usually decreased during the movement of the limb toward a target. The tremor of parkinsonism often persists with complete relaxation in bed whereas cerebellar tremor usually disappears. Some patients with basal ganglia disorders, such as Wilson disease, display coarse proximal static and kinetic limb tremors on maintaining the limb in various positions. In Wilson disease, holding both arms straight forward parallel to the floor in protraction and extension or abducted with the elbows flexed may elicit a coarse tremor of the limbs in abduction and adduction arising at the shoulders. The marked akinesia, rigidity, and dystonia in Wilson disease may help to distinguish this disease from cerebellar disturbances. Patients with essential tremor may have both proximal and distal static tremors. This tremor, however, is considerably more marked at the distal joints of the limb than the tremor of cerebellar disease. In addition, the adduction-abduction movements of individual fingers commonly seen in essential tremor usually do not occur with cerebellar disorders. The tremor of hyperthyroidism is principally a distal movement best demonstrated by having the patient maintain the limbs extended forward. A proximal kinetic tremor should not appear in hyperthyroidism. Kinetic tremors also can occur with neurologic disorders causing weakness, including corticospinal tract and anterior horn cell disease. These disorders can be distinguished by the demonstration of weakness and signs of spasticity or muscle wasting.

Cerebellar tremor occurs usually from cerebellar lateral zone disorders, affecting chiefly the ipsilateral limbs (Table 11). Midline cerebellar disease usually evokes either no tremor or tremor appearing bilaterally (see Table 5).

Check, Rebound, and Limb Weakness

Impaired check and excessive rebound are closely related signs of focal or widespread cerebellar damage.[68, 73] Several techniques can be used to test for these signs. With his arms outstretched forward, the patient is asked to maintain his limbs immobile in space while the examiner taps the wrists strongly enough to

Table 11. Kinetic tremor

Limbs Most Affected	Cerebellar Lesion					
	Left Hemisphere		Right Hemisphere		Vermis	
	Affected	% of Left	Affected	% of Right	Affected	% of Vermis
Left	11	24	4	10	4	11
Right	1	7	7	17	2	6
Both equally	6	13	5	12	10	28
Neither	27	60	25	61	20	55

displace the arms. The patient keeps his eyes shut and his hands pronated. A small displacement with rapid, accurate return to the original position occurs normally. With cerebellar damage, a light tap to the wrist results in a large displacement of the affected limb, followed by overshoot beyond the original position.[18, 37] Return to the original position is achieved by oscillation of the arm about its initial position. Wide excursion of the affected limb is the product of impaired check. Excessive rebound results in overshoot beyond the original position.

Impaired check can be assessed also by pulling forcefully on the patient's forearm while the patient flexes his elbow.[73] On releasing the forearm abruptly, the examiner will precipitate an unchecked contraction of the arm with the patient consequently striking his chest with his hand or wrist. This is generally termed the Stewart-Holmes sign. The basic phenomenon is an inability to stop abruptly an ongoing movement.

The rebound phenomenon originally described by Gordon Holmes[39] actually was unrelated to the excessive rebound of cerebellar disease. He observed that patients with spastic limbs had an excessive degree of recoil or rebound when an opposed flexion was released suddenly.[37] When opposition of a flexed spastic arm was released abruptly, the patient would check the flexion and extend the arm at the elbow inadvertently as if the arm were recoiling from the biceps flexion.[4] This rebound presumably reflected an imbalance or disparity in relaxation times between antagonistic muscles in a spastic limb. Patients with signs of cerebellar disease in a limb characteristically lacked this rebound phenomenon in the affected limb.[37, 73] Common usage of this term has distorted Holmes' original intent.

Limb weakness has been described with cerebellar lesions,[37, 38, 73, 76] but this results more from a deficit in organization and coordination of muscle activity than true weakness.

Ocular Motor Disorders

Lateral cerebellar disorders result in a number of ocular motor disturbances including those described in association with midline cerebellar diseases (gaze evoked nystagmus, rebound nystagmus, ocular dysmetria, and abnormalities of optokinetic nystagmus). Other ocular motor disorders in cerebellar disease cannot be localized clearly to the lateral cerebellar zones, appearing often in the presence of widespread cerebellar disease or in diseases involving both the cerebellum and the brainstem.

OPSOCLONUS. This is an ocular movement disorder in which the eyes constantly make random conjugate saccades of unequal amplitudes in all directions.[17, 69]

213

The abnormal eye movements are most marked immediately before and after a fixation. Patients with bursts of opsoclonus may notice no distortion of normal vision, but some report jumping of objects in the visual field as their eyes move erratically to and fro.[17] Cerebellar degeneration occurring as a remote effect of carcinoma and neuroblastoma usually are associated with this rare disorder.[11, 12]

OCULAR FLUTTER. Ocular flutter is an ocular motor disorder occurring either spontaneously or with changes in fixation. Rapid to-and-fro oscillations of the eyes develop abruptly, last for a few seconds, and disturb vision for the duration of the episode.[17] The frequency of attacks may increase with excitement. Unlike ocular dysmetria there is no stereotyped structure to the oscillations and the oscillations may develop with gaze directed straight ahead. Eccentric gaze is not important in the initiation of the flutter movements. A large variety of cerebellar diseases results in ocular flutter.

OCULAR BOBBING. In this disorder, both eyes intermittently dip abruptly downward through an arc of a few degrees. Following this movement, the eyes return synchronously to the primary position at a rate much slower than their rate of downward displacement. The movements usually are not as rhythmic as the movements in nystagmus and the fast movement downward with ocular bobbing is relatively slow compared to the fast component of the movement in vertical nystagmus. Ocular bobbing is usually associated with complete paralysis of spontaneous and reflex horizontal eye movements. The downward excursions in ocular bobbing occur only a few times each minute, a frequency suggesting a similarity to roving eye movements[26] With roving eye movements, the abrupt step-like activity of the saccadic eye movement is lost and the eyes seem to drift conjugately or dysconjugately. Ocular bobbing has been likened to roving eye movements without lateral gaze.[26] Thus, the vertical eye movements actually are fragments of roving movements, the brainstem structures essential for lateral gaze having been compromised or destroyed. The eyes can only drift up or down. Ocular bobbing appears with pontine lesions and occurs frequently following occlusion of the basilar artery.[26] Perhaps because of the inevitable compression of the pons with rapidly expanding cerebellar masses, ocular bobbing also occurs with acute cerebellar hemorrhages.

Although ocular bobbing is not a form of nystagmus, there is a true downbeat nystagmus developing with brainstem disease as well as with some hereditary cerebellar degenerative diseases.[8, 78, 79] With the eyes in the primary position, a typical jerk nystagmus with a fast component down occurs spontaneously. This downbeat nystagmus usually is attributed to disease at the cervicomedullary junction and occurs often with the Arnold-Chiari malformation.

OCULAR MYOCLONUS. This is a rhythmic, pendular or rotatory oscillation of the eyes associated with synchronous oscillation of the palate. Associated rhythmic oscillations can occur in the pharynx, larynx, tongue, and diaphragm. Ocular and palatal myoclonus can occur in association with lesions disrupting the connections between the cerebellar dentate nucleus, the red nucleus, and the inferior olivary nucleus.

GAZE APRAXIA. Gaze apraxia is a disorder of conjugate ocular deviation without paralysis of the muscles needed for the movement. Normal saccadic eye movements bring images to the fovea in one rapid movement.[22] The speed of this movement is constant in an individual for a given angular displacement of the eyes. In many patients with familial cerebellar degeneration,[17] these short rapid eye movements are slow or inaccurate and the smooth, constant sweep of the eyes involved in following objects is slowed or lost.[22] The main problem in these cases is an inability to initiate conjugate ocular deviation, a deficit so severe in some patients with the cerebellar degenerative disorder, ataxia telangiectasia, that an apraxia of gaze develops[8] (Fig. 7). The patient voluntarily cannot move the eyes laterally but accomplishes the movement by thrusting his head in the direction he wants his eyes to go. To look to the left he rotates his head rapidly to the left. Both eyes swing over to the right as part of the intact oculocephalic (doll's eye) reflex movement,[48] but with maximal rotation of the head to the left, the eyes literally are dragged to the left. Aligned on the new fixation point, the eyes drift back to the primary position of gaze as the patient slowly straightens his head. The object of this entire maneuver is to enable the patient to break the fixation on the original target and look at a different point.

Patients with diffuse cerebellar atrophy occasionally have inappropriately small saccadic eye movements which are termed hypometric saccades.[5] This disorder of saccadic eye movements is more characteristic of basal ganglia disorders, such as Parkinson disease, than of cerebellar disorders.

PARESIS OF CONJUGATE GAZE. Paresis of conjugate gaze may appear with rapidly evolving cerebellar mass lesions. This is especially common with cerebellar infarctions and hemorrhages, perhaps because of brainstem ischemia associated with these acute lesions. In one series of patients with cerebellar infarction, gaze palsies or sixth nerve palsies developed in 9 of 16 patients shortly after the onset of symptoms.[54] In another series, conjugate lateral gaze disorders developed in 9 of 13 patients with cerebellar hemorrhages.[27] Gaze paresis to the side of the cerebellar lesion occurred in 8 of these 9 cases and forced deviation of the eyes away from the side of the lesion appeared in 6 patients. Deviation of the eyes away from the side of the cerebellar damage often is helpful in making the diagnosis of cerebellar hemorrhage or infarction,[59] but deviation toward the involved side does occur in some patients with these lesions.[66]

NEUROLOGIC SIGNS OCCURRING IN CONJUNCTION WITH CEREBELLAR DISEASE

Papilledema

Increased intracranial pressure developing with cerebellar disease commonly produces papilledema.[46] Compression rostral to the cerebellum at the aqueduct of Sylvius or caudal and anterior at the foramina of Luschka and Magendie may block cerebrospinal fluid entry into the subarachnoid space. Many cerebellar tumors grow into the fourth ventricle and obstruct cerebrospinal fluid movement through this structure.[73] Medulloblastomas and ependymomas in children are particularly prone to invade the fourth ventricle extensively.[67, 71] Whereas pressure changes usually are gradual with neoplasms,[3] abrupt elevations of intracranial pressure develop with cerebellar hemorrhage or infarction.[27, 66, 74] Papilledema may appear within hours of an increase in intracranial pressure.[66] The course can be so rapid in patients with hemorrhages or infarctions, however, that they die from brainstem compression before papilledema develops. Inflammatory diseases affecting the cerebellum may lead to a ventriculitis with thick exudates obstructing the fourth ventricle foramina, thereby causing papilledema. Retrobulbar neuritis, as occurs with multiple sclerosis,[55] produces a clinical disorder sometimes confused with cerebellar tumor if other signs of posterior fossa disease are present;

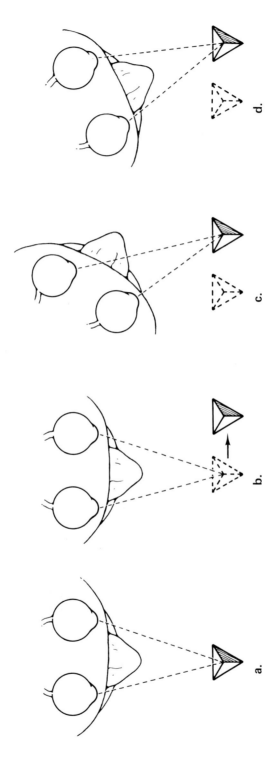

Figure 7. Gaze apraxia and head thrusting. a, The patient is looking at a target in the primary position. b, The target moves to the left; the patient cannot shift his gaze to the new position and continues to look at an imaginary target in the primary position. c, Fixation is shifted by turning the head rapidly in the direction of the target's movement. An oculocephalic reflex shifts the eyes as far to the right as they can go and head rotation continues until the eyes are dragged on-target. d, Fixed on the target in the new position, the eyes remain on-target as the head is slowly rotated back into its original position.

216

but the visual loss occasioned by optic neuritis should leave little question that pressure effects are not of primary importance in such patients. True papilledema is of no localizing value with cerebellar lesions and does not develop with strictly demyelinative or degenerative lesions of the cerebellum.

Altered Mentation

Alterations of mentation often develop in association with cerebellar lesions.[41, 45] The abnormalities vary in severity, ranging from forgetfulness to florid paranoid psychoses.[23, 45, 46] Alterations of mentation with cerebellar disease presumably do not result from the cerebellar lesion itself; rather, the disturbances are ascribed to the effects of hydrocephalus, cerebral degeneration, or brainstem compression.[3, 19, 35] In out series,[53] disorders of intellectual function occurred commonly. Twenty-four percent of patients had some alteration of consciousness ranging from lethargy to coma. Forty-one percent of patients evaluated for memory function had clear impairment. More than 10 percent of the patients had overt signs of psychosis, including visual hallucinations, depression, paranoid ideation, manic episodes, and confabulation. Memory deficits also occur frequently in cerebelloparenchymal disease and overt psychosis appears sporadically in association with cerebellar degenerative disease.[45]

Ophthalmoplegia

Ophthalmoplegia develops commonly in the comatose patient with cerebellar hemorrhage or infarction, but substantial brainstem compromise is apparent by the time this sign appears. Some forms of cerebellar degeneration are characterized by limited ophthalmoplegias,[63, 77] though these abnormalities may not result from the cerebellar lesion.[48] Some of these patients lose their ability to look down voluntarily while retaining good lateral gaze function.[63] In other patients, lateral gaze deteriorates before vertical gaze.[77] Selective impairment of saccades or rapid pursuit develops in some patients with partial ophthalmoplegias, presumably because of brainstem disease.

Facial Weakness

Facial weakness occurs in association with cerebellar disease, developing more often with hemisphere lesions than with midline lesions.[73] It is usually mild and limited to the lower portion of the face. This sign occurs commonly with focal cerebellar lesions,[3, 46] leading to the conclusion that it does not result simply from pressure or traction on the seventh cranial nerve. Traction clearly can produce palsies of the sixth cranial nerve, but in our series these were only half as frequent as facial weakness (see Table 5). The cause of this disorder is unclear.

Other Cranial Nerve Disorders

Traction on cranial nerves or direct involvement of nerves by a posterior fossa lesion may produce abducens palsies, hearing loss, and abnormal facial sensation.[3, 19] Schwannomas of the eighth cranial nerve are an especially common cause of cerebellar disturbances associated with dysfunction of multiple cranial nerves. A sixth nerve palsy[73] may occur with mass lesions in the cerebellum, not as a re-

217

sult of the cerebellar damage, but because of tension on the nerve produced by increased intracranial pressure or an expanding posterior fossa lesion (see Table 5).[46, 65] Diplopia develops when the palsy has an abrupt onset or is severe. With less complete lesions, diplopia may be apparent only on red glass testing. This test entails covering one eye with a translucent red material to allow the examiner to differentiate between the images seen with each eye. With the red glass over the eye with impaired sixth nerve function, a small light viewed by the patient will be seen as two images, one red and one white, located beside each other. On deviation of the eyes laterally toward the side of the paretic sixth nerve, the involved eye will not abduct normally and the red image will move farther laterally than the white image. This illusion reflects the fact that light falls on different regions of the retina in the two eyes. The red image appears to move where the eye is not moving. The degree of weakness may be too slight to observe as grossly dysconjugate gaze,[76] but the red glass test will provide evidence of the sixth nerve paresis.

Isolated dysfunction of the oculomotor and trochlear nerves does not occur characteristically with cerebellar lesions; involvement of these nerves generally indicates brainstem disease. An acute cerebellar hemorrhage may produce a small reactive pupil ipsilateral to the side of the hemorrhage,[27] but this probably represents a disorder of brainstem function.

Cerebellar Fits

Cerebellar fits are rare phenomena found in patients with large midline cerebellar tumors.[73] They do not represent seizure phenomena,[19, 73] but are decerebrate spasms with intermittent opisthotonos and rigidity.[76] Cerebellar fits may represent the human equivalent of the alpha rigidity described in animals with cerebellar and forebrain lesions (Chap. 7).

Catalepsy

A rarely mentioned sign of cerebellar damage is cerebellar catalepsy,[75] also termed the Babinski phenomenon. With the patient supine, both legs are flexed at the hips and knees. With extensive cerebellar damage, some patients will be able to remain immobile in this posture for protracted periods. Adventitial movements in the legs, normally apparent after a minute or two, do not develop on the side of the affected limb.

REFERENCES

1. ADAMS, R. D.: *Occlusion of the anterior inferior cerebellar artery.* Arch. Neurol. Psychiat. 49: 765, 1943.
2. AMASSIAN, V. E., AND RUDELL, A.: *When does the cerebellum become important in co-ordinating placing movements.* J. Physiol. 276:35p, 1978.
3. AMICI, R., AVANZINI, G., AND PACINI, L.: *Cerebellar Tumors,* in *Monographs in Neural Sciences,* Vol IV. Karger, Switzerland, 1976.
4. ANGEL, R. W.: *The rebound phenomenon of Gordon Holmes.* Arch. Neurol. 34:250, 1977.
5. ASCHOFF, J. C., AND COHEN, B.: *Changes in saccadic eye movements produced by cerebellar cortical lesions.* Exp. Neurol. 32:123, 1971.
6. BALOH, R. W., KONRAD, H. R., AND HONRUBIA, V.: *Vestibulo-ocular function in patients with cerebellar atrophy.* Neurology 25:160, 1975.

218

7. BIRD, T. D., AND SHAW, C. M.: *Progressive myoclonus and epilepsy with dentatorubral degeneration: a clinicopathological study of Ramsay-Hunt syndrome.* J. Neurol. Neurosurg. Psychiat. 41:140, 1978.

8. BALOH, R. W., YEE, R. D., AND BODER, E.: *Eye movements in ataxia-telangiectasia.* Neurology 28:1099, 1978.

9. BARBEAU, A.: *Cooperative study, phase two: statement of the problems.* Can. J. Neurol. Sci. 5:57, 1978.

10. BLACKWOOD W., DIX, M. R., AND RUDGE, P.: *The cerebral pathways of optokinetic nystagmus: a neuroanatomical study.* Brain 98:297, 1975.

11. BRAIN, L., AND WILKINSON, M.: *Subacute cerebellar degeneration associated with neoplasms.* Brain 88:465, 1965.

12. BRAY, P. F., ZITER, F. A., LAHEY, M, E., ET AL.: *The coincidence of neuroblastoma and acute cerebellar encephalopathy.* J. Pediat. 75:983, 1969.

13. BROWN, J. R.: *Localizing cerebellar syndromes.* JAMA 141:518, 1949.

14. BROWN, J. R.: *Degenerative cerebellar ataxias.* Neurology 9:799, 1959.

15. BROWN-SÉQUARD, C. E.: *Lectures on the diagnosis and treatment of the various forms of paralytic, convulsive, and mental affections IV.* Lancet 2:515, 1861.

16. CHALHUB, E. G.: *Neurocutaneous syndromes in children.* Ped. Clin. N. Am. 23:499, 1976.

17. COGAN, D. G.: *Ocular dysmetria; flutter-like oscillations of the eyes and opsoclonus.* Arch. Ophthal. 51:318, 1954.

18. DEJONG, R. N.: *The Neurologic Examination.* Harper & Row, New York, 1979.

19. DOW, R. S., AND MORUZZI, G.: *The Physiology and Pathology of the Cerebellum.* University of Minnesota Press, Minneapolis, 1958.

20. DUNCAN, G. W., PARKER, S. W., AND FISHER, C. M.: *Acute cerebellar infarction in the PICA territory.* Arch. Neurol. 32:364, 1975.

21. ECKER, A.: *Upward transtentorial herniation of the brainstem and cerebellum due to tumor of the posterior fossa.* J. Neurosurg. 5:51, 1948.

22. ELLENBERGER, C., KELTNER, J. L., AND STROUD, M. H.: *Ocular dyskinesia in cerebellar disease.* Brain 95:685, 1972.

23. FARMER, T. W., AND MUSTIAN, V. M.: *Vestibulocerebellar ataxia.* Arch. Neurol. 8:471, 1963.

24. FARWELL, J. R., DOHRMANN, G. J., AND FLANNERY, J. T.: *Intracranial neoplasms in infants.* Arch. Neurol. 35:533, 1978.

25. FEINDEL, W., PENFIELD, W., AND McNAUGHTON, F. L.: *The tentorial nerves and localization of intracranial pain in man.* Neurology 10:555, 1960.

26. FISHER, C. M.: *Ocular bobbing.* Arch. Neurol. 11:543, 1964.

27. FISHER, C. M., PICARD, E. H., POLAK, A., ET AL.: *Acute hypertensive cerebellar hemorrhage: diagnosis and surgical treatment.* J. Nerv. Ment. Dis. 140:38, 1965.

28. FISHER, J. D.: *Contributions illustrative of the functions of the cerebellum.* Am. J. Med. Sci. 23: 352, 1839.

29. GARDNER-THORPE, C., AND AL-MUFTI, S. T.: *Metastatic cerebellar abscess producing nerve deafness.* J. Neurol. Neurosurg. Psychiat. 32:360, 1969.

30. GAUTHIER, G. M., HOFFERER, J., HOYT, W. F., ET AL.: *Visual-motor adaptation.* Arch. Neurol. 36:155, 1979.

31. GESCHWIND, N.: *Current concepts: aphasia.* N. Engl. J. Med. 284:654, 1971.

32. GILBERT, G. J., McENTEE, W. J. III, AND GLASER, G. H.: *Familial myoclonus and ataxia.* Neurology 13:365, 1963.

33. GLASSCOCK, M. E. III: *The diagnosis and management of cerebello-pontine angle tumors.* J. Otolaryngol. 7:125, 1978.

34. GREENBERG, J., SKUBICK, D., AND SHENKIN, H.: *Acute hydrocephalus in cerebellar infarct and hemorrhage.* Neurology 29:409, 1979.

35. HEILMAN, K. M., AND VALENSTEIN, E.: *Mechanisms underlying hemispatial neglect.* Ann. Neurol. 5:166, 1979.

36. HEIMAN, T. D., AND SATYA-MURTI, S.: *Benign cerebellar hemorrhages.* Ann. Neurol. 3:366, 1978.

37. HOLMES, G.: *The Croonian lectures on the clinical symptoms of cerebellar disease and their interpretation.* Lancet 1:1177, 1922.

38. HOLMES, G.: *The Croonian lectures on the clinical symptoms of cerebellar disease and their interpretation.* Lancet 2:59, 1922.

39. HOLMES, G.: *The cerebellum of man.* Brain 62:1, 1939.

40. HOOD, J. D., KAYAN, A., AND LEECH, J.: *Rebound nystagmus.* Brain 96:507, 1973.

41. HORNABROOK, R. W.: *Kuru—a subacute cerebellar degeneration: The natural history and clinical features.* Brain 91:53, 1968.

42. HUNT, J. R.: *Dyssynergia cerebellaris progressiva—a chronic progressive form of cerebellar tremor.* Brain 37:247, 1914.

43. HUNT, J. R.: *Dyssynergia cerebellaris myoclonica—primary atrophy of the dentate system: A contribution to the pathology and symptomatology of the cerebellum.* Brain 44:490, 1921.

44. INGVAR, S.: *On cerebellar localization.* Brain 46:301, 1922.

45. KEDDIE, K. M. G.: *Hereditary ataxia, presumed to be Menzel type, complicated by paranoid psychosis, in a mother and two sons.* J. Neurol. Neurosurg. Psychiat. 32:82, 1969.

46. KESCHNER, M., AND GROSSMAN, M.: *Cerebellar symptomatology evaluation on the basis of intracerebellar and extracerebellar lesions.* Arch. Neurol. Psychiat. 19:78, 1928.

47. KIMMEL, D. L.: *Innervation of spinal dura mater and dura mater of the posterior cranial fossa.* Neurology 11:800, 1961.

48. KOEPPEN, A. H., AND HANS, M. B.: *Supranuclear ophthalmoplegia in olivopontocerebellar degeneration.* Neurology 26:764, 1976.

49. KOLODNY, E. H., HASS, W. K., LANE, B., ET AL.: *Refsum's syndrome.* Arch. Neurol. 12:583, 1965.

50. KONIGSMARK, B. W., AND WEINER, L. P.: *The olivopontocerebellar atrophies: A review.* Medicine 49:227, 1970.

51. LANDRIGAN, P. J., BERENBERG, W., AND BRESNAN, M.: *Behr's syndrome: familial optic atrophy, spastic diplegia and ataxia.* Develop. Med. Child. Neurol. 15:41, 1973.

52. LECHTENBERG, R., AND GILMAN, S.: *Localization of function in the cerebellum.* Neurology 28:376, 1978.

53. LECHTENBERG, R., AND GILMAN, S.: *Speech disorders in cerebellar disease.* Ann. Neurol. 3:285, 1978.

54. LEHRICH, J. R., WINKLER, G. F., AND OJEMANN, R. G.: *Cerebellar infarction with brain stem compression.* Arch. Neurol. 22:490, 1970.

55. LESSELL, S.: *Optic neuropathies.* N. Engl. J. Med. 299:533, 1978.

56. MACLEOD, P. M., WOOD, S., JAN, J. E., ET AL.: *Progressive cerebellar ataxia, spasticity, psychomotor retardation, and hexosaminidase deficiency in a 10 year old child: juvenile Sandhoff disease.* Neurology 27:571, 1977.

57. MANCALL, E. L., AND McENTEE, W. J.: *Alterations of the cerebellar cortex in nutritional encephalopathy.* Neurology 15:303, 1965.

58. MAURICE-WILLIAMS, R. S.: *Mechanism of production of gait unsteadiness by tumors of the posterior fossa.* J. Neurol. Neurosurg. Psychiat. 38:143, 1975.

59. McKISSOCK, W., RICHARDSON, A., AND WALSH, L.: *Spontaneous cerebellar hemorrhage.* Brain 83:1, 1960.

60. MILLER, R. G., PORTER, R. J., NIELSEN, S. L., ET AL.: *Von Hippel-Lindau's disease.* Can. J. Neurol. Sci. 3:29, 1976.

61. MORALES-GARCIA, C., CARDENAS, J. L., ARRIAGADA, C., ET AL.: *Clinical significance of rebound nystagmus in neuro-otological diagnosis.* Ann. Otol. Rhinol. Laryngol. 87:238, 1978.

62. MUSSEN, A. T.: *The cerebellum.* Arch. Neurol. Psychiat. 25:702, 1931.

63. NEVILLE, B. G. R., LAKE, B. D., STEPHENS, R., ET AL.: *A neurovisceral storage disease with vertical supranuclear ophthalmoplegia and its relationship to Niemann-Pick disease.* Brain 96:97, 1973.

64. OTT, K. H., KASE, C. S., OJEMANN, R. G., ET AL.: *Cerebellar hemorrhage: diagnosis and treatment.* Arch. Neurol. 31:160, 1974.

65. PLUM, F., AND POSNER, J. B.: *Diagnosis of Stupor and Coma.* F. A. Davis, Philadelphia, 1972.

66. REY-BELLET, J.: *Cerebellar hemorrhage: a clinicopathologic study.* Neurology 10:217, 1960.

220

67. RUBINSTEIN, L. J., AND NORTHFIELD, D. W. C.: *The medulloblastoma and the so-called "arach-noidal cerebellar sarcoma."* Brain 87:379, 1964.

68. SARNAT, H. B., AND NETSKY, M. G.: *Evolution of the Nervous System.* Oxford University Press, New York, 1974.

69. SELHORST, J. B., STARK, L., OCHS. A. L., ET AL.: *Disorders in cerebellar ocular motor control. I. Saccadic overshoot dysmetria.* Brain 99:497, 1976.

70. SELHORST, J. B., STARK, L., OCHS, A. L., ET AL: *Disorders in cerebellar ocular motor control. II. Macrosaccadic oscillation.* Brain 99:509, 1976.

71. SHUMAN, R. M., ALVORD, E. C., AND LEECH, R. W.: *The biology of childhood ependymomas.* Arch. Neurol. 32:731, 1975.

72. SINGH, N., RAO, S., AND BHUYAN, U. N.: *Reversible cerebello-cerebral disorder in primary hemochromatosis.* Arch. Neurol. 34:123, 1977.

73. STEWART, T. G., AND HOLMES, G.: *Symptomatology of cerebellar tumors. A study of forty cases.* Brain 27:522, 1904.

74. SYPERT, G. W., AND ALVORD, E. C., JR.: *Cerebellar infarction. A clinicopathological study.* Arch. Neurol. 32:357, 1975.

75. VICTOR, M., ADAMS, R. D., AND MANCALL, E. L.: *A restricted form of cerebellar cortical degeneration occurring in alcoholic patients.* Arch. Neurol. 1:579, 1959.

76. WEISENBURG, T. H.: *Cerebellar localization and its symptomatology.* Brain 50:357, 1927.

77. WOODS, B. T., AND SCHAUMBURG, H. H.: *Nigro-spino-dentatal degeneration with nuclear ophthalmoplegia.* J. Neurol. Sci. 17:149, 1972.

78. ZEE, D. S., FRIENDLICH, A. R., AND ROBINSON, D. A.: *The mechanism of downbeat nystagmus.* Arch. Neurol. 30:227, 1974.

79. ZEE, D. S., YEE, R. D., COGAN, D. G., ET AL.: *Ocular motor abnormalities in hereditary cerebellar ataxia.* Brain 99:207, 1976.

80. SCOTTI, G., SPINNLER, H., STERZI, R., ET AL.: *Cerebellar softening.* Ann. Neurol. 8:133, 1980.

CHAPTER 11

Dysarthria

CEREBELLAR DYSARTHRIA

Changes in the clarity, rhythm, and rate of speech develop with many cerebellar disorders.[14] The altered speech patterns from cerebellar disease collectively are termed dysarthria, but they are, in fact, a diverse group.[11] The variety of dysarthrias observed emphasizes the complexity of the systems responsible for the strictly motor phenomena of speech. Whatever form cerebellar dysarthria assumes, it is usually a composite of several categories of speech dysfunction. Common descriptors of dysarthric speech include scanning, slurring, staccato, explosive, hesitant, slow, altered accent, and garbled.

Scanning speech is the most easily recognized speech pattern associated with cerebellar disease. Charcot described this phenomenon in his discussion of patients suffering from multiple sclerosis.[12] He referred to scanning speech as a "peculiar difficulty of enunciation" with speech production slowed and words "measured or scanned." Patients with scanning speech produce syllables slowly and hesitate in the delivery of phrases, but they do not stammer or stutter. The basic defect is in the rhythm of speech, the flow from one word to the next.[24] These patients accentuate syllables or words inappropriately, omitting pauses where appropriate and adding pauses where unnecessary. Particular sounds may be labored over or slurred, especially labial phonemes.

The sum of the difficulties with the regulation of speech in cerebellar disease is called dysprosody.[13, 31] The grammar and meaning of the sentences are intact, but the more melodic elements of speech are deranged. The overall effect may be likened to an unpracticed student laboriously reading lines of poetry, making a special effort to decipher the rhythmic structure of the verse. The speech has an unnatural, impersonal, sing-song character. The dysprosody of cerebellar dysarthria may assume several forms.[13] In addition to scanning, slowed, and slurred speech, there is the equally distinctive explosive or hesitant speech.[38] The patient speaks with a staccato rhythm and speech volume has little meaningful modulation. The less common but more dramatic feature in some patients is a distortion of the customary accent. The patient seems to have newly acquired a foreign accent.[13] Despite difficulties with enunciation, patients with cerebellar disease do not produce paraphasias.[14] It is the intonation, accentuation, and melodic elaboration of speech that is disturbed. These are elements more akin to musical function than to verbal function.

Recent studies have characterized the elements of speech which are disturbed in patients with cerebellar damage.[11] Each element of the dysarthria is viewed in terms of the component parts, and these abnormal components are referred to as deviant dimensions.[11] Unfortunately, most studies of dysarthria have involved patients with chronic cerebellar diseases and the extent of the diseases has not been verified anatomically. Consequently, the precise limits of the cerebellar lesions are unknown.[11, 12] Dysarthria in patients with diseases considered on clinical examination to be limited to the cerebellum is characterized by 10 abnormalities. These are present to varying degrees in each patient and are: 1) imprecise consonants, a feature basic to all dysarthrias; 2) excess and equal stress, the inappropriate allocation of emphasis and accent; 3) irregular articulatory breakdown, the elision of syllables or phonemes; 4) distorted vowels; 5) harshness; 6) prolonged phonemes; 7) prolonged intervals; 8) monopitch; 9) monoloudness; and 10) slow rate. Viewed in terms of these deviant dimensions, scanning speech is a combination of excess and equal stress, irregular articulatory breakdown, prolonged phonemes, and prolonged intervals. The patients stress sounds inappropriately, drop some syllables, run word fragments together, prolong individual sounds, and leave inappropriate intervals between syllables and words. Additional characteristics in patients with cerebellar dysarthria include tremulous speech, nasal speech, and variable rate of speech.[6, 11, 22, 23] Speech volume occasionally will taper off to a whisper. Changes in breathing are not responsible for these alterations.[11]

Radiographic studies of tongue and mouth movements and measurements of voice patterns indicate an overall slowing of the rate and initiation of speech related movements in patients with some form of cerebellar dysarthria. In at least one patient[24] with the more common deviant dimensions of speech, the major deficit was in intonation rather than articulation. The actual muscle movements required for production of a sound were all present, but the speed with which they started and progressed was unduly slow for the desired sound. The cerebellar dysarthrias may result, in part, from a generalized hypotonia[24] which has been related to a disorder of muscle spindle function. With cerebellar damage, the control of muscle spindle sensitivity by fusimotor efferents is defective,[20] and this disturbance may lead to prolonged movements associated with articulation. Other general abnormalities of movement control from cerebellar dysfunction probably also contribute to the disorders of speech.

NONCEREBELLAR DYSARTHRIA

The dysarthria often described as "cerebellar"[22, 23] or "ataxic"[24] can occur with disease of forebrain structures without cerebellar damage.[6] Certain disturbances in the melody and rhythm of speech are fairly characteristic of cerebellar destruction, however,[14] and these disorders of prosody can be helpful in localizing a lesion to the posterior fossa. Other elements of speech are affected by disturbances in any one of several areas in the brain or brainstem.[18] Changes in the clarity or rate of speech provide little clue to the site of the central nervous system damage.

Slurred speech, as well as speech arrest, occurs with a lesion in the supplementary motor area of the cerebral cortex.[6] Dysarthria with inarticulate, intermittently explosive speech occurs commonly in pseudobulbar palsy from disease bilaterally in the cerebral hemispheres. Poorly modulated, monotonous, and often halting speech has long been recognized as typical of basal ganglia disorders[38]

224

such as Parkinson disease. Acceleration or arrest of speech and decreasing speech volume accompany electrical stimulation in the ventrolateral thalamus of patients. Decreased voice volume occurs with destruction of the globus pallidus and slurred speech can develop with bilateral thalamic lesions.[6] Disturbances in speech with damage to the ventrolateral nucleus of the thalamus are not surprising in view of the cerebellar projections to that area.[2] Entire systems of cerebellar control over speech are disconnected from cortical and subcortical terminals in the cerebrum by lesions in the thalamus.

LOCALIZATION OF SPEECH FUNCTION IN THE CEREBELLUM

Holmes found that men with gunshot and shrapnel wounds to their cerebellar hemispheres occasionally had dysarthria, but speech dysfunction in these cases was more apparent when both the hemispheres and the vermis were damaged.[21-23] He concluded that the vermal portion of the cerebellum is important in the regulation of speech. Holmes' opinion was in accord with the observations of Mills and Weisenburg[29, 35] on a patient with dysarthria of abrupt onset. Months after the development of dysarthria the patient died, and autopsy revealed changes in the superior cerebellum, especially the vermis. These pathologic changes were interpreted as the results of a hemorrhage. The superior vermis was virtually destroyed, leading the authors to conclude that this was the site responsible for the changes in speech. Holmes' work did not contradict this localization, but Holmes did note dysarthria associated with what appeared to be strictly hemispheric lesions. None of his patients had isolated vermal lesions.

Subsequent investigators have provided little clarification of the localization of speech functions in the cerebellum. Brown[9] concluded that dysarthria occurred in patients with bilateral cerebellar hemisphere damage, as well as those with generalized cerebellar damage. Years later[10] he noted in 26 patients with progressive cerebellar disease that dysarthrias developed at about the same point in the progression of the degenerative disease as limb ataxia. The structures important to limb movements, but not gait, seemed to be close to structures important in speech. By inference this moved the important locus for speech dysfunction into the cerebellar hemispheres and out of the vermis.

Victor, in studies cited by Brown,[11] doubted the importance of the superior vermis and the anterior portions of the anterior lobe in dysarthria. Victor examined numerous patients with extensive alcoholism related damage to these structures who had no speech dysfunction. In reviewing the case histories of 250 patients with cerebellar tumors, Amici and coworkers[4] found dysarthria in 8.5 percent of the cases and noted that dysarthria occurred most often in patients with damage to the paravermal and lateral elements of the hemispheres. Surgical descriptions defined the limits of damage caused by the tumors. There was no clear association of vermal destruction with the development of dysarthria.

Several other studies of various cerebellar lesions have implicated unilateral hemispheric disease in the development of speech disorders. A chart review of 21 patients with well documented cerebellar hemorrhage uncovered 7 patients with dysarthria, an incidence of 33 percent.[17] This study provided localization of the site of the hemorrhage in 18 of the 21 cases, with 11 of the 18 patients having primarily left hemisphere hemorrhages. In another study of patients with cerebellar hemorrhage,[7] dysarthria occurred in 8 of 9 patients, but all of the patients had rapidly evolving hemorrhages with damage to multiple brainstem nuclei. In a third study, 6 of 16 patients[28] with cerebellar hemispheric infarctions had dysarthria, and 5 of these 6 had marked left hemisphere damage. In a fourth study, dysarthria developed in 14 of 21 patients with cerebellar infarctions and, again, this high incidence of dysarthria coincided with a high incidence of primarily left hemisphere disease.[34] Sixty-eight percent of the entire group had left sided infarctions.

The inclusion of patients with extensive brainstem damage in studies of the association of cerebellar disease and speech disorders has probably led to confusion in understanding the role of the cerebellum in speech function. The rapid evolution of signs of neurologic disease in studies of cerebellar hemorrhage and some of cerebellar infarction is a major limitation to their usefulness in establishing sites responsible for the signs. Nevertheless, patients with cerebellar vascular disease can be helpful in understanding the localization of cerebellar speech functions, as shown by the following report.

Case Report

A 50-year-old, right handed, hypertensive woman abruptly developed a generalized headache and dizziness. These symptoms persisted for several hours, during which time both the patient and her relatives noticed progressive slurring of her speech. She was still awake and alert when she arrived at the hospital, but her headache and slurred speech had increased in severity. She had marked dysarthria but did not have scanning speech. She had no papilledema or nystagmus, but within an hour of her initial examination she developed dysconjugate gaze. Other cranial nerve functions were intact except for a slight right lower facial weakness and a questionably decreased right corneal reflex. Sensation was preserved to pinprick and strength was slightly better on the left than the right. The resistance to passive manipulation was decreased in the left limbs. The deep tendon reflexes were 2 + and symmetric.

While being examined, the patient became increasingly inattentive and then stuporous. Her deteriorating level of consciousness prompted an emergency computerized tomogram, which revealed dense, patchy lesions in the left paravermal area, interpreted as a hemorrhage. A suboccipital craniotomy was performed the same day and, when the meninges were incised, a strikingly edematous left cerebellar hemisphere protruded posteriorly. Some displacement of the vermis was apparent. There was no evidence grossly of damage to the vermis or the right hemisphere. The edematous portion of the left hemisphere was removed with suction, and about 10 ml of clotted blood was encountered and removed. No vermal tissue was removed and most of the left hemisphere remained intact. The lesion was interpreted as a hemorrhagic infarction.

Following the operation, the patient's speech remained slightly slurred for a few days before returning to normal. Coarse gaze-evoked nystagmus appeared on right, left, and upward gaze. Extraocular movements and pupillary reactions otherwise remained normal. She had a head tilt to the right. Movements of the left arm were ataxic and dysmetria was found in both of the left limbs. There was no past-pointing, excessive rebound, impaired check, or abnormal resistance to passive manipulation of the limbs. At no time did she develop papilledema or ocular dysmetria.

Despite the initial improvement, the patient became progressively obtunded at the end of the first week postoperatively. Hydrocephalus was discovered and a ventricular shunt was placed. A shunt infection developed within a few days, and the patient died during surgical efforts to revise the shunt. An autopsy was not performed.

In this patient, hemorrhagic infarction with edema in the left cerebellar hemisphere produced severe dysarthria. The prominence of dysarthria resulting from this lesion concurs with the experience in other patients with left hemisphere lesions.[27]

Recent Observations

Lechtenberg and Gilman[27] found 31 patients with dysarthria in a series of 162 cases of focal cerebellar disease studied retrospectively. An adequate description of speech was provided in 122 of the 162 patients. Speech patterns characteristic of cerebellar damage, as outlined by Brown and coworkers,[11] were sought in the patient records. The most commonly observed abnormalities were slurred, slowed, and scanning speech. These were the result of articulatory breakdown, excess and equal stress, imprecise consonants, prolonged phonemes, prolonged intervals, and slow rate. In accord with prior studies,[4] hemispheric lesions were associated with speech disorders more often than vermal lesions. Of the 31 patients with dysarthria, 22 had predominantly or exclusively left hemisphere lesions, and 2 had vermal disease. The association between left hemisphere disease and dysarthria was statistically significant.[27] The difference between the incidence of dysarthria in the right hemisphere group and the vermal group was not significant.

The evolution of speech disorders in patients with cerebellar damage also implicates the left cerebellar hemisphere. Patients with progressive lesions, such as tumors and recurrent abscesses, develop dysarthria as the lesion extends into the

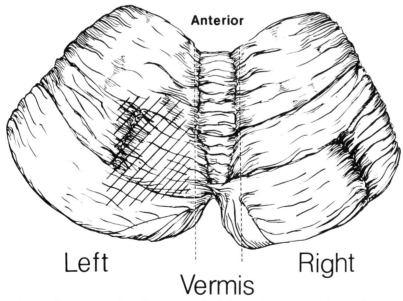

Figure 1. Schematic representation of areas over the left superior paravermal cerebellum most often damaged when dysarthria occurs as a sign of cerebellar disease. (From Lechtenberg and Gilman,[27] with permission.)

left hemisphere.[27] Patients with vermal disease requiring paravermal resections develop dysarthria on occasion after resection of the left paravermal area. The area of encroachment that repeatedly appears in patients with speech disorders is the superior paravermal segment of the left hemisphere about Larsell's lobules HVI and HVII (Fig. 1). This area receives inputs from auditory stimulation and from stimulation of the laryngeal nerve.[3, 26, 37] This area is in the cerebellar hemisphere,[4] an observation compatible with the concept that the cerebellar regulation of speech developed in phylogenetically recent cerebellar structures.[32] The intense involvement of a single cerebellar hemisphere in speech function follows the pattern seen in the cerebrum.[18, 19] The importance of the left cerebellar hemisphere in speech function was not found previously in large series of cases, probably because the investigators did not focus on the lateralization of speech function in the cerebellum.[4, 25]

An unexpected finding in the data of Lechtenberg and Gilman[27] is the association of speech function and the left side of the cerebellum (Fig. 1). The interconnections between the cerebral cortex and the cerebellar hemispheres are principally contralateral.[2, 8, 15, 16] The left cerebral hemisphere is the principal site of speech production in the right-handed person[18, 19] and the major interconnections of the hemisphere and the cerebellum are with the right cerebellar hemisphere. Even at the level of the thalamus,[38] damage to the left seems more important in the disruption of speech than damage to the right. Consequently, the speech disorder associated with cerebellar disease would be expected to result from lesions of the right rather than the left cerebellar hemisphere. An understanding of the importance of the left cerebellar hemisphere in speech results from consideration of the function of the right (nondominant) cerebral hemisphere in speech production.

DYSARTHRIA AND THE NONDOMINANT CEREBRAL HEMISPHERE

As mentioned earlier, the major components of cerebellar dysarthria relate to prosody, that is, the melodic aspects of speech. The conception and delivery of meaningful verbal symbols generally is facile and accurate. Thus, the choice of words, sequential patterning of speech, and other aspects of speech affected in aphasia are not altered with cerebellar disorders.[18, 19] The patient may complain of difficulty with enunciation, but there is no problem with word finding. Repetition is accurate except for elision of syllables, which may occur with irregular articulatory breakdown. The intonation, accentuation, and melodic transformations in a series of syllables or words are generated poorly. These more harmonic than sequential aspects of speech would best be served by structures with access to the nondominant hemisphere.[31]

Recognition of melody is a nondominant cerebral hemisphere function.[33] Damage to the right temporal lobe interferes with the perception of melodies whereas damage to the left temporal lobe impairs the appreciation of similarly presented numbers.[33] This lateralization of auditory functions apparently does not hold for professional musicians or even musically experienced listeners,[5] but is well established for the average right-handed person.[31] Specialized dichotic listening tests with nonverbal stimuli presented separately to each ear also have demonstrated a right cerebral advantage in storing nonverbal information.[30, 31] The musical functions of the cerebral hemispheres are complex and involve both the left and right sides,[36] however, the allegedly silent nondominant hemisphere plays a major role in at least harmonic aspects of musical function. Recovery of language in patients with damaged dominant hemispheres can be helped by melodic intonation of phrases,[1] a phenomenon consistent with the notion of a musically oriented non-dominant hemisphere.

Basic to every language is a set of melodic and harmonic rules which invest a string of words with additional meaning. An interaction between the speech dominant and tone perceptive hemispheres of the cerebrum must be basic to all spoken languages. The findings of Lechtenberg and Gilman[27] suggest that the left cerebellar hemisphere interacts with the nondominant right hemisphere in regulating the melody and rhythm of speech.

This view of the cerebrocerebellar interconnections in speech function could be reinforced by a sample of right cerebral hemisphere dominant patients with dysarthria and superior right paravermal damage. Such a collection of left handed subjects is not available in any series of patients with cerebellar lesions. Our study[27] included only ten left handed patients, seven with cerebellar hemisphere damage. Three of these had left sided lesions and five had right sided lesions. Two patients were dysarthric, one from the left hemisphere group and one from the right hemisphere group. The dysarthric left handed patient with right cerebellar hemispheric lesions had primarily superior paravermal involvement. The implication is that this patient had reversed dominance, but with so few patients available for study, this is conjecture.

We conclude that cerebellar damage can produce a variety of dysarthrias, with derangement of the melody, intonation, and harmonic coloring of speech. Excess stress, prolonged phonemes, elision of syllables, and inappropriate tone and volume often contribute to the distortion of speech. The most constant feature of these speech disorders is a disruption of the prosody of speech. There are no aphasic elements to these speech disorders. Although the present evidence implicates a focal lesion in the superior paravermal segment of the left cerebellar hemisphere in cerebellar speech disorders, it is unlikely that only one cerebellar locus could be responsible for all the facets of speech disorder occurring with cerebellar disease. More complete comprehension of cerebellar mechanisms in speech and the disorders of these mechanisms will emerge with further studies of the localization of focal cerebellar disease in patients with well documented speech disturbances.

REFERENCES

1. ALBERT, M. L., SPARKS, R. W., AND HELM, N. A.: *Melodic intonation therapy for aphasia.* Arch. Neurol. 29:130, 1973.

2. ALLEN, G. I., AND TSUKAHARA, N.: *Cerebrocerebellar communication systems.* Physiol. Rev. 54:957, 1974.

3. ALTMAN, J. A., BECHTEREV, N. N., RADIONOVA, E. A., ET AL.: *Electrical responses of the auditory area of the cerebellar cortex to acoustic stimulation.* Exp. Brain Res. 26:285, 1976.

4. AMICI, R., AVANZINI, G., AND PACINI, L.: *Cerebellar Tumors.* Monographs in Neural Sciences, Vol. IV. Karger, Switzerland, 1976.

5. BEVER, T. G., AND CHIARELLO, R. J.: *Cerebral dominance in musicians and nonmusicians.* Science 185:537, 1974.

6. BOTEZ, M. I., AND BARBEAU, A.: *Role of subcortical structures and particularly of the thalamus, in the mechanisms of speech and language.* Int. J. Neurol. 8:300, 1971.

7. BRENNAN, R. W., AND BERGLAND, R. M.: *Acute cerebellar hemorrhage: analysis of clinical findings and outcome in 12 cases.* Neurology 27:527, 1977.

8. BRODAL, A.: *Cerebrocerebellar pathways. Anatomical data and some functional implications.* Acta Physiol. Scand. (48 Suppl.) 51:153, 1972.

9. BROWN, J. R.: *Localizing cerebellar syndromes.* JAMA 141:518, 1949.

10. BROWN, J. R.: *Degenerative cerebellar ataxias.* Neurology 9:799, 1959.

11. BROWN, J. R., DARLEY, F. L., AND ARONSON, A. E.: *Ataxic dysarthria.* Int. J. Neurol. 7:302, 1970.

12. CHARCOT, J. M.: *Charcot on Diseases of the Nervous System.* Translated by G. Sigerson. The New Sydenham Society, London, Vol. 72, 1877.

13. COLE, M.: *Dysprosody due to posterior fossa lesions.* Trans. Am. Neurol. Assoc. 96:151, 1971.

14. DOW, R. S., AND MORUZZI, G.: *The Physiology and Pathology of the Cerebellum.* University of Minnesota Press, Minneapolis, 1958.

15. ECCLES, J. C.: *Circuits in the cerebellar control of movement.* Proc. Nat. Acad. Sci. 58:336, 1967.

16. EVARTS, E. V., AND THACH, W. T.: *Motor mechanisms of the CNS: cerebrocerebellar interrelations.* Rev. Physiol. 31:451, 1969.

17. FISHER, C. M., PICARD, E. H., POLAK, A., ET AL.: *Acute hypertensive cerebellar hemorrhage: diagnosis and surgical treatment.* J. Nerv. Ment. Dis. 140:38, 1965.

18. GESCHWIND, N.: *Disconnexion syndromes in animals and man.* Brain 88:237, 1965.

19. GESCHWIND, N.: *Case records of the Massachusetts General Hospital: case 15-1975.* N. Engl. J. Med. 292:852, 1975.

20. GILMAN, S.: *The mechanism of cerebellar hypotonia. An experimental study in the monkey.* Brain 92:621, 1969.

21. HOLMES, G.: *The symptoms of acute cerebellar injuries due to gunshot injuries.* Brain 40:461, 1917.

22. HOLMES, G.: *The Croonian lectures on the clinical symptoms of cerebellar disease and their interpretation.* Lancet 1:1177, 1922.

23. HOLMES, G.: *The Croonian lectures on the clinical symptoms of cerebellar disease and their interpretation.* Lancet 2:59, 1922.

24. KENT, R., AND NETSELL, R.: *A case study of an ataxic dysarthria: cineradiographic and spectrographic observations.* J. Speech Hearing Disorders 40:115, 1975.

25. KESCHNER, M., AND GROSSMAN, M.: *Cerebellar symptomatology evaluation on the basis of intracerebellar and extracerebellar lesions.* Arch. Neurol. Psychiat. 19:78, 1928.

26. LAM, R. L., AND OGURA, J. H.: *An afferent representation of the larynx in the cerebellum.* Laryngoscope 62:486, 1952.

27. LECHTENBERG, R., AND GILMAN, S.: *Speech disorders in cerebellar disease.* Ann Neurol. 3:285, 1978.

28. LEHRICH, J. R., WINKLER, G. F., AND OJEMANN, R. G.: *Cerebellar infarction with brain stem compression.* Arch. Neurol. 22:490, 1970.

29. MILLS, C. K., AND WEISENBURG, T. H.: *Cerebellar symptoms and cerebellar localization.* Am. Med. Assoc. J. 63:1813, 1914.

30. OSCAR-BERMAN, M., GOODGLASS, H., AND DONNENFELD, H.: *Dichotic ear-order effects with non-verbal stimuli.* Cortex 10:270, 1974.

31. ROSS, E. D., AND MESULAM, M.: *Dominant language functions of the right hemisphere? Prosody and emotional gesturing.* Arch. Neurol. 36:144, 1979.

32. SARNAT, H. B., AND NETSKY, M. G.: *Evolution of the Nervous System.* Oxford University Press, New York, 1974.

33. SHANKWEILER, D.: *Effects of temporal-lobe damage on perception of dichotically presented melodies.* J. Comp. Physiol. Psychol. 62:115, 1966.

34. SYPERT, G. W., AND ALVORD, E. C., JR.: *Cerebellar infarction. A clinicopathological study.* Arch. Neurol. 32:357, 1975.

35. WEISENBURG, T. H.: *Cerebellar localization and its symptomatology.* Brain 50:357, 1927.

36. WERTHEIM, N., AND BOTEZ, M. I.: *Receptive amusia: A clinical analysis.* Brain 84:19, 1961.

37. WOLFE, J. W.: *Responses of the cerebellar auditory area to pure tone stimuli.* Exp. Neurol. 36:295, 1972.

38. ZENTAY P. J.: *Motor disorders of the nervous system and their significance for speech. Part 1. Cerebral and cerebellar dysarthrias.* Laryngoscope 47:147, 1937.

CHAPTER 12

Degenerative Diseases

CLASSIFICATION

The development of a definitive classification of the degenerative diseases of the cerebellum has been difficult, chiefly because the mechanisms underlying most are unknown. Although some recently have been traced to metabolic causes,[13, 56, 80] attempts to characterize the biochemical changes in most have been unsuccessful.[8] Efforts to classify these diseases have relied upon clinical, pathologic, or genetic criteria.[7, 8, 72, 105] Each of these classifications has limitations, for invariably a large number of patients falls outside of well defined categories. Clinical classifications have had limited application because, as a disease evolves in a particular patient, traits justifying the inclusion of the disorder in one class of degenerative diseases may disappear as signs typical of another class evolve. Thus, the hyperreflexic patient becomes hyporeflexic, and the patient with normal eye movements develops gaze palsies. Neuropathologic findings have provided a useful method of classifying degenerative disease, but even access to the damaged tissues may not provide definitive information. The brain at death often has nonspecific changes in areas that were the most active sites of pathology years before the patient died. A useful classification of the degenerative disorders may arise from studies on genetic markers in these conditions,[54, 72] but such studies have yielded little information thus far. Current systems of classification cannot incorporate several widely observed phenomena, such as the coexistence of Friedreich disease, Roussy-Lévy syndrome, and Charcot-Marie-Tooth disease in the same extended families.[65, 69] These diseases share some features, but they are distinct entities pathologically. Their occurrence together provides evidence of a common biochemical basis or close genetic linkage.

We have classified the degenerative diseases of the cerebellum according to etiology insofar as possible. Since many of these diseases are transmitted genetically, our first two major subgroups consist of the diseases transmitted with recessive (see Table 1) and dominant (see Tables 2 and 3) inheritance patterns, respectively. A third subgroup consists of a miscellaneous collection of diseases due to metabolic (see Table 4) and storage (see Table 5) diseases as well as others without known cause. In organizing this presentation we have had to abandon some previous classifications [17, 23, 30, 46, 103] and use more current views of disease associations.[7, 11, 14, 22, 29, 39, 62] Considerable overlap exists between the subgroups in

231

our classification. Thus, several recessively inherited ataxias result from metabolic diseases and the olivopontocerebellar atrophies, largely inherited with dominant patterns, include a recessively inherited form. The progressive ataxias in association with epilepsy or myoclonus have been viewed as distinct entities,[51, 52] but this has never been established. Familial spastic ataxias[45] and olivocerebellar degenerations[46] clearly overlap considerably with the progressive, recessively inherited ataxias and olivopontocerebellar atrophy, but they are considered separately here.

CLINICAL PRESENTATION

Suspicion of a cerebellar degenerative disease usually arises when a patient develops progressive gait difficulty or limb ataxia. Tremors, clumsiness, and nystagmus appearing even in a few members of a family suggest a hereditary cerebellar degenerative disease, which usually is termed a hereditary ataxia. Hereditary ataxias pass through families in autosomal recessive or dominant patterns. The principal sites of the pathologic changes are the pons, spinal cord, and cerebellum.[28] Processes largely limited to the cerebellum are termed cerebelloparenchymal, those affecting spinal cord tracts are spinocerebellar, and those affecting the inferior olivary nuclei and pontine nuclei are olivopontocerebellar. Friedreich disease and similar progressive ataxias also are termed spinal ataxias because they have predominantly spinal cord pathology.[59] These designations are arbitrary. Minor damage to several different loci in the central nervous system occurs more often with these degenerative diseases than major pathology restricted to a single locus.

Most patients with progressive ataxias develop their first symptoms in adult life[28, 34, 63] and consequently all the common causes of death in adult life interrupt the frequently nonfatal disease process. In an early series of ataxic patients,[17] 70 percent of 103 patients developed signs of the progressive degenerative disease at 0 to 19 or 50 to 70 years of age. The younger end of the spectrum is composed largely of patients with Friedreich disease.[28] The adult group is a more diverse collection of degenerative disorders.[17, 23] For the nonjuvenile patient, the typical course starts at about 50 years of age with complaints of increasing difficulty in walking over the course of years. The patient seeks medical attention after several months or years of clumsiness, dysarthria, and tremor. At the initial evaluation, double vision, abnormal eye movements, vertigo, and impaired hearing are likely to be found. [17] Forgetfulness, impaired urinary control, and tinnitus are frequent complaints.[36] These and other symptoms may appear in other members of the family. Less commonly an extensive family history will uncover no other affected members in the family.[23] Subsequent generations may prove this apparently sporadic occurrence of the cerebellar degenerative disease to be just the first recognized case of a recessively inherited disorder. Some sporadic cases of ataxia are actually infectious or endocrine disorders, such as Creutzfeldt-Jakob disease or hypothyroidism.

Cerebellar degenerative diseases commonly evolve over the course of decades. An individual with cerebellar degeneration presenting initially with mild signs of limb incoordination later may develop disorders of ocular motor, sensory, and extrapyramidal function. Dementia can be an early[36] or terminal phenomenon.[23] Lesions in the central nervous system evolve with time just as the clinical exami-

Table 1. The recessively inherited progressive ataxias

Type	Tendon Reflexes	Age of Onset	Pathology Sites	Representative Diseases
1	Hyperreflexic	Congenital 0–6 months	Cerebrum Diencephalon Cerebellum	a. Marinesco-Sjoegren disease[3, 7, 71] b. Congenital ataxia with aniridia of Gillespie[7, 38] c. Spongy degeneration with pontocerebellar atrophy[102] d. Infantile Gaucher disease[101]
2	Hyperreflexic	Infantile 0–6 years	Cerebrum Cerebellum Posterior columns	a. Charlevoix-Saguenay disease[14] b. Troyer syndrome[24] c. Behr disease[49, 64] d. Ataxia telangiectasia[5, 6, 19, 74, 83, 94, 96, 97, 99] e. Familial cerebrotendinous xanthomatosis f. Infantile neuronal ceroid lipofuscinosis[39, 81] g. Niemann-Pick variant[78] h. Sandhoff disease[70, 80] i. Johnson-Chutorian hexosaminidase deficiency[56]
3	Hyporeflexic	Childhood 6–16 years	Cerebellum Posterior columns Corticospinal tracts	a. Friedreich disease[7, 8, 12, 21, 53, 69, 88] b. Refsum disease[2, 18, 61, 85, 86] c. Bassen-Kornzweig abetalipoproteinemia[9, 100] d. Gamma-glutamylcysteine synthetase deficiency[87] e. Nephronophthisis with progressive ataxia[84]
4	Hyporeflexic	Juvenile 16–25 years	Posterior columns Corticospinal tracts Peripheral nerves	Recessive Roussy-Lévy syndrome[31, 65, 69]
5	Normoreflexic	Adult	Cerebellum Brainstem	Olivopontocerebellar atrophy type II[7, 23, 62, 63, 82]

233

nation changes. Ataxia telangiectasia, for example, produces minor changes in the cerebellum of the one-year-old, but prominent deterioration of the cerebellum in the 20-year-old.[99]

THE RECESSIVELY INHERITED ATAXIAS

The ataxias inherited as autosomal recessive traits are a diverse group of diseases including two relatively frequent disorders, Friedreich disease and ataxia telangiectasia. A recently described method of classifying these diseases is based on the reactivity of the deep tendon reflexes.[7, 8, 17] The hyperreflexic, hyporeflexic, and normoreflexic categories denote fairly discrete forms of ataxia, some idiopathic and some with known metabolic bases (Table 1). There are two major forms of hyperreflexic ataxias, two hyporeflexic, and one normoreflexic. Associated features such as dementia, corticospinal tract disease, and posterior column disease help to differentiate the subgroups.[7] A fairly consistent relationship exists between the age of the patient at the time of onset of symptoms and the class of ataxia. Both the clinical features and the pathologic changes correlate well with the age of onset of the disease.[7] Infants developing a progressive ataxia are likely to be hyperreflexic, even if they appear floppy. Adults with ataxia are usually hyporeflexic or normoreflexic, even if they have increased resistance to passive manipulation of the limbs.

Type 1 Recessive Ataxias

The hyperreflexic progressive ataxias have signs largely referrable to the cerebrum, the corticospinal tracts, and the cerebellum. Both types 1 and 2 begin at birth or during the first years of life. Type 1 progressive ataxias generally are considered to be congenital defects, with evidence of ocular motor disturbances, psychomotor retardation, and spasticity in the first days or weeks of life.

Marinesco-Sjoegren Syndrome

This is a disorder affecting the newborn.[7] Marinesco's original patients were four siblings in a Rumanian family who had cataracts evident at birth, delayed psychomotor milestones from birth, and truncal and limb ataxia within the first years of life.[71] Strabismus and hypotonia occur in some neonates with this disorder and, with maturation, nystagmus and muscle wasting appear occasionally. Hyperreflexia is a fairly consistent feature of the disease. Plantar responses are extensor in about half the affected cases.[3] Kyphoscoliosis and foot deformities develop frequently. Patients with Marinesco-Sjoegren syndrome survive for decades, demonstrating profound dysarthria and truncal instability as adults. The few autopsies performed on patients with this disease show little pathology in the brain apart from a severely atrophic cerebellum.[71] Purkinje cell loss is virtually complete and granule cell depletion is associated with a marked gliosis.[3] The cerebellar atrophy is presumably a consequence of neural damage which appeared as the children matured in their first year of life.[71]

Congenital Ataxia with Aniridia

This disorder is virtually identical to the Marinesco-Sjoegren syndrome in its onset, signs, and course with the notable exception of abnormalities of the eyes.[3, 38] At birth, defects are apparent in the irides, giving the appearance of virtual aniridia. There are no cataracts. While infants, these patients exhibit considerable psychomotor retardation with delayed walking and poor cognitive development. Ataxia of the limbs and trunk appears within the first few years of life. The skeletal abnormalities seen in Marinesco-Sjoegren syndrome also appear in this disorder. Sensory deficits do not develop in either of these type 1 recessive ataxias even if the patient lives 40 or 50 years.[3, 38] The pathology in ataxia with aniridia is presumably similar to that found in Marinesco-Sjoegren syndrome, but this has not yet been established.

Spongy Degeneration with Pontocerebellar Atrophy

This disorder was described in twin brothers who had severe neurologic disorders from the first days of life, including progressive hypertonia, opisthotonic posturing, impaired vision, and recurrent seizures. They both died before eight months of age and at autopsy had spongy degeneration of the cerebrum, atrophy of the ventral pons, and demyelination of the pontocerebellar fibers.[102] Although Purkinje cells were still present, basket cells were lost and the granular layer was vacuolated. The dentate nucleus was relatively intact. Abnormal inclusions appeared in the Purkinje cells and some glial cells. It was speculated that the nervous system changes began before birth. Although this disorder results from extensive central nervous system damage, it is included with the recessively inherited ataxias because the cerebellar degeneration is a prominent component of the process.

Infantile Gaucher Disease

This is a congenital storage disorder with prominent cerebellar changes presenting pathologic, genetic, and temporal features in common with the other type 1 recessive ataxias.[101] Within the first months of life, the affected infant has apparent spasticity and opisthotonic posturing. Ocular motor deficits, such as bilateral estropia, may develop even earlier. Psychomotor retardation is apparent during the first year of life and the child may die with uncontrollable seizures before the second year of life.[101] Systemic signs of Gaucher disease include bone marrows filled with Gaucher cells, splenomegaly, lymphadenopathy, and interstitial chest infiltrates. The course of this disorder is usually so rapid that the infant has little opportunity to display complex cerebellar deficits, despite the prominent loss of cerebellar structures on autopsy examination. Focal neuronal degeneration occurs in the caudate, thalamus, lateral cuneate, and pontine nuclei as well as in cerebellar structures. Focal loss of Purkinje cells and gliosis in the molecular layer are prominent.[101]

Type 2 Recessive Ataxias

The type 2 ataxias are apparent within the first years of life, but definitive diagnosis often requires the evolution of the disease over decades. Posterior column disease is typical of patients in this group, with cerebral and cerebellar pathology developing in the majority of cases. Hyperreflexia occurs during much of the course of these diseases. None of these diseases presents exclusively as a cerebellar disorder, but signs of cerebellar involvement are prominent in all of them.

Charlevoix-Saguenay Ataxia

This disorder appeared in an isolated region of Quebec in two counties adopted as the eponym for this disease.[14] All of the affected patients had abnormalities of gait from the time they first tried to walk. Frequent falls and poor dexterity were obvious in infancy, but deficits in truncal stability usually did not progress until adolescence. Nystagmus on lateral and vertical gaze developed in infancy or early childhood and pursuit eye movements were consistently defective, resulting in dysmetric saccades on attempted conjugate pursuit. Other abnormalities included hypotonia, impaired vibration and position sense, hyperreflexia, extensor plantar responses, distal muscle atrophy, pes cavus, bowel and bladder incontinence, vertigo, facial asymmetry, and choreoathetotic movements.[14] Sensory nerve action potentials were altered, showing both a decrease in amplitude and slowing.[14] A high incidence of mitral valve prolapse occurred in this group, but these patients did not develop the lethal cardiomyopathy or the spinal scoliosis seen in Friedreich disease. The absence of lethal cardiac disease accounts for survival of these patients decades longer than patients with Friedreich disease.

The Troyer Syndrome

This is another recessively inherited ataxia appearing in isolated enclaves such as the Amish communities in the United States.[24] This degenerative disease exhibits most of the characteristics prominent in Charlevoix-Saguenay disease, including a gait disorder beginning in infancy or childhood, generalized hyperreflexia, distal muscle atrophy, pes cavus, and dysarthria. Kyphoscoliosis develops frequently. A progressive spastic paraparesis develops, distinguishing this recessive disorder from other type 2 progressive ataxias. Dementia is an early feature of the Troyer syndrome. Affected individuals live into their fourth and fifth decade, usually developing emotional lability and paranoid psychoses.[24] The psychosis is not a response to the neurologic disability; the psychiatric dysfunction is adequately stereotyped to be viewed as a sign of the degeneration.[24] Cardiac abnormalities have not been found with the Troyer syndrome.[24] The general absence of systemic disorders in this syndrome undoubtedly contributes to the longevity of affected individuals.

Behr Disease

This disorder is similar in many ways to Refsum disease.[64] It begins in infancy and soon thereafter produces largely static signs of ataxia, spasticity, mental retardation, visual loss, and posterior column sensory loss.[49] The ataxia in Behr disease is mild, the neuropathy often is not evident clinically, and associated defects include hearing loss, dysarthria, and nystagmus.[64] The hyperreflexia of Behr disease helps distinguish it from Refsum disease. Pathologic changes include atrophy of the optic nerves, disruption of the laminar arrangements of neurons in the lateral geniculate bodies, and focal dropout of Purkinje cells in the cerebellum with sparing of the granule cells.[49] Axonal spheroids are scattered throughout the lateral geniculate nuclei and other thalamic nuclei. Rare spheroids appear in the dentate nuclei.

236

Ataxia Telangiectasia (Louis-Bar Syndrome)

This relatively common spinocerebellar degeneration is usually recognized in childhood or infancy although definite signs of the disease can be found shortly after birth. It is a multisystem disease with defects most apparent in the nervous and immune systems. Despite this widespread dysfunction, genetic studies suggest that this recessive disorder is determined by a single gene.[97] It is the disturbance of cerebellar function which usually brings the patient to medical attention.

The neurologic disturbances in ataxia telangiectasia follow a fairly consistent clinical course. Side-to-side tremors of the head occur when the patient is a few months old and an unstable gait develops when the child first attempts walking. Coarse nystagmus is a prominent early sign. Limb tremors develop over subsequent years, and the child's speech becomes slowed, slurred, and scanning as ataxia in all limbs increases. The patients are hyperreflexic early in the course of the disease but become hyporeflexic later. Vibration and position sense are lost in the first decade of life. Choreoathetosis occurs in older children and ataxia in the arms is well developed before adolescence. As the patient enters adolescence, peripheral neuropathy and anterior horn cell disease may appear.[19] At this stage the development of dystonic posturing, myoclonic jerks, and kinetic tremors limits the child's motor performance.[74] Power and muscle tone remain intact, though eventually the distal limb muscles waste and contractures develop. Voluntary eye movements are impaired, but doll's eye movements are normal.[99] A gaze apraxia appears in many of these patients, with typical headthrusting movements shifting the eyes from one point of fixation to another.[5] Although some fast saccades can be produced with caloric stimulation of the labyrinth, optokinetic nystagmus usually is absent and both eyes drift in the direction of the slow component. Spontaneous rotatory and downbeat nystagmus are seen in older patients when the patient looks straight ahead. Saccadic eye movements, when present at all, are clearly hypometric.[5] Pursuit movements are slowed, and catch-up saccades occur in some patients. Dementia occurs in adolescence and, once apparent, progresses relentlessly. Death occurs in adolescence from infection or neoplasm.

The cutaneous manifestations of ataxia telangiectasia evolve in concert with the neurologic disorders.[96] Telangiectasias appear in the eyes on the bulbar conjunctivae within the first decade of life. Cutaneous telangiectasias develop within years of the conjunctival vascular anomalies, affecting the malar.eminences, ear lobes, upper chest, and antecubital fossae. Cutaneous telangiectasias are associated with tortuous cerebellar blood vessels only in rare patients;[74] intracranial arteriovenous malformations are not characteristic of this disease. Additional skin lesions include seborrheic dermatitis, eczema, senile keratosis, and even basal cell carcinoma.[99] Patches of hyperpigmentation or hypopigmentation occur in the areas affected by the telangiectasias.

Immune system defects are responsible for terminal diseases in most patients with ataxia telangiectasia. Defects of both cellular and humoral immunity are prominent, and malignant transformation of lymphoid tissue is common.[83] The alteration on chromosome 14 seen in some patients with leukemia also develops in patients with ataxia telangiectasia, but this is probably an effect of the immune deficits rather than a cause.[97] IgA and IgE deficiences, as well as production of abnormal IgM, may contribute to the development of infections.[99] Eighty-five percent of patients with ataxia telangiectasia have recurrent infections of the middle ear, nasal sinuses, and lungs.[96] Chronic hepatitis affects many patients,[97] perhaps reflecting vulnerability to viral as well as bacterial infections. Poor cell mediated immunity and a decrease in the T-cell population enhances the patient's susceptibility to infectious agents.[19]

The frequent association of insulin-resistant hyperglycemia with ataxia telangiectasia is evidence of a defect in receptor affinity for insulin.[6] Sixty percent of patients are affected by this glucose intolerance and, although receptor blocking is the obvious explanation, no inhibitor has been found.[6] All of these patients have elevated serum alpha-fetoprotein,[97] a protein characteristic of embryonic tissue and not normally present in children.

The basic defect in ataxia telangiectasia is unknown. It has not been determined whether it is a generalized disorder of the mesoderm and tissues developing in concert with the mesoderm, an autoimmune reaction to antigens common to both the thymus and nervous system, or a chromosomal disturbance with multisystem effects.[97] A susceptibility to viral infection could cause the damage usually found on chromosome 14, and that susceptibility could be traced back to thymic damage. What is the primary defect and what is secondary damage remains a major question. Some investigators[74] suspect that the aberrant immune system causes or permits the central nervous system degeneration. An autoimmune reaction in the brain should be fairly obvious, but a decreased resistance to normally benign viruses could cause slow, subtle destruction.

Autopsy studies have revealed multiple sites of nervous system disease in patients with ataxia telangiectasia. Peripheral nerves show fibrosis with mild loss of nerve fibers[74] and skeletal muscles show signs of denervation. The cerebellum is the principal site of degeneration and the vermis shows this degenerative change much more than the hemispheres. Purkinje cell loss, basket cell depletion, internal granular layer thinning, and slight atrophy of the molecular layer are apparent in all folia.[19] The dentate and other deep nuclei are intact in most patients, but occasional cases bear dentate neuron loss.[74] The inferior olivary nucleus and pontine nuclei are normal. Demyelination develops in the posterior columns and, rarely, in the dorsal spinocerebellar tracts.[94, 96] Clarke's column is unaffected. Characteristically lesions are not found in the meninges, cerebrum, brainstem, basal ganglia, thalamus, or hypothalamus.

Familial Cerebrotendinous Xanthomatosis
Infantile Neuronal Ceroid Lipofuscinosis
Niemann-Pick Variant

These are neuronal storage diseases presenting with prominent signs of cerebellar and cerebral dysfunction with hyperreflexia. Other storage diseases causing cerebellar pathology are presented in Table 5. These disorders are discussed in Chapter 16.

Sandhoff Disease

This is a metabolic disorder from deficiencies in N-acetyl-β-hexosaminidase A and B which lead to the accumulation of globoside in visceral cells and a generalized increase in GM_2 ganglioside. The disorder presents with progressive mental, motor, and visual loss from the first months of life.[80] Most patients have a macular cherry-red spot, myoclonic seizures, and a spastic quadriparesis. Although death usually occurs in the first few years of life with typical Sandhoff disease,[57] one ataxic patient was 10 years old when examined.[70] He had dementia, dysarthria, kinetic tremor, dysdiadochokinesis, and hemiparesis. A pneumoencephalogram revealed a shrunken cerebellum.

Johnson and Chutorian Hexosaminidase Deficiency

This results in a similar but less severe clinical disorder than Sandhoff disease. Further discussion of these disorders appears in Chapter 16.

Type 3 Recessive Ataxias

The hyporeflexic or areflexic ataxias, which are grouped together into the type 3 and type 4 recessive ataxias, develop in older age groups than the hyperreflexic ataxias. Group 3 ataxias affect patients in childhood, and group 4 ataxias affect patients in the late stages of adolescence or in early adulthood.

Friedreich Disease

This is a progressive ataxia with a fairly uniform clinical presentation and course. All races are affected and it is slightly more common in the male sex. The disease usually appears before puberty,[8] although some cases do appear after 20 years of age[21] and, in rare cases, the age of onset may be 25 years.[69] The mean duration of the disease is 24 years.[69] Gait difficulty is usually the presenting complaint,[8] though the child first may complain of weakness and easy fatiguability. Vertigo is a rare complaint. If the patient is examined at this stage, ataxia is found to be worse in the legs than in the arms. The patient performs poorly on heel-to-shin testing, but dysmetria is slight or absent on finger-to-nose testing. Succession deficits are prominent in the legs. Vibration sense and position sense are faulty in the lower limbs, but sensation is otherwise intact at this stage. The deep tendon reflexes uniformly are decreased or absent and the plantar responses are extensor.

As the child grows older, the gait ataxia progresses without remission and dysarthria begins to appear. Within two years of the initial symptoms of clumsiness and staggering, pes cavus foot deformities and kyphoscoliotic spinal deformities usually develop.[8] Gaze evoked nystagmus occurs in more than half the patients;[69] optic atrophy, retinitis pigmentosa, and sensory neuropathy occur commonly. Many patients have abnormal ocular motility, with opsoclonus and ocular dysmetria described in much of the affected population. Despite the chronic nature of this disease, however, rebound nystagmus, spontaneous nystagmus, and periodic alternating nystagmus do not appear.[75] These types of nystagmus occur with other chronic cerebellar diseases and brainstem lesions.[21, 48] Their absence probably reflects the limited damage to brainstem and cerebellar parenchyma in Friedreich disease. Although dementia usually is not a prominent feature, minor intellectual difficulties, irritability, paranoid ideation, and even frank hallucinations occur in some adolescents affected by the disease.[59]

A number of medical disorders appear in patients with Friedreich disease. Abnormalities of bilirubin level have been detected in many,[7] but there is no evidence that this is a basic feature of the disease. There may be a linkage between Friedreich disease genes and a hyperbilirubinemia gene, such as in Gilbert disease.[7] Diabetes mellitus has been reported in patients with Friedreich disease,

239

though less than 10 percent of patients have this disturbance. A hypertrophic cardiomyopathy occurs in a large majority of patients. Electrocardiographic abnormalities appear in over 90 percent of patients with Friedreich disease, and cardiomyopathy without ataxia occurs in relatives of these patients.[53] The initial symptoms of the cardiac disorder are palpitations and dyspnea on exertion. The patients do not develop angina pectoris.[69] Right ventricular hypertrophy is common, whereas valvular heart disease and coarctation of the aorta are rare.[53] The cardiomyopathy is progressive and accounts for the deaths of most of these patients. Death is usually between 26 and 36 years of age.[53]

The electroencephalogram in Friedreich disease usually is normal, but nerve conduction studies are abnormal. Sensory nerve conduction is virtually absent in the legs and slowed in the arms.[8, 69] Motor fiber conduction and muscle fiber potentials evoked on electromyography are normal. Nerve biopsy and autopsy studies show a decrease in the number of large myelinated fibers in the posterior nerve roots and the peripheral nerves. Fine myelinated fibers are preserved. This peripheral nerve involvement is a constant feature and provides the link with other neuropathic disorders, such as Charcot-Marie-Tooth disease and Roussy-Lévy syndrome, which occur in families with Friedreich disease.[69]

Pathologic changes in Friedreich disease are primarily in the posterior columns, ventral and dorsal spinocerebellar tracts, and crossed corticospinal tracts (Fig.

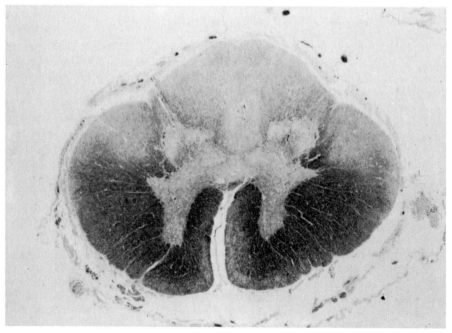

Figure 1. A histologic section of the spinal cord of a 25-year-old woman with Friedreich disease. The patient was one of 8 siblings, 3 of whom developed the disease. The disease began at age 4 in this patient and progressed until the patient became confined to bed by her neurologic disorder. Examination 6 years before death revealed ataxia of the extremities, absent deep tendon reflexes, extensor plantar responses, and absent position sense in the lower extremities. The spinal cord shows degenerative changes in the posterior and lateral columns with involvement of the spinocerebellar and corticospinal tracts. The fibers of the posterior root show degenerative changes (luxol fast blue-cresyl violet-eosin stain).

240

1).[69] Clarke's column also may be atrophied and sclerotic. The inferior olivary nuclei and the corticopontocerebellar tracts uniformly are intact.[114]

Friedreich disease is considered currently to be the product of an inborn error of metabolism inherited in an autosomal recessive pattern. The primary metabolic defect is unknown,[69] even though many abnormal enzyme and substrate levels have been detected. Alpha lipoprotein composition is abnormal,[7] an observation of possible consequence in ultimately explaining the evolution of the cardiac lesions. Oxidation of pyruvate is slow in Friedreich disease following a glucose load.[8] Attempts to localize the metabolic basis for this defect have incriminated lipoamide dehydrogenase,[75] an enzyme important in pyruvate metabolism. Fifty percent[88] of patients with Friedreich disease have deficient pyruvate oxidation in muscle slices and skin fibroblasts. Platelets from these patients have low activity levels for the enzyme regenerating the oxidized lipoyl moiety of pyruvate dehydrogenase and alpha-ketoglutarate dehydrogenase, lipoamide dehydrogenase.[88] Kinetic assays of lipoamide dehydrogenase have been used recently for carrier detection.[112] Despite these findings, an abnormality of lipoamide dehydrogenase has not been considered to be the fundamental defect in Friedreich disease.[12, 111] Glutamic acid, gamma-aminobutyric acid, and aspartic acid are decreased in the cerebellum of patients with Friedreich disease.[111] These abnormalities may reflect the primary defect in the disease.[111]

A syndrome similar to Friedreich disease occurs with autosomal dominant inheritance.[69] This syndrome has a later age of onset and a longer survival. Signs appear in the third decade and patients survive into their fifth and sixth decade. The myriad forms assumed by the olivopontocerebellar atrophies[62] suggest that this is probably a variant of the dominant olivopontocerebellar degenerations, rather than a disorder in any way related to Friedreich disease.

Refsum Disease (Heredopathia Atactica Polyneuritiformis)

This is a type 3 recessively inherited ataxia associated with abnormal phytanic acid metabolism.[85] The result is an increase in serum and tissue levels of phytanic acid, which probably interferes with normal myelin production.[2] The disorder begins in childhood with clumsiness and a gait disorder.[86] A progressive visual disorder occurs, with symptoms of night blindness or photophobia.[61] A progressive sensorineural hearing loss may appear early in the disease. Other sensory deficits are minor,[2] although three out of four affected adults will have sensory deficits in the legs.[86] Neurologic examination reveals a severe ataxia of gait, limb dysmetria, dysdiadochokinesis, nystagmus, a peripheral neuritis, and an atypical retinitis pigmentosa or a salt and pepper pattern of retinal degeneration.[61] Less constant features are dysarthria, anosmia, pupillary abnormalities, and skeletal anomalies. The cerebrospinal fluid protein usually is elevated to several hundred milligrams per deciliter.[2] Nerve conduction studies show slowing and electromyography indicates denervation.[61]

Refsum disease shares many features with Friedreich disease.[2] In addition to the signs of cerebellar disorder and the temporal course of the disease, both are associated with pes cavus and scoliosis and often with a hypertrophic cardiomyopathy. Cardiac deaths are not nearly so common in Refsum disease as in Friedreich disease, but arrhythmias are the probable cause of death in many patients with Refsum disease.[61, 86] Additional findings at autopsy include lesions in both brainstem and cerebellar pathways[61] associated with phytanic acid accumulation in myelin sheaths.[2] The white matter about the inferior olivary nuclei has considerable loss of myelin, and similar changes occur around the dentate nuclei in the cerebellum. Purkinje cell loss is moderate, but the cerebellar cortex otherwise is fairly well preserved.

Abetalipoproteinemia

This is a type 3 ataxia identified readily by an abnormal lipoprotein profile and the presence of acanthocytes on peripheral blood smear. The disease was described by Bassen and Kornzweig, whose original patient was an adolescent Jewish girl with central and peripheral scotomas producing very limited vision.[9] The visual disorder developed from a pigmentary degeneration of the retina with macular involvement. She had other neurologic deficits, including a peripheral neuropathy, with impaired touch and vibration sense and a progressive ataxia.[9] Both truncal and limb ataxia developed along with kinetic tremors, impaired check, pendular reflexes, and clumsy finger movements. This child differed little from patients with Friedreich disease. Indeed, autosomal recessive inheritance was suggested by the fact that the parents were first cousins. The clue that this adolescent girl had another disease was the crenated or spiked appearance of her red blood cells on a smear of her peripheral blood.[9]

Neurologic symptoms seen in subsequent patients have varied little from this initial description. Gait and limb ataxia appear consistently during childhood in affected individuals. The disease progresses as the patient becomes an adult and dysarthria, loss of position sense, hyporeflexia, and extensor plantar responses are well developed late in the disease.[100] This is still a rare disorder, but the red blood cell changes are so unique for an ataxic syndrome that the diagnosis can be reached relatively easily. Some patients with abetalipoproteinemia have the intestinal disorder sprue associated with retinitis pigmentosa and ataxia.[3] Rare patients with acanthocytosis and ataxia have normal betalipoprotein levels.[100] Pathologic changes affect both the central and the peripheral nervous system. Aside from demyelination in peripheral nerves, the degenerative changes accounting for the ataxia involve both the spinal cord and cerebellum. Both spinocerebellar and posterior column tracts show degeneration. The cerebellar cortex has considerable neuronal loss late in the disease.

Gamma-Glutamylcysteine Synthetase (GGCS) Deficiency

This disease is characterized by a recessively inherited progressive ataxia with peripheral neuropathy, pes cavus, hyporeflexia, and signs of posterior column dysfunction. GGCS deficiency leads to a decrease of reduced glutathione.[87] Glutathione is an important hydrogen receptor and, when reduced, an essential reducing agent important as a free radical scavenger in many metabolic pathways. Patients with this inborn error of metabolism have a complex aminoaciduria as well as a high probability of developing a hemolytic anemia. Symptoms of this disease begin in the third and fourth decades with slowly progressive gait difficulty and clumsiness. Dysarthria as well as prominent limb dysmetria appear as the disease evolves over the ensuing years. Myoclonus and areflexia are relatively late signs of the disease. Pes cavus may develop and myopathy may be associated with the ataxia. The relatively late onset differentiates this metabolic disorder from other type 3 recessive ataxias. As in Friedreich disease and Refsum disease. cardiomyopathy develops at an early age in patients with this disease.

Nephronophthisis with Progressive Ataxia

This is a rare and poorly defined syndrome in which a progressive ataxia and retinal pigmentary degeneration develop in children with kidney disease.[84] The patient has a rapidly progressive interstitial nephritis and retinitis pigmentosa which result in renal failure and blindness before puberty. An unstable gait appears by the age of five years, and poor limb coordination is prominent. Coarse horizontal nystagmus accompanies the reduced visual acuity. Dysmetria and dysdiadochokinesis progress with the evolution of the disease over a few years. Renal disease limits the survival of these patients.

Type 4 Recessive Ataxia

Roussy-Lévy Syndrome

This is a slowly progressive, recessively inherited ataxia associated with a severe peripheral neuropathy. The disorder is similar in many respects to Friedreich disease and may appear in families with this disease.[31, 69] The disease shows a marked similarity to Charcot-Marie-Tooth disease also, prompting the speculation the Roussy-Lévy syndrome is not a distinct entity.[31, 65] Although this issue has not been resolved, we have continued to classify the Roussy-Lévy syndrome as an entity separate from Friedreich disease because of the severe neuropathy and the more indolent course in the Roussy-Lévy syndrome.

The disease begins in childhood with a gait disorder, but in occasional cases the onset is delayed until middle age. Deficits in balance and dexterity progress slowly over the course of years.[65] Early in the course of the disease, clinical examination reveals a wide based gait, impaired limb coordination, hypotonia, hyporeflexia or areflexia in the legs, nystagmus, pes cavus, atrophy of the distal muscles, and a distal sensory loss. Tremor commonly occurs, but it is a static, rather than a kinetic, tremor. As the disease progresses, patients develop areflexia, an extensive peripheral sensory loss, atrophy of proximal and distal muscles, kyphoscoliosis, and impaired position and vibration sense. Although the neuropathology underlying this disorder is unknown, peripheral nerve biopsies in these patients reveal a hypertrophic neuropathy of the Dejerine-Sottas type.

Type 5 Recessive Ataxia

The normoreflexic progressive ataxias consist of the recessively inherited olivopontocerebellar degenerations which develop in adult life. These are discussed in the following section as the type II olivopontocerebellar atrophies.

THE DOMINANTLY INHERITED AND SPORADIC ATAXIAS

Progressive ataxias may have autosomal recessive patterns of inheritance, autosomal dominant inheritance, or nonfamilial patterns of appearance. The five types of autosomal recessive ataxias are relatively consistent in presentation and course when compared to the dominant and sporadic ataxias[7, 45, 62] (Table 2). Most degenerative disorders of the cerebellum transmitted in a dominant pattern have associated damage in the olivary nuclei and the pons (Figs. 2, 3, 4). Consequently these are termed the olivopontocerebellar atrophies[62] (Table 3).

243

Table 2. The dominantly inherited ataxias

Olivopontocerebellar degeneration
  types I, III, IV, V
Familial spastic ataxia
Olivocerebellar degeneration of Holmes
Idiopathic paroxysmal ataxia
Vestibulocerebellar ataxia
Familial ataxia with photomyoclonus and lipomas

Olivopontocerebellar Atrophy

Many patients with ataxia have pathologic changes in the olivary nuclei, pons, and cerebellum which justify their being grouped together into the olivopontocerebellar atrophies.[105] Dejerine and Thomas provided the first autopsy documentation of this disease, but they were incorrect in their impression that this is a nonfamilial disorder.[23] Indeed, inheritance has proved to follow an autosomal dominant pattern in most cases. Criteria for subgroups in this diverse group of illnesses have been provided by ocular motor abnormalities, mode of inheritance, ages of onset, degrees of disability, and associated systemic disease. Konigsmark and Weiner devised the most comprehensive classification[62] by using both Greenfield's criteria of hereditary or sporadic and Becker's divisions into dominant, re-

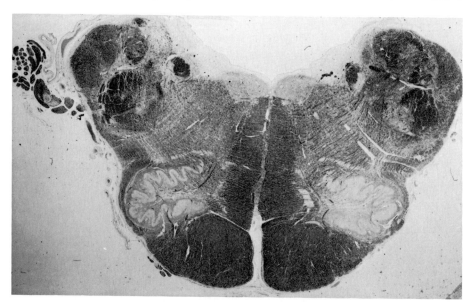

Figure 2. Olivopontocerebellar degeneration. The patient was a 54-year-old man who developed ataxic movements of the upper limbs, worse on the right, and an ataxia of gait at age 47. Examination about 6 months after the onset revealed a static tremor of the arms, slowness of rapid alternating movements, ataxic movements of the lower extremities, and an ataxic gait. The deep tendon reflexes were hyperactive and the plantar responses were flexor. Subsequently the patient's vision became impaired and he developed severe dysarthria and difficulty swallowing. Examination at age 54 revealed worsening of the kinetic tremor of the upper extremities, absent deep tendon reflexes except for the ankle jerks, and flexor plantar responses. The histologic section is a low magnification view of the brainstem showing loss of myelinated fibers and atrophy of the inferior olives (luxol fast blue-cresyl violet-eosin stain).

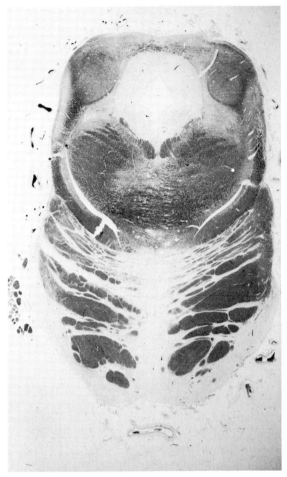

Figure 3. Olivopontocerebellar degeneration. A section of the pons showing loss of transverse fibers and atrophy of the pontine nuclei. Same case as in Figure 2 (luxol fast blue-cresyl violet-eosin stain).

cessive, and atypical types. They classed the majority of described families with olivopontocerebellar atrophy into five major groups.[62] Even with this classification, however, each ataxic family described by different authors tends to be disturbingly unique. The families described by Schut,[91] for example, exhibited so many different ataxic syndromes that Konigsmark and Weiner placed this kindred in a class of its own. Treatment with physostigmine has reduced the ataxia of several forms of the olivopontocerebellar atrophies, as well as Friedreich disease and cerebelloparenchymal degeneration.[12, 58] Thus, at least therapeutically, there may be more similarity between these disorders than is apparent on a pathologic or clinical basis. Investigations of enzymatic abnormalities in patients with olivopontocerebellar atrophy have not progressed as far as those in patients with Friedreich disease. Recent studies have shown an abnormality of the enzyme glutamate dehydrogenase in tissues of patients with olivopontocerebellar atrophy.[113] The significance of this finding is not clear as yet.

245

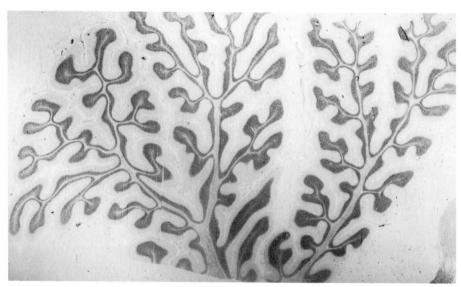

Figure 4. Olivopontocerebellar degeneration. A section of the cerebellar folia showing loss of myelinated fibers. Same case as in Figure 2 (luxol fast blue-cresyl violet-eosin stain).

Type I Olivopontocerebellar Atrophy

This is a dominantly inherited disorder appearing in the third and fourth decade of life and characterized by dysarthria, impaired ocular movements, a gait disorder, limb ataxia, disturbed position and vibration sense, hyperreflexia, and choreiform movements. This is known also as Menzel's type[105] after the physician who described a patient with gait ataxia, kinetic tremor, head tremors, involuntary choreiform movements, and sensory deficits appearing in middle age.[62] Cerebellar atrophy in this individual largely spared the vermis and inferior cerebellar structures, but the inferior olivary nuclei and basis pontis had severe neuronal loss. Other families have appeared with more substantial choreiform movements,[26, 60] often leading to premorbid difficulties in distinguishing this disease from Huntington disease; however, mentation characteristically is intact in this disorder. Dysarthria evolves from slurred or monotonous to explosive and high pitched speech.[23] Position sense and vibration sense are impaired and the deep tendon reflexes are hyperactive. Death in the sixth or seventh decade results from inanition or respiratory infection.

Ophthalmoplegia is characteristic of this disease in some families and rare in others.[26] In one large Scottish family[60] saccadic eye movements were impaired selectively. These patients were unable to initiate the saccadic eye movements necessary for conjugate eye deviation, but slow pursuit movements were intact. This was a supranuclear disturbance; oculocephalic reflexes and ocular deviation on caloric stimulation were present. These patients were atypical in minor respects, showing absent deep tendon reflexes and severe titubation, but they were well within the spectrum of type I olivopontocerebellar atrophies. Another family[92] with similarly affected eye movements had vertical gaze preserved with complete loss of horizontal gaze. All saccadic eye movements were lost on voluntary gaze, as well as on optokinetic and caloric stimulation. Dementia with the

Table 3. Olivopontocerebellar degeneration

Type	Eponym	Inheritance	Principal Findings	Principal Pathology
I	Menzel	Autosomal dominant	Gait and limb ataxia Head and limb tremor Dysarthria Choreiform movements Impaired vibration and position sense	Atrophy of cerebellar folia, dentate nuclei, inferior olives, substantia nigra, spinal cord long tracts
II	Fickler-Winkler	Autosomal recessive	Gait and limb ataxia Limb tremor Normal sensation No choreiform movements	Atrophy of cerebellar folia, inferior olives, normal dentate, substantia nigra, spinal cord
III		Autosomal dominant	Visual loss Gait ataxia Limb tremor Supranuclear gaze palsy Dementia	Atrophy of pontine nuclei, inferior olives, Purkinje cells, retinal degeneration
IV	Schut-Haymaker	Autosomal dominant	Impaired vibration and position sense Gait ataxia Bulbar palsies Dysarthria Kinetic tremor	Atrophy of cerebellar cortex, inferior olives, cerebellar peduncles, cranial nuclei IX, X, XII
V		Autosomal dominant	Parkinsonism Ophthalmoplegia Gait ataxia Dementia	Atrophy of cerebellar cortex, basal ganglia, inferior olive, ocular motor nuclei, pontine nuclei, cerebral cortex

early loss of recent memory and the late appearance of a vegetative state occurred commonly in this kindred. Autopsy examination confirmed the conclusion that the oculomotor dysfunction was supranuclear. Ocular motor nuclei III, IV, and VI and the medial longitudinal fasciculus were normal.[92]

Although type I olivopontocerebellar atrophy presents a reasonably uniform clinical pattern, the range of presentations and courses may cause difficulty in arriving at the correct diagnosis before autopsy when an extensive family history is unavailable. A large kindred described by Perry and his associates[82] was classified as type IV on clinical grounds until autopsy material on some members of the family proved to be much more characteristic of type I. Symptoms appeared at an unusually young age, 20 to 30 years, and rapidly progressive gait ataxia soon became associated with dysarthria, but without extensive limb dysmetria. Dementia was prominent in some family members. A provocative biochemical finding in Perry's kindred[82] was altered aspartic acid levels in the cerebellum. Taurine also was elevated in the cerebellar cortex and dentate nucleus. Aspartic acid, gamma-aminobutyric acid, and homocarnosine were reduced in the cerebellar cortex and dentate.[82] Aspartic acid is thought to act as an excitatory synaptic transmitter in climbing fiber synapses with Purkinje cell dendrites. The pathologically proven loss of cerebellar climbing fibers in this degenerative disorder may be linked to the decreased level of aspartic acid.[82]

Autopsy findings in type I degeneration are diverse, but some features appear repeatedly. The common findings include diffuse atrophy of cerebellar folia, loss of cerebellar white matter, depletion of dentate neurons, inferior olivary nucleus atrophy, and reduced numbers of neurons in the substantia nigra.[62, 92] The posterior columns, corticospinal tracts, and dorsal spinocerebellar tracts may have pathologic changes. Neuronal loss is severe in the basis pontis and atrophy of the middle cerebellar peduncle accounts for much of the apparent pontine wasting. The granular layer necrosis found in some patients is usually a postmortem artifact.[1]

This form of olivopontocerebellar atrophy has been studied with HLA typing and linkage analysis.[54] A locus consistently associated with the ataxia can be identified on chromosome 6, and there is a high probability of linkage with the HLA locus. The presence of the "ataxia gene"[54] can be predicted with 90 percent accuracy. Type I olivopontocerebellar atrophy is a relatively homogeneous entity, and genetic studies with other progressive ataxias are not likely to be so straightforward.

Type II Olivopontocerebellar Atrophy (The Fickler-Winkler Type)

This disorder is similar to type I except for a recessive pattern of inheritance and the absence of sensory abnormalities, reflex changes, and choreiform movements.[62] Barbeau classified this disorder as a type 5 progressive recessive ataxia.[7] Adult patients develop dysarthria, a gait disorder, limb ataxia, kinetic tremor, and a head tremor. The sensory examination and the deep tendon reflexes are normal. This is the only recessive form of olivopontocerebellar atrophy, making it easy to recognize when the family history of disease is available and autopsy studies on one member of the family have been performed. Pathologically there is no tract degeneration in the spinal cord, and the substantia nigra and dentate nuclei have no neuronal loss. Cerebellar folial atrophy is more marked in the hemispheres than the vermis, with neuronal loss most apparent in the Purkinje cell layer. The inferior olives and base of the pons also have neuronal depletion.[62]

Type III Olivopontocerebellar Atrophy

This is a dominantly inherited disorder characterized by severe retinal degeneration in association with ataxia.[62] Optic atrophy may appear with type I disease, but the visual disorder is more severe with type III disease. The age of onset is variable, ranging from 5 to 40 years even within a single kindred.[55] In one series with signs appearing in the first few years of life,[66] gait ataxia, dysarthria, and kinetic tremors developed in parallel with visual loss. Dementia is an inconstant sign. Ophthalmoplegia develops in some families with retinal degeneration and ataxia,[55] but this disturbance of gaze is a supranuclear palsy and is not accompanied by ptosis. Spasticity and choreiform movements are characteristic of some families[62] and may be pronounced. The duration of survival is as variable as the age of onset. Pathologically, the pontine nuclei are atrophic, the inferior olivary nuclei have extensive neuronal loss, and Purkinje cells are depleted throughout the cerebellum, with the exception of the ventral vermis. The cerebellar cortex is normal and the granular cell layer of the cerebellum is well preserved. The substantia nigra and locus ceruleus commonly are affected. The spinal cord typically shows no abnormality or only mild atrophy of the posterior columns and spinocerebellar tracts.[62] Examination of the eyes reveals an atypical retinitis pigmentosa or degeneration of the papillomacular bundle.[55, 105] Retinal disease often includes adhesions of the retina to the choroid with loss of pigment epithelium.

Type IV Olivopontocerebellar Atrophy

This is a dominantly inherited ataxia with prominent sensory deficits and impairment of multiple lower brainstem nuclei.[62] The disease begins in the third or fourth decade with an ataxia and, as the disease progresses, vibration sense and position sense are lost. Disturbances of swallowing and speech appear. On neuropathologic examination, cerebellar cortical cell loss and inferior olivary nucleus degeneration resemble that found in the other olivopontocerebellar atrophies, but the nuclei in the basis pontis are affected variably. The cerebellar peduncles are severely atrophied. The twelfth cranial nerve is affected commonly, and the ninth and tenth are involved occasionally.

In Schut's early study of a kindred with olivopontocerebellar degeneration,[91] the only truly consistent features were a dominant mode of inheritance and initial signs of gait difficulty. The 45 patients that he described had either hyperactive or hypoactive reflexes, and some patients appeared to have a disorder indistinguishable from Friedreich disease. Schut believed that members of each generation developed the disease at an earlier age, but much of this information was based on the reports of surviving relatives and this phenomenon of anticipation has not been described in any large series since 1950. Twenty-five years after the initial study of this type IV kindred, a reevaluation[63] of the members previously described and examination of additional symptomatic family members showed evolution of signs to include spasticity, muscular atrophy, markedly impaired vibration and position sense, optic atrophy, and supranuclear ocular motor disorders.

Cerebellar biopsies obtained on two patients with type IV olivopontocerebellar atrophy, 28 and 41 years of age, confirmed the findings of neuronal loss in the cerebellar cortex.[63] Also present in at least these two patients were findings suggestive of viral particles consisting of vermiform tubules, resembling paramyxovirus nucleocapsids, in association with crystalline inclusions. There has been no other evidence of this disease having a viral basis.

Type V Olivopontocerebellar Atrophy

This dominantly inherited disease is characterized by ataxia in association with parkinsonism, ophthalmoplegia, and dementia. Unlike type III, the ophthalmoplegia results from a lower motor neuron disorder rather than a supranuclear palsy.[107] Both lateral and vertical gaze are impaired. The lower motor neuron component of the syndrome is an important clinical clue in distinguishing this entity from the progressive supranuclear palsy of Steele, Richardson and Olszewski. The age of onset varies from the first to the fifth decade of life. An ataxia of gait along with an expressionless face, dementia, rigidity, and extensor plantar responses appear early in the course. Neuropathologic examination reveals that the cerebellar changes are limited to the cortex with substantial loss of Purkinje cells, but the dentate nucleus is normal.[22] The basal ganglia are severely involved with most neuronal loss in the substantia nigra and milder changes in the lenticular and caudate nuclei. In addition to loss of neurons in the base of the pons and the inferior olive, there is atrophy of the cerebral cortex and the ocular motor nuclei.

249

Type V olivopontocerebellar atrophy is a multisystem degenerative disease. Categorizing it with the olivopontocerebellar atrophies is arbitrary and probably ascribes undue importance to one facet of the disease. Indeed, one kindred with all the major clinical features of this disease in 11 members was found to have no major olivary nucleus damage in the one patient autopsied.[107] The dentate nucleus in this family member was severly atrophic and changes in the cerebellar cortex were not extensive. This was described as a nigrospinodentatal degeneration with ophthalmoplegia.

Most of the features of type V olivopontocerebellar degeneration appear in a dominantly inherited degenerative disease found in the Azores Islands. In the extensive kindred[22] studied with this disorder, a phenomenon occurs similar to that found with the recessively inherited progressive ataxias. The age of the patient at the onset of symptoms often is correlated with the course the disease will follow. If a gait disorder begins in the first decade of life, dysarthria, dystonia, scoliosis, pes cavus, and hyperreflexia commonly appear by the second decade. In these children, the corticospinal tract disease and extrapyramidal deficits are more prominent than the cerebellar deficits. Progressive external ophthalmoplegia appears when the disease begins in childhood or adolescence.[22] In older relatives of these patients with symptoms developing in middle age or later, cerebellar deficits and distal muscle atrophy are more prominent than the corticospinal or ocular motor signs. Dementia may develop in either the younger or the older patients. Although this pattern of early onset of corticospinal tract disease or late onset of cerebellar disease had many exceptions, it was evident from this kindred that what is almost certainly the same disease may have remarkably different symptoms and courses in different individuals.

Other types of olivopontocerebellar atrophy appear occasionally that do not fit into types I to V. Many sporadic cases have proven to be type II, because the autosomal recessive inheritance pattern produces affected individuals quite irregularly.

Familial Spastic Ataxia

Patients with dominantly inherited cerebelloparenchymal disease and spasticity but little if any brainstem disease constitute a less homogenous group than patients with olivopontocerebellar disease. This collection of spastic ataxias has been labeled the "familial spastic ataxias" and consists of a conglomerate of degenerative diseases not fitting entirely into the schemes devised by Barbeau[7] and Konigsmark and Weiner.[62] Some of the kindreds included with the familial spastic ataxias[45] can be integrated into these classifications, however, and regrouping of other kindreds previously considered unrelated[17, 30] may justify discarding this designation in the future. The designation of familial spastic ataxia has much of the ambiguity once inherent in the disease termed "Marie's ataxia."[54] The families constituting Marie's ataxia are now recognized to have been a heterogeneous collection of olivopontocerebellar atrophies and cerebelloparenchymal diseases.

The familial spastic ataxias have inheritance patterns and clinical courses similar to the olivopontocerebellar atrophies[62] and pathologic changes characteristics of the recessively inherited progressive ataxias.[7] However, different families and even different generations in the same families affected by this disorder have variable courses and signs. The disorder presents with cerebellar dysfunction in the form of gait difficulty or dysarthria in the fourth, fifth, or sixth decades of life.[45] Ocular motor disorders may be especially prominent early in the course of the disease. For example, ocular dysmetria and spontaneous down-beating nystagmus were present uniformly in one family with gait ataxia and limb dysmetria developing in most affected individuals in the fifth decade.[108] As the disease evolves over 10 to 15 years from the time of onset, other ocular motor abnormalities appear, including poor pursuit, hypometric saccades, gaze evoked nystagmus, and slow saccades.[45] Many patients develop a progressive hearing loss and tinnitus.[21] Hyperreflexia is a prominent sign in the familial spastic ataxias,[45] and this finding alone helps distinguish these idiopathic cerebelloparenchymal disorders from clinically similar diseases with established endocrine or metabolic bases such as hypothyroidism, Refsum disease, and abetalipoproteinemia. Optic atrophy, ptosis, ophthalmoparesis, and abnormal pupillary responses may appear during the course of the illness. Dementia occurs within months or years after the appearance of signs of cerebellar disease. The severity of the intellectual deficit ranges from mild memory loss to profound dementia. Kinetic tremors generally develop late in the clinical course.[45] Sensory loss is notably absent or minor. The duration of the illness from onset to death is usually decades. Symptoms of cerebellar, corticospinal tract, and ocular disease advance slowly and unremittingly throughout the course.

On neuropathologic examination the cerebellum shows major abnormalities.[45] Purkinje cell loss is prominent in the anterior and superior portions of the cerebellum. The dentate nuclei have more neuronal loss and gliosis than the other cerebellar nuclei. The flocculus and the posterior inferior cerebellar structures are largely free of degenerative changes. The brainstem usually shows little or no degeneration, inadequate even to account for the abnormalities of ocular motor function. Although the olivary nuclei are not significantly degenerated in this disease, the olivocerebellar fibers often are depleted. In the spinal cord, significant anterior horn cell loss may occur. The spinocerebellar tracts and the posterior columns are usually demyelinated, changes reminiscent of Friedreich disease. Demyelination of the corticospinal tracts appears in some individuals, but it is not a constant feature.

Olivocerebellar Degeneration of Holmes

Gordon Holmes described a kindred with degeneration of the inferior olive and the cerebellum in a pattern that initially was named cerebello-olivary.[46] At the time of his report the diversity of cerebellar atrophies and the possible causes of these disorders were largely unknown.[52] Indeed, the cerebello-olivary atrophy of Holmes was mistakenly considered a distinct entity because it was presumed to be dissimilar to the olivopontocerebellar atrophies in its mode of inheritance. At the time the olivopontocerebellar degenerations were thought to be sporadic.[23] Despite this misconception, the designation of the olivocerebellar atrophies as a distinct entity has proved to be appropriate, since additional cases have been described.

Weber described[103] a group of women with signs of a dominantly inherited ataxia and pathologic evidence of cerebelloparenchymal disease. These patients developed gait ataxia and dysarthria in the fifth, sixth, and seventh decades of life. Limb ataxia appeared as the disease evolved. Autopsy examination of one member revealed prominent wasting of the superior aspect of the cerebellum,

251

especially in the folia of the vermis and adjacent tissue. Purkinje cell loss was widespread, but the dentate and other deep cerebellar nuclei appeared fairly normal.[103] There was obvious depletion of neurons in the dorsal half of the inferior olivary nuclei, a degenerative change that Weber explained as a remote effect of the cerebelloparenchymal neuronal loss.

Hoffman and associates[44] encountered a family subsequently which had much in common with the kindred described by Weber, including pathologic changes intermediate between cerebelloparenchymal disease and olivopontocerebellar degeneration. This dominantly inherited ataxia appeared in the sixth decade of life with a slowly progressive gait disorder and dysarthria. Nystagmus, sensory loss, and signs of extrapyramidal neuronal disease did not develop, but difficulty in swallowing appeared as a late complication. Dysphagia also appeared in Weber's kindred.[103] Dementia and labile affect occurred sporadically, but many patients complained of subtle difficulties with memory, especially recent memory. Life spans were normal for these patients and at autopsy generalized cerebellar atrophy was striking.[44] Pontine nuclei, spinocerebellar tracts, and cerebellar peduncles were normal. The olivary nuclei appeared grossly normal, but microscopic examination revealed Weber's finding of limited loss of neurons in the inferior olivary nuclei, localized by Hoffman to the dorsal and medial neurons of the nuclei. The deep cerebellar nuclei had no prominent changes except for minor neuronal loss in the dentate nucleus. As in Weber's cases, the most severe atrophy of the cerebellar folia was over the superior and anterior aspects of the cerebellum. Enough individual cases have appeared with these clinical and pathologic features to suggest a distinct category of cerebellar degeneration designated olivocerebellar disease. Additional familial cases have been described,[30] and sporadic cases of olivocerebellar atrophy have been linked to neoplasms, especially of the lymphoid system.[50]

Idiopathic Paroxysmal Ataxia

Ataxias inherited as autosomal dominant traits need not be progressive. An idiopathic paroxysmal ataxia develops in some families in which there is little evidence of increasing cerebellar deficits.[40, 106] The disorder appears in infancy with frequent episodes of gait ataxia, titubation, nystagmus, and clumsiness, which persist into adult life with the added features of paroxysmal dysarthria, oscillopsia, vertigo, and vomiting. With the dysarthria and clumsiness, the patient has complex nystagmus and ocular motor abnormalities.[106] The attacks last minutes to hours and may be precipitated by a physical or emotional strain. The electroencephalogram between attacks is normal. Longevity is not affected by this disorder even though it starts in infancy. Age does not diminish the frequency of the attacks. Patients with this disease often are thought to have a psychiatric disorder. Their problems are neurologic, however, as shown by 1) the stereotyped and unequivocal signs of cerebellar dysfunction during the attack and 2) the uniform response to treatment with the carbonic anhydrase inhibitor, acetazolamide. Even when treated in a blind fashion with placebo and acetazolamide, the patient responds only to the carbonic anhydrase inhibitor with complete cessation of the attacks. In relating this syndrome to suspected pyruvate metabolism disorders in Friedreich disease,[88] some authors suggest that the acetazolamide acts by reducing brain lactate and pyruvate as it induces a local acidosis.

252

Vestibulocerebellar Ataxia

Vestibulocerebellar ataxia[36] is an episodic ataxia with autosomal dominant inheritance which differs from other idiopathic paroxysmal ataxias in its late onset and progressive course. Attacks of vertigo, diplopia, and gait ataxia lasting minutes to months appear in adult life and are usually accompanied by an insidiously progressive cerebellar dysfunction. After two or three decades of recurrent episodes of ataxia, many affected individuals develop kinetic tremors, staggering gait, and titubation permanently.[36] Life span is unaffected by this disorder.

Familial Ataxia with Photomyoclonus and Lipomas

Ataxia may appear in combination with a variety of neurologic and systemic disorders. One striking example of this is a kindred described by Ekbom[33] of five generations with an ataxia inherited as an autosomal dominant trait. As in other ataxias with a dominant inheritance, the age of onset was in the fourth decade and gait ataxia was the earliest sign. Dysarthria and kinetic tremors in the arms appeared early in this group. Nystagmus as well as other ocular signs were absent. These patients had prominent dementia usually expressed as memory loss, apathy, and depression. The unusual feature of this kindred was that all members of the family had myoclonic responses to photic stimulation.[33] The myoclonus was similar to that seen with other rare cerebellar diseases, such as the Ramsay Hunt syndrome and Unverricht's disease.[51, 52] Also unusual for an ataxic syndrome was the development of lipomas on the nape of the neck between the shoulders or on the upper back in most of the members of the kindred affected by the ataxia.[33]

MISCELLANEOUS ATAXIAS

Ataxias with Metabolic and Other Diseases

Intermittent ataxias develop with several metabolic diseases, including disturbances of pyruvate metabolism (Table 4), Hartnup disease, branched-chain ketonuria, and storage diseases (Table 5).[13, 27, 68] Patients with pyruvate decarboxylase deficiency develop paroxysmal ataxia just as early in life as patients with idiopathic ataxia; however, the episodes of ataxia occur more frequently with the idiopathic form.[13] Pyruvate decarboxylase deficiency is distinct from other causes of elevated serum pyruvic acid which are associated with progressive ataxia. Unlike pyruvicacidemia[64] from other sources, the signs of pyruvate decarboxylase deficiency are not improved with excess thiamine.

Disorders of pyruvic acid metabolism appear frequently in patients with ataxias of various types. There is evidence of abnormal pyruvate metabolism in the reces-

Table 4. Ataxias with disordered pyruvate metabolism

Friedreich disease
Charlevoix-Saguenay syndrome
Recessive Roussy-Lévy syndrome
Idiopathic pyruvicacidemia with alaninuria
Pyruvate decarboxylase deficiency

Table 5. Storage disorders producing cerebellar pathology

Neuronal ceroid lipofuscinosis
Niemann-Pick variant
Infantile Gaucher disease
Sandhoff disease
Johnson-Chutorian hexosaminidase deficiency
Adult hexosaminidase deficiency
Lafora body disease
Familial cerebrotendinous xanthomatosis
Juvenile Tay-Sachs disease

sive ataxias of Charlevoix-Saguenay and Roussy-Lévy[7] and the evidence of aberrant pyruvate metabolism in Friedreich disease is substantial.[88] Blass[12] estimates that nearly 50 percent of patients with ataxic syndromes have abnormal pyruvate metabolism. Pyruvic acid metabolism may even be involved in branched-chain ketonuria. The pyruvate decarboxylase complex is located on the inner mitochondrial membrane and pyruvate transport to this site may be inhibited by metabolites accumulating with branched-chain ketonuria.[76] Patients with the intermittent form of this disease have anorexia, vomiting, unsteady gait, and apathy first appearing between 10 months and 2 years of life. Symptoms recur episodically for years, and at death the principal evidence of cerebellar disease is diffuse abnormalities in myelin about the dentate nuclei.[76]

Paroxysmal ataxia occasionally develops with other diseases affecting the cerebellum such as multiple sclerosis[73] and, in these patients as with the idiopathic form, ataxia and dysarthria may be precipitated by hyperventilation or emotional stress.[29] Transient ischemic attacks of course are the most likely explanation for transient ataxia in the elderly.[77]

Cerebellar Disorders with Myoclonus and Epilepsy

The Ramsay Hunt Syndrome (Dentatorubral Degeneration)

In 1914 Ramsay Hunt[51] described three patients with slowly progressive kinetic tremor, intermittent myoclonus, and ataxia, who had neither nystagmus nor vertigo. One of these patients proved to have degeneration of the dentate nucleus, the superior cerebellar peduncles, Clarke's column, the posterior columns, and the spinocerebellar tracts.[37, 52] Patients with similar deficits appearing in adolescence had red nucleus changes,[11] prompting the designation dentatorubral degeneration or Ramsay Hunt syndrome.[109] Epilepsy was not a feature of the syndrome as proposed initially by Ramsay Hunt, but he subsequently[52] found a few patients similar to his original cases developing a seizure disorder in association with their progressive tremors.

Cases of myoclonus and ataxia without epilepsy may represent any one of several degenerative disorders,[37] and it has not been determined whether cases with epilepsy represent a distinct entity or syndrome. The dyssynergia cerebellaris myoclonica of Ramsay Hunt is at best a designation for the idiopathic or poorly defined classes of disease resulting in ataxia, myoclonus, and epilepsy in relatively young adults. The diagnosis should be limited to patients with extensive dentato-

254

rubral and spinocerebellar degeneration associated with cerebral cortical degeneration.[11] This excludes patients with corticospinal tract disease, cardiomyopathy, and scoliosis.

Progressive Cerebellar Dyssynergia with Myoclonus and Epilepsy

Several diseases lead to a progressive cerebellar disorder in association with myoclonus and epilepsy, including Lafora body disease, Creutzfeldt-Jakob disease, cerebral lipidosis, neuroblastoma, chronic progressive encephalitis following rubella infection, and lipofuscinosis. There is also an idiopathic form of progressive cerebellar dyssynergia with myoclonus and epilepsy. The neuropathologic changes in these disorders usually are widespread in the central nervous system. Lafora body disease is a neurologic disorder characterized by progressive myoclonus, ataxia, kinetic tremors, and dementia, resulting in death within a few years of the onset.[11, 41] Inclusion bodies of fairly typical appearance can be found in both brain and muscle, and the cerebellum shows extensive damage, especially in the dentate nucleus.[41] Creutzfeldt-Jakob disease is a progressive disorder affecting adults and causing dementia, myoclonus, ataxia, and seizures.[89] The disease results from a slow virus infection of the central nervous system. Cerebral lipidoses are ascribed to limited, though not necessarily known, enzymatic defects. Cerebral lipidoses also may produce myoclonus, epilepsy, and ataxia. Neuroblastomas may cause an encephalopathy with myoclonus. In this disorder, neuropathologic changes occur prominently in the dentate nuclei.[110] Chronic progressive encephalitis following rubella infection in childhood may cause ataxia, myoclonus, and seizures.[98, 104] Lipofuscinosis was described in a middle aged man with progressive ataxia, myoclonus, and epilepsy.[81] The deterioration from the patient's initial clumsiness and myoclonic jerks to death took only six years. Lipofuscin distended the dendrites of all cerebellar neurons, and Purkinje cells were decreased in number. There was a history of similarly affected relatives, suggesting a sporadic or autosomal recessive pattern.

The ages of the affected patients in the diseases listed above span several decades, even though the signs and symptoms of the diseases are similar. For several of these disorders dysarthria is an early sign and limb dysmetria, kinetic tremors, and severe truncal myoclonus develop in parallel with intellectual disorders. This course occurs whether the disease is idiopathic or caused by Lafora body disease or lipidosis.

In idiopathic cases of progressive cerebellar dyssynergia the electroencephalogram shows bilateral spike discharges and intermittent rhythmical slowing.[41, 79] There may be generalized irregular slow waves and reduced alpha wave activity. Spikes are not necessarily coincident with the myoclonic jerks.[11]

There is evidence that the idiopathic form of progressive cerebellar dyssynergia with myoclonus and epilepsy may be transmitted as an autosomal recessive trait, for the offspring of first cousins have developed this same pattern of disease with relatively high frequency.[79] Seizure-free relatives of patients affected by myoclonus and epilepsy with ataxia occasionally have Friedreich disease[93] and some patients with the typical features of a fatal progressive ataxia with myoclonus and epilepsy have exhibited pathologic features of Friedreich disease.[109]

Autopsy findings in some sporadic cases of progressive cerebellar dyssynergia with myoclonus and epilepsy are highly suggestive of a subacute spongiform encephalopathy, such as that seen in Creutzfeldt-Jakob disease.[93] The pathologic findings in other patients with this "syndrome" of dyssynergia with myoclonus and epilepsy are as diverse as the backgrounds of the patients manifesting it.[11, 81, 93] Progressive cerebellar dyssynergia with myoclonus and epilepsy most likely represents a common response to progressive neuronal damage when that damage has a predilection for elements associated with the cerebellum.

Remote Effects of Carcinoma, Neuroblastoma, and Other Neoplasms

Cerebellar degeneration occurs as a remote effect of neoplasms outside the central nervous system. The basis for this is unknown. Signs of cerebellar degeneration may appear before local evidence of a neoplasm develops or long after the neoplasms is recognized and treated.[15] The cerebellar deficits evolve over days or months and, although the progression of symptoms may stop as abruptly as it begins, the losses are largely irreversible.[43] No tumor has a selective propensity for inciting this cerebellar damage, but in adults, lung, breast, uterine, and ovarian carcinomas[15, 43] and, in children, neuroblastomas[16, 95] have produced this remote effect with slightly increased frequency when compared with other neoplasms. Rapidly progressive degeneration occurs rarely with Hodgkin disease.[25, 50]

The clinical disorder appearing with all these tumors is characteristic of a destructive cerebellar lesion and has no clinical features to distinguish it from infectious or neoplastic diseases of the cerebellum. Signs of severe cerebellar damage may develop over the course of a few days.[95] Deficits include dysarthria, titubation, limb dysmetria, and hyporeflexia. Opsoclonus is one of the more striking signs of cerebellar degeneration in some of the patients with the remote effects of neoplasms.[32, 35] Myoclonic jerks and gait ataxia accompany the opsoclonus[110] and nausea and vomiting with changes in position develop days or weeks afterwards.[90] Vertigo was a prominent early symptom in a series of five affected adults, but limb or gait ataxia eventually overshadowed all other deficits in all these patients.[43] Deafness occurs occasionally, and persistent dementia is especially common in children.[16] Infantile polymyoclonus may start with the very abrupt onset of violent persistent skeletal muscle activity and generalized irritability.[32] With or without cerebellar disease, patients with carcinoma may have sensory disturbances, progressive external ophthalmoplegia, and muscle atrophy.[43] Although waxing and waning or resolving deficits have been described in some children after neuroblastoma resection,[95] most experience indicates that the deficits arising with neuroblastoma, as with adult carcinoma, will persist after excision of the lesion.[16] Radiotherapy of the neuroblastoma does not affect myoclonus substantially, but ACTH therapy may abruptly stop both the myoclonus and ocular oscillations.[32]

Disorders of cerebellar function resulting from the remote effects of neoplasms can evolve over months and, if the history and examination suggest a destructive cerebellar lesion, primary neoplastic or infectious etiologies must be considered before the syndrome can be ascribed to the remote effect of a carcinoma or neuroblastoma.[47] In children and infants at risk for neuroblastoma, a chest x-ray, intravenous pyelogram, abdominal x-ray, skeletal survey, bone marrow aspirate, and urinary catecholamine estimation are appropriate when ataxia and opsoclonus are unexplained by gross pathology in the cerebellum. Adults with cerebellar degenerative and carcinoma will have transient abnormalities in cerebrospinal fluid protein in fewer than half the cases.[43]

On neuropathologic examination of patients with cerebellar degeneration due to the remote effects of neoplasms, there is astrocytic proliferation in the medulla and pons,[90] but the most striking changes are in the cerebellum. With carcinomas, Purkinje cell loss is widespread and substantial; the molecular layer is slightly thinned and the granular layer may be depleted.[15] The dentate and olivary nuclei are normal. Cerebellar parenchymal changes occur in variable association with demyelination of the superior cerebellar peduncles,[43] microglial proliferation in the cerebral white matter, degeneration of ocular motor and other cranial nerve nuclei, and spinal cord demyelination.[15] Anterior horn cell damage and pyramidal tract degeneration also occur in some patients.[15] Plasmacytic and lymphocytic infiltrates about blood vessels in the cerebellum develop with this progressive degeneration.[32, 50] Pathologic findings with neuroblastoma are even more strikingly limited to the cerebellum. In addition to scattered Purkinje cell loss, the major lesion is demyelination and gliosis about and within otherwise normal dentate nuclei.[110]

Multiple Sclerosis

In patients with multiple sclerosis, plaques of demyelination appear commonly in the cerebellum and in cerebellar pathways. Patients affected by this disease rarely have only signs of cerebellar disease; only 6 percent of multiple sclerosis plaques occur in the cerebellum,[73] multiple central nervous system sites of involvement are common, and the cerebrum and brain stem are involved more commonly than the cerebellum. Plaques of demyelination in the cerebellum occur in any site in the white matter and at different sites with the passage of time. Although the etiology of this disease is unknown, an immune disorder is a possibility and patients with multiple sclerosis have a disproportionate incidence of HLA-A3 histocompatibility antigen.[67]

Multiple sclerosis is characterized by exacerbations and remissions. Spasticity, ataxia, visual loss, sensory disturbance, and urinary dysfunction are the dominant signs of this disorder.[10, 20] Gait difficulty suggestive of cerebellar dysfunction is a presenting complaint in 14 percent of multiple sclerosis patients with more than one symptom at the time of their first apparent disease episode.[73] Indeed, gait difficulty rarely appears as an isolated complaint. Truncal ataxia, limb tremors, and titubation all commonly occur together in this disease.[4] Nystagmus of various types occurs both with ataxia and independently.[73] Dysarthria may appear as little more than diminished clarity in speech or as notably explosive, staccato speech. Optic neuritis in association with scanning speech, ocular dysmetria, limb ataxia, or dysdiadochokinesis is strong evidence of multiple sclerosis.[67] The diagnosis may be made with a high degree of confidence when these signs occur together. Signs of cerebellar disease occurring with a bilateral internuclear ophthalmoplegia are also virtually pathognomonic of multiple sclerosis.

The initial examination of the multiple sclerosis patient will reveal signs of cerebellar dysfunction in at least 37 percent of cases.[73] Ataxia of gait is the manifestation of cerebellar involvement in the majority of patients and tremors are the principal manifestation in the minority. Early involvement of the cerebellum indicates a poor outlook. Forty-one percent of patients ultimately dying prematurely or suffering severe disability as a direct result of their disease had signs of cerebellar dysfunction among their initial deficits.[73]

Limb and gait ataxia occasionally is paroxysmal, lasting only minutes or hours

257

or recurring repeatedly over the course of a month.[29] Well established cases of multiple sclerosis may have recurrent attacks of dysarthria or limb dysmetria 40 to 50 times daily for months or years.[35] These attacks may be related to emotional stress or hyperventilation but their form is so stereotyped for each individual that a seizure disorder at a cerebellar or brainstem level is suggested.[42] Supporting this notion is the observed efficacy of carbamazepine, an anticonvulsant, in some patients with this disorder.

Although there is little treatment for this disease, there are clearly agents exacerbating the signs of cerebellar dysfunction in the affected patient. A variety of psychopharmacologic agents, such as the benzodiazepines, will increase the severity of the ataxia.[10] ACTH does not affect the level of function ultimately reached after an exacerbation of multiple sclerosis, but it does speed whatever recovery will occur.[67] The kinetic tremors and action myoclonus seen with multiple sclerosis are not so likely to remit as are the optic neuritis and other cranial nerve lesions occurring in this disease.[10] Signs of cerebellar disease may persist for protracted periods or they may become permanent.

REFERENCES

1. ALBRECHTSEN, R.: *The pathogenesis of acute selective necrosis of the granular layer of the human cerebellar cortex.* Acta Neuropathol. 37:31, 1977.
2. ALEXANDER, W. S.: *Phytanic acid in Refsum's syndrome.* J. Neurol. Neurosurg. Psychiat. 29:412, 1966.
3. ALTER, M., TALBERT, O. R., AND CROFFEAD, G.: *Cerebellar ataxia, congenital cataracts and retarded somatic and mental development.* Trans. Am. Neurol. Assoc. 87:91, 1962.
4. ASCHOFF, J. C., CONRAD, B., AND KORNHUBER, H. H.: *Acquired pendular nystagmus with oscillopsia in multiple sclerosis: a sign of cerebellar nuclei disease.* J. Neurol. Neurosurg. Psychiat. 37:570, 1974.
5. BALOH, R. W., YEE, R. D., AND BODER, E.: *Eye movements in ataxia telangiectasia.* Neurology 28:1099, 1978.
6. BAR, R. S., LEVIS, W. R., RECHLER, M. M., ET AL.: *Extreme insulin resistance in ataxia telangiectasia.* N. Engl. J. Med. 298:1164, 1978.
7. BARBEAU, A.: *Cooperative study, phase two: statement of the problems.* Can. J. Neurol. Sci. 5:57, 1978.
8. BARBEAU, A.: *Friedreich's ataxia 1978 — an overview.* Can. J. Neurol. Sci. 5:161, 1978.
9. BASSEN, F. A., AND KORNZWEIG, A. L.: *Malformation of the erythrocytes in a case of atypical retinitis pigmentosa.* Blood 5:381, 1950.
10. BAUER, H. J.: *Problems of symptomatic therapy in multiple sclerosis.* Neurology 28 (Suppl.):8, 1978.
11. BIRD, T. D., AND SHAW, C. M.: *Progressive myoclonus and epilepsy with dentatorubral degeneration: a clinicopathological study of the Ramsay-Hunt syndrome.* J. Neurol. Neurosurg. Psychiat. 41:140, 1978.
12. BLASS, J. P.: *Disorders of pyruvate metabolism.* Neurology 29:280, 1979.
13. BLASS, J. P., AVIGAN, J., AND UHLENDORF, B. W.: *A defect in pyruvate decarboxylase in a child with an intermittent movement disorder.* J. Clin. Invest. 49:423, 1970.
14. BOUCHARD, J. P., BARBEAU, A., BOUCHARD, R., ET AL.: *Autosomal recessive spastic ataxia of Charlevoix-Saguenay.* Can. J. Neurol. Sci. 5:61, 1978.
15. BRAIN, L., AND WILKINSON, M.: *Subacute cerebellar degeneration associated with neoplasms.* Brain 88:465, 1965.
16. BRAY, P. F., ZITER, F. A., LAHEY, M. E., ET AL.: *The coincidence of neuroblastoma and acute cerebellar encephalopathy.* J. Pediatr. 75:983, 1969.
17. BROWN, J. R.: *Degenerative cerebellar ataxias.* Neurology 9:799, 1959.

18. CAMMERMEYER, J.: *Refsum's disease*, in Vinken, P. J., and Bruyn, G. W. (eds.): *Handbook of Neurology*, Vol 21. American Elsevier Publishing, New York, 1975, pp. 231 – 263.

19. CHALHUB, E. G.: *Neurocutaneous syndromes in children*. Ped. Clin. North Amer. 23:499, 1976.

20. CLEMENTE, C. D.: *Neurophysiologic mechanisms and neuroanatomic substrates related to spasticity*. Neurology 28 (Suppl.):40, 1978.

21. COGAN, D. G.: *Ocular dysmetria; flutter-like oscillations of the eyes and opsoclonus*. Arch. Ophthal. 51:318, 1954.

22. COUTINHO, P., AND ANDRADE, C.: *Autosomal dominant system degeneration in Portuguese families of the Azores Islands*. Neurology 28:703, 1978.

23. CRITCHLEY, M., AND GREENFIELD, J. G.: *Olivopontocerebellar atrophy*. Brain 71:343, 1948.

24. CROSS, H. E., AND MCKUSICK, V. A.: *The Troyer syndrome—a recessive form of spastic paraplegia with distal muscle wasting*. Arch. Neurol. 16:473, 1967.

25. CURRIE, S., HENSON, R. A., MORGAN, H. G., ET AL.: *The incidence of the nonmetastatic neurological syndromes of obscure origin in the reticuloses*. Brain 93:629, 1970.

26. CURRIER, R. D., GLOVER, G., JACKSON, J. F., ET AL.: *Spinocerebellar ataxia: study of a large kindred*. Neurology 22:1040, 1972.

27. DANCIS, J., HUTZLER, J., AND ROKKONES, T.: *Intermittent branched chain ketonuria. Variant of maple-syrup-urine disease*. N. Engl. J. Med. 276:84, 1967.

28. DAWSON, D. M.: *Ataxia in families from the Azores*. N. Engl. J. Med. 296:1529, 1977.

29. DECASTRO, W., AND CAMPBELL, J.: *Periodic ataxia*. JAMA 200:892, 1967.

30. DOW, R. S., AND MORUZZI, G.: *The Physiology and Pathology of the Cerebellum*. University of Minnesota Press, Minneapolis, 1958.

31. DYCK, P. J.: *Inherited neuronal degeneration and atrophy affecting peripheral motor, sensory, and autonomic neurons*, in Dyck, P. J., Thomas, P. K., Lambert, E. H. (eds.): *Peripheral Neuropathy*. W. B. Saunders Co., Philadelphia, 1975, pp. 825 – 867.

32. DYKEN, P., AND KOLÁŘ, O: *Dancing eyes, dancing feet: Infantile polymyoclonia*. Brain 91:305, 1968.

33. EKBOM, K.: *Hereditary ataxia, photomyoclonus, skeletal deformities and lipoma*. Acta Neurol. Scand. 51:393, 1975.

34. ELLENBERGER, C., KELTNER, J. L., AND STROUD, M. H.: *Ocular dyskinesia in cerebellar disease*. Brain 95:685, 1972.

35. ESPIR, M. L. E., WATKINS, S. M., AND SMITH, H. V.: *Paroxysmal dysarthria and other transient neurological disturbances in disseminated sclerosis*. J. Neurol. Neurosurg. Psychiat. 29:323, 1966.

36. FARMER, T. W., AND MUSTIAN, V. M.: *Vestibulocerebellar ataxia*. Arch. Neurol. 8:471, 1963.

37. GILBERT, G. J., MCENTEE, W. J., III, AND GLASER, G. H.: *Familial myoclonus and ataxia*. Neurology 31:365, 1963.

38. GILLESPIE, F. D.: *Aniridia, cerebellar ataxia and oligophrenia in siblings*. Arch. Ophthal. 73: 338, 1965.

39. GREENWOOD, R. S., AND NELSON, J. S.: *Atypical neuronal ceroid-lipofuscinosis*. Neurology 28: 710, 1978.

40. GRIGGS, R. C., MOXLEY, R. T., III, LAFRANCE, R. A., ET AL.: *Hereditary paroxysmal ataxia: response to acetazolamide*. Neurology 28:1259, 1978.

41. HARRIMAN, D. G. F., MILLAR, J. H. D., AND STEVENSON, A. C.: *Progressive familial myoclonic epilepsy in three families: Its clinical features and pathological basis*. Brain 78:325, 1955.

42. HARRISON, M., AND MCGILL, J. I.: *Transient neurological disturbances in disseminated sclerosis: A case report*. J. Neurol. Neurosurg. Psychiatr. 32:230, 1969.

43. HENSON, R. A., RUSSELL, D. S., AND WILKINSON, M.: *Carcinomatous neuropathy and myopathy. A clinical and pathological study*. Brain 77:82, 1954.

44. HOFFMAN, P. M., STUART, W. H., EARLE, K. M., ET AL.: *Hereditary late-onset cerebellar degeneration*. Neurology 21:771, 1971.

45. HOGAN, G. R., AND BAUMAN, M. L.: *Familial spastic ataxia: Occurrence in childhood*. Neurology 27:520, 1977.

46. HOLMES, G.: *A form of familial degeneration of the cerebellum*. Brain 30:466, 1907.

47. HOOD, J. D., KAYAN, A., AND LEECH, J.: *Rebound nystagmus.* Brain 96:507, 1973.

48. HORNABROOK, R. W.: *Kuru—A subacute cerebellar degeneration. The natural history and clinical features.* Brain 91:53, 1968.

49. HOROUPIAN, D. S., ZUCKER, D. K., MOSHE, S., ET AL.: *Behr syndrome: a clinicopathologic report.* Neurology 29:323, 1979.

50. HORWICH, L., BUXTON, P. H., AND RYAN, G. M. S.: *Cerebellar degeneration in Hodgkin's disease.* J. Neurol. Neurosurg. Psychiat. 29:45, 1966.

51. HUNT, J. R.: *Dyssynergia cerebellaris progressiva—a chronic progressive form of cerebellar tremor.* Brain 37:247, 1914.

52. HUNT, J. R.: *Dyssynergia cerebellaris myoclonica—Primary atrophy of the dentate system: A contribution to the pathology and symptomatology of the cerebellum.* Brain 44:490, 1921.

53. HUXTABLE, R. J.: *Cardiac pharmacology and cardiomyopathy in Friedreich's ataxia.* Can. J. Neurol. Sci. 5:83, 1978.

54. JACKSON, J. F., CURRIER, R. D., TERASAKI, P. I., ET AL.: *Spinocerebellar ataxia and HLA linkage.* N. Engl. J. Med. 296:1138, 1977.

55. JAMPEL, R. S., OKAZAKI, H., AND BERNSTEIN, H.: *Ophthalmoplegia and retinal degeneration associated with spinocerebellar ataxia.* Arch. Ophthalmol. 66:247, 1961.

56. JOHNSON, W. G., AND CHUTORIAN, A. M.: *Inheritance of the enzyme defect in a new hexosaminidase deficiency disease.* Ann. Neurol. 4:399, 1978.

57. JOHNSON, W. G., CHUTORIAN, A., AND MIRANDA, A.: *A new juvenile hexosaminidase deficiency disease presenting as cerebellar ataxia: clinical and biochemical studies.* Neurology 27:1012, 1977.

58. KARK, R. A. P., BLASS, J. P., AND SPENCE, M. A.: *Physostigmine in familial ataxias.* Neurology 27:70, 1977.

59. KEDDIE, K. M. G.: *Hereditary ataxia, presumed to be of the Menzel type, complicated by paranoid psychosis, in a mother and two sons.* J. Neurol. Neurosurg. Psychiat. 32:82, 1969.

60. KOEPPEN, A. H., AND HANS, M. B.: *Supranuclear ophthalmoplegia in olivopontocerebellar degeneration.* Neurology 26:764, 1976.

61. KOLODNY, E. H., HASS, W. K., LANE, B., ET AL.: *Refsum's syndrome.* Arch. Neurol. 12:583, 1965.

62. KONIGSMARK, B. W., AND WEINER, L. P.: *The olivopontocerebellar atrophies: A review.* Medicine 49:227, 1970.

63. LANDIS, D. M. D., ROSENBERG, R. N., LANDIS, S. C., ET AL.: *Olivopontocerebellar degeneration.* Arch. Neurol. 31:295, 1974.

64. LANDRIGAN, P. J., BERENBERG, W., AND BRESNAN, M.: *Behr's syndrome: familial optic atrophy, spastic diplegia and ataxia.* Develop. Med. Child. Neurol. 15:41, 1973.

65. LAPRESLE, J., AND SALISACHS, P.: *Roussy-Lévy syndrome,* in Vinken, P. J., and Bruyn, G. W. (eds.): *Handbook of Clinical Neurology,* vol 21. American Elsevier Publishing Co., New York, 1975, pp. 171–179.

66. LEEUWEN, M. A., AND VAN BOGAERT, L.: *Hereditary ataxia with optic atrophy of the retrobulbar neuritis type, and latent pallido-Luysian degeneration.* Brain 72:340, 1949.

67. LESSELL, S.: *Optic neuropathies.* N. Engl. J. Med. 299:533, 1978.

68. LONSDALE, D., FAULKNER, W. R., PRICE, J. W., ET AL.: *Intermittent cerebellar ataxia associated with hyperpyruvic acidemia, hyperalaninemia, and hyperalaninuria.* Pediatrics 43:1025, 1969.

69. LUBOZYNSKI, M. F., AND ROELOFS, R. I.: *Friedreich's ataxia.* Southern Med. J. 68:757, 1975.

70. MACLEOD, P. M., WOOD, S., JAN, J. E., ET AL.: *Progressive cerebellar ataxia, spasticity, psychomotor retardation, and hexosaminidase deficiency in a 10 year old child: juvenile Sandhoff disease.* Neurology 27:571, 1977.

71. MAHLOUDJI, M.: *Marinesco-Sjoegren syndrome,* in Vinken, P. J., and Bruyn, G. W. (eds.): *Handbook of Clinical Neurology,* vol 21. American Elsevier Publishing Co., New York, 1975, pp. 555–561.

72. MATSON, G. A., SCHUT, J. W., AND SWANSON, J.: *Hereditary ataxia. Linkage studies in hereditary ataxia.* Ann. Human Genet. 25:7, 1961.

260

73. McALPINE, D., LUMSDEN, C. E., AND ACHESON, E. D.: *Multiple Sclerosis. A Reappraisal.* The Williams and Wilkins Co., Baltimore, 1972.

74. McFARLIN, D. E., STROBER, W., AND WALDMANN, T. A.: *Ataxia-telangiectasia.* Medicine 51: 281, 1972.

75. MONDAY, L. A., LEMIEUX, B., ST-VINCENT, H., ET AL.: *Clinical and electronystagmographic findings in Friedreich's ataxia.* Can. J. Neurol. Sci. 5:71, 1978.

76. MOSER, H. W.: *Maple syrup urine disease (branched chain ketonuria)* in Vinken, P. J., Bruyn, G. W. (eds.): *Handbook of Neurology,* vol 29. American Elsevier Publishing Co., New York, 1977, pp. 53–85.

77. NARITOMI, H., SAKAI, F., AND MEYERS, J. S.: *Pathogenesis of transient ischemic attacks within the vertebrobasilar arterial system.* Arch. Neurol. 36:121, 1979.

78. NEVILLE, B. G. R., LAKE, B. D., STEPHENS, R., ET AL.: *A neurovisceral storage disease with vertical supranuclear ophthalmoplegia and its relationship to Niemann-Pick disease.* Brain 96: 97, 1973.

79. NOAD, K. B., AND LANCE, J. W.: *Familial myoclonic epilepsy and its association with cerebellar disturbance.* Brain 83, 618, 1960.

80. OONK, J. G. W., VAN DER HELM, H. J., AND MARTIN, J. J.: *Spinocerebellar degeneration: Hexosaminidase A and B deficiency in two adult sisters.* Neurology 29:380, 1979.

81. PALLIS, C. A., DUCKETT, S., AND PEARSE, A. G. E.: *Diffuse lipofuscinosis of the central nervous system.* Neurology 17:381, 1967.

82. PERRY, T. L., CURRIER, R. D., HANSEN, S., ET AL.: *Aspartate taurine imbalance in dominantly inherited olivopontocerebellar artophy.* Neurology 27:257, 1977.

83. PETERSON, R. D. A., AND GOOD, R. A.: *Ataxia-telangiectasia.* Birth Defects 4:370, 1968.

84. POPOVIĆ-ROLOVIĆ, M., ČALIĆ-PERIŠIĆ, N., BUNJEVAČKI, G., ET AL.: *Juvenile nephronophthisis associated with retinal pigmentary dystrophy, cerebellar ataxia, and skeletal abnormalities.* Arch. Dis. Child. 51:801, 1976.

85. RAKE, M., AND SAUNDERS, M.: *Refsum's disease: A disorder of lipid metabolism.* J. Neurol. Neurosurg. Psychiat. 29:417, 1966.

86. REFSUM, S.: *Heredopathia atactica polyneuritiformis (phytanic acid storage disease),* in VINKEN, R. J., BRUYN, G. W. (eds.): *Handbook of Neurology,* vol. 21. American Elsevier Publishing Co., New York, 1975, pp. 181–230.

87. RICHARDS, F., II, COOPER, M. R., PEARCE, L. A., ET AL.: *Familial spinocerebellar degeneration, hemolytic anemia, and glutathione deficiency.* Arch. Int. Med. 134:534, 1974.

88. RODRIGUEZ-BUDELLI, M., AND KARK, P.: *Kinetic evidence for a structural abnormality of lipoamide-dehydrogenase in two patients with Friedreich ataxia.* Neurology 28:1283, 1978.

89. ROOS, R., GAJDUSEK, D. C., AND GIBBS, C. J., JR.: *The clinical characteristics of transmissible Creutzfeldt-Jakob disease.* Brain 96:1, 1973.

90. ROSS, A. T., AND ZEMAN, W.: *Opsoclonus, occult carcinoma, and chemical pathology in dentate nuclei.* Arch. Neurol. 17:546, 1967.

91. SCHUT, J. W.: *Hereditary ataxia.* Arch. Neurol. Psychiat. 63:535, 1950.

92. SEARS, E. S., HAMMERBERG, E. K., NORENBERG, M. D., ET AL.: *Supranuclear ophthalmoplegia and dementia in olivopontocerebellar atrophy: a clinicopathologic study.* Neurology 25:395, 1975.

93. SKRE, H., AND LÖKEN, A. C.: *Myoclonus epilepsy and subacute presenile dementia in heredoataxia.* Acta Neurol. Scandinav. 46:18, 1970.

94. SOLITARE, G. B.: *Louis-Bar's syndrome (ataxia-telangiectasia).* Neurology 18:1180, 1968.

95. SOLOMON, G. E., AND CHUTORIAN, A. M.: *Opsoclonus and occult neuroblastoma.* N. Engl. J. Med. 279:475, 1968.

96. STRICH, S. J.: *Pathological findings in three cases of ataxia-telangiectasia.* J. Neurol. Neurosurg. Psychiat. 29:489, 1966.

97. TEPLITZ, R. L.: *Ataxia telangiectasia.* Arch. Neurol. 35:553, 1978.

98. TOWNSEND, J. J., BARINGER, J. R., WOLINSKY, J. S., ET AL.: *Progressive rubella panencephalitis.* N. Engl. J. Med. 292:990, 1975.

261

99. TRUMAN, J. T.: *Case records of the Massachusetts General Hospital.* N. Engl. J. Med. 292: 1231, 1975.

100. URICH, H.: *Diseases of peripheral nerves,* in BLACKWOOD, W., AND CORSELLIS, J. A. N. (eds.): *Greenfield's Neuropathology.* Edward Arnold Ltd, London, 1976, pp. 689–770.

101. VERITY, M. A., AND MOUTASIR, M.: *Infantile Gaucher's disease: Neuropathology, acid hydrolase activities and negative staining observations.* Neuropädiatr. 8:89, 1977.

102. VUIA, O.: *Congenital spongy degeneration of the brain (Van Bogaert-Bertrand) associated with micrencephaly and ponto-cerebellar atrophy.* Neuropädiatr. 8:73, 1977.

103. WEBER, F. P., AND GREENFIELD, J. G.: *Cerebello-olivary degeneration: An example of heredofamilial incidence.* Brain 65:220, 1942.

104. WEIL, M. L., ITABASHI, H. H., CREMER, N. E., ET AL.: *Chronic progressive panencephalitis due to rubella virus simulating subacute sclerosing panencephalitis.* N. Engl. J. Med. 292:994, 1975.

105. WEINER, L. P., KONIGSMARK, B. W., STOLL, J., JR., ET AL.: *Hereditary olivopontocerebellar atrophy with retinal degeneration.* Arch. Neurol. 16:364, 1967.

106. WHITE, J. C.: *Familial periodic nystagmus, vertigo and ataxia.* Arch. Neurol. 20:276, 1969.

107. WOODS, B. T., AND SCHAUMBURG, H. H.: *Nigro-spino-dentatal degeneration with nuclear ophthalmoplegia.* J. Neurol. Sci. 17:149, 1972.

108. ZEE, D. S., YEE, R. D., COGAN, D. G., ET AL.: *Ocular motor abnormalities in hereditary cerebellar ataxia.* Brain 99:207, 1976.

109. ZEIGLER, D. K., VAN SPEYBROECH, N. W., AND SEITZ, E. F.: *Myoclonic epilepsia partialis continua and Friedreich ataxia.* Arch. Neurol. 31:308, 1974.

110. ZITER, F. A., BRAY, P. F., AND CANCILLA, P. A.: *Neuropathologic findings in a patient with neuroblastoma and myoclonic encephalopathy.* Arch. Neurol. 36:51, 1979.

111. BARBEAU, A., AND DAVIGNON, J.: *Biochemical changes in Friedreich's ataxia.* Trans. Am. Neurol. Assoc. 104:52, 1979.

112. KARK, R. A. P., RODRIGUEZ-BUDELLI, M., PERLMAN, S., ET AL.: *Preclinical diagnosis and carrier detection in ataxia associated with abnormalities of lipoamide dehydrogenase.* Neurology 30:502, 1980.

113. PLAITAKIS, A., NICKLAS, W. J., AND DESNICK, R. J.: *Glutamate dehydrogenase deficiency in three patients with spinocerebellar ataxia: A new enzymatic defect?* Trans. Am. Neurol. Assoc. 104:54, 1979.

114. GREENFIELD, J. G.: *The Spino-Cerebellar Degenerations.* Blackwell, Oxford, England, 1954.

CHAPTER 13

Cerebellar Anomalies

AGENESIS

Malformation of the cerebellum usually occurs in association with other anomalies in the brain, especially in the hindbrain. Although some patients with cerebellar malformations are asymptomatic and even careful clinical testing may fail to reveal any signs of neurologic dysfunction, most patients with cerebellar anomalies have substantial evidence of brainstem and cerebellar disease.[10, 18, 27] Agenesis, the complete absence of the cerebellum, is extremely rare in infants surviving more than a few months. A small nodule of residual cerebellar tissue may be the only evidence of a cerebellar anlage and, when present, this structure can be found over or about the fourth ventricle.[31] A recently described family included three sons with cerebellar dysgenesis that was virtually complete, and congenital hydrocephalus.[26] The infants survived for several months and then expired. At autopsy, there were clumps of uniform immature cells scattered about, overlying the fourth ventricle. There was no area of organized neural elements that could be interpreted as part of the cerebellum. Other anomalies in the infants included absence of the foramina of Luschka and Magendie. As in most cases of cerebellar dysgenesis, other parts of the brain were abnormal. Other children of both sexes born to the same parents were normal, suggesting that this total agenesis had sex-linked recessive transmission.

Agenesis of a portion of the cerebellum is more common than complete agenesis. The involved structure often is the vermis or a hemisphere,[31] which may be lacking completely in sporadic cases.[15] An absent hemisphere will be reflected in the brainstem by atrophy of the contralateral inferior olivary nucleus,[31] an indication that some anomalies found with cerebellar dysgenesis may, in fact, result from the cerebellar abnormality.

THE JOUBERT SYNDROME

Vermal agenesis appears as part of several different disorders.[15] The Joubert syndrome is one of them and consists of vermal agenesis with episodic hyperpnea.[21] Infants with partial or complete vermal agenesis have episodes of rapid breathing at rates up to 180 per minute,[5] occasionally alternating with periods of apnea lasting 5 to 12 seconds,[21] with no associated abnormalities of their arterial blood gases. Breathing is normal during sleep. Other prominent findings in these patients are mental retardation, pendular or rotatory eye movements, hypotonia, and incoordination. In addition to the cerebellar anomalies, more than half the infants with this syndrome have other midline central nervous system malformations such as meningoencephaloceles and neuronal heterotopias. In the posterior fossa, the fourth ventricle usually is enlarged without any upward displacement of the transverse sinuses and tentorium cerebelli. The vermis may be completely absent or partially absent. When the vermis is only partially absent, invariably it is the anterosuperior aspect that remains. This can be explained embryologically since the elements forming the vermis start as lateral plates which approach each other over the roof of the fourth ventricle and fuse in the midline. This fusion begins at the most anterior limit of the cerebellar elements and progresses inferiorly. Consequently, the anterior vermis is the earliest vermal element formed. Any insult to or disruption in the genetic determination of cerebellar development resulting in the arrest of cerebellar formation early in embryogenesis would prevent the appearance of the posterior inferior vermis.

OTHER FORMS OF DYSGENESIS

Rare forms of cerebellar dysgenesis include various types of hypoplasia (Table 1). A small but largely complete cerebellum often is found in patients with Down syndrome.[15] In contrast to Down syndrome, an early injury destroying much of a cerebral hemisphere in an otherwise normal patient will produce a hypoplastic contralateral cerebellar hemisphere.[31] This is often called sympathetic cerebellar hypoplasia to indicate that the cerebellar anomaly is a consequence of events elsewhere in the brain. Hypoplasia may be limited to specific fiber systems, such as pontoneocerebellar hypoplasia.[31] This malformation involves the ventral pons, which is small and depleted of its nuclei, and the afferent cerebellar fibers, which are largely absent. The folia may have limited development as in other hypoplastic syndromes, and this will give the cerebellum a smooth or microgyric appearance. Patients with all of these dysgenetic or hypoplastic cerebellar disorders are symptomatic for either cerebellar deficiency or for associated neurologic deficits. Postural abnormalities, limb dysmetria, or focal hypotonia may reflect the hindbrain malformations.

THE DANDY-WALKER MALFORMATION

Hydrocephalus in association with a posterior fossa cyst and dysgenesis of the cerebellum was first described by Sutton in 1887.[29] Dandy and Blackfan[11] subsequently described an additional case and Taggart and Walker[30] ascribed these abnormalities to atresia of the foramina of Luschka and Magendie. The entity

Table 1. Syndromes with cerebellar dysgenesis

Joubert's hyperpnea
Down syndrome
Dandy-Walker anomaly
Arnold-Chiari anomaly
Sympathetic cerebellar hypoplasia
Pontoneocerebellar hypoplasia

264

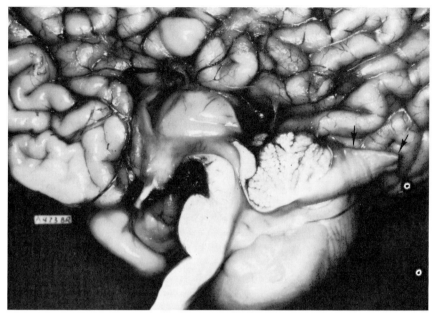

Figure 1. Dandy-Walker malformation. A sagittal section of the brain of an 8-month-old male infant noted to have a large head at 3 weeks of age. Examination at 4 months revealed an enlarged head, dilated veins over the cranium, and bilateral extensor plantar responses. The specimen contained an encephalocoele of the fourth ventricle, with marked enlargement of the ventricle. The roof of the ventricle (arrows) consists of a thin strip of vermis that was continuous with an extensive, paper-thin, transparent membrane. The tip of the strip of vermis has been cut off (right arrow). The anterior parts of the cerebellum are continuous across the midline but the posterior parts are separated into two halves connected in the midline only by the strip of vermis and the thin membrane. The corpus callosum is absent.

usually designated the Dandy-Walker malformation, however, is more than dysgenesis of the cerebellum; it need not be associated with hydrocephalus, and it may appear without atresia of the foramina of Luschka or Magendie.[18] The more constant features of the Dandy-Walker malformation are a hypoplastic vermis, a posterior fossa cyst (Figs. 1, 2, and 3), enlargement of the fourth ventricle, enlargement of the posterior fossa, abnormally high placement of the tentorium cerebelli, and elevation of the transverse sinuses.[17, 18] It is primarily the inferior portion of the vermis which is absent. The posterior fossa cyst forms from the fourth ventricle above the median aperture, the opening in the roof of the fourth ventricle that becomes the foramen of Magendie.

The large number of nervous system anomalies associated with the Dandy-Walker malformation provides evidence of brain dysgenesis extending beyond the posterior fossa (Table 2). These include agenesis of the corpus callosum (Fig. 1), heterotopias or islands of misplaced glial tissues (Fig. 4), spinal defects, renal malformations, polydactyly, fused hypothalami, and agenesis of the brainstem pyramids.[10] Hydrocephalus commonly, but not invariably, occurs with the Dandy-Walker malformation. Sixty-eight percent of patients with the major features of partial absence of the cerebellar vermis and a posterior fossa cyst continuous with the fourth ventricle have other malformations in the brain.[18] Twenty-five percent of the patients with anomalies in areas of the brain outside the cerebellum and

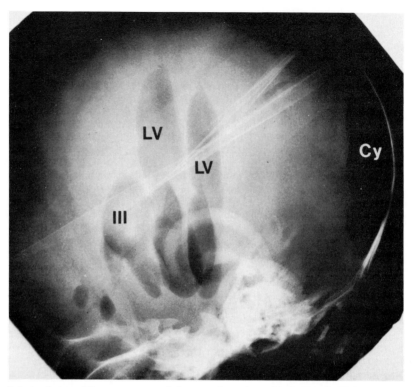

Figure 2. Lateral view of the pneumoencephalogram of a patient with the Dandy-Walker malformation. A large posterior fossa cyst (Cy) is in communication with enlarged lateral ventricles (LV) and an enlarged third ventricle (III).

fourth ventricle have congenital malformations outside the central nervous system.[18] This diversity of associated congenital malformations suggests that the Dandy-Walker anomaly is a spectrum of closely related malformations rather than a single entity.

The primary events accounting for the Dandy-Walker malformation have not been determined, but a developmental error occurring early in embryonic life must be responsible. Atresia of structures previously formed, as from cystic dilatation of the fourth ventricle, cannot account for the findings. The basic defect is malformation of the rostral part of the roof of the fourth ventricle.[17] The dorsal part of the neural tube does not follow its normal pattern for elaboration of cerebellar structures. In the embryo, the roof of the fourth ventricle is formed by a membrane, divided in the middle by the developing choroid plexus. Above the primitive plexus is the rostral membranous area and below it is the caudal membranous area. Normally the rostral membranous area is incorporated into the vermis which forms with the fusion of two lateral cerebellar elements in the midline over the membranous area and the choroid plexus. The caudal membranous area elaborates a median aperture early in its development, and this is the basis for later foramina. This chain of events provides a fully formed cerebellum overlying a perforate fourth ventricle with the choroid plexus lying within. The full sequence probably relies on cues from both the surrounding neural tissue and me-

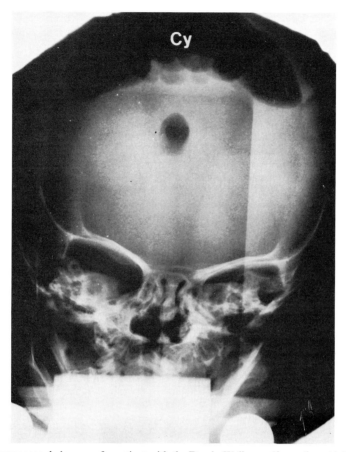

Figure 3. Pneumoencephalogram of a patient with the Dandy-Walker malformation. Air in the posterior fossa outlines the lateral extent of the posterior fossa cyst (Cy).

sodermal structures. The abnormally high tentorium cerebelli and sinuses reflect an arrest in the normal descent of the embryonic elements forming these structures. This mesodermal anomaly probably develops from vulnerability to the same insult that disrupts neuronal tissue development.

Autopsy findings agree with the notion that the Dandy-Walker malformation results from abnormal development rather than atresia of structures previously formed.[17] The posterior fossa structures found in patients with the typical malformations include fragments of cerebellum and choroid plexus overlying the attenuated membrane of the fourth ventricular cyst. Fusion of the cerebellar elements over the rostral membranous area and the resultant introduction of the embryonic choroid plexus into the fourth ventricle apparently do not occur. Considered as a divergence from normal embryonic maturation, the Dandy-Walker malformation must arise in the sixth to seventh week of embryonic life.[17]

A substantial percentage of patients with the Dandy-Walker malformation are stillborn or die shortly after birth with hydrocephalus.[11] If hydrocephalus does not develop, the malformation may go undetected throughout life. Clinical signs of the malformation usually appear in infancy with the onset of a progressive hydroceph-

267

Table 2. Dandy-Walker malformation

Major features
   Posterior fossa cyst
   Dysgenesis of cerebellar vermis
   High tentorium cerebelli
   Enlarged posterior fossa
   Elevation of the transverse sinuses

Commonly occurring CNS features
   Hydrocephalus
   Agenesis of the corpus callosum
   Atresia of foramina of Luschka and Magendie
   Neuronal and glial heterotopias
   Agenesis of cerebellar flocculi and tonsils
   Gyral anomalies of the cerebrum

Occasional CNS features
   Malformation of the inferior olives
   Aqueductal stenosis
   Microcephaly
   Posterior fossa lipoma
   Fusion of the hypothalami
   Syringomyelia
   Cystic dilatation of the third ventricle
   Agenesis of the brainstem pyramids
   Infundibular hamartoma

Associated non-neural defects
   Spinal dysplasia
   Polydactyly
   Renal defects
   Cleft palate

alus.[18] Nausea and vomiting appear as nonspecific signs of the increased intracranial pressure, and a feeding disturbance may occur together with vomiting. In older children and adults, deficits appearing abruptly or insidiously include ocular palsies, visual loss, hearing loss, gait instability, and nystagmus.[10] Symptoms and signs on occasion may develop over the course of years. One of Taggart and Walker's original cases had headaches and vomiting for 2 years prior to the precipitous deterioration of neurologic function.[30] That child abruptly lost the ability to walk independently and had a wide based gait, generalized hypotonia and hyporeflexia, and papilledema when examined at 5 years of age.[30] Mental retardation has been reported in several patients living long enough to allow an assessment of psychomotor development.[11, 30] These retarded patients probably had a low grade congenital hydrocephalus or multiple central nervous system anomalies. In one study of 9 patients with fourth ventricular anomalies and hydrocephalus, the oldest survivor was only 23 years old.[10] The oldest reported patient with Dandy-Walker malformation was 72 years old when his anomaly was first discovered, and at that age he remained asymptomatic.[17]

Radiographic studies assist the diagnosis. Skull x-rays occasionally show elevation of the imprint of the lateral sinuses and thinning of the ballooned occipital bone. Computerized tomography or ventriculography demonstrate the cyst in the

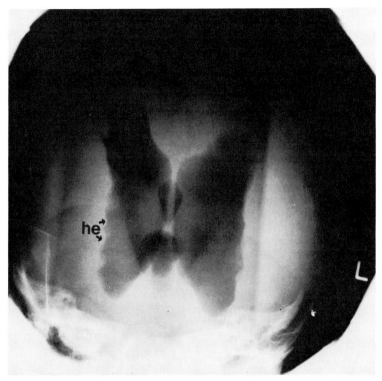

Figure 4. Pneumoencephalogram of a patient with the Dandy-Walker malformation. The lateral ventricles are shaped abnormally because of hydrocephalus, hypoplasia of the corpus callosum, and heterotopias in the lateral walls of the ventricles (he).

fourth ventricle and the elevated tentorium, as well as hydrocephalus, vermal hypoplasia, and agenesis of the corpus callosum (Figs. 5 to 8). When discovered this anomaly should be handled with as little intervention as feasible. The limited deficits appearing in many patients with an extensive posterior fossa cyst and a very hypoplastic cerebellar vermis support the notion of limiting the extent of surgery; shunting procedures usually provide the maximum benefit.

Hydrocephalus is the major clinical problem in the simplest cases of Dandy-Walker malformation. Children asymptomatic except for increased intracranial pressure may develop normally with ventriculoperitoneal shunting. A fourth ventricular cyst and malformed cerebellum are not fatal or even severely disabling lesions when they occur by themselves. Unfortunately, most with Dandy-Walker malformation have numerous complicating conditions, limiting both their psychomotor development and their viability.

THE CHIARI MALFORMATIONS

The Chiari malformations are anomalies of the hindbrain with major pathologic features in both the brainstem and the cerebellum. Chiari originally divided these anomalies, in association with hydrocephalus, into four types (Table 3).[7, 8] Type 1 consisted of displacement of the cerebellar tonsils into the upper cervical canal

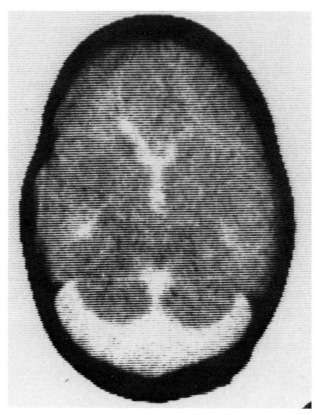

Figure 5. CT scan of a patient with the Dandy-Walker malformation. The cerebellar vermis is absent and the lateral aspects of the cerebellum are hypoplastic.

with no change in the position of the medulla. Type 2 was a complex and variable combination of brainstem and cerebellar anomalies with caudal displacement of the medulla and pons and extension of the vermis into the upper cervical canal. In type 3 the cerebellum was herniated into a high cervical meningocele, and type 4 consisted of generalized hypoplasia of the cerebellum. The type 2 anomaly subsequently was named the Arnold-Chiari malformation, even though its essential features all had been described in 1883 by Cleland[9] in a discussion of hydrocephalus, anencephaly, and encephalocele. Arnold's description of a case of Chiari malformation without hydrocephalus noted the downward displacement of the cerebellum in association with spina bifida, but left the hindbrain anomaly largely undescribed.[3]

The Chiari malformations result from abnormalities of embryonic development. At least with type 2, they probably occur earlier in embryogenesis than the disturbances producing Dandy-Walker anomalies.[17] The type 2 malformation is the best studied of the Chiari malformations and the most amenable to treatment. This malformation has assorted central nervous system structural defects associated with it, some of which produce symptoms in infancy and others which are silent until late adult life. The course is largely unpredictable, but surgery can minimize the deficits in some patients with the Chiari anomalies.

270

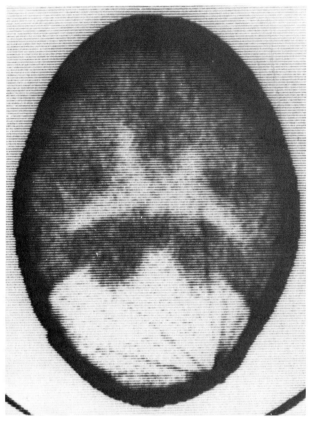

Figure 6. CT scan of a patient with the Dandy-Walker malformation. The posterior fossa contains little more than a large cyst. The abnormal configuration of the lateral ventricles reflects dysgenesis of the corpus callosum.

Type 1 Chiari Malformation

In the type 1 or so-called "adult" Chiari malformation, the cerebellar tonsils are herniated chronically into the foramen magnum and may extend a few segments down the cervical canal (Figs. 9 and 10).[2] Hydrocephalus (Fig. 11), syringomyelia, syringobulbia, or an imperforate foramen of Magendie commonly are found with this anomaly.[13] The progressive sensory and motor deficits of syringomyelia can be the first indications of a hindbrain anomaly.[2, 4] Signs of brainstem dysfunction develop occasionally, but symptoms evolve slowly, and their course is measured in months or years.[4] Gaze palsies, dysarthria, and other disorders of cranial nerve function may appear in childhood and persist. Paroxysmal symptoms develop in 75 percent of cases.[14] These include headaches, dizziness, blurred vision, vomiting, vertigo, and nonsyncopal drop attacks. Positional changes, coughing, sneezing, or straining at stool all may precipitate symptoms. These symptoms probably reflect brainstem or vertebrobasilar artery compression with changes in the intracranial pressure. Posterior fossa decompression eliminates all the symptoms.[2]

271

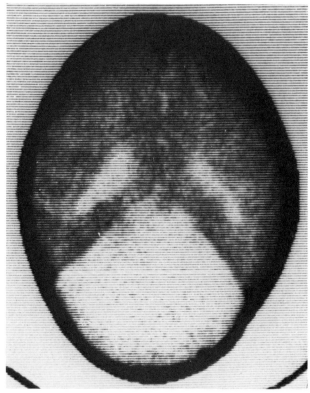

Figure 7. CT scan of a patient with the Dandy-Walker malformation. The superior extent of the posterior fossa cyst is devoid of cerebellar tissue.

Type 2 Chiari (Arnold-Chiari) Malformation

Type 2 Chiari malformation is an anomaly of both the cerebellum and the brainstem (Table 4, Fig. 12). There is caudal displacement of the medulla oblongata, often with a step-like deformity of the cervicomedullary junction.[16] The brainstem may lie so low that the lower cranial nerves must course upward through the foramen magnum before pursuing their normal course.[28] The cerebellar vermis extends to or below the foramen magnum. Vermal herniation may extend down to the thoracic cord level. Hydrocephalus develops in many patients with the type 2 malformation.[23] The posterior fossa characteristically is small, the tentorium cerebelli is low, and spina bifida often is present. When spina bifida does occur, the patient usually has an associated myelomeningocele and hydrocephalus.[16] The conus medullaris may sit low in the spinal canal with little or no filum terminale between the end of the cord and its sacral attachment. This low-lying cord is called tethered, but the implication that the cord's terminal attachment is pulling it down or keeping it down in the spinal canal is inaccurate. In some individuals, the first few cervical spinal roots do course upward, rather than downward, to their outlet foramina in the spinal column, but this is evidence of a cervicomedullary anomaly rather than an indication of a tautly stretched spinal cord. Other features usually found in patients with hindbrain anomaly include basilar impression of the

272

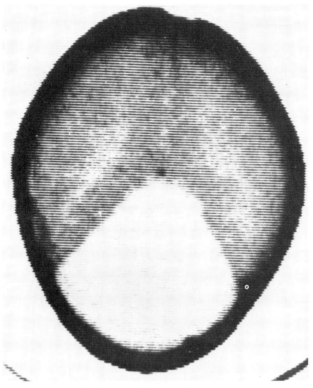

Figure 8. CT scan of a patient with the Dandy-Walker malformation. The tentorium cerebelli is placed abnormally high and most of the posterior volume of the skull is occupied by the posterior fossa cyst.

skull, cervical spine malformation, mesencephalic spur formation, attenuation of the falx cerebri, fenestration of the septum pellucidum, an enlarged interthalamic connection, and hydromyelia.[1, 9, 16, 24] Aqueductal stenosis, cerebral microgyria, intraventricular heterotopias, hypoplasia of the tentorium cerebelli, and dilatation of the foramina of Monro[17, 24] also occur.

The presenting symptoms and signs in the patient with type 2 malformation

Table 3. Chiari malformations

Type 1
    Cerebellar tonsils herniated into foramen magnum
      (no caudal displacement of medulla)

Type 2
    Cerebellar vermis displaced caudally
      (caudal displacement of medulla and pons)

Type 3
    Cerebellar herniation into high cervical meningocele
      (caudal displacement of medulla)

Type 4
    Cerebellar hypoplasia

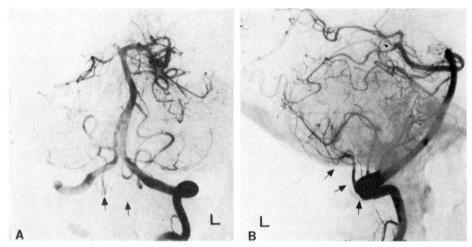

Figure 9. Chiari type 1 malformation. The patient was a 67-year-old man complaining of loss of fine control of the hands and numbness in the fingertips of five years duration. Examination revealed decreased pinprick sensation in a shawl like distribution extending from C_2 through T_3 bilaterally. The deep tendon reflexes were intact and the plantar responses were extensor. A, Vertebral arteriogram in the anteroposterior (transfacial) view. The branches of the posterior inferior cerebellar artery extend downward through the foramen magnum (arrows). B, A lateral view of the vertebral angiogram shown in A demonstrating the tonsillohemispheric branch (arrows) of the left posterior inferior cerebellar artery passing down to the lower margin of the C_1 segment (lowest arrow).

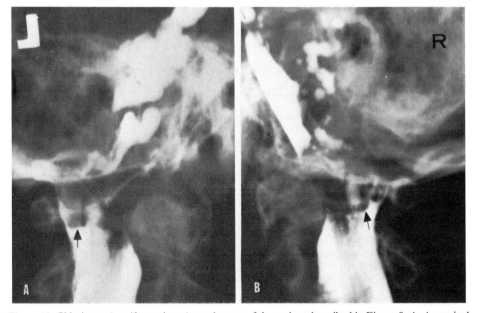

Figure 10. Chiari type 1 malformation. A myelogram of the patient described in Figure 9. A, A cervical myelogram with the left side of the body downward. The contrast material outlines the cerebellar tonsils which protrude down to the C_1 region (arrow). B, The same myelogram with the patient's right side down showing protrusion of the cerebellar tonsils down to the C_1 level (arrows).

274

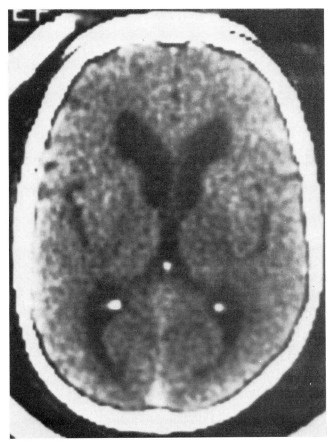

Figure 11. Chiari type 1 malformation. CT scan of the patient described in Figure 9. The scan shows mild generalized ventricular dilatation.

vary with the assortment of anomalies in the individual. Respiratory stridor and feeding disorders in the neonate occasionally are the earliest signs of an anomalous brainstem.[28] If hydrocephalus develops, the usual manifestations of increased intracranial pressure will overshadow other signs. Headache, lethargy, visual changes, and confusion are likely to be prominent. With a myelomeningocele, the deformity overlying the spine will signal a central nervous system malformation at birth. Although this may be occult in rare individuals, in many children the defect extends over several cord segments.[16] If hydrocephalus or myelomeningocele are not present, the presenting symptoms will be pain about the occiput, neck, or arms.[27] Usually, this is a diffuse, burning discomfort, not conforming to a dermatomal pattern. It may be exacerbated on neck movements and may become unremitting. Headaches, especially with exertion, also develop and are located primarily at the base of the skull. Positional vertigo, hand weakness, and gait difficulty often prompt the initial visit to a physician. The gait usually is spastic rather than ataxic, and careful examination will uncover associated muscle atrophy in the arms or hands. In 20 percent of patients with the Chiari 2 anomaly, this segmental atrophy, spastic weakness, and variable dysesthesia are accompanied by a dissociated

275

Table 4. Chiari type 2 malformation

Major features
Medulla oblongata caudally displaced
Cerebellar vermis caudally displaced
Small posterior fossa
Low tentorium cerebelli

Common features
Cerebellar vermis displaced into cervical canal
Hydrocephalus
Elongated fourth ventricle
Beaked cervicomedullary junction
Spina bifida
Meningomyelocele
Tethered spinal cord
Attenuated falx cerebri
Fenestrated septum pellucidum
Enlarged interthalamic connection
Conical tectal plate
Cephalad course for cervical roots
Dilated foramina of Monro

Occasional features
Aqueductal stenosis
Spina bifida occulta
Cerebellar demyelination
Intraventricular heterotopias
Hypoplasia of the tentorium cerebelli
Cerebral microgyria
Craniolacunia
Aqueductal forking
Cyst of the foramen of Magendie
Hemivertebrae
Diastematomyelia
Partial obliteration of the great cerebral fissure
Atlanto-occipital fusion
Klippel-Feil syndrome

Visceral anomalies
Cardiovascular malformations
Imperforate anus

sensory loss in a cloak or cape distribution,[27] indicating a central cervical cord lesion. Ten percent have a combination of gait or limb ataxia, dysarthria, nystagmus, and signs of corticospinal tract disease.[27] Forty-three percent of the patients without hydrocephalus or myelomeningocele have some form of nystagmus and about 28 percent have palatal weakness.[27]

The mean age of onset of symptoms in Arnold-Chiari patients free of hydrocephalus is 38 years.[27] Patients with myelomeningocele are likely to receive the diagnosis of Chiari type 2 malformation shortly after birth; patients destined to have hydrocephalus usually develop this complication by the time of birth or shortly thereafter. The progression of hydromyelia in the central spinal cord may appear with or without hydrocephalus, but it is invariably symptomatic.[25] Brain-

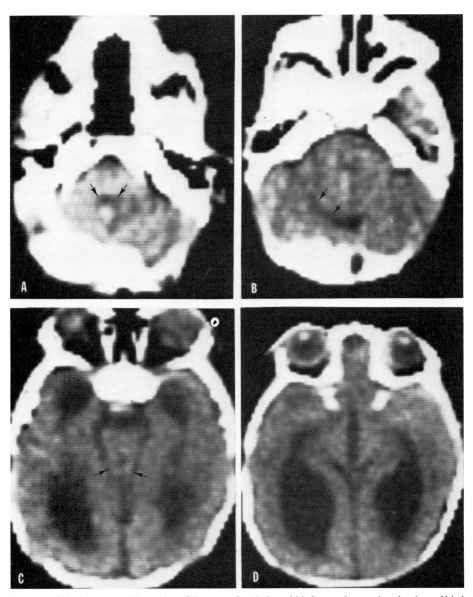

Figure 12. Chiari type 2 malformation. CT scans of a 12-day-old infant male noted at the time of birth to have a large thoracolumbar myelomeningocele. Examination revealed flaccid paralysis of the lower extremities with anesthesia to pinprick below the level of T_6 bilaterally. The deep tendon reflexes were intact in the upper extremities and absent in the lower. A, Low placement of the fourth ventricle (arrows). B, Hollow appearance of the clivus with a low cerebellar fissure (arrows). C, "Beaked" appearance of the tectum (arrows) and enlarged lateral ventricles. D, Enlarged lateral ventricles, particularly the occipital horns.

stem compromise is more variable. Impaction of the brainstem in the foramen magnum may be unsuspected until the patient suddenly develops respiratory stridor from bilateral vocal cord paralysis.[25] Indeed, 38 percent of patients with Arnold-Chiari malformation who have hydrocephalus develop a clinical syndrome of impaction of the brainstem at the foramen magnum.[27] When fully developed this includes headache, gait ataxia, nystagmus, dysphagia, limb weakness, impaired sensation, and spasticity.

The array of malformations found in the Arnold-Chiari anomaly has fostered an equal assortment of theories on its origin. The most likely cause of this anomaly is an insult to the neural tube during the development of the structures which are subsequently malformed.[23] Placing this event at about the time of neural tube closure would mean a pathogenetic defect occurring in the fourth or fifth week of embryonic life.[17] Early theories that an intrauterine hydrocephalus was responsible for most features of the Chiari type 2 anomaly ignored the substantial number of patients without hydrocephalus.[3, 23] The foramina of Luschka and Magendie clearly are patent in 75 percent of patients with Arnold-Chiari malformation.[23] A theory that hindbrain malformations resulted from a tethered spinal cord had to be discarded when the Arnold-Chiari malformation was described in embryos before the cord began its normal ascent in the spinal column.[17]

Treatment of the type 2 Chiari anomaly can often improve neurologic function. Shunting is appropriate when hydrocephalus develops, but for patients without hydrocephalus who become symptomatic, suboccipital craniectomy may provide relief. In 60 adults with Arnold-Chiari malformation, suboccipital decompression improved 65 percent of patients for up to 14 years.[27] The poorest results occur with signs of central cord disease.[27] Some surgeons[25] recommend wide incision of cervical hydromyelia by a posterolateral myelotomy to allow drainage of the cyst and limit the pressure increase in the central canal of the spinal cord. A plug at the inferior limit of the hydromyelia also may help prevent further destruction of the central spinal cord. These techniques have not been proven to be effective.

Diagnosis of the type 2 Chiari malformation usually is simplest with myelography. An air myelogram may be necessary to determine whether hydromyelia is present. The deformity of the cervicomedullary junction may be too small to visualize with a pantopaque myelogram, but the low lying vermis or vermal herniation should be apparent. Skull films will show basilar impression, atlanto-occipital fusion, or any of the other cervical spine anomalies appearing with the malformation. Vertebral angiography usually is not helpful, but the caudal loop of the posterior inferior cerebellar artery may assume an unusually low descent with this anomaly.[25]

Types 3 and 4 Chiari Malformations

Type 3 Chiari malformations are disturbances in the formation of both the hindbrain and the occipital bone. The cerebellum is small and positioned abnormally about a kinked brainstem. The medulla oblongata is flattened and appears to have remained split in development, again suggesting a disturbance in neural tube closure during embryogenesis as the etiology.[12] The defective roof plate apparently does not allow the normal inward rotation of the inferior vermis and choroid plexus. Fetuses with this anomaly usually are not viable enough to come to term.

Type 4 Chiari malformations are no longer considered a distinct entity.[2] Cases falling into this group are now considered as cerebellar hypoplasia or dysgenesis.

278

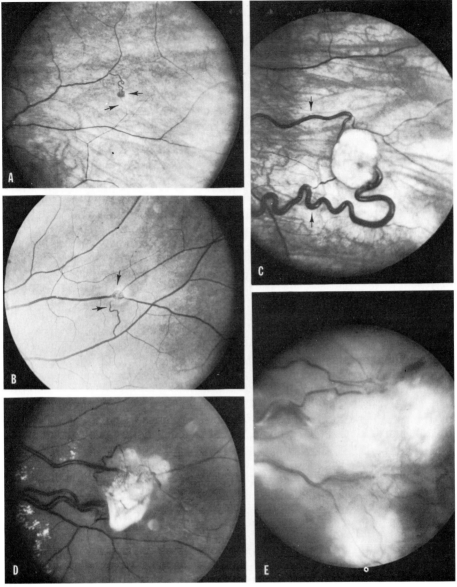

Figure 13. Retinal abnormalities of patients with von Hippel-Lindau syndrome showing the progression of the disorder if untreated. A, The fundus of a 15-year-old male showing an early angioma (upper arrow) receiving its arteriolar supply from below (lower arrow). Only slight vascular dilatation is visible and there are no distinct signs of leakage. The vein leading from the angiomatous formation is more tortuous than normal and is slightly dilated. B, The fundus of a 16-year-old female, the sister of the patient whose fundus is shown in A. This shows a somewhat more advanced angioma (upper arrow) that happens to sit on the branching site of a peripheral retinal vein. The arteriole supplying the lesion from below (lower arrow) is enlarged and tortuous. The angioma shows signs of leakage which appear as a white halo in the photograph. C, Another area of the fundus of the patient shown in A. This shows a more advanced angioma with its arterial supply entering from above (upper arrow) and a dilated vein emerging from below (lower arrow). The angiomatous malformation is no longer visible because of the accumulation of old blood or fatty exudate in its capsule. D, The fundus of a 24-year-old male showing more extensive evidence of leakage with involvement of the vitreous and surrounding retina. The veil over the lesion results from a collection of blood or exudate in the vitreous. The small patchy exudates on the left side of the lesion are deep within the retina and indicate extensive involvement in the process. E, The fundus of a 14-year-old male showing extensive accumulation of old blood or exudate in the vitreous from an advanced retinal angioma. There is considerable irregular neovascularization in the fundus near the angioma.

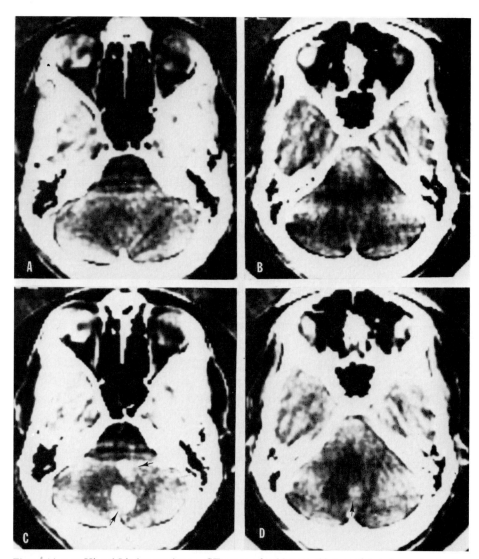

Figure 14. von Hippel-Lindau syndrome. CT scans of a 22-year-old man who underwent operative removal of a cerebellar hemangioblastoma 10 years before this study. A retinal angioma was treated with coagulation 5 years later. He presented with intermittent nausea, vomiting, lightheadedness, episodic dimness of vision, and staggering. Examination revealed only an ataxia of gait. A and B, CT scans through the cerebellum before infusion showing only slightly decreased attenuation in the left cerebellar hemisphere. C and D, CT scans with infusion showing two midline lesions enhanced by infusion in the region of the inferior vermis (arrows).

THE VON HIPPEL-LINDAU SYNDROME

The von Hippel-Lindau syndrome is the association of cerebellar hemangioblastomas with retinal angiomas and visceral cysts or tumors. It is a familial disorder with transmission by an autosomal dominant factor with variable penetrance.[19] The cerebellar hemangioblastoma is the usual source of the initial symptoms and the most common cause of death.[19] The management of this syn-

280

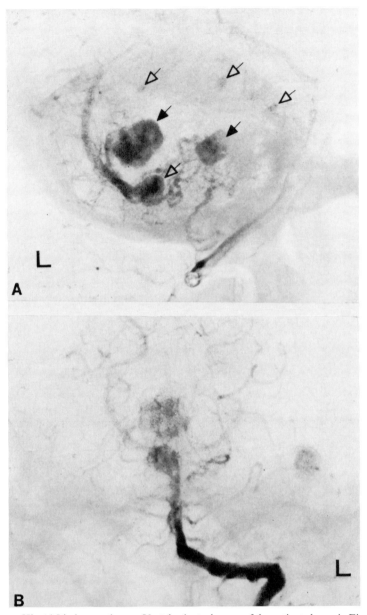

Figure 15. von Hippel-Lindau syndrome. Vertebral arteriogram of the patient shown in Figure 14. The two hemangioblastomas seen on CT scans are indicated with filled arrows. Other angiomas not seen with the CT scan are shown with open arrows. A is a lateral view and B is a frontal view.

drome is based upon the aggressive treatment of individual disorders as they arise.

The most common neurologic disorders arising in von Hippel-Lindau disease are blindness from retinal tumors (Fig. 13), symptoms of cerebellar or brainstem dysfunction from posterior fossa hemangioblastoma (Figs. 14 and 15), and evidence of disease in the adrenals, pancreas, epididymis, or kidney. Cysts and angiomas develop in these and other abdominal organs, but bilateral pheochromocy-

281

tomas also appear in certain kindreds (Table 5).[19] Most of these abdominal organ disorders, as well as gross cerebellar dysfunction, appear about the fourth decade of life.[17] The most serious of the kidney disorders, renal cell carcinomas, are manifest later in life.[19] Up to 60 percent of patients with other signs of the disorder have clearly manifest hemangioblastomas of the cerebellum,[19] but this may be an underestimate reflecting the uncertain course and etiology of these posterior fossa tumors.

Hepatic cysts, renal adenomas, and epididymal adenomas develop in less than 20 percent of patients, while pancreatic, renal, and epididymal cysts are found in more than 50 percent.[19] The retinal and cerebellar tumors are similar if not identical histologically and both appear to be circumscribed neoplasms. The retinal tumors may present as glaucoma or retinal detachment.[6] Retinal hemangioblastomas prove to be bilateral in 50 percent of patients with any feature of the von Hippel-Lindau syndrome, and 20 percent of patients with other major features of the syndrome have retinal tumor.[22] Tumors in the cerebellum are multiple in only 10 percent of cases. Syringomyelia is an additional complication in at least 25 percent of patients,[19] but this develops consistently in association with brainstem or spinal cord hemangioblastomas.

Table 5. von Hippel-Lindau syndrome

Major features
Retinal angiomas
Cerebellar hemangioblastoma
Renal cell carcinoma
Renal cysts
Pheochromocytoma
Pancreatic cysts
Epididymal cysts
Erythrocytosis

Common features
Pancreatic adenomas
Epididymal adenomas
Syringomyelia
Brainstem hemangioblastoma
Spinal cord hemangioblastoma
Hepatic angiomas
Renal angiomas
Hepatic cysts
Renal adenomas

Rare features
Cerebellar cysts
Splenic cysts
Lung cysts
Omental cysts
Skeletal hemangiomas
Adrenal cortical angiomas
Adrenal cortical adenomas
Sympathetic paraganglioma
Ovarian cyst
Ovarian angioma

Cerebellar hemangioblastomas are the source of initial symptoms in 40 percent of patients.[19] The most common presentation is headache, vertigo, and vomiting.[22] Visual changes are the first problem in 10 percent of the cases.[19] A catastrophic hemorrhage into a cerebellar hemangioblastoma may be both the presentation and the termination of the disease. In those surviving the cerebellar tumor and the early development of pheochromocytomas, renal cell carcinoma is likely to be the fatal illness. Renal cell carcinoma develops metastases in half the patients and accounts for death in over a third.[19] The renal tumor may appear in the fifth decade of life, after surgical resection of the cerebellar lesions has provided a dormant picture for years. The cerebellar tumors themselves are often a problem, not because of metastases, but because of recurrences. A recurrence at the same site or a new site will develop in at least 15 percent of patients.[20] Another complicating feature of this tumor is erythrocytosis. The elevated hemoglobin concentration in the blood of affected individuals complicates both the surgical treatment of their lesions and their postoperative course.

Diagnosis of this syndrome is simplest when a family history of similar disease is available. The discovery of retinal angiomas or cerebellar hemangioblastomas should prompt an investigation of adrenal function and a search for renal cell carcinoma. This means both endocrine investigations of catecholamine production and an intravenous pyelogram or computerized tomogram of the abdomen. The cerebellar hemangioblastomas appear as dense uptakes on radionuclide brain scan and as enhancing masses on computerized tomograms of the brain. Characteristically the tumors lie in contact with the pial lining of the cerebellum, especially about the posterolateral aspects of the organ.[6]

REFERENCES

1. ADELOYE, A.: *Mesencephalic spur (beaking deformity of the tectum) in Arnold-Chiari malformation.* J. Neurosurg. 45:315, 1976.

2. APPLEBY, A., FOSTER, J. B., HANKINSON, J., ET AL.: *The diagnosis and management of the Chiari anomalies in adult life.* Brain 91:131, 1968.

3. ARNOLD, J.: *Myelocyste, Transposition von Gewebskeimen und Symbodie.* Beitr. Pathol. Anat. 16:1, 1894.

4. BANERJI, N. K., AND MILLAR, J. H. D.: *Chiari malformation presenting in adult life.* Brain 97: 157, 1974.

5. BOLTSHAUSER, E., AND ISLER, W.: *Joubert syndrome: episodic hyperpnea, abnormal eye movements, retardation and ataxia, associated with dysplasia of the cerebellar vermis.* Neuropädiatr. 8:57, 1977.

6. CHALHUB, E. G.: *Neurocutaneous syndromes in children.* Ped. Clin. N. Amer. 23:499, 1976.

7. CHIARI, H.: *Über Veränderungen des Kleinhirns infolge von Hydrocephalie des Grosshirns.* Dtsch. Med. Wochenschr. 17:1172, 1891.

8. CHIARI, H.: *Über Veränderungen des Kleinhirns, der Pons und der Medulla oblongata infolge von congenitaler Hydrocephalie des Grosshirns.* Denkschr. Akad. Wissensch. Wien. 63:71, 1896.

9. CLELAND, J.: *Contribution to the study of spina bifida, encephalocele, and anencephalus.* J. Anat. Physiol. 17:257, 1883.

10. D'AGOSTINO, A. N., KERNOHAN, J. W., AND BROWN, J. R.: *The Dandy-Walker syndrome.* J. Neuropath. Exp. Neurol. 22:450, 1963.

11. DANDY, W. E., AND BLACKFAN, K. D.: *Internal hydrocephalus: An experimental, clinical, and pathological study.* Am. J. Dis. Child. 8:406, 1914.

12. DEREUCK, J., AND THIENPONT, L.: *Fetal Chiari's type III malformation.* Child's Brain 2:85, 1976.

13. DOBKIN, B. H.: *The adult Chiari malformation.* Bull. L. A. Neurol. Soc. 42:23, 1977.

14. DOBKIN, B. H.: *Syncope in the adult Chiari anomaly.* Neurology 28:718, 1978.

15. DOW, R. S., AND MORUZZI, G.: *The Physiology and Pathology of the Cerebellum.* University of Minnesota Press, Minneapolis, 1958.

16. EMERY, J. L., AND MACKENZIE, N.: *Medullo-cervical dislocation deformity (Chiari II deformity) related to neurospinal dysraphism (meningomyelocele).* Brain 96:155, 1973.

17. GARDNER, E., O'RAHILLY, R., AND PROLO, D.: *The Dandy-Walker and Arnold-Chiari malformation.* Arch. Neurol. 32:393, 1975.

18. HART, M. N., MALAMUD, N., AND ELLIS, W. G.: *The Dandy-Walker syndrome.* Neurology 22: 771, 1972.

19. HORTON, W. A., WONG, V., AND ELDRIDGE, R.: *Von Hippel-Lindau disease.* Arch. Intern. Med. 136:769, 1976.

20. JEFFREYS, R.: *Clinical and surgical aspects of posterior fossa haemangioblastoma.* J. Neurol. Neurosurg. Psychiat. 38:105, 1975.

21. JOUBERT, M., EISENRING, J., ROBB, J. P. ET AL.: *Familial agenesis of the cerebellar vermis.* Neurology 19:813, 1969.

22. MILLER, R. G., PORTER, R. J., NIELSEN, S. L. ET AL.: *Von Hippel-Lindau's disease.* Can. J. Neurol. Sci. 3:29, 1976.

23. PEACH, B.: *The Arnold-Chiari malformation.* Arch. Neurol. 12:527, 1965.

24. PEACH, B.: *Arnold-Chiari malformation.* Arch. Neurol. 12:613, 1965.

25. RHOTON, A. L.: *Microsurgery of Arnold-Chiari malformation in adults with and without hydromyelia.* J. Neurosurg. 45:473, 1976.

26. RICCARDI, V. M., AND MARCUS, E. S.: *Congenital hydrocephalus and cerebellar agenesis.* Clin. Genet. 13:443, 1978.

27. SAEZ, R. J., ONOFRIO, B. M., AND YANAGIHARA, T.: *Experience with Arnold-Chiari malformation, 1960 to 1970.* J. Neurosurg. 45:416, 1976.

28. SIEBEN, R. L., HAMIDA, M. B., AND SHULMAN, K.: *Multiple cranial nerve deficits associated with the Arnold-Chiari malformation.* Neurology 21, 673, 1971.

29. SUTTON, J. B.: *The lateral recesses of the fourth ventricle: Their relation to certain cysts and tumors of the cerebellum, and to occipital meningocele.* Brain 9:352, 1887.

30. TAGGART, J. K., AND WALKER, A. E.: *Congenital atresia of the foramens of Luschka and Magendie.* Arch. Neurol. Psychiat. 48:583, 1942.

31. URICH, H.: *Malformations of the nervous system, perinatal damage and related conditions in early life,* in Blackwood, W., and Corsellis, J. A. N. (eds.): *Greenfield's Neuropathology.* Edward Arnold Publishers, London, 1976, pp. 361–469.

CHAPTER 14

Vascular Disease

THE BLOOD SUPPLY TO THE CEREBELLUM

The vertebrobasilar arterial system provides the only significant source of blood for the cerebellum (Fig. 1). Two vertebral arteries enter the skull by way of the foramen magnum and pierce the dura mater on either side of the medulla oblongata. After ascending in the groove between the pyramids and the inferior olives, they unite at the lower margin of the pons to form the basilar artery. At the level of the midbrain, rostral to the level of the third cranial nerve, the basilar artery bifurcates terminally to form the two posterior cerebral arteries (Fig. 2). The posterior cerebral arteries connect with the posterior communicating arteries, which form part of the circle of Willis and comprise the major link between the anterior intracranial system of the carotids and the posterior system of the vertebrals. The posterior communicating arteries occasionally are major vessels, but more commonly they are vestigial. There are other anastomoses between the vertebrobasilar and carotid systems. Two branches of the anterior inferior cerebellar artery, the internal auditory artery and the labyrinthine artery, anastomose with the carotid circulation through the temporal bone and the middle ear.[25] The branches of the vertebral and basilar arteries are variable, but the usual major branches are the posterior inferior cerebellar artery, the anterior inferior cerebellar artery, and the superior cerebellar artery.

The posterior inferior cerebellar artery usually arises from the vertebral artery alongside the medulla, sometimes branching from the vertebral artery on one side and from the basilar artery on the other side.[21] The posterior inferior cerebellar artery originates laterally and courses cranially to loop about the foramen of Luschka. From there it continues inferiorly and medially, passing between the brainstem and the cerebellar tonsils, sending branches into the fourth ventricle to supply the choroid plexus and to the inferior vermis to supply its cortex[21] (Fig. 3). Other branches provide the major blood supply to the inferior aspect of the cerebellar cortex, extending up to the primary horizontal fissure.[20] As the vessel passes over the medulla and onto the cerebellar surface it divides into lateral and medial branches, the lateral branches supplying the lower two-thirds of the gracile lobule and a major portion of the inferior semilunar lobule. The medial branches supply part of the biventral lobule as well as the inferior vermis, medial inferior semilunar lobule, and the lateral medulla oblongata. The posterior inferior cere-

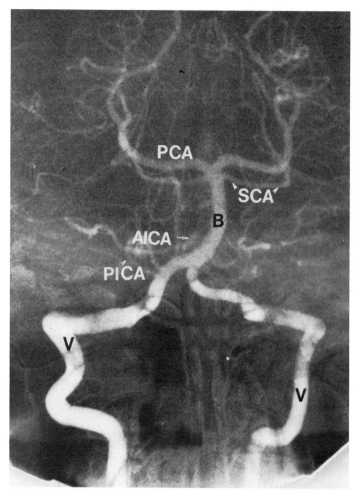

Figure 1. Anteroposterior projection of a vertebral angiogram in the arterial phase. The two vertebral arteries (V) form the basilar artery (B) and at least one of the posterior inferior cerebellar arteries (PICA) arises from the vertebral. The anterior inferior cerebellar artery (AICA) arises from the basilar artery and extends laterally. There are two superior cerebellar arteries (SCA) and two posterior cerebral arteries (PCA) arising from the basilar artery.

bellar artery branches supply the dentate, interposed, and fastigial nuclei deep in the substance of the cerebellum. Minor branches also go to the restiform body.[29]

The anterior inferior cerebellar artery arises from the basilar artery, but it too is variable in its site of origin and degree of development.[1] The most common origin is about 1 cm rostral to the junction of the vertebral arteries. It may arise in common with the internal auditory artery or independent of this vessel.[20] The anterior inferior cerebellar artery courses backward, inferior to the seventh and eighth cranial nerves, passing under the flocculus, supplying the anterior and inferior surfaces of the cerebellum. Its position in the cerebellopontine angle makes it a useful indicator of eighth nerve tumors or mass lesions in the region of the cerebellopontine angle. The artery gives off separate internal auditory and labyrinthine arteries

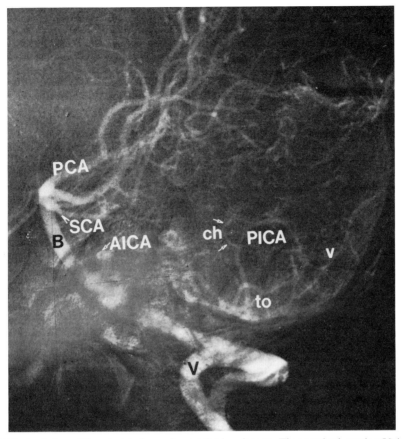

Figure 2. Lateral view of the arterial phase of a vertebral angiogram. The vertebral arteries (V) join just below the pons to form the basilar artery (B) which terminates in the pair of posterior cerebral arteries (PCA). The superior cerebellar arteries (SCA) arise from the basilar artery just below the posterior cerebral arteries, but the course of these vessels (SCA) is obscured by supratentorial branches of the posterior cerebral arteries. The temporal bone obscures much of the anterior inferior cerebellar artery (AICA), but a large part of the posterior inferior cerebellar artery (PICA) is apparent, including choroidal (ch), vermian (v), and tonsillar (to) branches.

before sending a recurrent branch to the lateral cerebellum.[25] Branches distribute to the inferior and middle cerebellar peduncles, the flocculus, the biventer, the inferior semilunar lobule, and the superior semilunar lobules.[1] Much of the blood provided by this artery supplies the structures about the cerebellopontine angle. A small branch of the anterior inferior cerebellar artery near its origin supplies the fifth cranial nerve as well as the nucleus of the fifth cranial nerve.[21] Another branch extends to the inferolateral pontine tegmentum.

The superior cerebellar artery is the last branch before the bifurcation of the basilar artery into the posterior cerebral arteries. This vessel lies below the oculomotor nerve and it runs along the superior aspect of the cerebellum. The left superior cerebellar artery often provides a single superior vermian artery[20] descending along the midline of the vermis. Other branches of both superior cerebellar arteries lie along the anterior margin of the cerebellar hemispheres and the

287

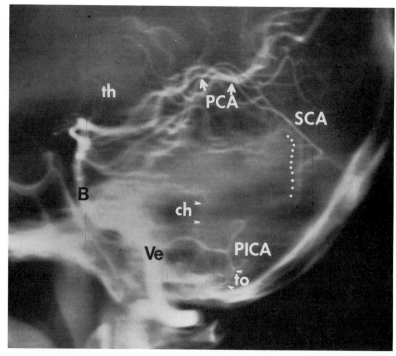

Figure 3. An autotomogram of the arterial phase of a vertebral angiogram with good visualization of the vertebral artery (Ve) and basilar artery (B). The posterior inferior cerebellar artery (PICA) has prominent tonsilar branches (to) and much less distinct choroidal branches (ch). The superior cerebellar artery (SCA) runs just superior and posterior to a fine plexus of vessels (outlined by the white dots) defining the vermian cortex. The posterior cerebral artery (PCA) is supratentorial throughout its course even through the superior cerebellar artery seems to loop above it in this projection. Fine thalamic vessels (th) and medial choroidal arteries are visible.

middle cerebellar peduncle. Branches extend to the anterior and posterior quadrangular lobules, the superior semilunar lobules, and all of the deep cerebellar nuclei.

All of the major branches of the vertebral and basilar arteries are highly anastomotic. Connections between the posterior inferior, anterior inferior, and superior cerebellar arteries are common and unpredictable. In addition, there are marked variations in the sizes and distributions of these vessels, as well as occasional anomalous vessels. In fetal development the trigeminal artery provides the vascular supply to the hindbrain. The trigeminal artery, which arises from the internal carotid artery at the level of the first embryonic aortic arch,[20] may persist as a communication between the internal carotid and the basilar artery in the adult (Fig. 4). A persistent vessel at the level of the second embryonic aortic arch will produce an anomalous hypoglossal artery in the adult (Fig. 5).

The venous drainage of the cerebellum merges superiorly with that of the cerebrum (Figs. 6 and 7). The superior vermian vein courses upward to the tentorium cerebelli and enters the great cerebral vein of Galen.[27] The dorsal and dorsolateral surfaces of the hemisphere are drained by superior and inferior posterior cerebellar veins which connect with the superior petrosal and transverse sinuses superiorly and the marginal or sigmoid sinuses inferiorly (Fig. 8). Of some help in de-

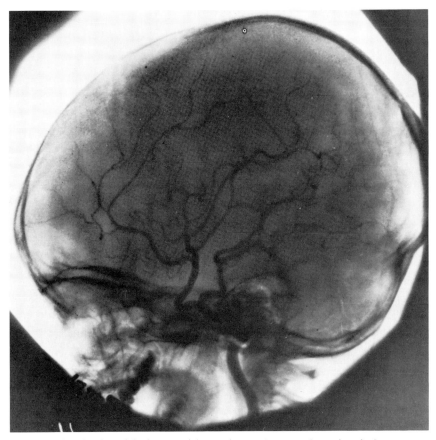

Figure 4. Lateral projection of the intracranial vasculature. An anomalous trigeminal artery connects the internal carotid artery to the basilar artery.

tecting cerebellopontine angle masses is the petrosal vein of Dandy which lies ventrolaterally, ascending from the floccular region, running dorsally to the trigeminal nerve. This vessel may drain to the superior or inferior petrosal sinus and is commonly displaced with large masses in the cerebellopontine angle.

ISCHEMIC DISEASES OF THE CEREBELLUM

The most common types of vascular disease affecting the cerebellum are infarction and hemorrhage, both of which may present with similar symptoms and cause death within hours to days[29, 46, 48] if not recognized and treated early.[40] Cerebellar infarctions are much less common than cerebellar hemorrhages; the anastomotic character of blood vessels in the posterior fossa[20] probably accounts for the low incidence of infarctions.[29] The brainstem and cerebellum usually are damaged together with occlusion or malformation of a major vessel in the vertebrobasilar system. The pattern of deficits developing with a branch occlusion often is so consistent that it allows recognition of the particular vessel involved.

289

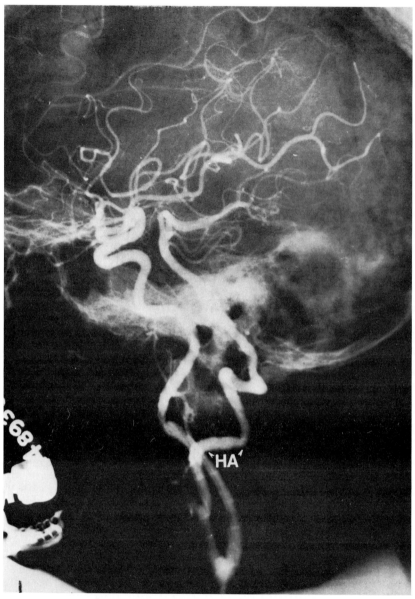

Figure 5. Lateral projection of the intracranial vasculature. An anomalous hypoglossal artery (HA) arises from the external carotid and connects the carotid artery system with the basilar artery system.

Transient Ischemic Attacks

A transient ischemic attack in the vertebrobasilar arterial system (the posterior circulation) consists of an episode of focal neurologic symptoms and signs with abrupt onset and complete resolution within 24 hours. The symptoms and signs result from the dysfunction of structures in the posterior fossa.

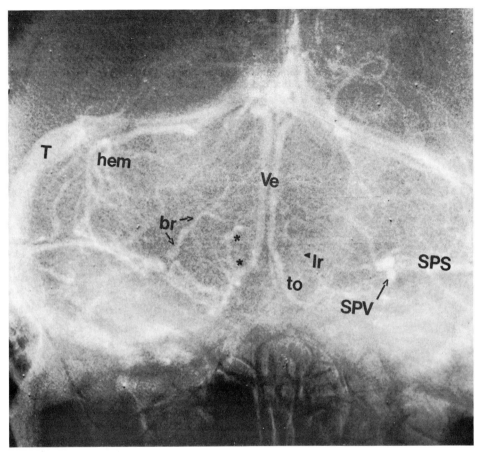

Figure 6. Venous phase of a vertebral angiogram demonstrating drainage from midline and lateral cerebellar structures. A pair of vermian veins (Ve) is supplied by tonsillar branches (to) as well as a prominent branch hooking about the pyramis on one side (**). A large plexus of hemispheric veins (hem) drains into the transverse sinus (T) and the midline vein of Galen. Other fairly constant structures include the brachial veins (br) which course over the brachium conjunctivum and brachium pontis and the vein to the lateral recess of the fourth ventricle (lr). The superior petrosal sinus (SPS) is fed by the superior petrosal vein (SPV).

Pathogenesis

The cause of transient ischemic attacks in the posterior circulation is unresolved.[47] The attacks may result from several etiologies which share the common element of inadequate perfusion of this part of the brain. Atherosclerotic heart disease and other disorders associated with occlusive vascular disease, including diabetes mellitus and hypertension, occur with a high incidence in patients with transient ischemic attacks.[35, 39] This observation has led to the conclusion that signs of vertebrobasilar insufficiency result from narrowing of the vertebral and basilar arteries or from emboli in the arteries from atherosclerotic plaques. Additional causes of ischemia include anemia, polycythemia, vertebral artery compression from cervical spondylosis, postural hypotension, and other causes of transient hypotension.[39] All these factors may be involved in vertebrobasilar in-

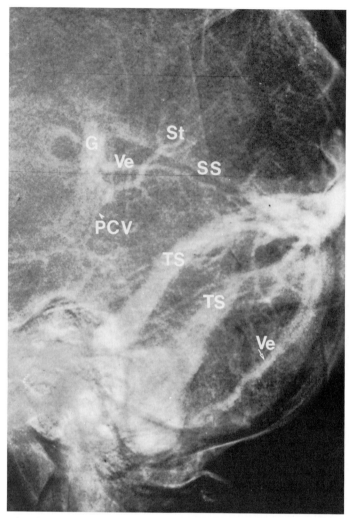

Figure 7. Lateral projection of a normal vertebral angiogram in the venous phase. Large vermian veins (Ve) drain into the vein of Galen (G) along with a precentral vein (PCV). Supratentorial veins (St) drain into the vein of Galen along with the infratentorial vessels. The straight sinus (SS) is largely washed out in this film, but the transverse sinuses (TS) can be seen on both sides of the posterior fossa.

sufficiency, but recent studies of blood flow in the posterior fossa of symptomatic patients indicate that a failure of autoregulation is the most important factor.[39] The normal individual responds to abrupt changes in posture with systemic and local alterations in vascular resistance which maintain a constant level of perfusion through various parts of the brain. The patient with vertebrobasilar transient ischemic attacks has impaired autoregulation and this impairment increases as the patient develops more ischemic episodes. Even in the absence of overt postural hypotension, 70 percent of patients with vertebrobasilar insufficiency will have ischemic episodes associated with postural changes.[39] The dysautoregulation may be a consequence of ischemic damage to the posterior fossa structures regulating

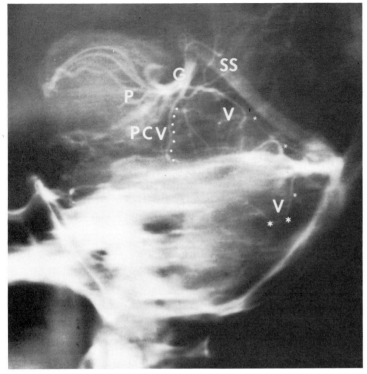

Figure 8. A midline autotomogram of the posterior fossa during the venous phase of a vertebral angiogram showing vermian veins (V) draining into the great cerebral vein of Galen (G), which itself drains into the straight sinus (SS). The high resolution of midline structures allows visualization of small vessels from the area of the pineal (P) and of the large precentral vein (PCV). The course of the precentral vein is outlined by the small white dots. The course of the vermian veins is outlined by small asterisks (*) with the two large asterisks indicating the hook of the vein at the level of the pyramis.

vascular tone and thereby produce transient neurologic signs when coupled with ongoing vascular occlusive disease. The notion that thromboembolism in the posterior circulation causes transient ischemic attacks may prove partly accurate, with the sequela of the thromboembolism including the dysautoregulation which seems to be basic to the occurrence of the ischemic episode.[39]

Symptoms and Signs

Most of the symptoms and signs of vertebrobasilar ischemic attacks reflect brainstem dysfunction rather than cerebellar or cerebral disorders. Vertebrobasilar transient ischemia produces vertigo, episodic deafness, syncope, transient blurring of vision, and unsteadiness of gait.[39] Diplopia, limb ataxia, and even bilateral limb weakness or sensory deficits also occur commonly.[35] Dysphagia, bilateral field defects, and tinnitus are less common.[6] Occipital headache frequently accompanies these transient signs and symptoms, making difficult the distinction between vertebrobasilar insufficiency and complicated migraine in the posterior circulation.[39]

The most common symptom of transient ischemia in the posterior circulation is vertigo or dizziness, a phenomenon reported in as much as 90 percent of affected individuals.[39] Vertigo alone is not evidence of a vertebrobasilar ischemic episode, however, since this is associated commonly with disease of the labyrinth or the eighth cranial nerve. Visual disturbances develop in about half the patients and fully one-fifth have other signs of cranial nerve dysfunction. Rarest amongst the signs of vertebrobasilar insufficiency are transient dementia and transient global amnesia.

Course

Transient ischemic attacks occur twice as often in the carotid system as in the vertebrobasilar system, but the risks associated with ischemic attacks in either system are similar.[6] Although retrospective studies[38] have demonstrated a higher incidence of infarction following carotid attacks than following vertebrobasilar attacks, prospective studies[6, 49] reveal no significant difference in the incidence of infarction following either type of ischemic episode. About one-third of the patients in either group develop completed strokes after one or more transient ischemic episodes, the percentage in the carotid group being slightly higher than that in the vertebrobasilar group.[49] The risk of stroke is greatest just after the occurrence of an ischemic episode, with 24 percent of those patients who will ultimately have a stroke after vertebrobasilar insufficiency having their infarction within one month of the attack. There may be a slight increase in the frequency of transient ischemic attacks just prior to the development of a fixed deficit,[5] a phenomenon probably tied to progressive inadequacies in the vertebrobasilar system as the basis for both the ischemic attacks and the infarction. Slight changes in position may coincide with the abrupt conversion of an ischemic episode into a fixed deficit.[5] The development of a fixed deficit does not necessarily indicate that transient ischemic attacks in the vertebrobasilar system will cease.[3] A few percent of patients with well documented vertebrobasilar occlusions will have transient neurologic deficits involving functions not interrupted by the infarction. The vascular obstruction responsible for the infarction is presumed to provide emboli which spread distal to the occlusion.[3] In most cases, transient ischemic attacks do cease with the appearance of a fixed deficit, but some patients spontaneously stop having ischemic episodes without developing an infarction and without any medical or surgical intervention.

Therapy

MEDICAL. There is no consensus on the value of medical therapy for transient ischemic attacks.[3, 49] Risk factors such as hypertension, diabetes, and cigarette smoking should be identified and handled appropriately. The medication used most often now is aspirin, although its efficacy remains controversial. Other medications commonly used include papaverine and warfarin. Papaverine is used as a vasodilating agent with variable results.[39] Warfarin is an effective anticoagulant that inhibits thrombus formation in patients with vertebrobasilar insufficiency, but it has little influence on the risk of stroke in patients with transient ischemic attacks.[49] The increased risk of a fatal hemorrhagic stroke in the patient developing an infarct while on anticoagulation is another argument against this mode of therapy. Since the recent onset of ischemic attacks or their increasing frequency may be associated with an increased short term incidence of completed strokes, anticoagulants are probably of some use in individuals with these developments, at least during the high risk period of the first month after the development of the signs. The limited effectiveness of anticoagulation supports the notion that dysautoregulation in the vertebrobasilar circulation is of central importance in the pathogenesis of vertebrobasilar insufficiency.[39]

SURGICAL. The vertebral arteries ascend through foramina in the transverse processes of the cervical vertebrae for most of their course. This bony mantle makes them much less accessible than the carotid arteries and may be a major factor in the poor results usually obtained with endarterectomy of these vessels. If surgery on the vertebral arteries has any effect, it is to increase slightly the short term occurrence of infarctions,[49] but this procedure has largely been abandoned. Presuming that the basic problem in many patients with vertebrobasilar insufficiency is thrombotic occlusion of the vertebrals or basilar artery, some surgeons have attempted to increase blood flow to the posterior circulation by correcting partial occlusions in the anterior circulation. Patients with vertebrobasilar disease submitting to carotid endarterectomy in fact do more poorly than patients suffering vertebrobasilar transient ischemic attacks not subjected to intervention.[35] The presumed advantages of increasing the flow through the internal carotid artery in patients with vertebrobasilar insufficiency[35] depend upon effective shunting of increased volume to the posterior circulation by way of the posterior communicating artery. The lack of success with carotid endarterectomy may reflect partly the ineffectiveness of the posterior communicating artery to compensate for disease of the vertebrobasilar vessels in most affected individuals. The risks and poor results of surgery weigh against the hypothetical gains from increased flow through the circle of Willis.[48]

One situation improved by surgery or anticoagulation is recurrent transient ischemic attacks in the patient with complete obstruction of the vessel implicated.[3, 11] Emboli are presumably formed in and dispersed from the cul-de-sac above the occlusion. Surgical elimination of the cul-de-sac or chronic anticoagulation reduces the formation of clots responsible for the emboli.

Microsurgical procedures for anastomosing the ascending branch of the occipital artery to the posterior inferior cerebellar artery are being used to treat some patients with vertebrobasilar transient ischemic attacks, but the usefulness of this technique is not yet established.[47] If this external carotid anastomosis can by-pass evolving vertebral artery thromboses, it should curtail the development of vertebrobasilar stroke.

Prognosis

Patients with recurrent transient ischemic attacks who develop fixed deficits are likely to do better eventually than patients developing infarctions in the distribution of the vertebrobasilar system without any premonitory signs.[5] The deficits in patients with preceding attacks are less likely to persist indefinitely and may resolve completely within weeks or months. A permanent deficit is more likely when the infarction occurs within days of a transient ischemic attack, an observation which suggests that such ischemic attacks are in fact part of the infarction. Infarctions preceded by transient ischemic attacks are more likely to be fatal than infarctions developing remotely from or independent of vertebrobasilar ischemic attacks.[6] This does not indicate that transient ischemic attacks are a grave prognostic sign. In fact the long term prognosis for patients with transient ischemic attacks in the distribution of the vertebrobasilar arteries with or without treatment is relatively benign.[39] The principal cause of death in all patients with transient ischemic attacks is cardiac disease.[6, 49]

Cerebellar Infarction

Etiology and Pathogenesis

Thrombosis, rather than embolism, accounts for most basilar artery occlusions and the majority of intracranial vertebral artery occlusions.[7] Eighty percent of vertebrobasilar occlusions results from atherosclerosis.[7] Emboli from the heart are carried less commonly in the vertebrobasilar system than in the carotid system. In addition to embolic and thrombotic events in the vertebrobasilar system, infarction may develop from rare causes of intracranial ischemia, such as complicated migraine,[11, 40, 49] trauma,[39] and infection.[36] The most frequent site of infarction is the posteroinferior half of one cerebellar hemisphere.[12, 48] There is no clear predilection for one side of the cerebellum over the other.[12, 29]

Symptoms and Signs

The early symptoms of cerebellar infarction are fairly consistent. Common complaints include difficulty with standing or walking, nausea and vomiting, dizziness or vertigo, slurred speech, and clumsiness.[28] Headache precedes all other symptoms by days or weeks in some patients, and the pain characteristically is frontal or occipital.[29] Headache appeared initially in only four of Sypert and Alvord's 28 cases,[48] but it was present almost invariably in the 16 cases reviewed by Lehrich and coworkers.[29] Mentation may be impaired early in the course.[29] Vertigo may recur for days prior to the development of a fixed deficit. The initial complaints may be episodic, though an acute onset with multiple complaints from the start is more typical.[12] The onset of symptoms is abrupt in one-third of patients.[29] With progression of the signs and symptoms, the majority of patients develop abducens or gaze palsies which limit gaze toward the side of the infarction. Gaze evoked nystagmus increases with ocular deviation toward the side of the damage. Facial palsies also are common but dysfunction of other cranial nerves typically is absent unless brainstem structures are infarcted.[29] When brainstem infarction appears coincident with cerebellar infarction, as in the lateral medullary infarction of Wallenberg, the signs of brainstem disease overshadow the cerebellar deficits.

Course

Marked fluctuations in the deficits are likely over the first few days or weeks. Hydrocephalus develops in a substantial percentage of patients with cerebellar infarction[22, 29] and impaired cognitive function or consciousness appears in about half the patients with hydrocephalus.[10, 48, 50] Tonsillar herniation with obstruction of cerebrospinal fluid flow at the level of the fourth ventricle is responsible for the hydrocephalus, at least in some cases. As edema develops around the infarction, transtentorial herniation of the cerebellum may compromise posterior cerebral artery perfusion and result in impaired vision or cortical blindness from occipital lobe ischemia.[14]

Diagnostic Studies

The etiologic factors involved in both transient ischemic attacks and strokes in the majority of patients cannot be determined.[35, 39] Indeed, even recognizing infarction as the basis for the patient's symptoms may be difficult. Examination of the posterior fossa by computerized tomography reveals decreased density in the area of the infarction if the lesion is large enough to be resolved.[51] Often, however, the results of computerized tomography with infarction in the posterior fossa are unreliable. The development of hydrocephalus usually can be detected with computerized tomography. Examination of the cerebrospinal fluid by lumbar puncture early in the evolution of a cerebellar infarction presents the hazard of precipitating herniation of the cerebellum through the foramen magnum. In addition, the cerebrospinal fluid shows no abnormalities early in the course of cerebellar infarctions in almost all cases.[29] Vertebrobasilar angiography may be helpful in the diagnosis, though the results occasionally are ambiguous. Electroencephalography may show focal slowing over occipital or temporal leads or diffuse slowing.[10] More commonly the record is normal or suggestive of hydrocephalus.

Therapy

Small infarctions of the cerebellum can be managed without surgery. When an extensive cerebellar infarction is recognized, however, exploration of the posterior fossa and resection of the necrotic cerebellar tissue are essential.[12, 29] Survival without decompression of the area is unlikely.[40] Mortality approaches 80 percent if the patient becomes comatose or stuporous, but this figure falls to 50 percent if the patient is operated upon before obtundation occurs.[22] Treatment with high dose corticosteriods and hyperosmolar agents may slow the progression of the lesion enough to allow surgery, but they are not a reliable alternative to surgery. A suboccipital craniectomy to explore the posterior fossa is a substantial neurosurgical procedure for a patient suspected of having a brainstem infarction. The decision to operate rests heavily on the clinical diagnosis. If predominantly cerebellar disease is suspected in a patient stable enough to survive the operation, surgery clearly is indicated. Unfortunately, the course in many patients is so rapid that surgery never becomes an option.

Prognosis

In the rapidly progressive case, the infarcted cerebellum becomes edematous (Fig. 9) and soon exceeds the volume of the posterior fossa. With this swelling, tonsillar herniation results and cardiorespiratory failure follows.[29] Death from brainstem compression is a frequent outcome of infarction, especially if the disorder is not recognized early and surgical decompression is delayed.[29] In Sypert and Alvord's series of 28 cases of cerebellar infarction, 15 patients died within 12 hours of the onset of coma.[48] The mortality for the first 48 hours was 15 percent and death occurred within three to six days after the development of symptoms in all patients who succumbed. Not all cerebellar infarctions are fatal, but when the outcome is fatal, the initial deterioration usually is very rapid.

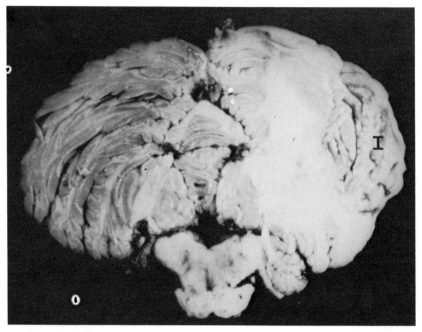

Figure 9. A coronal section of the cerebellum and brainstem of an 81-year-old women with a left superior cerebellar hemisphere infarction (I). The patient's initial symptom was slurred speech. The superolateral aspect of the hemisphere is necrotic and edematous. The superior cerebellar artery was apparent over the right hemisphere and unidentifiable over the left hemisphere.

The Occlusion of Vertebrobasilar Artery Branches

Infarction in the distribution of the vertebrobasilar system may cause one of several characteristic syndromes. The vessel involved determines the syndrome manifested. Basilar artery occlusion produces diverse signs of brainstem disease, whereas posterior inferior cerebellar artery occlusion evokes rather stereotyped symptoms and signs. Superior cerebellar and anterior inferior cerebellar arteries have less constant territories of supply and are uncommonly the sites of occlusions.

Basilar Artery Occlusion

Headache, vertigo, and confusion progress rapidly to coma with complete basilar artery occlusion. Thrombi and emboli are presumed to be the most common bases for basilar artery occlusions,[7] but the disorder occurs frequently in patients with hypertension.[2] Anastomoses between the cerebellar arteries and even between the cerebellar vessels and the leptomeningeal vessels are common,[16] and hypertension is thought to restrict the anastomoses between these vessels.[2] By reducing the collateral flow to the cerebellar vessels, hypertension makes the patient much more susceptible to vertebrobasilar ischemia. Consistent with this increased susceptibility is the observation that transient ischemic attacks occur almost invariably prior to basilar artery occlusion.[16]

Signs of basilar artery occlusion include dysarthria, pupillary abnormalities, ocular motor defects, facial paresis, hemiplegia or tetraplegia, and variable pares-thesias.[16] The *locked-in syndrome* develops in as much as 10 percent of patients and up to 60 percent are obtunded or comatose by the time they arrive at the hospital.[2, 5] This high incidence of early coma reflects the frequent involvement of the rostral segment of the basilar artery. Penetrating branches from this part of the artery supply the paramedian pontine tegmental gray matter and infarction of this region results in coma. The rostral vertebral artery is the principal site of occlusion in 40 percent of patients with basilar artery occlusion.[2] Coma vigile or akinetic mutism appear in occasional patients with disease in this area.[16]

Most patients die within 2 to 5 days.[16] Survivors may linger for weeks or months in an apparently awake, but minimally responsive state. This high fatality rate is tied to the extensive involvement of brainstem rather than cerebellar structures.

Vertebral Artery Occlusion

The symptoms associated with vertebral artery disease vary with the importance of the vessel affected and the patency of the other vertebral artery. Gradually progressive obstruction of one vessel may be virtually asymptomatic if the other vertebral artery previously has provided the bulk of the flow to the posterior fossa. Abrupt occlusion of the vertebral artery providing the major flow may produce signs and symptoms typical of occlusion of the basilar artery or the posterior inferior cerebellar artery. Evidence of disease in these distal vessels presumably results from thrombus extension or emboli from the principal thrombus.[5] Dysarthria, diplopia, impaired hearing, gait ataxia, quadriplegia, and ocular bobbing all may appear with an obstruction to blood flow through the vertebral artery. Acutely the patient may complain of headache, nausea, vomiting, facial weakness, and double vision.[50] In quite a large number of children and young adults presenting with these complaints there is a history of cervical spine trauma, either as a result of accidental injury or chiropractic manipulation.[50] The diagnosis is established readily by arteriography and the course depends largely on the distal vessels involved. If the vertebral artery occluded is the sole source of flow for the ipsilateral posterior inferior cerebellar artery, the extent of cerebellum infarcted may be considerable. The cerebellum, brainstem, and occipital cortex are all likely sites for distal embolization, and the extent to which these structures are involved determines the prognosis following the vertebral artery occlusion.

PICA Occlusion

The posterior inferior cerebellar artery (PICA) is likely to produce cerebellar deficits with occlusion either near its origin or more distally (Table 1). Proximal obstruction or occlusion of the medial branch of the posterior inferior cerebellar artery gives rise to the lateral medullary syndrome of Wallenberg.[44] This is characterized by an ipsilateral Horner syndrome (miosis, ptosis, and decreased facial sweating), gait ataxia, nystagmus, palatal weakness, impaired ipsilateral facial pain and corneal reflexes, and impaired pain and temperature sensations over the contralateral side of the body.[44] Additional signs of cerebellar dysfunction are variably present. The patient often complains of nausea, vomiting, diplopia, vertigo, difficulty swallowing, and clumsiness.[12, 44]

The symptoms and signs in the lateral medullary syndrome can be understood

Table 1. Posterior inferior cerebellar artery occlusion

Ipsilateral signs
　Limb ataxia
　Horner's syndrome
　Impaired facial pain and temperature sensation
　Kinetic tremor
　Dysarthria

Contralateral signs
　Impaired pain and temperature sensation over body

Nonlateralizing signs
　Gait ataxia
　Nystagmus
　Vomiting
　Bradycardia

by considering the structures perfused by the posterior inferior cerebellar artery. The lateral elements of the cerebellum are affected less commonly than vermal structures because the lateral branches of the posterior inferior cerebellar artery anastomose with the superior cerebellar and anterior inferior cerebellar arteries.[12, 21] Touch, position sense, vibration sense, stereognosis, two-point discrimination, and pain on deep pressure are preserved. This reflects sparing of the medial lemniscus, which is supplied by the anterior spinal artery or other branches from the vertebral arteries.[21] The area of the medulla supplied by the medial branch of the posterior inferior cerebellar artery extends from the middle of the hypoglossal nucleus caudally to the inferior cerebellar peduncle cranially. The structures supplied include the reticular substance with its sympathetic tracts; the nucleus ambiguus, which provides innervation to the palate and pharyngeal musculature; the solitary nucleus and its tract; the trigeminal nucleus and its descending tract; and the spinothalamic, olivocerebellar, and dorsal and ventral spinocerebellar tracts.[21] The source of the observed nystagmus[12] is debatable, but it may reflect damage to the vestibular nuclei or to brainstem connections with the vestibular nuclei.[24] Unilateral paralysis of a vocal cord and other pharyngeal musculature may produce difficulty with speech. Involvement of the visceral afferent fibers from the vagus nerve may cause bradycardia,[4] but usually this is not significant clinically. With more extensive cerebellar involvement, there may develop ipsilateral kinetic tremor, dysmetria, and past-pointing. Unless infarction of the cerebellum causes marked edema and brainstem compression, these patients generally are awake and aware of their deficits. With extensive cerebellar infarction the course is more precipitous and the prognosis is poor. The infarction may become hemorrhagic and tonsillar herniation can ensue.[12] Without hemorrhage, the infarction may produce edema and a resultant obstructive hydrocephalus. This is likely to have lethal consequences.

AICA Occlusion

Anterior inferior cerebellar artery (AICA) occlusion is notably uncommon.[48] When it occurs the patient develops ataxia of the ipsilateral limbs as well as a

Table 2. Anterior inferior cerebellar artery occlusion

Ipsilateral signs
　Limb ataxia
　Horner's syndrome
　Deafness
　Facial paralysis
　Decreased corneal reflex
　Impaired pain and temperature sensation on face

Contralateral signs
　Partial impairment of pain and temperature sensation over body

Nonlateralizing signs
　Vertigo
　Vomiting
　Dysarthria
　Nystagmus

lower motor neuron facial palsy and complete nerve deafness ipsilateral to the lesion (Table 2). The patient commonly complains of vertigo, tinnitus, nausea, vomiting, and dysarthria.[21] A Horner syndrome, decreased facial pain, and decreased corneal reflex all develop on the side of the affected vessel. As with posterior inferior cerebellar artery occlusion, gaze evoked nystagmus appears acutely.[1] Facial sensation may be spared because of an independent vessel arising from the basilar artery on the pons to supply the fifth cranial nerve and its nucleus.[21] Limb ataxia ipsilateral to the occluded vessel is usually prominent and may be accompanied by kinetic tremors.[1] Ipsilateral hypotonia and excessive rebound also are likely to develop. The prognosis with occlusion of the anterior inferior cerebellar artery depends largely upon the extent of brainstem damage associated with the cerebellar infarction. A terminal branch occlusion of the artery may produce little more than long term cerebellar deficits, whereas a more proximal occlusion may lead to extensive brainstem infarction, cerebellar necrosis, obstructive hydrocephalus, and death.

Superior Cerebellar Artery Occlusion

Superior cerebellar artery occlusion occurs much less commonly than vertebral, basilar, or posterior inferior cerebellar artery occlusions, but it may develop along with basilar artery occlusion.[2] Even without basilar artery involvement, the area of cerebellar infarction resulting from superior cerebellar artery occlusion may be large enough to be life threatening (Fig. 10). The patient is likely to have tinnitus, dizziness, visual disturbances, and speech difficulty with the onset of the ischemia.[5] Ipsilateral limb ataxia often is associated with choreiform movements.[1] Brainstem involvement will be apparent, producing an ipsilateral Horner syndrome, decreased pain and temperature sense over the contralateral face and body, and impaired hearing. Facial weakness is slight if present at all[1] (Table 3). The prognosis depends on the same factors important in other cerebellar branch occlusions, specifically, the extent of cerebellum infarcted and the severity of the brainstem disease.

301

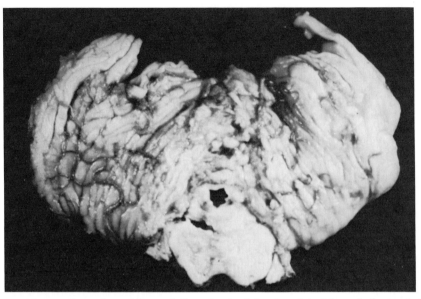

Figure 10. The superior surface of the cerebellum showing infarction of the left cerebellar hemisphere following occlusion of the left superior cerebellar artery.

CEREBELLAR HEMORRHAGE

Etiology and Pathogenesis

Bleeding into the cerebellum occurs with systemic disorders and local disease. Both men and women are affected, the highest incidence of cerebellar hemorrhage occurring in the fifth, sixth, and seventh decades of life. A slight preponderance of men in some series reflects the higher incidence of hypertension in this group.[40] An estimated 10 percent of all intracranial hemorrhages are cerebellar,[23] and the majority of these cerebellar hemorrhages are associated with chronic hypertension.[18, 46] Although hypertension is the most common causative factor, anticoagulant therapy and intrinsic coagulation defects also may produce hemorrhage into the cerebellum, as well as in other parts of the brain. Vascular malformations,[31, 43] neoplasms, infection, and trauma account for most of the other cases of cerebellar hemorrhage.

Table 3. Superior cerebellar artery occlusion

Ipsilateral signs
  Limb dysmetria
  Choreiform movements
  Horner syndrome

Contralateral signs
  Partial deafness
  Loss of pain and temperature sensation over face and body
  Possible hemifacial weakness

Cranial trauma may result in bleeding into the cerebellum even when the blow is not to the back of the head. Shearing forces to the base of the skull can tear vessels in the cerebellum. Trivial trauma may precipitate the hemorrhage, especially if there is an underlying capillary angioma or some other type of vascular malformation. A variety of tumors arising within the cerebellum or spreading metastatically to the cerebellum may bleed without evident cause.[33] Among the primary tumors, hemangioblastomas are highly likely to cause hemorrhage. Among metastatic tumors, bronchogenic carcinoma, rhabdomyosarcoma, and malignant melanoma can cause cerebellar bleeding.[40] Cerebellar infarction rarely becomes hemorrhagic as it evolves. When this occurs it becomes manifest by the sudden deterioration of a mildly impaired patient. Syphilis was considered a relatively common cause of cerebellar hemorrhage in the preantibiotic era,[36] but it is rarely an etiologic consideration now. Mycotic aneurysms developing with infections may lead to hemorrhage in this part of the brain, but this too is uncommon.

Symptoms and Signs

Early diagnosis is essential for the effective treatment of the lesion, but the early recognition of a hemorrhage often is difficult. Cerebellar hemorrhage and infarction often present with identical symptoms. Headache occasionally is helpful in distinguishing between these two causes of cerebellar catastrophe, for it occurs more consistently with hemorrhage.[29, 48] The sudden onset of occipital headache with vomiting, dizziness, and gait difficulty is most characteristic of a hemorrhage.[42, 46] Gait or truncal ataxia develops more frequently than limb ataxia but both are common. With a hemorrhage in the hemisphere, ipsilateral limb dysmetria or past-pointing develops.

Gaze palsies and facial palsies are associated with the limb ataxia in over two-thirds of the patients who can be tested for these signs.[42] Difficulty with conjugate lateral gaze usually is ipsilateral to the side of the hemorrhage. An abducens palsy on the side of the hemorrhage prevents the patient from abducting that eye in some cases; in others there is only a tendency to deviate the eyes away from the side of the hemorrhage. About one-third of patients with cerebellar hemorrhage will be comatose by the time of their hospital admission.[34] These patients usually have total ophthalmoplegia on initial examination.[42] Miotic pupils, gaze evoked horizontal nystagmus, decreased corneal reflexes, neck stiffness, dysarthria, and vertigo occur in the awake patients.[18, 34, 42, 46] Forced deviation of the eyes[18, 46] or the head[36] toward the unaffected side is observed in many patients with hemorrhage into the cerebellar hemisphere. Ocular bobbing occurs rarely and is associated with hemorrhages that extend to the midline.[17] McKissock[34] suggested that a triad of constricted pupils, periodic respiration, and fixed deviation of the eyes away from the side of the lesion may help in the diagnosis of cerebellar hemorrhage, but these and many of the other signs observed with cerebellar hemorrhage are, in fact, signs of brainstem dysfunction.[45] This same triad would be likely to develop with lower pontine hemorrhage, and the patient at risk for cerebellar hemorrhage, the hypertensive male, also is at risk for pontine hemorrhage. The diagnosis is even more difficult with a vermal hemorrhage. Symptoms and signs with a midline cerebellar hemorrhage are nonspecific and often misleading.[46] Obstructive hydrocephalus or massive intraventricular bleeding developing with a vermal hemorrhage will produce signs of both brainstem dysfunction and cerebral cortical dysfunction.

303

Only 3 of 24 cases of cerebellar hemorrhage or infarction received an accurate diagnosis on admission in one Canadian study.[40] Misdiagnosis may occur with trauma, when epidural or subdural hematomas are misconstrued as intraparenchymal lesions. From a therapeutic point of view this is of little consequence since a wide suboccipital craniectomy is advisable for each of these possibilities. Infratentorial subdural hematomas occur with only 9 percent of the frequency of supratentorial subdural hematomas, but coincident intracerebral and subdural collections do occur with trauma.[9] Even with severe cranial trauma, subdural collections in the posterior fossa develop in only 0.67 percent of patients.[8] A lucid period may intervene between the time of the trauma and the disturbance of consciousness with both subdural and epidural hematomas.

The greatest diagnostic problems develop in patients with few or no signs specifically indicating cerebellar disease. The clinical presentations with hemorrhages in the cerebellum, pons, thalamus, and putamen may be similar. Fisher noted some ocular features helpful in localizing the lesion.[17, 18] With putamenal hemorrhage, the eyes deviate toward the side of the lesion rather than away as in cerebellar hemorrhage. Other signs, such as corticospinal tract deficits, must be relied upon to determine the side of the lesion. With a thalamic hemorrhage, the eyes often deviate downward, vertical gaze is impaired, and the pupils are small and unreactive. With pontine hemorrhages the pupils are often pinpoint, but remain responsive. Ocular bobbing may occur.[17, 18]

Diagnostic Studies

Computerized tomography is the most helpful advance in the diagnosis of cerebellar hemorrhages since the initial description of this disorder. The higher density of blood compared to brain allows rapid recognition of a posterior fossa hemorrhage. Lumbar puncture is hazardous and can only demonstrate the presence of blood in the subarachnoid space, and arteriography has been of little assistance in most studies.[34, 40] Ventriculography can be used to visualize the posterior fossa mass, but the amount of time and extent of manipulation of the patient required in this test make it unfeasible. Computerized tomography, in contrast, can allow the clot to be visualized within minutes without invasive techniques.

Therapy and Prognosis

Much of our present knowledge concerning the course of patients with cerebellar hemorrhage was gathered prior to the advent of CT scans. Cerebellar hemorrhage has been considered a rapidly fatal disease, with a mortality exceeding 80 percent in untreated patients.[18, 22, 23, 42] Autopsy studies[36] reveal that death from cerebellar hemorrhage usually occurs within a week after the onset of symptoms. Survivors of cerebellar hemorrhage have been a clinical curiosity,[37] but in recent decades there has been an increasing number of reported survivors.[15, 19, 23, 30] In Fisher's review of 21 cases of cerebellar hemorrhage, all but one of the fatal cases died within 32 hours of symptom onset.[18] Only 9 of 56 patients discussed by Ott and coworkers[42] survived the hemorrhage without surgery. Although the overall mortality of patients operated on exceeds 50 percent,[22] the likelihood of survival increases if surgery is attempted before the patient becomes stuporous or comatose.[34, 42] Seventy percent of patients awake or only drowsy at the time of operation survive.[42]

The use of CT scans in the diagnosis and treatment of patients with cerebellar hemorrhage has begun to change our view of this disorder. The diagnosis can be made with greater certainty and small hemorrhages can be detected. Little and others[30] withheld surgery and observed patients with cerebellar hemorrhages confirmed with computerized tomography when there was little or no evidence of brainstem compromise. The hematomas in four such patients were less than 3 cm in diameter. All four patients survived without surgery. Other investigators recently also have managed cerebellar hemorrhages without surgical intervention and without clinical residua by monitoring the patients with clinical observation and CT scans.[15, 19] At present surgery should be considered if the patient develops hydrocephalus or a deteriorating level of consciousness or both. Hydrocephalus can result from obstruction of the fourth ventricle or aqueduct by the blood clot, or by compression from blood within the cerebellum or the edematous cerebellar tissue. Some patients can be managed without surgery, but the criteria for predicting which patients will do well without resection of the lesion have yet to be established.

Case Presentation

The following patient illustrates the course often resulting from cerebellar hemorrhage:

A 61-year-old right-handed woman with several years' history of hypertension and alcoholism developed left sided headache and slurred speech shortly after awakening in the morning. Her family noted her altered speech and took her to an emergency room immediately. En route to the hospital, her left leg became stiff and weak and she became lethargic. On arrival at the hospital she was drowsy but responded appropriately on initial questioning. Within minutes of arriving she developed a right gaze preference, unintelligibly slurred speech, increased tone in both legs, and extensor plantar responses bilaterally. Her blood pressure was 190/120. She had no papilledema and her pupils were equal, regular, and reactive to light. The corneal reflexes were decreased bilaterally but no other cranial nerve deficits were evident. There was a left hemiparesis which evolved into bilateral decorticate posturing as the patient became less responsive. Within a few hours of arrival she was responding only to painful stimuli. A CT scan revealed a left cerebellar hemorrhage and enlarged ventricles (Fig. 11 and 12). At suboccipital craniectomy, a hematoma in the left cerebellar hemisphere was evacuated. The blood clot was largely inferior, extending from the midhemisphere medially. It did not involve the vermis or the right hemisphere.

After surgery the patient awoke and had slow, hoarse speech. A right gaze preference persisted and there was slight left lateral rectus muscle paresis. Nystagmus was not present. Left lower facial weakness was slight but unequivocal. Other cranial nerve functions were preserved. The right arm was slightly weak, but sensation was normal in all limbs. She had no dysmetria or past-pointing in her arms, but she had slight difficulty with heel-to-shin testing in both legs. The resistance to passive manipulation and reflexes were normal. Over subsequent days she continued to improve and was discharged within several weeks of admission.

This patient's hypertension accounted for the cerebellar hemorrhage, though her alcoholism may have contributed. Liver disease was not a prominent element in her illness, but a mild coagulopathy developed with her alcoholism. The early development of dysarthria, which cleared with resection of the inferior hemisphe-

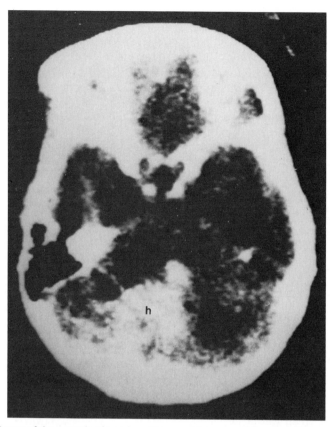

Figure 11. CT scan of the posterior fossa in a 61-year-old woman with a large intracerebellar hemorrhage (h). The patient complained of headache and slurred speech for several hours before developing progressive lethargy. The density to the left of the midline, extending into the midline, appeared without contrast enhancement. At surgery, the blood clot was limited to the left cerebellar hemisphere. The vermis was shifted to the right.

ric mass, is in accord with current notions of the localization of speech disorder.[28] As described in Chapter 11, dysarthria is thought to develop with damage to the superior paravermal aspect of the left hemisphere. Although this area was compromised, it was not destroyed, thereby allowing speech to return to normal after the hematoma was evacuated. Papilledema was absent, a common observation with cerebellar hemorrhage, possibly explained by the rapidity of the course.[40] The gaze preference was toward the undamaged hemisphere, and the facial weakness was ipsilateral to the damage. Thus, both of these signs adhered to the expected patterns. The right hemiparesis probably reflected compression of the corticospinal tract in the pons or medulla as the cerebellar mass pushed the brainstem forward.

VASCULAR MALFORMATIONS

Vascular malformations in or about the cerebellum usually are discovered at the time of hemorrhage, but may present clinically as space occupying lesions prior to

306

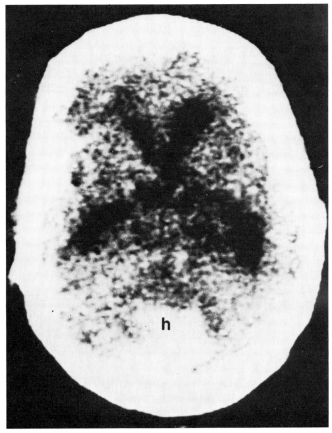

Figure 12. CT scan with good visualization of the lateral ventricles in patient with an acute cerebellar hemorrhage (h). Marked hydrocephalus reflects obstruction of the fourth ventricle by the hemorrhage.

a hemorrhage or after the hemorrhage. The types of vascular malformations affecting the cerebellum are the same as elsewhere in the brain.[32] Aneurysms may develop on any of the major vessels in the posterior fossa, but occur most commonly on the vertebral[43] and basilar arteries. Angiomas in the cerebellum may be venous, arterial, or mixed in character. Arteriovenous malformations may increase in size as the patient matures; blood vessels become larger and patterns of blood shunting may shift.

Aneurysms

Aneurysms of the posterior fossa account for 8 to 15 percent of all intracranial aneurysms.[13] Most posterior fossa aneurysms occur at the bifurcation of the basilar artery into the posterior cerebral arteries or along the basilar artery itself. The mode of presentation of aneurysms in the posterior fossa is determined by the size, type, and location of the aneurysm. Usually the patient is more than 20 years of age at the onset of symptoms.[13] The initial manifestation may consist of a subarachnoid hemorrhage, and in this case the patient will lose consciousness or be-

307

come confused following complaints of severe headache, nausea, vomiting, and photophobia.[25] These manifestations of subarachnoid hemorrhage do not indicate the site of the lesion, but if ataxia and dysarthria accompany these other symptoms and signs, it is most likely that the responsible aneurysm is on the basilar artery.[13] Aneurysms of the vertebral artery may cause bleeding into or compression of the cerebellum.[43] A large aneurysm of a cerebellar branch artery near its junction with the basilar artery occasionally produces a cerebellopontine angle syndrome with impaired hearing, facial weakness, and limb ataxia on the side of the lesion. Less than 1 percent of aneurysms occurs on the anterior inferior cerebellar artery[25] and these usually appear as cerebellopontine angle masses. In this situation, traction on cranial nerves arising from the medulla produces focal deficits suggestive of brainstem infarction or tumor.

The course in many patients is protracted. Recurrent episodes of loss of consciousness and headache may occur over the course of years.[13] With repeated hemorrhages and local reaction to the hemorrhages about the roof of the fourth ventricle, an obstructive hydrocephalus may develop. The problem usually initiating medical attention, however, is progressive brainstem dysfunction;[43] the cerebellum is involved infrequently.

Once an aneurysm is suspected, arteriography is indicated since it is the only reliable method of recognizing the malformation. If the aneurysm can be visualized, a surgical approach is advisable.[25, 43] This may involve difficult surgery, especially with large basilar artery aneurysms. If a cerebellar hematoma is associated with the aneurysmal hemorrhage, the intracerebral clot should be evacuated early in the management of the disorder.

Arteriovenous Malformations

Arteriovenous malformations with artery to vein shunting represent the retention of an embryonic arteriovenous network. These occur both in and about the cerebellum, presenting more often in men than women by a ratio of 2 to 1.[26] Only 5 to 10 percent of all intracranial arteriovenous malformations develop in the posterior fossa,[32] but these often are accessible to surgery. They become manifest by the occurrence of hemorrhage[32, 44] or progressive signs of neurologic disease in the second, third, and fourth decades of life.[41] Cerebellar hemorrhage is the most common initial cause of symptoms and signs. Clinically it is difficult to distinguish a bleeding arteriovenous malformation from a bleeding angioma, aneurysm, hemangioblastoma, or venous malformation in the posterior fossa.[21] The patient with a vascular malformation acutely develops headache, dizziness, nausea, vomiting, diplopia, dysarthria, photophobia, and other signs dependent upon the posterior fossa structures damaged. The course may be slowly progressive, episodic, or catastrophic, this being largely a function of whether the malformation is slowly expanding, causing recurrent small hemorrhages, or presenting with a massive hemorrhage. If the patient does survive the first hemorrhage, the vascular malformation may be quiescent for years.[32] Despite this relatively benign prognosis, the risks associated with recurrent hemorrhages mandate resection of the lesion when that is feasible.

The diagnostic evaluation of a patient suspected of having a cerebellar arteriovenous malformation has been simplified by computerized tomography. The CT scan with enhancement will reveal the malformation in over 80 percent of cases.[26] Plain x-rays usually show no abnormality, but in 10 percent of the patients calcifications can be seen in the arteriovenous malformations. Surgical resection of the anomaly often can be performed without leaving major neurologic disorders.[26] Embolization of the anomaly with spheres or glue may facilitate resection of the lesion. Brainstem vascular malformations are not as readily treatable as those limited to the cerebellum because the abnormal vessels may be an integral part of the brainstem vascular supply.[31]

REFERENCES

1. ADAMS, R. D.: *Occlusion of the anterior inferior cerebellar artery.* Arch. Neurol. Psychiat. 49: 765, 1943.

2. ARCHER, C. R., AND HORENSTEIN, S.: *Basilar artery occlusion.* Stroke 8:383, 1977.

3. BARNETT, H. J. M.: *Delayed cerebral ischemic episodes distal to occlusion of major cerebral arteries.* Neurology 28:769, 1978.

4. BRODAL, A.: *The Cranial Nerves.* Blackwell Scientific Publications, Oxford, 1969.

5. CAPLAN, L. R.: *Occlusion of the vertebral or basilar artery. Follow-up analysis of some patients with benign outcome.* Stroke 10:277, 1979.

6. CARTLIDGE, N. E. F., AND WHISNANT, J. P.: *Carotid and vertebral-basilar transient cerebral ischemic attacks.* Mayo Clin. Proc. 52:117, 1977.

7. CASTAIGNE, P., LHERMITTE, F., GAUTIER, J. C., ET AL.: *Arterial occlusions in the vertebrobasilar system.* Brain 96:133, 1973.

8. CIEMBRONIEWICZ, J. E.: *Subdural hematoma of the posterior fossa.* J. Neurosurg. 22:465, 1969.

9. CLITHEROW, N. R., FOWLER, A., AND SEDZIMIR, C. B.: *Combined intracerebellar and posterior fossa subdural hematomas.* J. Neurosurg. 30:744, 1969.

10. DEREUCK, J., AND VANDER-EEKEN, H.: *Cerebellar infarction and internal hydrocephalus.* Acta Neurol. Belg. 78:129, 1978.

11. DEVIVO, D. C., AND FARRELL, F. W., JR.: *Vertebrobasilar occlusive disease in children.* Arch. Neurol. 26:278, 1972.

12. DUNCAN, G. W., PARKER, S. W., AND FISHER, C. M.: *Acute cerebellar infarction in the PICA territory.* Arch. Neurol. 32:364, 1975.

13. DUVOISIN, R. C., AND YAHR, M. D.: *Posterior fossa aneurysms.* Neurology 15:231, 1965.

14. ECKER, A.: *Upward transtentorial herniation of the brainstem and cerebellum due to tumor of the posterior fossa.* J. Neurosurg. 5:51, 1948.

15. FEIJOO DE FREIXO, M., JIMINEZ GARCIA, M., AND GALDOS ALCELAY, L.: *Cerebellar hemorrhage: Nonsurgical forms.* Ann. Neurol. 6:84, 1979.

16. FIELDS, W. S., RATINOV, G., WEIBEL, J., ET AL.: *Survival following basilar artery occlusion.* Arch. Neurol. 15:463, 1966.

17. FISHER, C. M.: *Ocular bobbing.* Arch. Neurol. 11:543, 1964.

18. FISHER, C. M., PICARD, E. H., POLAK, A., ET AL.: *Acute hypertensive cerebellar hemorrhage: diagnosis and surgical treatment.* J. Nerv. Ment. Dis. 140:38, 1965.

19. FREEMAN, J. W., KENNEDY, R. M., AND PETTY, S. S.: *Prognosis of nonoperated cerebellar hemorrhage.* Ann. Neurol. 4:389, 1978.

20. GILLILAN, L. A.: *Anatomy and embryology of the arterial system of the brainstem and cerebellum,* in VINKEN, P. J., BRUYN, G. W. (eds.): *Handbook of Clinical Neurology,* vol. 11, American Elsevier Publishing Co, New York, 1972, pp. 24–44.

21. GOODHART, S. P., AND DAVISON, C.: *Syndrome of the posterior inferior and anterior inferior cerebellar arteries and their branches.* Arch. Neurol. Psychiat. 35:501, 1936.

22. GREENBERG, J., SKUBICK, D., AND SHENKIN, H.: *Acute hydrocephalus in cerebellar infarct and hemorrhage.* Neurology 29:409, 1979.

23. HEIMAN, T. D., AND SATYA-MURTI, S.: *Benign cerebellar hemorrhages.* Ann. Neurol. 3:366, 1978.

24. HOOD, J. D., KAYAN, A., AND LEECH, J.: *Rebound nystagmus.* Brain 96:507, 1973.

25. JOHNSON, J. H., AND KLINE, D. G.: *Anterior inferior cerebellar artery aneurysms.* J. Neurosurg. 48:455, 1978.

26. KELLY, J. J., JR., MELLINGER, J. F., AND SUNDT, T. M., JR.: *Intracranial arteriovenous malformations in childhood.* Ann. Neurol. 3:338, 1978.

27. KRAYENBUHL, H., AND YASARGIL, M. G.: *Radiological anatomy and topography of the cerebral veins,* in Vinken, P. J., and Bruyn, G. W. (eds.): *Handbook of Clinical Neurology,* vol. 11. American Elsevier, New York, 1972, pp. 65–101.

28. LECHTENBERG, R., AND GILMAN, S.: *Speech disorders in cerebellar disease.* Ann. Neurol. 3:285, 1978.

29. LEHRICH, J. R., WINKLER, G. F., AND OJEMANN, R. G.: *Cerebellar infarction with brainstem compression.* Arch. Neurol. 22:490, 1970.

30. LITTLE, J. R., TUBMAN, D. E., AND ETHIER, R.: *Cerebellar hemorrhage in adults.* J. Neurosurg. 48:575, 1978.

31. LOGUE, V., AND MONCKTON, G.: *Posterior fossa angiomas.* Brain 77:252, 1954.

32. LUSINS, J., AND SENCER, W.: *Posterior fossa vascular malformations. Long-term follow-up.* N.Y. State J. Med. 76:416, 1976.

33. MANDYBUR, T. I.: *Intracranial hemorrhage caused by metastatic tumors.* Neurology 27:650, 1977.

34. MCKISSOCK, W., RICHARDSON, A., AND WALSH, L.: *Spontaneous cerebellar hemorrhage.* Brain 83:1, 1960.

35. MCNAMARA, J. O., HEYMAN, A., SILVER, D., ET AL.: *The value of carotid endarterectomy in treating transient cerebral ischemia of the posterior circulation.* Neurology 27:682, 1977.

36. MICHAEL, J. C.: *Cerebellar apoplexy.* Am. J. Med. Sci. 183:687, 1932.

37. MILLS, C. K., AND WEISENBURG, T. H.: *Cerebellar symptoms and cerebellar localization.* Am. Med. Assoc. J. 63:1813, 1914.

38. MOHR, J. P.: *Transient ischemic attacks and the prevention of strokes.* N. Eng. J. Med. 299:93, 1978.

39. NARITOMI, H., SAKAI, F., AND MEYER, J. S.: *Pathogenesis of transient ischemic attacks within the vertebrobasilar arterial system.* Arch. Neurol. 36:121, 1979.

40. NORRIS, J. W., EISEN, A. A., AND BRANCH, C. L.: *Problems in cerebellar hemorrhage and infarction.* Neurology 19:1043, 1969.

41. ODOM, G. L., TINDALL, G. T., AND DUKES, H. T.: *Cerebellar hematoma caused by angiomatous malformations.* J. Neurosurg. 18:777, 1961.

42. OTT, K. H., KASE, C. S., OJEMANN, R. G. ET AL.: *Cerebellar hemorrhage: diagnosis and treatment.* Arch. Neurol. 31:160, 1974.

43. PAULSON, G., NASHOLD, B. S., AND MARGOLIS, G.: *Aneurysms of the vertebral artery.* Neurology 9:590, 1959.

44. PERLO, V. P., SCULLY, R. E., AND PLANK, C.: *Case records of the Massachusetts General Hospital.* N. Engl. J. Med. 287:1291, 1972.

45. PLUM, F., AND POSNER, J. B.: *Diagnosis of Stupor and Coma.* F. A. Davis Co., Philadelphia, 1972.

46. REY-BELLET, J.: *Cerebellar hemorrhage: a clinicopathologic study.* Neurology 10:217, 1960.

47. SUNDT, T. M., AND PIEPGRAS, D. G.: *Occipital to posterior inferior cerebellar artery bypass surgery.* J. Neurosurg. 48:916, 1978.

48. SYPERT, G. W., AND ALVORD, E. C., JR.: *Cerebellar infarction. A clinicopathological study.* Arch. Neurol. 32:357, 1975.

49. TOOLE, J. F., YUSON, C. P., JANEWAY, R. ET AL.: *Transient ischemic attacks: A prospective study of 225 patients.* Neurology 28:746, 1978.

50. ZIMMERMAN, A. W., KUMAR, A. J., GADOTH, N. ET AL.: *Traumatic vertebrobasilar occlusive disease in childhood.* Neurology 28:185, 1978.

51. SCOTTI, G., SPINNLER, H., STERZI, R., AND VALLAR, G.: *Cerebellar softening.* Ann. Neurol. 8:133, 1980.

CHAPTER 15

Infections

BACTERIAL DISEASE

Cerebellar damage occurs with generalized central nervous system infections in relatively few patients.[27] If a meningoencephalitis does result in permanent deficits, dementia, spastic paresis, or a seizure disorder are more likely sequelae than limb dysmetria or gait ataxia.[18, 28, 29] Patients surviving pneumococcal meningitis occasionally develop truncal ataxia, but in most cases this appears to be secondary to vestibular damage rather than cerebellar damage.[27] Consequently, focal signs of cerebellar dysfunction occurring with bacterial infection must be considered the result of a cerebellar abscess until proven otherwise.

Bacterial damage to the cerebellum was fairly common in the preantibiotic era.[2] This was from focal cerebellitis or an abscess developing with chronic mastoiditis.[21, 26] The incidence of abscess in the cerebellum has not changed since the introduction of antibiotics[2] and the proportion of brain abscesses developing in this structure has remained relatively high. Ten to eighteen percent of all brain abscesses are still in the cerebellum.[2, 21, 26]

Most cerebellar abscesses develop from infections in or adjacent to the central nervous system (Fig. 1), but 5 to 10 percent of all cerebellar abscesses result from spread of more remote infections.[2, 11] Spread from contiguous structures may occur by the enlargement of purulent foci or by retrograde septic thrombophlebitis.[26] The lung and heart are the most likely sources of bacteria when a source in the central nervous system is not apparent.[26] Cerebellar dysfunction does occur even without abscess formation[27] in childhood bacterial meningitis, especially when the infecting organism is *Hemophilus influenzae*, but this is rare.[28] Those described with acute meningitis followed by persistent ataxia have all been survivors of the infection and less than four years of age.[27]

Cerebellar abscesses usually present with signs of increased intracranial pressure rather than limb ataxia or gait dysfunction.[11, 22] The most common initial complaint with an abscess in the cerebellum is headache,[21] and this symptom has little localizing value. Focal signs of cerebellar dysfunction may appear as the abscess enlarges, but evidence of brainstem compression is just as likely.[22] Obtundation or cranial nerve deficits are likely to appear as the disease evolves.[14, 22] Although papilledema is uncommon,[21] facial weakness and hearing loss may ap-

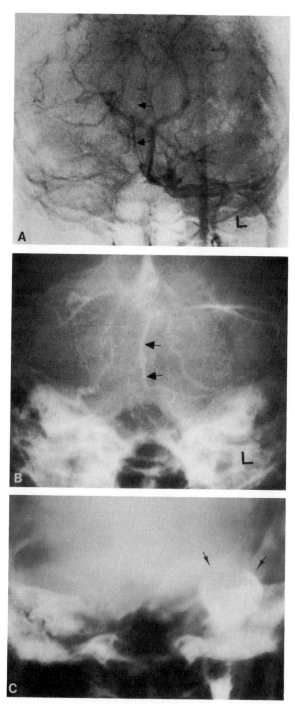

Figure 1. Contrast studies in an 18-year-old male with an abscess in the left cerebellar hemisphere following mastoiditis on the left. A, The arterial phase of a vertebral arteriogram showing the inferior vermian branch of the posterior inferior cerebellar artery shifted to the right (arrows). B, The venous phase of the study showing stretching of the inferior vermain vein to the right (arrows). C, The abscess cavity is demonstrated by insertion of barium into the cavity (arrows).

312

pear with compression of cranial nerves VII and VIII[11] and dysconjugate gaze develops with compromise of the VIth nerve.

Cerebellar abscesses need to be distinguished from extraparenchymal and non-pyogenic lesions.[17] Signs of cerebellar disease can appear with an epidural abscess compressing the cerebellar cortex.[22] Tuberculomas and other granulomas may evolve in the cerebellum with signs and symptoms indistinguishable from tumor. All these lesions present considerable diagnostic difficulties, especially since there is no consistent clinical profile for an abscess. In 17 cases of cerebellar abscess,[21] only 4 patients had fever and 3 had papilledema. Lumbar puncture may reveal an elevated cerebrospinal fluid protein or elevated cell count, but these changes are notoriously inconstant.[18, 22] Moreover, lumbar puncture should be avoided when brain abscess is suspected.[18, 26] Computerized tomography will help in the diagnosis, especially if a ring of enhancement with contrast medium develops around the necrotic hypodense area (Fig. 2). This is not pathognomonic of abscess and the diagnosis rests ultimately with biopsy of the lesion. Failure to detect and treat this

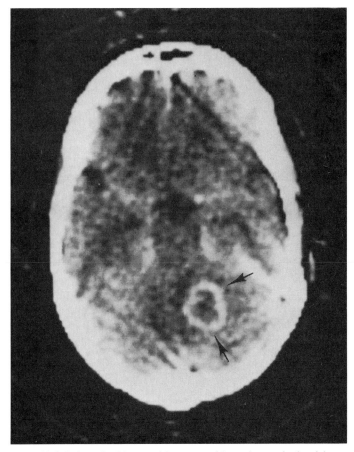

Figure 2. CT scan with infusion of a 54-year-old woman with an abscess in the right cerebellar hemisphere. An enhancing ring lesion appears in the medial portion of the right cerebellar hemisphere (arrows) obliterating the fourth ventricle. The abscess proved to be due to nocardia.

313

lesion effectively leads to death from spread of the infection[14] or from brainstem compromise.[2]

Cerebellar abscess requires surgery for effective treatment.[2] Even after posterior fossa decompression and abscess resection, the mortality with this lesion is about 14 percent,[14, 21] however, both the mortality and morbidity after surgery for patients with cerebellar abscess is better than that for patients with cerebral abscess.[22] Some complications such as seizure disorders are unlikely and neurologic sequelae after evacuation of the abscess are likely to be minor.[22] Resection of the lesion is essential, despite the vulnerability of most responsible organisms to antibiotics. Antibiotics alone cannot halt the progression of this disease reliably,[12, 18] regardless of the organism responsible for the abscess. Streptococcus, Staphylococcus, and Proteus organisms grow from most cerebellar abscesses,[22] a selection of organisms reflecting the high incidence of spread from the ear.[21, 26] If only antibiotic treatment is employed or the abscess is drained through a burr hole, the early mortality more than doubles.[14] Mortality also increases if the patient is unconscious or if meningitis is apparent at the time of posterior fossa surgery.[14] The mortality figures with cerebellar abscess have not changed since the advent of antibiotics.[2, 14] Despite previous evidence indicating the need for surgical therapy of cerebellar abscesses, it is possible that some abscesses may be treated without surgical drainage. The advent of CT scanning has made it possible to reassessed the effective modes of therapy in this condition as in cerebellar hemorrhage. The following case illustrates the course of a cerebellar abscess in a young patient.

Case Presentation

A 2½-year-old right handed girl became lethargic and unsteady on her feet over the course of a few days. She had had bilateral otitis media nine months previously and suspicion of a recurrent ear infection prompted a myringotomy the day prior to admission. She was admitted with vomiting and dysconjugate gaze. On initial examination she was irritable and stuporous. Her speech was limited to single words and simple phrases, but she had no dysarthria. Neck stiffness and a positive Brudzinski sign were present. The right tympanic membrane was bulging, but she was afebrile. Papilledema was evident in the left fundus. The right eye deviated to the left and nystagmus developed on right lateral gaze. Her right hand was clumsy and a kinetic tremor appeared on reaching for objects. Her gait was severely ataxic, with repeated falling to the right. She had no areas of decreased response to painful stimuli. Deep tendon reflexes were increased on the left and the plantar responses were both extensor. She was generally hypotonic.

Skull x-rays demonstrated widened sutures, but normal mastoid air cells. A lumbar puncture yielded cloudly cerebrospinal fluid with an elevated opening pressure, 8 polymorphonuclear cells and 4 mononuclear cells per cubic millimeter, a sugar of 76 mg/dl, and a protein of 10 mg/dl. Gram negative cocci were recognized on staining the fluid. These findings were considered adequately suggestive of an abscess to prompt ventriculography which showed enlarged third and lateral ventricles and a fourth ventricle displaced to the left. Suboccipital craniectomy revealed a right cerebellar hemisphere abscess extending up to the tentorium cerebelli. The abscess cavity was 3 cm by 4 cm and the bulk of the abscess was anterior and superior in the hemisphere. Pus aspirated from the lesion grew gram-positive cocci, later identified as hemolytic streptococci. Postoperative recovery was rapid. An ataxic gait was the only sign of neurologic disease one week after surgery, and this, too, had greatly improved.

VIRAL INFECTIONS

Transient signs of cerebellar dysfunction may develop with some viral exanthems affecting the central nervous system.[7, 13] Epidemic parotitis from mumps is a viral illness capable of major central nervous system involvement[29] which also produces signs of cerebellar disease. This is not a manifestation of the aqueductal stenosis or hydrocephalus which may follow mumps encephalitis,[29] but it is rather a more specific effect on cerebellar systems.[7] Patients with hindbrain anomalies appear to be especially susceptible to cerebellar manifestations with mumps infection.[10] Presumably, a poorly developed cerebellum is compromised further by the exanthem. A rapidly fatal deterioration, characterized by prominent gait and limb ataxia, also occurs with mumps infection in patients with neurovisceral storage disorders.[23]

The Epstein-Barr virus produces a wide variety of neurologic disorders, some of which have prominent signs of cerebellar dysfunction.[15] In a large series of patients with Epstein-Barr infection manifest as typical infectious mononucleosis, signs of neurologic involvement developed in 7.3 percent of patients.[13] Serious neurologic complications were rare, occurring in about 1 percent of cases of infectious mononucleosis.[13] Manifestations of cerebellar dysfunction include dysarthria, gait ataxia, nystagmus, and occasional limb ataxia. A lymphocytic meningitis or encephalomyelitis develops in some of these patients.[15] The rare patient who dies has degeneration of Purkinje cells as well as mononuclear cell infiltration of the cranial nerves, spinal nerve roots, and peripheral nerves.[13] Signs and symptoms of the neurologic disease are not necessarily coincident with the hepatic, lymphatic, and splenic manifestations of the infection.[15] Signs may appear coincident with the systemic illness or after a delay of up to two weeks. Diffuse slowing appears in the electroencephalogram in one-third of all patients with neurologic symptoms.[13] These are unusual rather than typical cases and cerebellar changes in the standard Epstein-Barr viral infection may be absent. Little more than headache or neck stiffness will develop in the majority of symptomatic patients.[13]

Rabies is a considerably more malignant viral disease showing histologic changes in the cerebellum. Although this usually presents with altered mentation and no signs of cerebellar involvement,[3] the disease is associated with microscopic changes in cerebellar neurons. Eosinophilic inclusion bodies in Purkinje cells with basophilic stippling, Negri bodies, are virtually pathognomonic for rabies, although these same inclusions have appeared in Reye syndrome.[6] The cerebellum is the most common site of Negri bodies, with these inclusions appearing in 59 percent of patients with fatal infections.[8] The second most common site is the hippocampus, perhaps because of the direct communication between the cerebellum and this part of the cerebrum.[1] Why the cerebellar cells are typically affected in this way without actual loss of Purkinje cells is unknown.

Chronic progressive panencephalitis with prominent cerebellar signs develops after rubella infection.[31] Children with this disorder may be born with multiple anomalies from in utero rubella; but, despite the cataracts, sensorineural hearing loss, cardiac abnormalities, and microcephaly apparent at birth, their deficits generally remain stable for the first years of life. By early adolescence, seizures may herald the onset of a slowly progressive psychomotor deterioration.[30] Less severe initial signs of the chronic panencephalitis include changes in speech clarity, mild gait difficulty, or clumsiness. These deficits are unremitting, usually evolving over the course of years. Mentation deteriorates along with gait, speech, and coordination.[31] The patients usually develop hyperreflexia with nystagmus, myoclonus, dysmetria, dysdiadochokinesis, titubation, and choreiform movements within a few years of the initial signs of the chronic encephalitis. Terminally, these children have a profound dementia, are unable to walk, and may have an internuclear ophthalmoplegia.[30] Death from inanition, infection, or uncontrollable seizures occurs before 25 years of age, the course of the illness sometimes extending as much as 9 years. Autopsy may reveal a fairly normal size cerebrum with a severely atrophic cerebellum.[31] There is loss of white matter in the cerebrum and microglial nodules in the thalamus and pons, but the cerebellum has severe loss of Purkinje cells, thinning of the granular layer, loss of white matter, and microglial nodules.[30] There are numerous iron and calcium deposits in vessels of the cerebral cortex and the molecular layer of the cerebellum. Although this syndrome has been described with congenital rubella, the cerebellar atrophy is not characteristic of the nonprogressive congenital infection.[30] The similarity of this illness to subacute sclerosing panencephalitis is apparent and their pathogenesis may be the same. As in subacute sclerosing panencephalitis, the cerebrospinal fluid IgG immunoglobulin is elevated,[31] but serum and cerebrospinal fluid titers for antibody to rubella are elevated also.[30]

SLOW VIRUS INFECTIONS

Transmissible virus infections are known to result in dementia with gait difficulty appearing in adult life and progressing to severe behavioral disturbances, rigidity, myoclonus, visual disturbances, and signs of cerebellar dysfunction. The best understood of these slow viral infections are kuru and Creutzfeldt-Jakob disease, both of which produce a subacute spongiform encephalopathy. These are classified as slow infections because of the delay of months or years between exposure to the virus and the development of symptoms. The course of the disease is subacute with the interval from onset to death usually extending from four months to two years.[9, 16]

Kuru

This is a degenerative disease of the cerebellum, signaled in 70 percent of patients by progressive gait difficulty.[16] The Fore islanders subject to this uniformly fatal illness ascribed it to sorcery and their name for the disease means "trembling with fear."[16] The distribution of affected individuals[16] was a distinctive feature in this illness which led to the discovery that it was an infection transmitted by ritual cannibalism. Most affected individuals were women in the childbearing age group or children under 15 years of age. These same individuals were most involved during the cannibalistic rituals in handling the brains of individuals who had expired with the disease. The neurologic deficits, course, and pathology in kuru are similar to those in Creutzfeldt-Jakob disease,[5, 16, 25] though patients with kuru show early and prominent signs of cerebellar disease.[16] Tremors in the legs appear

316

early in over 20 percent of kuru victims,[16] and gait difficulty invariably dominates the clinical picture. Patients generally suspect they have the disorder when their gait deteriorates and stumbling develops. Early in the course of the disease the affected individual develops a stooped posture with the trunk stiffly inclined forward and the feet set widely apart. Over the course of months, individual steps become more irregular in terms of both speed and distance covered. Slurred speech develops apace with arm ataxia. Within a year or two speech may be unintelligible, and independent gait, impossible. Titubation and truncal ataxia interfere with sitting as well as standing. Before the patient is virtually immobilized by the motor deficits, he commonly exhibits considerable hostility and anger. This leads to assaultive behavior with little or no provocation. Depression replaces paranoia and hostility as cognitive deficits become more apparent. Profound dementia develops as the patient reaches a terminal state.[16] Victims of kuru usually die with inanition or intercurrent infections.

Creutzfeldt-Jakob Disease

In this disease 55 percent of patients have signs of cerebellar dysfunction.[25] The disease usually begins with memory loss, occasional perseveration, and mild anomic aphasia.[4] Dementia evolves over the course of months. The cognitive disturbance and complaints of visual hallucinations[5] may raise the question of psychiatric illness before the true nature of this disease is recognized. Depression, paranoia, and withdrawal may be prominent signs for weeks or months, but a neurologic evaluation at the time these affective disorders are prominent will reveal hyperreflexia, extensor plantar responses, agnosia, dysgraphia, and mild limb ataxia. Myoclonus, exaggerated startle reactions, and signs of extrapyramidal disorder are likely to appear before signs of cerebellar dysfunction. Occasionally the signs of cerebellar disease dominate the clinical picture from the beginning. The initial signs of cerebellar dysfunction include gait ataxia, kinetic tremors, dysdiadochokinesis, decomposition of movement, hypotonia, and nystagmus. Often patients with this disease develop hypokinesia, bradykinesia, choreoathetoid movements, rigidity, and dystonia. Signs of corticospinal tract lesions and anterior horn cell disease may develop. Impaired vision occurs in about 50 percent of patients.[4] The mean duration of the illness is about 6 to 7 months[20] and the cause of death is most often systemic infection.[25] The relentless progression of the disease results in a terminally mute, akinetic patient.

The electroencephalogram helps in the diagnosis of Creutzfeldt-Jakob disease (Fig. 3). Early in the course, the EEG has slow, polyrhythmic activity.[19] The slowing may be focal[25] but the pattern evolves into rhythmic bursts of high voltage triphasic complexes on a generally slow background.[19] Periodic spikes or sharp waves may coincide with myoclonic jerks.

In the subacute spongiform encephalopathies there is no correlation between the duration of the illness and the pathologic changes in the brain. In both kuru and Creutzfeldt-Jakob disease, there are three characteristic pathologic changes in the brain: 1) status spongiosus, 2) proliferation of hypertrophied astrocytes, and 3) neuronal loss.[5] A fine meshed vacuolation affects most of the cerebral cortex to a greater extent than the subcortical structures. The cerebellar cortex has vacuolation of the molecular layer, with a generalized increase in the number of astrocytes and a prominent depletion of the granule cells.[4] Purkinje cells typically are well preserved. The spongy change in the cortex and molecular layer is probably

317

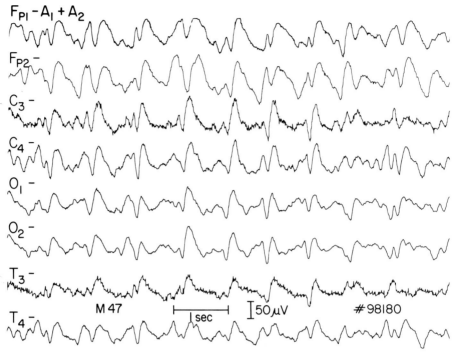

Figure 3. Electroencephalographic tracing from a 47-year-old male with Creutzfeldt-Jakob disease. The patient had 4½ months of visual blurring, disorientation, gait difficulty, and episodes of confusion. Examination revealed dementia, nystagmus, dysmetria of arm and leg movements, a broad based ataxic gait, hyperactive deep tendon reflexes, and positive snout, grasp, and suck reflexes. The EEG shows 1.5 cycle per second rhythmic sharp and slow wave complexes maximal in the frontal and central areas. The patient was alert at the time of this tracing. Electrode placement corresponds to the international classification.

from the accumulation of fluid in dendrites and astrocytic processes, with subsequent disruption of the cell membranes. Early neuropathologic accounts of kuru and Creutzfeldt-Jakob disease described histologic differences between them which included "barred" bodies[24] and PAS-positive plaques[25] in victims of kuru alone, but at least the PAS-positive plaques are now recognized as characteristic of both kuru and Creutzfeldt-Jakob disease.[4] Cerebellar degenerative changes occur in 53 percent to as much as 100 percent of patients with well documented Creutzfeldt-Jakob disease.[20] In some patients the cerebellar changes are atypical in that Purkinje cell loss is prominent and filamentous intranuclear inclusions develop in the remaining Purkinje cells. In these patients, loss of granule cells is slight and glial proliferation is intense.[20]

Status spongiosus appears in all three layers of the cerebellar cortex. The subcortical white matter is moderately demyelinated and some axons in the granular layer are greatly distended with homogeneous material producing a characteristic torpedo-like shape. These axonal torpedoes are processes of the Purkinje cells. The PAS-positive plaques are most abundant in the vermis and they have radially oriented fibers at their periphery.[5] These plaques appear in the granular cell layer, subcortical white matter, and the molecular layer.

318

REFERENCES

1. ALLEN, G. I., AND TSUKAHARA, N.: *Cerebrocerebellar communication systems.* Physiol. Rev. 54:957, 1974.

2. BELLER, A. J., SAHAR, A., AND PRAISS, I.: *Brain abscess. Review of 89 cases over a period of 30 years.* J. Neurol. Neurosurg. Psychiat. 36:757, 1973.

3. BERNSTEIN, C. A., AND STEVENSON, L. D.: *Human rabies.* J. Neuropathol. Exp. Neurol. 12:169, 1953.

4. BROWNE, T. R.: *Case records of the Massachusetts General Hospital—Case 43-1977.* N. Eng. J. Med. 297:930, 1977.

5. CHOU, S. M., AND MARTIN, J. D.: *Kuru-plaques in a case of Creutzfeldt-Jakob disease.* Acta Neuropathol. (Berl.) 17:150, 1971.

6. DERAKHSHAN, I.: *Is the Negri body specific for rabies.* Arch. Neurol. 32:75, 1975.

7. DOW, R. S., AND MORUZZI, G.: *The Physiology and Pathology of the Cerebellum.* University of Minnesota Press, Minneapolis, 1958.

8. DUPONT, J. R., AND EARLE, K. M.: *Human rabies encephalitis.* Neurology 15:1023, 1965.

9. GAJDUSEK, D. C., GIBBS, C. J., JR., ASHER, D. M., ET AL.: *Precautions in medical care of, and in handling materials from patients with transmissible virus dementia (Creutzfeldt-Jakob disease).* N. Eng. J. Med. 297:1253, 1977.

10. GARDNER, E., O'RAHILLY, R., AND PROLO, D.: *The Dandy-Walker and Arnold-Chiari malformations.* Arch. Neurol. 32:393, 1975.

11. GARDNER-THORPE, C., AND AL-MUFTI, S. T.: *Metastatic cerebellar abscess producing nerve deafness.* J. Neurol. Neurosurg. Psychiat. 32:360, 1969.

12. GARFIELD, J.: *Management of supratentorial intracranial abscesses. A review of 200 cases.* Br. Med. J. 2:7, 1969.

13. GAUTIER-SMITH, P. C.: *Neurological complications of glandular fever (infectious mononucleosis).* Brain 88:323, 1965.

14. GRIFFITH, H. B.: *Factors in the mortality of cerebellar abscess.* J. Neurol. Neurosurg. Psychiat. 31:89, 1968.

15. GROSE, C., HENLE, W., HENLE, G., ET AL.: *Primary Epstein-Barr virus infections in acute neurologic diseases.* N. Eng. J. Med. 292:392, 1975.

16. HORNABROOK, R. W.: *Kuru-A subacute cerebellar degeneration. The natural history and clinical features.* Brain 91:53, 1968.

17. KONIGSMARK, B. W., AND WEINER, L.P.: *The olivopontocerebellar atrophies: A review.* Medicine 49:227, 1970.

18. LECHTENBERG, R., SIERRA, M. F., PRINGLE, G. F., ET AL.: *Listeria monocytogenes: Brain abscess or meningoencephalitis.* Neurology 29:86, 1979.

19. MAYER, V., OROLIN, D., MITROVÁ, E., ET AL.: *Transmissible virus dementia. I. An unusual space and time clustering of Creutzfeldt-Jakob disease and of other organic presenile dementia cases.* Acta Virol. 22:146, 1978.

20. MITROVÁ, E., MAYER, V., AND OROLIN, D.: *Transmissible virus dementia. II. Neurohistology of three, geographically clustered cases of Creutzfeldt-Jakob disease.* Acta Virol. 22:154, 1978.

21. MORGAN, H., AND WOOD, M. W.: *Cerebellar abscesses: a review of seventeen cases.* Surg. Neurol. 3:93, 1975.

22. MORGAN, H., WOOD, M. W., AND MURPHY, F.: *Experience with 88 consecutive cases of brain abscess.* J. Neurosurg. 38:698, 1973.

23. NEVILLE, B. G. R., LAKE, B. D., STEPHENS, R., ET AL.: *A neurovisceral storage disease with vertical supranuclear ophthalmoplegia and its relationship to Niemann-Pick disease.* Brain 96:97, 1973.

24. PEAT, A., AND FIELD, E. J.: *An unusual structure in Kuru brain.* Acta Neuropathol. (Berl.) 15:288, 1970.

25. ROOS, R., GAJDUSEK, D. C., AND GIBBS, C. J., JR.: *The clinical characteristics of transmissible Creutzfeldt-Jakob disease.* Brain 96:1, 1973.

26. SAMSON, D. S., AND CLARK, K.: *A current review of brain abscess.* Am. J. Med. 54:201, 1973.

27. SCHWARTZ, J.F.: *Ataxia in bacterial meningitis.* Neurology 22:1071, 1972.

28. SELL, S. H. W., MERRILL, R. E., DOYNE, E. O., ET AL.: *Long-term sequelae of Hemophilus influenzae meningitis.* Pediatr. 49:206, 1972.

29. TIMMONS, G. D., AND JOHNSON, K. P.: *Aqueductal stenosis and hydrocephalus after mumps encephalitis.* N. Eng. J. Med. 283:1505, 1970.

30. TOWNSEND, J. J., BARINGER, J. R., WOLINSKY, J. S., ET AL.: *Progressive rubella panencephalitis.* N. Eng. J. Med. 292:990, 1975.

31. WEIL, M. L., ITABASHI, H. H., CREMER, N. E., ET AL.: *Chronic progressive panencephalitis due to rubella virus simulating subacute sclerosing panencephalitis.* N. Eng. J. Med. 292:994, 1975.

CHAPTER 16

Metabolic Disorders

Systemic metabolic disorders can disturb both cerebellar structure and function. Most of these disorders do not involve the cerebellum specifically, but affect it along with the other components of the central nervous system. The symptoms resulting from these disorders vary, depending upon the localization of the major effects of the disorder. Symptoms and signs of cerebellar dysfunction may be the most obvious disorder of neural function but rarely constitute the only disorder. A number of metabolic disorders affect the cerebellum, including: hypoxia and ischemia; hyperthermia; toxicity resulting from heavy metals, drugs, alcohol, and hepatic disease; disorders of enzyme function, including trace metal deficiency, vitamin deficiency, specific enzyme disturbances, and storage diseases; amino acid deficiencies; and endocrine disorders.

HYPOXIA, ISCHEMIA, AND HYPERTHERMIA

For all practical purposes, there are no stores of oxygen in the brain. Consequently, a decline of cerebral blood flow below a critical level results in cerebral hypoxia. Essentially all states of central nervous system ischemia are associated with hypoxia. In contrast, central nervous system hypoxia from reduced delivery of oxygen can occur without ischemia. The end result of central nervous system hypoxia is a decline in the rate of oxidative metabolism and this leads to a decline of metabolic energy stores, particularly ATP. Vital cellular functions become compromised due to lack of energy, cell membrane pumps cannot operate, ion leaks occur, and the intracellular ionic, enzymatic, and pH environment becomes compromised severely. Secondary membrane damage can result from these changes. Depending upon the severity of hypoxia, central nervous system tissues manifest lowered functional activity or death. The specific symptoms and signs occurring clinically vary depending upon the site of the major disturbance. The effects of cerebrovascular disease often lead to focal cerebellar injury, as discussed in Chapter 14. Generalized hypoxia can affect all portions of the central nervous system; however, neurons of Ammon's horn in the hippocampus and Purkinje cells throughout the cerebellar cortex are among the most sensitive elements to the effects of anoxia.[31] Specific signs of cerebellar dysfunction usually are overshadowed by the generalized cerebral dysfunction associated with hypoxic states.

321

Hyperthermia enhances the rate of metabolism and this depletes the central nervous system energy stores. If the hyperthermia is sufficiently severe and protracted, cellular activity cannot compensate for the decreased energy stores and the result, as in severe hypoxic states, is a progressive decrease of cellular functional activity, and ultimately, tissue death. Neuronal elements in the cerebellum are highly sensitive to hyperthermia.[50] Even transient hyperthermia produces Purkinje cell depletion, granule cell rarefaction, and generalized gliosis. Experimentally induced focal cerebellar hyperthermia leads to marked changes in cerebellar function.[15, 50]

TOXINS

Heavy Metals

Heavy metal accumulation in the central nervous system leads to neuronal damage and death. Heavy metals become concentrated in certain organs and injure the cells in these organs. Excessive ingestion of lead, for example, leads to the accumulation of lead in many tissues, but especially vulnerable tissues include the kidney and the central nervous system. Heavy metals incorporated within cells affect membranes specifically involved in metabolism, particularly the mitochondria. Accumulation of metal leads to the progressive inhibition of metabolic activity. The result is a progressive decline of the metabolic energy stores needed to drive cellular activity and, as in the case of hypoxia, ultimate damage to cellular function and structure.

Toxicity with thallium and lead can affect cerebellar function specifically. Thallium toxicity may result from the ingestion of rat poison or from exposure to thallium in industry. Thallium toxicity can cause ataxia, tremors, choreoathetosis, as well as seizures, peripheral neuropathy, and cranial nerve palsies.[3] The clinical signs that appear initially in the affected patient vary greatly from one individual to the next. With acute thallium ingestion the patient has considerable gastrointestinal distress. Vomiting and diarrhea develop within hours after the ingestion of a large dose of the poison.[39] Systemic effects of thallium are widespread, with toxicity especially prominent in the kidneys and vasomotor regulatory systems. Tachycardia develops as the patient slips into shock and high output heart failure can lead to death. The dehydration and electrolyte disturbances produced by the gastrointestinal disorder also may be fatal.

Chronic poisoning with small doses of thallium over the course of days or weeks leads to alopecia and characteristic nervous system dysfunction. Both central and peripheral nervous systems are affected. Headache, probably resulting from cerebral edema,[39] is likely to be the patient's first symptom of nervous system involvement. A peripheral nerve disorder develops consisting of a painful, symmetric distal neuropathy associated with prominent dysautonomia. Sleep disturbances invariably are present, with complaints of drowsiness during the day and restlessness at night. Paranoia, apathy, and irritability precede frank hallucinations in patients who develop cognitive and affective disorders. The widespread cerebellar disorder resulting from thallium intoxication is reflected in limb ataxia and tremors. Pathologically, the cerebellar lesions involve principally the neural elements.[22] Multilamellar cytoplasmic bodies and altered mitochondria appear in most cerebellar neurons. The glia are largely unaffected, except for extensive edema in the white matter.[39] Demyelination is less prominent a feature than axonal degeneration in both the central and peripheral nervous systems.[3]

The diagnosis of thallium toxicity can be made by obtaining urinary levels of the substance. Much of the damage incurred with thallium poisoning can be corrected with elimination of the toxin from the body. With an acutely lethal dose, this may require hemodialysis as well as cathartic agents and gastric lavage.[39]

Other heavy metals causing a generalized encephalopathy, such as lead, also may affect cerebellar function.[15] Lead encephalopathy in rat pups produces widespread interstitial edema in the cerebellum with attendant gait ataxia.[20] The capillary structure in the cerebellum has a special vulnerability to lead[20] and Purkinje cell damage has been documented after lethal lead encephalopathy. The basis for the metabolic effects of lead on the cerebellar vessel walls is unknown.[20] Children with lead poisoning develop a staggering gait and limb tremors, but it is not known whether these disorders result from cerebellar lesions.[15]

Drugs

The ingestion of a large number of drugs can lead to symptoms and signs of central nervous system dysfunction and some drugs evoke prominent signs of cerebellar disorder. Drugs generally have specific effects on specific enzyme systems. Many drugs and their metabolic products have different and highly specific binding sites in cellular membranes. Barbiturates, for example, affect mitochondria in a specific site. Some drugs, such as certain gaseous anesthetics, bind to the lipid layers of myelin as well as to cellular membranes. Microsomal enzyme systems have specific drug metabolizing sites. These systems can be altered with chronic drug treatment.

Transient symptoms of cerebellar dysfunction commonly occur during anticonvulsant therapy.[17] Gait ataxia, dysarthria, clumsiness, and nystagmus are likely to develop as serum drug levels approach the toxic range, and to remit as drug levels fall.[41] Some patients treated chronically for seizure disorders have progressive deficits that do not remit with discontinuation of the drug. After decades of episodic symptoms, persistent gait ataxia, kinetic tremors, dysarthria, generalized hypotonia, and nystagmus may increase insidiously.[17] The ataxia may be severe enough to interfere with functional gait.[17] This occurs most often with chronic phenytoin use,[14] regardless of the adequacy of seizure control. Cerebellar changes with chronic phenytoin use include Purkinje cell loss, an increase of Bergmann glia cells, sparse granular cells, and diffuse edema.[41] Basket cell axons and other neuronal elements in the cerebellum are preserved. Electron microscopic studies[14] of the granule cell layer show that the major changes are in the cellular processes. Membranous cytoplasmic bodies similar to those seen in the lipidoses are found in both the remaining Purkinje cells and the Bergmann glial cells.[14] These morphologic changes have been attributed to the effects of chronic administration of anticonvulsant drugs, however, this issue is controversial. Some investigators have concluded that hypoxia from seizures accounts for these changes. The evidence bearing upon this controversy is discussed in Chapter 18.

Phenobarbital, also used as an anticonvulsant, can cause signs of cerebellar dysfunction which largely remit with discontinuation of the drug. Primidone, an anticonvulsant in large part metabolized to phenobarbital, also can produce ataxia and nystagmus independent of the phenobarbital level.[4]

Alcohol

Alcohol ingestion, both acute and chronic, results in symptoms and signs of cerebellar dysfunction. The slurred speech of acute alcohol intoxication is a transient phenomenon which clears as the blood alcohol level falls. The broad-based, staggering gait with acute intoxication becomes a chronic feature with repeated alcohol abuse; a broad-based, rhythmic, unsteady gait usually develops after years of alcoholism. The abnormality of stance and gait is the principal complaint of patients with progressive cerebellar deficits associated with alcoholism.[1, 18] This deficit develops over the course of weeks or months and is encountered more often in men than women.[2] The difficulty can evolve slowly but insidiously, rapidly but with subsequent stabilization, or erratically with episodic exacerbations.[52] Progression of the deficit usually is associated with continued alcohol ingestion coupled with poor nutrition. It is not at all uncommon for the signs of cerebellar dysfunction to stabilize after a few weeks or months,[2] especially if the patient's diet improves.

The principal disturbance of gait is in the sequencing of movement for climbing or stepping.[47] Attempts to place the feet accurately are frustrated repeatedly by an overshoot dysmetria of each leg. The trajectory of each step is in error and the result is a very unstable gait. Individual leg ataxia is much worse than arm ataxia.[52] Over the course of years the gait takes on a rigid, stiff-legged appearance that clears when leg movements are conducted in a lying position.[1] The gait ataxia itself is accentuated by tasks demanding rapid postural adjustments, such as walking in tandem. Titubation may appear later in the course of alcoholic cerebellar degeneration,[13] with as much as 25 percent of patients exhibiting truncal or head tremor at some point in their disease.[1] The gait ataxia and titubation are not affected by having the patient's eyes open or shut.[13]

Alcoholic cerebellar degeneration typically causes substantial gait changes with little permanent effect on speech or ocular motor function;[47] in contrast to other progressive degenerations, most patients do not develop nystagmus or dysarthria.[2] Only 25 percent of affected individuals develop tremors of the head or limbs.[1] If tremor does occur, it is invariably exacerbated on maintaining postures. The bulk of patients with nystagmus in association with the gait difficulty have other residua of Wernicke encephalopathy pointing to disease extending well beyond the cerebellum. Hypotonia, ocular dysmetria, kinetic tremors, and arm dysmetria are not at all typical of the strictly cerebellar disease.[1]

Alcoholic cerebellar degeneration probably results from nutritional deficiency rather than the direct effects of alcohol.[2] The transient effects of alcohol probably reflect transient changes in brain metabolism and neurotransmitter levels associated with alcohol ingestion. Brain concentrations of cyclic GMP fall sharply after a single dose of alcohol with the most marked changes occurring in the cerebellum, a phenomenon which persists after tolerance for ethanol appears in other structures.[19] With chronic ethanol intoxication, dopamine and norepinephrine levels increase in the brain while gamma-aminobutyric acid levels fall.[19] Thiamine deficiency probably is responsible for much of the neuronal damage found in the chronic alcoholic.[2] The signs of cerebellar dysfunction developing wih the thiamine deficiency state of Wernicke encephalopathy are no different from those seen with chronic alcoholism.[18] Although patients with alcohol related cerebellar degeneration may not show the confabulation, ophthalmoplegias, and peripheral

324

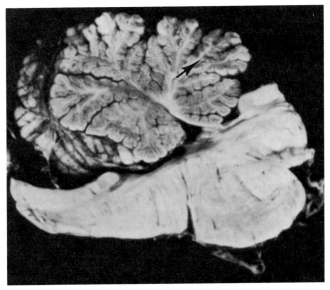

Figure 1. Alcoholic cerebellar degeneration. A midline section through the cerebellum and brainstem of a 66-year-old man with a 15 year history of alcoholism and poor nutrition. There is marked atrophy of the folia in the anterosuperior vermal region. The arrow points to the most severely affected folia.

neuropathy characteristic of other thiamine deficiency states, this probably reflects the degree of deficiency rather than its absence.

The pathologic changes in the cerebellum with chronic alcoholism and thiamine deficiency also are indistinguishable.[2, 47] The cerebellum has atrophy of all layers in the anterosuperior vermis (Fig. 1).[52] Purkinje cells are decreased to absent over the anterior vermis.[2] Neuronal loss may be prominent also in the dentate and inferior olivary nuclei.[18] The cerebellar hemispheres are involved much less often than the vermis,[52] an observation consistent with the primarily axial dysfunction occurring with chronic alcoholism. There is neuronal loss in the cerebellum with both Wernicke disease and alcohol related cerebellar degeneration, accounting for the largely irreversible nature of the deficits. With Wernicke encephalopathy, the ocular motor abnormalities may clear fairly completely with thiamine administration while the gait ataxia proves more refractory.[2] The patient surviving an episode of Wernicke encephalopathy may be left with a gait disorder resembling that seen in alcoholic cerebellar degeneration.[2]

Alcoholism can affect the central nervous system also through hepatic toxicity. Alcohol induced cirrhosis and hepatic diseases of many different types are associated with central nervous system disorders. Indeed, hepatic coma is the most common terminal event in all forms of liver disease.[12] Cerebral and cerebellar dysfunctions probably result from the failure of hepatic function to break down and clear large numbers of substances that can interfere with central nervous system function. Ammonia arising in the colon from bacterial activity has been implicated as the cause of hepatic encephalopathy.[12] Hepatic function converts the ammonia to urea, allowing clearance of the toxin from the blood. In hepatic failure this does not occur. In addition, glutamine accumulates in the central nervous system, as evidenced by increased levels in the cerebrospinal fluid.[49] Disturbed indole metabolism produces substances which also may contribute to dysfunction of the brain.[12] Although these abnormalities are known to occur in hepatic failure, it is now generally recognized that other substances, some yet to be characterized, are responsible for changes in the brain with liver failure.[7]

With deteriorating hepatic function, mild obtundation or somnolence are likely to be the first indications of central nervous system dysfunction.[42] Occasionally the patient is excitable at the onset of the disorder. Titubation, asterixis, dysarthria, dysmetria, gait ataxia, choreoathetosis, and dementia may appear as the patient's encephalopathy progresses.[49] Additional signs of neurologic disorder may appear over the course of hours, days, or weeks, depending upon the rapidity of hepatic deterioration.[42] Myoclonus, as well as generalized seizures, may appear as the nervous system deficits intensify. An initial increase in deep tendon reflex activity is followed by areflexia as the patient becomes comatose.[42] Hyperventilation and hyperthermia develop during the stage of coma, presumably on the basis of brain dysfunction. Respiratory failure is likely to develop abruptly. The outcome of hepatic encephalopathy is unpredictable even when the patient is in coma with no spontaneous breathing.[42] Even at that stage, complete recovery is possible. Cerebellar as well as cerebral signs of dysfunction may become permanent deficits if the bout of hepatic failure is protracted or recurrent.[49] The treatment of hepatic encephalopathy involves support of the patient's respiratory, cardiovascular, and renal systems while an effort is made to reduce the toxin load in the blood. Neomycin or lactulose installation into the intestine is still a mainstay of treatment.

Although experimental animals develop spongiform changes in the depths of the cerebellar folia, human brains rarely show these changes with hepatic encephalopathy.[7] Cerebellar changes are much the same as pathologic changes elsewhere in the brain with protracted hepatic failure. The cerebellar cortex at worse displays diffuse degeneration of neurons or patchy loss of myelin and neuronal elements throughout the structure.[49] Alzheimer type II astrocytes are prominent in the cerebellum as elsewhere.

DISORDERS OF ENZYMATIC FUNCTION

Trace Metal Deficiency

The functions of many enzyme systems depend upon the presence of trace amounts of minerals such as zinc and manganese. If these minerals are not present in adequate amounts, the enzyme systems cannot function at normal rates. The result is a decrease of metabolic activity. Many of the minerals required in trace amounts for normal metabolism become toxic if present in excessive quantities. Deficiencies of trace minerals are not commonly recognized as the basis for cerebellar dysfunction. One instance in which a trace mineral deficiency coincided with signs of cerebellar disease was inadvertently produced with zinc depletion. Patients fed histidine as an experimental treatment for progressive systemic sclerosis developed depressed serum zinc levels and increased urinary zinc excretion.[23] With these ion changes, several neurologic abnormalities occurred. The patients complained of anorexia, changes in taste and smell, and irritability. They

326

developed paranoid ideation, as well as gait and limb ataxia. The ataxia increased as long as the drug was continued and dysarthria and kinetic tremors appeared. All these disturbances subsided with zinc supplements, even when the histidine was not discontinued, and all disappeared when the histidine was stopped.[23] The presumed cerebellar dysfunction evidenced by ataxia, dysarthria, and kinetic tremors may have resulted from zinc depletion or the combination of low zinc levels with elevated histidine levels.

Vitamin Deficiency

Vitamins serve as cofactors for enzymatic reactions. The absence of a cofactor results in the slowing and eventual cessation of these reactions. The metabolic disturbance resulting from the absence of a specific cofactor varies depending upon the specific reactions that require the cofactor. Experimental deficiencies of particular vitamins have uncovered special cerebellar vulnerability to a few compounds. With thiamine deficiency in rats, the animals become severely ataxic.[37] This is presumed to result from the sensitivity of the cerebellum to decreased serotonin stores, secondary to the thiamine deficiency.[37] These animals have decreased uptake of serotonin in the cerebellum, a metabolic disorder of particular importance since there are serotonergic terminals in the cerebellum. Administering reserpine to these animals, thereby preventing serotonin storage,[9] exacerbates the signs of thiamine deficiency.

Some infants with feeding disorders develop cerebellar edema and necrosis with marked Purkinje cell loss.[30] Similar damage occurs in the chick cerebellum when the animals have diets restricted in alpha-tocopherol,[30] but this is not clearly an essential element in the human. A variety of other substrate or cofactor abnormalities may be the basis for this infantile disease.

Signs of cerebellar dysfunction develop in some individuals with severe malnutrition, which leads invariably to multiple vitamin deficiencies.[30] Although the cerebellum, like the brainstem, has a particular vulnerability to thiamine deficiency,[37] this is not the only factor involved in patients with malnutrition. For example, a nonalcoholic man dying with inanition developed truncal instability and gait ataxia as the first evidence of brain dysfunction.[30] His primary problem was malabsorption associated with intestinal disease, but the neurologic manifestations of this illness included gait difficulty, gaze-evoked nystagmus, and a progressive external ophthalmoplegia. Autopsy examination revealed substantial cerebellar lesions to account for the gait disorder. All neuronal elements in the cerebellum were affected in a pattern reminiscent of cerebellar degeneration from chronic alcoholism.[52] The cortex of the vermis and the anterosuperior portions of the cerebellar hemispheres in particular were necrotic. Almost all the Purkinje cells and their processes were lost. The molecular layer was completely depleted of neurons and the granule cell population was reduced. In addition to neuronal loss, there was demyelination in the subcortical white matter.[30] As in alcoholics,[52] the flocculonodular lobule was preserved. Deep white matter and nuclei were normal. Other changes in the brain included bilateral necrosis in periventricular and periaqueductal gray matter. Lesions similar to those seen in Wernicke disease were apparent in the mamillary bodies and brainstem structures.[30] Cerebral cortical areas were unremarkable.

327

Enzyme Disturbances and Storage Disorders

Deficiencies of specific enzymes usually result from genetic disturbances. In most diseases recognized clinically, only a single enzyme is deficient or absent.[26] Deficiency of the enzyme affects the synthetic mechanisms of the cell by slowing the production of particular substances. Complete absence of the enzyme leads to the failure of synthesis of the substances. The result usually is an accumulation of a precursor material involved in the metabolic pathway. The accumulation of substances is manifested clinically as storage disorders. Lysosomal enzymes often are involved in these storage disorders. These enzymes participate in the breakdown of cellular components that need to be resynthesized on a regular basis. The breakdown products are retrieved by the cell for the synthesis of new components.

Enzyme deficiencies may be quite specific for cerebellar pathways and forms of spinocerebellar degeneration. Sandhoff disease, a hexosaminidase A and B deficiency state, is one such disorder[35] already discussed in Chapter 12 in the context of hereditary degenerative cerebellar diseases. In the older literature[15] a similar predilection was noted for the juvenile form of Tay-Sach's disease, a designation which undoubtedly included many of the cases of hexosaminidase deficiency of the Sandhoff type.[35] Both of these disorders give rise to GM_2 ganglioside accumulation.[35]

Some enzymatic disorders produce nonspecific vacuolization and demyelination in the cerebellum as well as the cerebrum and spinal cord. Phenylketonuria produces disordered myelination rather than a true neuronal disorder.[29, 46] This is by no means a specifically cerebellar disease.

Systemic storage diseases may produce cerebellar symptomatology indirectly. Patients with hemochromatosis are known occasionally to develop gait ataxia, slurred speech, kinetic tremor, and limb ataxia.[48] Since the cerebellum invariably is normal in patients with hemochromatosis and the liver usually is cirrhotic, an hepatic encephalopathy probably causes the signs of cerebellar dysfunction.[48, 49] Widespread cerebral and cerebellar degeneration develops with some cases of infantile Gaucher's disease.[51] This is due to a deficiency of acid-betaglucosidase with the resultant accumulation of glucocerebroside in the brain. The prominent signs in the first months of life include spasticity, hyperreflexia, opisthotonos, seizures, and loss of vision. Lymphadenopathy and splenomegaly appearing early in life suggest a storage disorder. Although ataxia usually is not apparent in this infantile degenerative disease, hyperreflexia appears early, just as in the type 1 recessively inherited ataxias. The lipid accumulating in brain neurons can be demonstrated with periodic acid-Schiff stain. The cerebellum shows vacuolization of Purkinje cells and astrocytosis of the white matter.

Gait and limb ataxia, progressive psychomotor retardation, action myoclonus, and seizures appearing in infants may be the principal manifestations of a more poorly defined lipidosis, infantile neuronal ceroid lipofuscinosis.[36, 40] Patients with this disorder have a typical type 2 recessively inherited ataxia with hyperreflexia and dementia.[45] Microcephaly invariably is present. Visual loss develops by 1 year of age owing to optic atrophy. Myoclonus is prominent by 18 months of age, and by 3 years of age the child is usually mute and vegetative with an isoelectric EEG.[40] Peripheral nerve disease is not evident on electromyographic and nerve conduction studies. Neuronal ceroid lipofuscinosis also may present at widely different ages with limb ataxia, gait disorder, dysarthria, kinetic tremors, and myoclonus. Seizures and progressive dementia are more typical of the disease when it occurs in early life.[21] Neuropathologic changes include widespread neuronal damage, with extensive loss of Purkinje cells, granule cells, and dentate neurons. Although there is abnormal material stored throughout the brain, the cerebellar component of the damage is prominent. The principal pathologic feature is an excessive accumulation of granular lipopigment in the neurons above the area occupied by the cell nucleus.[21] This probably results from a disturbance in lipid metabolism resulting in increased lipid peroxidation.

A similar disorder in slightly older children is often called the Niemann-Pick variant. Patients with this disease develop ataxia, dementia, rigidity, spasticity, vertical supranuclear ophthalmoplegia, and seizures before the age of 10 years.[32] Unlike the infants with ceroid lipofuscinosis, vision is normal. The optic fundus has normal pigmentation. On neuropathologic examination, the cerebellum is the most abnormal brain structure grossly. There is widespread loss of both Purkinje cells and granule cells. Lipid inclusions distend most of the residual cerebellar cells.[34] Distinctive in these patients are foamy histiocytes in the bone marrow, unlike any seen in Niemann-Pick disease, but some have sphingomyelin greatly increased in the spleen.[32] The "sea-blue" histiocytes and visceral storage disease associated with this metabolic disorder emphasize the systemic nature of this progressive ataxia.

A specific enzyme dysfunction is known for Sandhoff hexosaminidase deficiency, and yet even this biochemical abnormality is not sufficient to understand fully this cerebellar ataxia. A slowly progressive, recessively inherited ataxia without the dementia and seizures frequent in Sandhoff disease develops in the juvenile group affected by Johnson-Chutorian[24] hexosaminidase B deficiency and in the adult group described by Oonk and his associates.[35] Biochemically these disorders are overlapping,[35] but clinically there is milder cerebellar dysfunction with the Johnson-Chutorian and adult types. One four year old had 18 months of increasing gait and truncal ataxia with kinetic tremors in the arms.[25] He had no dementia, but as in patients with Sandhoff disease, there was a macular cherry red spot. Adults with hexosaminidase A and B deficiency have an even more benign progressive ataxia[35] which may produce no substantial signs until the third decade of life.

A progressive spastic ataxia occurs with cerebrotendinous xanthomatosis, an autosomal recessive disorder.[16] This rare familial disease is characterized by juvenile cataracts, enlargement of the tendons, dementia, limb and gait ataxia, and other more variable signs of neurologic disease. The first symptoms of this disorder commonly occur in early adult life or later. The course of the illness is relatively slow and progressive ataxia may be a fairly late sign. Dementia occurs in the second decade of life and the patient may survive into his fourth decade.[16] Scoliosis, pes cavus, impaired sensation, palatal myoclonus, and disease of the long tracts may appear in later stages of the illness. There is excessive cholestanol in the cerebellum as well as the serum of these patients. Although cerebrotendinous xanthomatosis results from a generalized disorder of lipid metabolism, signs of brain dysfunction and specifically cerebellar dysfunction are prominent.

AMINO ACID DEFICIENCIES

Certain amino acids must be ingested with food since they cannot be synthesized by the body. A deficiency of these essential amino acids leads to the inability to synthesize certain proteins. The result is a protein deficiency with the loss of specific functions. Cerebellar ataxia may appear reversibly with disorders of amino acid metabolism[11] such as Hartnup disease.[33] This is corrected by nicotinamide,[43] but the ataxia is not secondary to a true deficiency of that vitamin. The disorder is responsive to excessive nicotinamide probably by compensating for inefficient handling of normally adequate nicotinamide supplies to the cerebellum.[43]

A reversible cerebellar disorder also occurs in children with idiopathic pyruvicacidemia.[28] When stressed by illness or injury, the patient develops progressive ataxia, vertigo, nystagmus, dysarthria, and confusion which remits within a few days. Pyruvicuria and alaninuria increase together with the ataxia. The probable metabolic disorder is a partial block in the oxidative decarboxylation of pyruvic acid.[5, 28] This disorder differs from pyruvate decarboxylase deficiency[6] in its response to thiamine. With idiopathic pyruvicaciduria, large doses of thiamine will reverse the cerebellar ataxia.[28] Self-limited episodes of ataxia, irritability, and obtundation occur with a variant of maple syrup urine disease. The episodes appear coincident with exacerbations of the branched-chain ketonuria.[11] There is no treatment for this disorder of amino acid metabolism.

ENDOCRINE DISORDERS

Most metabolic functions are controlled by circulating hormones and depend upon the concentrations of these substances as well as the available receptor sites of the cells influenced by these substances. Disturbances of metabolic function occur when diseases of the organ producing the hormone result in excessive or inadequate amounts of the hormone. The central nervous system effects of endocrine disorders are secondary to diseases of the organs producing the hormone. Correction of the endocrine disturbance restores neural function to normal.

Hyperthyroidism may produce kinetic tremors, choreoathetosis, and seizures, but these neurologic disorders are not usually mistaken for cerebellar disease. Hypothyroidism is the endocrine disturbance most clearly associated specifically with cerebellar dysfunction.[44] A true cerebellar gait ataxia may develop over a period of months to years in the adult with chronic hypothyroidism. Ataxia occasionally may be the first sign of hypothyroidism. Although the arms are less affected than the legs, all limbs have kinetic tremors, dysmetria, and dysdiadochokinesis. Deafness and dysarthria appear occasionally. The cerebrospinal fluid protein is increased. All these deficits are reversed at least partly with replacement therapy for the hypothyroidism. The pathologic basis for this dysfunction is not well established,[8] but there is probably some loss of Purkinje cells and gliosis in the cerebellum.[38] The cellular changes are most severe over the anterosuperior aspects of the vermis.[44] Despite these findings on neuropathologic examination, thyroid replacement provides a striking therapeutic effect, even after several years of disturbed cerebellar function.[10]

REFERENCES

1. ADAMS, R. D.: *Nutritional cerebellar degeneration*, in Vinken, P. J., and Bruyn, G. W. (eds.): *Handbook of Clinical Neurology*, vol. 28. American Elsevier Publishing Co., New York, 1976, pp. 271–284.
2. ADAMS, R. D., AND VICTOR, M.: *Principles of Neurology*. McGraw-Hill, New York, 1977.

3. BANK, W. J., PLEASURE, D. E., SUZUKI, K., ET AL.: *Thallium poisoning.* Arch. Neurol. 26:456, 1972.

4. BERMAN, P. H.: *Management of seizure disorders with anticonvulsant drugs: current concepts.* Pediat. Clin. North Amer. 23:443, 1976.

5. BLASS, J. P.: *Disorders of pyruvate metabolism.* Neurology 29:280, 1979.

6. BLASS, J. P., AVIGAN, J., AND UHLENDORF, B. W.: *A defect in pyruvate decarboxylase in a child with an intermittent movement disorder.* J. Clin. Invest. 49:423, 1970.

7. CAVANAGH, J. B.: *Liver bypass and the glia,* in Plum, F. (ed.): *Brain Dysfunction in Metabolic Disorders.* Raven Press, New York, 1974, pp. 13–38.

8. CLOS. J., AND LEGRAND, J.: *Effects of thyroid deficiency on the different cell populations of the cerebellum in the young rat.* Brain Res. 63:450, 1973.

9. COOPER, J. R., BLOOM, F. E., AND ROTH, R. H.: *The Biochemical Basis of Neuropharmacology.* Oxford University Press, New York, 1974.

10. CREMER, G. M. GOLDSTEIN, N. P., AND PARIS, J.: *Myxedema and ataxia.* Neurology 19:37, 1969.

11. DANCIS, J., HUTZLER, J., AND ROKKONES, T.: *Intermittent branched chain ketonuria. Variant of maple-syrup-urine disease.* N. Eng. J. Med. 276:84, 1967.

12. DAVIDSON, C. S.: *Treatment of alcoholic liver disease,* in Schaffner, F., Sherlock, S., and Leevy, C. M. (eds.): *The Liver and Its Diseases.* Intercontinental Medical Book Corp., New York, 1974, pp. 268–272.

13. DEJONG, R. N.: *The Neurologic Examination.* Harper & Row, New York, 1979.

14. DEL CERRO, M. P., AND SNIDER, R. S.: *Studies on Dilantin intoxication.* Neurology 17:452, 1967.

15. DOW, R. S., AND MORUZZI, G.: *The Physiology and Pathology of the Cerebellum.* University of Minnesota Press, Minneapolis, 1958.

16. FARPOUR, H., AND MAHLOUDJI, M.: *Familial cerebrotendinuous xanthomatosis.* Arch. Neurol. 32:223, 1975.

17. GHATAK, N. R., SANTOSO, R. A., AND McKINNEY, W. M.: *Cerebellar degeneration following long-term phenytoin therapy.* Neurology 26:818, 1976.

18. GILROY, J., AND MEYER, J. S.: *Medical Neurology.* Macmillan Publishing Co., New York, 1975.

19. GOLDSTEIN, D. B.: *Progress in the study of ethanol's actions in the brain,* in Seixas, F. A. (ed.): *Currents in Alcoholism,* vol. III. Grune and Stratton, New York, 1977, pp. 3–21.

20. GOLDSTEIN, G. W., AND DIAMOND, I.: *Metabolic basis of lead encephalopathy,* in Plum, F. (ed.): *Brain Dysfunction in Metabolic Disorders.* Raven Press, New York, 1974, pp. 293–304.

21. GREENWOOD, R. S., AND NELSON, J. S.: *Atypical neuronal ceroid-lipofuscinosis.* Neurology 28:710, 1978.

22. HASSAN, M., ASHRAF, I., AND BAJPAI, V. K.: *Electron miscroscopic study of the effects of thallium poisoning on the rat cerebellum.* Forensic Sci. 11:139, 1978.

23. HENKIN, R. I., PATTEN, B. M., RE, P. K. ET AL.: *A syndrome of acute zinc loss.* Arch. Neurol. 32:745, 1975.

24. JOHNSON, W. G., AND CHUTORIAN, A. M.: *Inheritance of the enzyme defect in a new hexosaminidase deficiency disease.* Ann. Neurol. 4:399, 1978.

25. JOHNSON, W. G., CHUTORIAN, A., AND MIRANDA, A.: *A new juvenile hexosaminidase deficiency disease presenting as cerebellar ataxia: clinical and biochemical studies.* Neurology 27:1012, 1977.

26. KOLODNY, E. H., HASS, W. K., LANE, B., ET AL.: *Refsum's syndrome.* Arch. Neurol. 12:583, 1965.

27. LIVERSEDGE, L. A., AND EMERY, V.: *Electroencephalographic changes in cerebellar degenerative lesions.* J. Neurol. Neurosurg. Psychiat. 24:326, 1961.

28. LONSDALE, D., FAULKNER, W. R., PRICE, J. W., ET AL.: *Intermittent cerebellar ataxia associated with hyperpyruvic acidemia, hyperalaninemia, and hyperalaninuria.* Pediatr. 43:1025, 1969.

29. MALAMUD, N.: *Neuropathology of phenylketonuria.* J. Neuropath. Exp. Neurol. 25:254, 1966.

30. MANCALL, E. L., AND McENTEE, W. J.: *Alterations of the cerebellar cortex in nutritional encephalopathy.* Neurology 15:303, 1965.

31. MARGERISON, J. H., AND CORSELLIS, J. A. N.: *Epilepsy and the temporal lobes.* Brain 89:499, 1966.

32. NEVILLE, B. G. R., LAKE, B. D., STEPHENS, R., ET AL.: *A neurovisceral storage disease with vertical supranuclear ophthalmoplegia and its relationship to Niemann-Pick disase.* Brain 96:97, 1973.

33. NOAD, K. B., AND LANCE, J. W.: *Familial myoclonic epilepsy and its association with cerebellar disturbance.* Brain 83:618, 1960.

34. NORMAN, R. M., FORRESTER, R. M., AND TINGEY, A. H.: *The juvenile form of Niemann-Pick disease.* Arch. Dis. Child. 42:91, 1967.

35. OONK, J. G. W., VAN DER HELM, H. J., AND MARTIN, J. J.: *Spinocerebellar degeneration: Hexosaminidase A and B deficiency in two adult sisters.* Neurology 29:380, 1979.

36. PALLIS, C. A., DUCKETT, S., AND PEARSE, A. G. E.: *Diffuse lipofuscinosis of the central nervous system.* Neurology 17:381, 1967.

37. PLAITAKIS, A., NICKLAS, W. J., AND BERL, S.: *Thiamine deficiency: selective impairment of the cerebellar serotonergic system.* Neurology 28:691, 1978.

38. PRICE, T. R., AND NETSKY, M. G.: *Myxedema and ataxia.* Neurology 16:957, 1966.

39. PRICK, J. J. G.: *Thallium poisoning,* in Vinken, P. J., Bruyn, G. W. (eds.): *Handbook of Clinical Neurology,* vol. 36. American Elsevier Publishing Co. New York, pp. 239–278.

40. RAPOLA, J., AND HALTIA, M.: *Cytoplasmic inclusions in the vermiform appendix and skeletal muscle in two types of so-called neuronal ceroid lipofuscinosis.* Brain 96:833, 1973.

41. RAPPORT, R. L. II, AND SHAW, C. M.: *Phenytoin-related cerebellar degeneration without seizures.* Ann. Neurol. 2:437, 1977.

42. REDEKER, A. G.: *Fulminant hepatitis,* in Schaffner, F., Sherlock, S., Leevy, C. M., (eds.): *The Liver and its Diseases.* Intercontinental Medical Book Corp., New York, 1974, pp. 149–155.

43. ROSENBERG, L. E.: *Vitamin-responsive inherited diseases affecting the nervous system,* in Plum, F. (ed.): *Brain Dysfunction in Metabolic Disorders.* Raven Press, New York, 1974, pp. 263–272.

44. ROSMAN, N. P.: *Neurological and muscular aspects of thyroid dysfunction in childhood.* Pediatr. Clin. North Am. 23:575, 1976.

45. SANTAVUORI, P., HALTIA, M., RAPOLA, J. ET AL.: *Infantile type of so-called neuronal ceroid-lipofuscinosis.* J. Neurol. Sci. 18:257, 1973.

46. SILBERBERG, D. H.: *Phenylketonuria metabolites in cerebellum culture morphology.* Arch. Neurol. 17:524, 1967.

47. SILFVERSKIÖLD B. P.: *Cortical cerebellar degeneration associated with a specific disorder of standing and locomotion.* Acta Neurol. Scand. 55:257, 1977.

48. SINGH, N., RAO, S., AND BHUYAN, U. N.: *Reversible cerebello-cerebral disorder in primary hemochromatosis.* Arch. Neurol. 34:123, 1977.

49. SMITH, W. T.: *Intoxications, poisons and metabolic disorders,* in Blackwood, W., and Corsellis, J. A. N. (eds.): *Greenfield's Neuropathology* Year Book Medical Publishers, Chicago, 1976, pp. 148–193.

50. SNIDER, R. S., THOMAS, W., AND SNIDER, S. R.: *Focal brain hyperthermia. I. The cerebellar cortex.* Experientia 34:479, 1078.

51. VERITY, M. A., AND MONTASIR, M.: *Infantile Gaucher's disease: Neuropathology, acid hydrolase activities and negative staining observations.* Neuropädiatr. 8:89, 1977.

52. VICTOR, M., ADAMS, R. D., AND MANCALL, E. L.: *A restricted form of cerebellar cortical degeneration occurring in alcoholic patients.* Arch. Neurol. 1:579, 1959.

CHAPTER 17

Neoplasms

Tumors of the cerebellum are common and often treatable. They can affect people at every age (Table 1), and the prognosis with each tumor is highly specific for the tumor type. Early accurate identification of the pathologic process is important, for some tumors can be treated adequately to achieve a complete cure with early intervention. Other tumors can be treated sufficiently to alter the length and quality of the patient's survival.

Neoplasms may arise from the proliferation of elements within the cerebellum, by extension from adjacent structures, or by metastasis of a remote tumor. The most common intraparenchymal tumors are the medulloblastomas, astrocytomas, metastatic tumors, and ependymomas.[1, 19] Angioreticulomas, sarcomas, and other gliomas probably are variants of these basic tumor types. The choroid plexus papilloma should be considered a form of ependymoma rather than a distinct tumor type.[39] Lymphomas,[62] neuroblastomas,[58] and gangliocytomas[50] are the rarest of the primary cerebellar tumors. Hemangiomas are not rare,[61] but some controversy surrounds the issue of whether or not they are truly neoplastic when they occur in the cerebellum. Hemangioblastomas, which must be distinguished from hemangiomas, clearly represent primary neoplasms of the cerebellum. The common extraparenchymal tumors are the meningiomas and schwannomas, which can produce tissue damage by compressing or invading the cerebellum.

Difficulties with the neuropathologic criteria for distinguishing tumor types, such as the distinction between medulloblastoma and sarcoma,[3, 29] have led to problems in determining the precise incidence of the various tumors. Nevertheless, metastatic tumors, astrocytomas, and medulloblastomas rank as the most common cerebellar tumors (Tables 1 and 2). Metastatic tumors occur most commonly after middle age whereas astrocytomas and medulloblastomas appear most frequently in childhood, accounting for one-third of all intracranial neoplasms in children.[6, 19]

SYMPTOMS AND SIGNS

Cerebellar tumors frequently produce symptoms of neurologic disease early in life and with striking rapidity. About one-third of all patients with cerebellar tumors develop symptoms and signs of disease within the first decade of life.[1] One-fourth of all patients have symptoms that begin less than 2 months prior to the

Table 1. Age distribution of cerebellar tumors in study of 162 patients

Age (yrs.)	Metastasis	Astrocytoma	Medulloblastoma	Hemangioblastoma	Schwannoma	Meningioma	Ependymoma	Other
0–2	0	1	2	0	0	0	1	0
2–5	0	6	4	0	0	0	0	0
5–10	0	8	4	0	0	0	0	2
10–20	0	16	5	1	0	0	0	1
20–30	0	3	7	0	0	0	0	1
30–40	1	1	1	0	1	1	0	0
40–60	36	3	0	3	1	1	0	3
Over 60	13	2	0	2	4	3	1	2

time they come to medical attention, and one-fourth have complaints extending over more than 6 months. The duration of the history with astrocytomas is usually longer than with medulloblastomas or ependymomas.[6] The shortest duration of symptoms associated with cerebellar tumors occurs in adults with metastatic disease.[1]

As with tumors affecting other components of the central nervous system, the symptoms and signs developing with any cerebellar tumor reflect the site of the lesion rather than the type of lesion.[16, 32] The most frequent presenting symptoms with any cerebellar tumor are headache and difficulty with standing and walking.[1, 6, 19] More than 90 percent of patients have difficulty with gait or stance early in their disease.[1, 44] The presenting symptoms also vary with the age of onset of the disorder. The infant with a cerebellar tumor may present to the physician with restlessness, irritability, or lethargy.[19] An enlarging head, head tilt, neck stiffness, and vomiting, however, may be the first evidence of cerebellar tumor in the infant.[6]

The neurologic signs resulting from cerebellar tumors are similar to those resulting from other types of cerebellar disease[27, 44] and are described in detail in Chapter 10. Nystagmus, hypotonia, dysmetria, and papilledema develop early in the course with most cerebellar tumors.[16] Papilledema appears in about three-fourths of all patients with cerebellar neoplasms about the time of the initial diagnosis and optic atrophy develops if the papilledema is chronic.[6] Although this is a

Table 2. Location of cerebellar neoplasms in study of 162 patients

Type	Total	Location Vermis	Location Hemisphere
Metastases	50	5	45
Astrocytomas	40	15	25
Medulloblastomas	23	14	9
Schwannomas	6	0	6
Hemangioblastomas	6	1	5
Meningiomas	5	0	5
Ependymomas	2	2	0
Other (Undifferentiated or rare)	9	4	5

common sign, often reflecting obstructive hydrocephalus at the level of the fourth ventricle, it is not invariably present, even with large tumors. The signs of cerebellar tumor generally are nonspecific in infants. Papilledema occurs in only 16 percent of infants under the age of 18 months.[19] Hypotonia is apparent in 11 percent of infants and ataxia occurs only in 7 percent.[19]

A cerebellar neoplasm should be suspected when the patient presents with frontal or occipital headaches associated with nausea, vomiting, an unsteady gait, and clumsiness.[23] Unilateral limb ataxia, diplopia, rebound nystagmus, titubation, pendular reflexes, dysarthria, and kinetic tremors may all be elicited on examination as supporting evidence of a destructive cerebellar lesion.[52] A long history of hearing loss associated with signs of ipsilateral cerebellar disease occurs typically with an acoustic schwannoma.[13] The early appearance of vomiting, listlessness, and irritability associated with focal motor or sensory deficits in a limb suggests an ependymoma or medulloblastoma seeding in the subarachnoid space from its origin in the posterior fossa.[56] Vertigo appears often with a cerebellar tumor,[12] but it is too nonspecific to implicate the cerebellum when it appears as an isolated symptom. Labyrinthitis or brainstem disease may produce vertigo with nausea and vomiting, but when the vertigo is associated with dysarthria or limb dysmetria, a cerebellar neoplasm is clearly implicated. Associated diseases may provide insight into the cause of the patient's symptoms. A patient with known lung carcinoma who abruptly develops oscillopsia and gait ataxia,[57] for example, must be presumed to have metastatic disease in the cerebellum, even though oscillopsia is a relatively uncommon sign of cerebellar disease. Rapidly evolving tumors may produce ocular dysmetria or mild facial weakness, but such disorders of ocular and other cranial nerve functions may prove to be secondary to brainstem compression from the rapidly expanding posterior fossa mass.

A common problem in the diagnosis of cerebellar tumors is that the lesion may produce few localizing signs. In many cases the signs will reflect only an increase in intracranial pressure from ventricular obstruction.[44] The signs of cerebellar dysfunction may be minimal,[8] but the signs which are observed usually reflect whether the tumor is in the hemisphere or the vermis and whether the superior or the inferior parts of the cerebellum are damaged.[16] Compensatory processes can mask much of the dysfunction produced by a slowly evolving lesion. Despite the principle that progressive lesions produce progressive symptomatology, patients with cerebellar tumors may have remitting and recurring signs.[1, 16]

DIAGNOSTIC STUDIES

The investigation of patients with suspected cerebellar tumors has been simplified greatly by computerized tomography of the brain. Most posterior fossa neoplasms are more dense or less dense than adjacent brain tissue, a characteristic which allows good resolution of a tumor without additional radiographic maneuvers. Tumors isodense with the affected cerebellum may appear more dense after the intravenous injection of contrast material. Tumors that are not vascular or do not enhance with contrast material for other reasons may be revealed by a shift of the fourth ventricle or an asymmetry in the cerebellar hemispheres. Highly cystic astrocytomas are readily distinguished from hemorrhages because of their differing densities, even though both would appear as largely avascular masses on arteriography. Meningiomas, choroid plexus papillomas, and hemangioblastomas all may have marked density enhancement after intravenous dye administration.

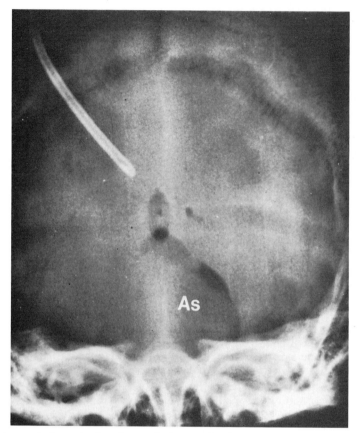

Figure 1. Anteroposterior projection of a ventriculogram allowing visualization of a large fourth ventricle tumor (As) which proved to be a subependymal astrocytoma.

Apart from computerized tomography, ventriculography is most specific for cerebellar neoplasms (Fig. 1) and angiography can be helpful. In ventriculograms the posterior half of the third ventricle may appear foreshortened with cerebellar neoplasms that cause transtentorial herniation of the cerebellum. The pineal gland is displaced upward in about 33 percent of patients with infratentorial gliomas.[17] The fourth ventricle may be shifted or obstructed. Arteriography (Fig. 2) can demonstrate stretching of posterior fossa vessels about the mass, but the normal variation in posterior fossa arteries makes interpretation of these studies difficult and highly specialized. A very large mass may result in the displacement of the straight sinus upward and backward and flattening of the curve of the vein of Galen.[17] A tumor blush may persist into the venous phase of the angiogram (Fig. 3).

The plain skull film and electroencephalogram usually provide little assistance in the diagnosis of cerebellar tumors. In many cases, however, plain skull radiograms may reveal split sutures in young children or thinning of the dorsum sella turcica in older patients with increased intracranial pressure. In the absence of computerized tomography, Tc 99m radionuclide brain scan is a fairly good indicator of posterior fossa neoplasms. The electroencephalogram is of limited value in the diagnosis of cerebellar tumors. Increased intracranial pressure may be re-

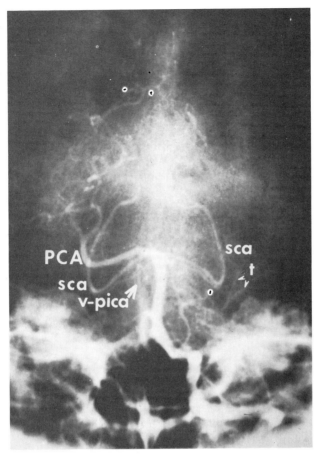

Figure 2. A vertebral angiogram with several abnormal features. The bilaterally paired superior cerebellar arteries (sca) are a normal variant, but the pair on the left is shifted superiorly by a tumor (t) lying beneath. The tumor is fed by the vessels indicated by small white arrows. The vermian branch of the posterior inferior cerebellar artery (v-pica) is shifted to the right. Only the right posterior cerebral artery was visualized (PCA) with this injection.

flected in high amplitude generalized slowing or intermittent, rhythmic slowing of electroencephalographic activity, but 24 percent of children with posterior fossa tumors have normal electroencephalograms.[6] Lumbar puncture is contraindicated in patients suspected of cerebellar tumor because of the hazard of precipitating cerebellar herniation.

THERAPY

The principal treatments available for cerebellar neoplasms are surgery and irradiation.[7, 20, 37, 51] Surgical techniques[7] allow extensive explorations of the posterior fossa and surgery alone may provide cures for some circumscribed lesions.[37] Even when the suspected tumor is not treatable, surgery will supply tissue for a definite diagnosis. Some cerebellar tumors, such as medulloblastomas, are highly sensitive to radiation therapy.[20, 51] Current efforts at chemotherapy for posterior fossa tumors have been disappointing. Methotrexate was used in the past for

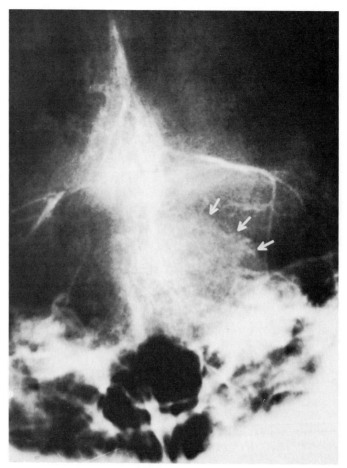

Figure 3. The venous phase of a vertebral angiogram showing a large tumor blush (arrows). The tumor was a meningioma in the left cerebellopontine angle.

treating primary posterior fossa tumors, but an unacceptable number of patients developed a leukoencephalopathy with subependymal necrosis.[49] Areas not irradiated showed necrosis, demonstrating that this was not the cumulative effect of combining chemotherapy and radiotherapy. Methotrexate alone was the responsible agent. Currently, cerebral tumors are being treated with the lipid soluble agents, lomustine, carmustine, and semustine, but the usefulness of these drugs in the treatment of cerebellar tumors remains unestablished.[49]

INTRAPARENCHYMAL TUMORS

Medulloblastoma

Incidence

Medulloblastomas occur in both children and adults, but the incidence and pattern of disease in these two groups are different. Medulloblastomas account for 25 percent of all brain tumors in childhood.[20] In this age group, the medulloblastoma

338

is primarily a midline tumor, extending into the vermis and the fourth ventricle.[10, 52, 53] It is one of the most malignant tumors of childhood, accounting for 10 percent of all malignant tumors in children and occurring twice as often in male children as in female children.[6, 52] In adults, medulloblastoma accounts for less than 5 percent of all brain tumors.[51] The adult medulloblastoma usually extends laterally into the hemispheres[10] and symptoms appear prior to vermal extension.[52] Tabulation of all patients with medulloblastoma as a group, irrespective of age, reveals that more than 80 percent occur in the midline.[10] There are occasional histologic differences between the adult and childhood medulloblastoma,[51, 53] probably because the tumor is affected by the maturity of the brain tissue it invades.[43]

Pathology

The medulloblastoma may be of glial origin,[20] but its behavior and morphology favor a neuroectodermal origin.[45, 53] Cushing and Bailey postulated that the tumor arises in hypothetical cells capable of differentiating into either glial or neural elements. Later studies of cell features, however, indicated that a precursor cell arises in the normally transient external granular layer.[45, 52] Cells in this layer appear to arise in the cerebellum near the posterior medullary velum and spread over the surface of the organ before differentiating and migrating into the internal granular layer.[53] Although there is no unequivocal evidence of neuronal structures in the medulloblastoma, the granule cells of the cerebellum have much the same size and form as medulloblastoma cells.[43] In children up to the age of 1 year, there is a persistent external granular layer in the vermis along the roof of the fourth ventricle. These infantile granule cells may be the source of medulloblastoma cells. If so, this would account for the exceedingly high incidence of these tumors in the first few years of life. Embryonic rests or granule cell transformations later in life may be the source of cells for medulloblastomas in the adult.[45]

The notion that medulloblastomas arise from granule cells is supported by the posterior medial cerebellar location of the tumor in more than 80 percent of cases.[52] The anterior medullary velum is involved by virtually all medulloblastomas lying anteriorly[47] and the posterior medullary velum is impinged upon by 75 percent of all medulloblastomas.[52] The anterior velum forms the roof of the fourth ventricle superiorly. It consists of a thin layer of white matter extending to the inferior colliculus of the midbrain, continuous with the white matter of the cerebellum.[47] The similarly structured posterior medullary velum provides part of the inferior roof of the fourth ventricle. If medulloblastomas originate from cells in the external granular layer, the medulloblastoma stands as the most poorly differentiated of any neuroectodermal tumor.[47]

Grossly the medulloblastoma appears solid and whitish or reddish gray, with deceptively distinct margins (Fig. 4).[52] Histologically the medulloblastoma is a very cellular tumor[10] with varied patterns of cell alignment (Fig. 5). Cells invariably extend beyond the apparent limits of the tumor. The tumor cells are small lymphocytoid cells with round or ovoid deeply staining nuclei.[38, 43] The chromatin pattern is diffuse and the cytoplasm is scant and usually eosinophilic. Bizarre or heterogeneous nuclei are notably absent[52] and there are rare neuroglial fibrils interspersed with the tumor cells. Overall the tumor appears similar to reticulum cell sarcoma, but there is no reticulin between the cells. These tumors are also similar in cell structure to neuroblastomas, though the absence of synaptic complexes makes the distinction between these tumor types relatively simple. Deep in the white matter of the cerebellum the tumor cells may arrange themselves along

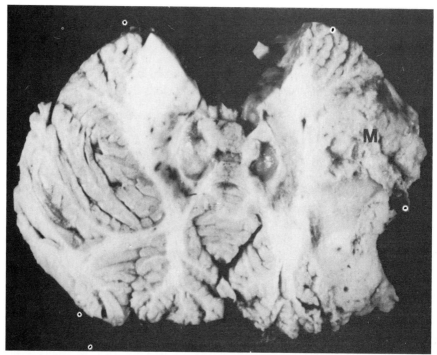

Figure 4. A coronal section through the cerebellum of a 25-year-old man with a medulloblastoma (M) invading and destroying much of the left cerebellar hemisphere. Headaches preceded the discovery of this tumor by 2 years. Blurred vision for 2 weeks prompted the neurologic investigation that uncovered the tumor. The patient survived 3 years from the time of diagnosis and underwent two surgical resections and a full course of radiotherapy. Microscopic examination of the ventricular walls revealed seeding of the medulloblastoma, despite the irradiation.

pre-existing tissue structures, consequently producing spindle shaped chains of cells or closely packed lobules.[43, 47] This pattern persists even after destruction of normal cerebellar tissue.

Oligodendroglia and myelin sheaths are destroyed rapidly by the tumor. Macroscopic or microscopic cysts form in 16 percent of all medulloblastomas.[52] In some areas, the tumor cells form rosettes around central areas packed with the microvilli and cytoplasmic processes that cover the cells. This rosette formation is similar to normal cerebellar granule cell behavior and appears in neuroblastomas as well.[43] Some authors distinguish between a "cerebellar arachnoid sarcoma" and medulloblastoma, but the fine structure of the two tumors is similar.[3, 38, 43, 53] The "arachnoid sarcoma" is more common in older children and adults and usually appears on the surface of the brain.[10] Characteristically it has abundant reticulin-like material and islands of pale cells. Rosettes or pseudorosettes are not present and the tumor is usually well circumscribed. Most of these atypical features probably reflect an interaction with the leptomeningeal elements invaded by the tumor.[53] On electron microscopic examination[43] the reticulin associated with the "arachnoid sarcoma" does not appear to be the same material as the reticulin found in extracerebellar sarcomas. Designating some medulloblastoma-like tumors as "sarcomas" is a distinction of limited value and probably will be abandoned.

340

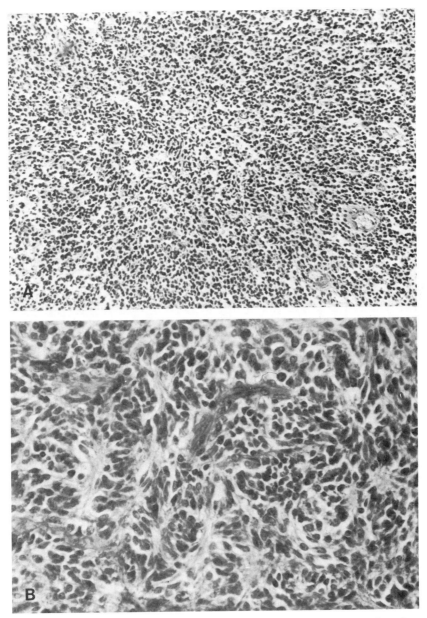

Figure 5. Microscopic sections of medulloblastomas from 2 patients. A, Low power view of a medulloblastoma showing large numbers of closely packed small lymphocytoid cells with round or ovoid deeply staining nuclei. B, Higher power view of a medulloblastoma showing arrays of small primitive neural cells, often radiating from vessels by fine, short processes. The tumor shows some differentiation toward young glial cells (phosphotungstic acid hematoxylin stain). The patient with this tumor, a 3-year-old male, developed vomiting, an awkward gait, and pain in the back of the neck. Examination revealed papilledema and a broad based gait with a tendency to fall backward. At operative exploration the tumor filled the fourth ventricle.

Medulloblastoma is a true malignancy, giving rise to metastatic disease both in and out of the central nervous system.[10, 64] Metastases occur in lymphatic tissue, lung, liver, kidney, spleen, pancreas, bone, ovary, parotid, muscle, and various tissues in the mediastinum. This extra-axial spread of the tumor is unusual, but dissemination of the tumor cells intra-axially along the ventricular system and about the central nervous system in the subarachnoid space is common.[20, 52] As many as 83 per cent of medulloblastomas have subarachnoid seeding to some extent.[18, 53] Intraventricular seeding of tumor is more characteristic of ependymoma than of medulloblastoma.[18, 47] Supratentorial metastases of medulloblastoma often are associated with a progressive hydrocephalus. Tumor metastases along the surface of the spinal cord produce a "candle-dripping" appearance on myelographic examination.[20] This spread of tumor throughout the central nervous system will produce unpredictable signs of tissue damage. Cranial nerves, spinal roots, spinal cord long tracts, and periventricular nuclear complexes all may be affected by focal accumulations of tumor cells. After ventriculoperitoneal shunts for hydrocephalus, metastases from the primary medulloblastoma may appear in the peritoneum, clearly aided in their spread by the shunt.[3] The mode of dissemination to other tissues is still unknown. Presumably the lymphatics are involved in some cases, especially those where there is lymph node involvement, and hematogenous spread may be responsible for many of the bone metastases. Bone expansion appears with medulloblastoma metastases and new periosteal bone accumulates. Lesions often are lytic and painful.[36]

Symptoms and Signs

The symptoms of medulloblastoma are variable in both their rapidity of onset and their severity. Headache, nausea, and vomiting usually develop over the course of 4 to 6 weeks before the patient comes to medical attention.[6] In a series of more than 100 patients with medulloblastoma, 85 percent had preoperative histories of less than 6 months.[52] The headache and vomiting usually are much worse in the morning and may be associated with blurred vision. Younger children may develop a slowly progressive head tilt and an abrupt deterioration in milestones of psychomotor development. Running and eventually walking are impaired. Adults may first manifest the tumor by changes in affective or cognitive function. Severe depression, presumably resulting from cerebral dysfunction with increased intracranial pressure, may occur.[51] Signs of cranial nerve dysfunction are often the first clear evidence of a destructive posterior fossa mass, and ocular motor function occasionally is disturbed as the tumor expands or seeds in the subarachnoid space.[47] Tinnitus, deafness, photophobia, drop attacks, and even amenorrhea may develop as the deficits progress.[45] Because the tumor is more likely to be in the midline in children, progressive limb ataxia largely limited to one side of the body is unlikely to occur in children and is more characteristic of the adult with medulloblastoma. Facial weakness is also more likely to develop in the adult with the more laterally placed tumor, and this sign occurs in more than 40 percent of affected adults.[45] As the tumor enlarges the patient's course usually changes suddenly with the development or rapid progression of an obstructive hydrocephalus. Much of the gait difficulty and confusion occurring in these patients may disappear with correction of the increased intracranial pressure alone.[56] Without treatment this lesion is likely to be fatal within a matter of months from the appearance of the first signs.

Therapy

Surgery is necessary both to obtain tissue for tumor identification and to decompress the posterior fossa, but it cannot provide a cure or even extended palliation. Some neurosurgeons approach these tumors by attempting a biopsy through a burr hole rather than with a suboccipital craniectomy.[3] This approach to the tumor does not affect the outcome significantly, but it does have the limitation of requiring further surgery if the preoperative impression is not accurate and the tumor proves to be an astrocytoma.

The medulloblastoma is highly radiosensitive.[20] In situ eradication of the tumor with a total dose to the posterior fossa of 5,000 rads is a reasonable expectation, but the inclination of the tumor to seed the subarachnoid space[48] necessitates irradiation of the entire craniospinal axis. With brain, posterior fossa, and spinal cord irradiation, apparent cures of medulloblastoma have been achieved.[20, 51] Patients surviving more than three years are often free of any tumor cells, and the five year survival with radiotherapy may be as high as 50 percent.[29] The disadvantages of radiation include bone marrow depression in young adults and the late development of thyroid carcinoma in children. Hair loss invariably occurs, but the loss is only transient for most patients. Skin reactions occur unpredictably, and with current radiation dose schedules they are uncommon. Kyphoscoliosis may develop if spinal cord irradiation damages spinal epiphyses. All effects considered together, the benefits of irradiation greatly outweigh the disadvantages.

Some chemotherapeutic agents have been used as part of the treatment regimen for medulloblastoma. Vincristine and lomustine administered for the treatment of peritoneal metastases following ventriculoperitoneal shunt have been reported to cause some shrinkage of the metastatic mass.[33] In other cases with bone metastases, combinations of vincristine and cyclophosphamide[36] have resulted in decreased pain from the affected bones within days of administration and evidence of reossification in these bones.[36] Other attempts at chemotherapy have included vincristine, prednisone, and carmustine in the treatment regimen.[38] All of these chemotherapeutic trials have resulted in only temporary palliation.

Prognosis

Life expectancy with medulloblastoma is about 9 months from the onset of symptoms if the tumor is left untreated.[29] Despite the use of meticulous surgical techniques, the tumor cannot be removed from the cerebellum or the fourth ventricle without leaving some residual cells. Even if the tumor were adequately circumscribed to allow a gross surgical resection, the tendency to spread in the central nervous system would limit the true cures to a small fraction of patients. Hemorrhage into the cerebellar tumor may be the terminal event (Fig. 6).

The "cerebellar arachnoid sarcomas" have a higher probability of being completely resected than the more typical medulloblastomas.[53] The "arachnoid sarcoma" is a variant of the medulloblastoma with peaks of incidence in the first and third decades of life whereas the more typical medulloblastoma occurs in highest incidence at about 6 years of age.[29] Identical approaches to these two tumor types result in a better survival for the group with the "arachnoid sarcoma" type medulloblastoma.[18, 53] A series of 201 cases with surgery and irradiation used to treat the medulloblastomas revealed an average survival after surgery of 18 months for the typical medulloblastoma and of 51 months for the "arachnoid sarcoma."[10] The

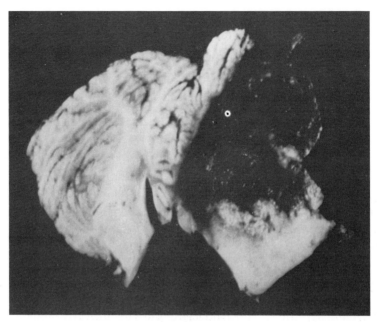

Figure 6. A coronal section through the cerebellum of a 29-year-old woman with a medulloblastoma invading the right cerebellar hemisphere. The patient developed headache, nausea, vomiting, dizziness, and right hand clumsiness over the course of 2 weeks at the age of 20. Despite recurrence of the tumor within 6 years of its original excision, the patient survived 9 years. Total irradiation to the posterior fossa approached 10,000 rads. The terminal event was a hemorrhage into the tumor. The friable tumor is still apparent at the lower margin of the blood clot.

"arachnoid sarcoma" type occurred primarily in adults, a group which had an average survival of 50 months regardless of the type of medulloblastoma.

Comparing patients under 10 years of age with those over 10 years of age, Miles and coworkers[45] found that 67 percent of the older group survived more than one year as opposed to only 33 percent of those under 10 years of age (Fig. 7). Survival is, of course, shortened when metastases develop.[33] Women and girls did better in Miles' series[45] when they were compared as a group with men and boys. The best survival with optimum treatment appeared in female patients between 10 and 20 years of age. The mean duration of survival in this group is nearly 5 years. In another study, five year survival reached 16 percent for the adult group, compared to 1 percent for patients under 16 year of age, but these patients clearly received inadequate postoperative irradiation.[29]

Case Presentation

The following case is presented to illustrate a typical mode of onset and progression in an adolescent with a medulloblastoma.

A 14-year-old right-handed girl complained of occipital headache for several months, with the most severe pain and occasional vomiting occurring in the morning. She had increasing gait difficulty and clumsiness in her right hand. She developed transient episodes in which her vision appeared gray. Speech became nasal and syncope occurred. Her handwriting deteriorated over the month prior to admission and she noticed less "force" in her voice. Her family complained that

344

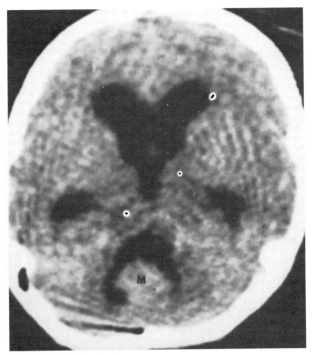

Figure 7. CT scan without contrast enhancement in a 10-year-old boy with a 9 week history of occipital headaches, vomiting, blurred vision, dizziness, and right head tilt. A large midline medulloblastoma (M) extended into the fourth ventricle and produced substantial hydrocephalus.

she had become reticent and withdrawn. On initial examination she was alert and cooperative, but her memory was impaired. She retained new information poorly and had a limited digit span of four forward and three backward. She had papilledema bilaterally, minor flattening of the right nasolabial fold, ocular dysmetria with gaze to the right, and gaze-evoked nystagmus with lateral and upward gaze. Her head was tilted to the left. Her gait was broad-based and unsteady, with falling to the left on attempted tandem gait. Decomposition of movement, impaired check, and excessive rebound were limited to the right arm. Dysmetria was more apparent in the right arm than the right leg, and succession deficits were apparent in both the right arm and the left. The deep tendon reflexes were generally decreased.

Computerized tomography revealed a large posterior fossa mass in the midline, extending up to the tentorium cerebelli and into the right hemisphere (Fig. 8). There was enhancement of the mass with contrast material. A ventriculoperitoneal shunt was placed three days prior to surgery, but the patient was not affected substantially by this procedure. Suboccipital craniectomy uncovered a medulloblastoma filling the fourth ventricle and infiltrating much of the vermis. The inferior vermis was split and the tumor partially resected. Extension into the ventricular aspects of the hemispheres was much more prominent on the right. The tumor did not extend through the vermis to its cortical surface. Radiotherapy to the posterior fossa, whole brain, and spinal axis was administered after the surgery.

Six months after surgery the patient had intact memory and mentation, normal speech, no papilledema, and slight ataxia in the right arm. She had gaze-evoked

345

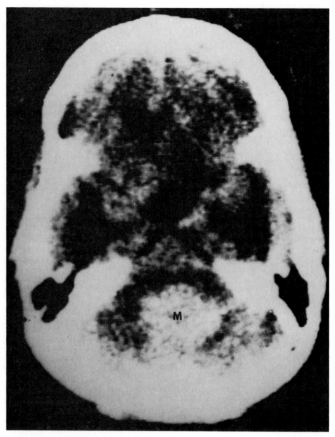

Figure 8. CT scan with contrast enhancement of a midline medulloblastoma (M). The patient was a 14-year-old girl who complained of occipital headaches and vomiting for several months prior to developing intermittently blurred vision, progressive gait difficulty, and right sided clumsiness. At surgery, the tumor was largely limited to the vermis with extension into the fourth ventricle.

nystagmus on right lateral gaze and minimal spontaneous upbeat nystagmus. The deep tendon reflexes were pendular on the right.

This adolescent patient responded in a fairly typical fashion to surgical and radiation therapy of a large medulloblastoma. The improved mentation after surgery preceded completion of the radiation treatment, indicating that it responded in part to relief of the obstructive hydrocephalus. Her limb ataxia and nystagmus would be expected to decrease further with time, though focal deficits indicative of cerebellar damage can persist indefinitely after subtotal resection and irradiation of a medulloblastoma.

Astrocytoma

Incidence

Cerebellar astrocytomas are circumscribed, slowly growing tumors, developing most often in childhood (Fig. 9). The age of onset for symptomatic tumors ranges from under 2 years of age to over 20 but in most cases falls between these limits.

346

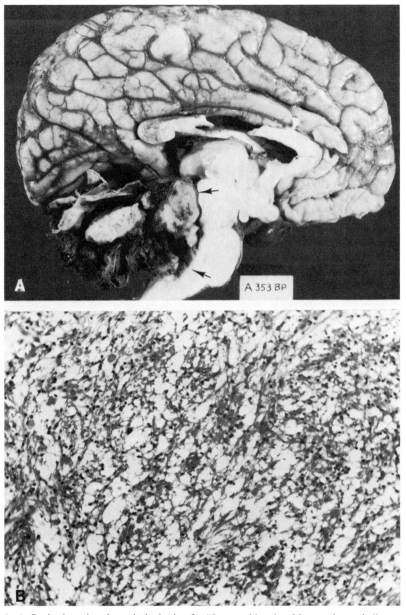

Figure 9. A, Sagittal section through the brain of a 15-year-old male with a cystic cerebellar astrocytoma compressing the midbrain (upper arrow) and invading the fourth ventricle (lower arrow). The patient was mentally retarded and had generalized neurofibromatosis with cafe-au-lait spots and soft skin tumors. At age 11 he developed headaches, vomiting, intermittent paresis of the left arm, and an ataxic gait. Examination revealed ataxic movements of the left limbs, mild weakness of the right limbs, and a wide based ataxic gait. A suboccipital craniectomy at age 11 revealed a large, firm tumor which proved to be an astrocytoma. The patient expired at age 15. B, Microscopic section of a cerebellar astrocytoma showing typical pilocytic features with compact areas of fibrillated fusiform cells and long, thin nuclei often arranged in parallel bands. There are prominent bundles of glial fibrils separated by spongy areas (phosphotungstic acid hematoxylin stain).

Cerebellar astrocytomas account for 8 percent of all gliomas and 30 percent of childhood gliomas,[35] ranking in some series as the most common infratentorial tumor of childhood.[23] They differ from cerebral astrocytomas in both morphology and behavior, although astrocytomas of the sort developing supratentorially occasionally appear in the cerebellum.[21] In rare cases,[35] a typical cerebellar astrocytoma will transform over the course of years to an anaplastic astrocytoma of the cerebral type.

Pathology

Based upon microscopic features, astrocytomas usually are divided into *protoplasmic, gemistocytic, fibrillary, piloid* or *pilocytic,* and *anaplastic* or *malignant.*[4, 25, 37, 60] The cellular appearance, cytoplasmic mass, staining qualities, and cellular arrangement characterize each of these tumor types. An alternative to this classification system is Kernohan's grading system in which the grade of tissue malignancy is estimated from the heterogeneity of nuclei, areas of necrosis, prevalence of mitotic figures, cellular pleomorphism, and blood vessel changes. Astrocytomas arising in the cerebellum do not conform well to either system of classification. Tissue appearing to be grade III or relatively malignant in Kernohan's system is likely to behave as benignly as a grade I or unequivocally benign tumor when it is found in the cerebellum. When cerebellar astrocytomas are separated into the histologic types used to describe cerebral astrocytomas, the cerebellar tumors appear to fit best into the group designated piloid or pilocytic (Fig. 9B). This classification, however, is inadequate to distinguish between the forms of cerebellar astrocytoma.

The typical pilocytic astrocytoma has compact areas of fibrillated fusiform cells, with long, thin nuclei, often arranged in parallel bands.[25, 37] Because this tumor appears most often in childhood, it is known also as the juvenile pilocytic astrocytoma.[25] It has features of the fibrillary or fibrous astrocytoma group and a clear distinction is not always made between these two forms of astrocytoma.[4] The fibrillary astrocytoma has coarse or fine fibrils which stain specifically with the PTAH method. These fibers are distributed generously throughout the tumor. Large globular cells wih eccentric nuclei, characteristic of the gemistocytic astrocytoma, are not likely to be found in the cerebellar astrocytoma, but the highly cystic matrix typical of the protoplasmic astrocytoma may be found in areas of the cerebellar tumor.

The inadequacy of the pilocytic designation to distinguish between various forms of cerebellar astrocytoma and the inaccuracy of the malignancy grading system in predicting the course of cerebellar astrocytomas prompted the separation of cerebellar astrocytomas into three categories.[25] The first type of juvenile pilocytic astrocytoma conforms precisely to the benign homogeneous appearance of the classic pilocytic astrocytoma; the second type is similar to the pilocytic astrocytoma, but also has prominent bundles of glial fibrils separated by spongy areas; the third type is indistinguishable from the anaplastic cerebral gliomas which have endothelial hyperplasia, giant cells, and atypical nuclei. The anaplastic form of cerebellar astrocytoma differs from the cerebral type; in the cerebellum the tumor usually is well circumscribed and noninvasive.[14] Any of these three types can exhibit inconsistently occurring features with no malignant prognosis, including eosinophilic hyaline droplets, dense fibrillary areas interspersed with microcysts, and foci of oligodendroglioma cells.[22] Irregular masses seen with hematoxy-

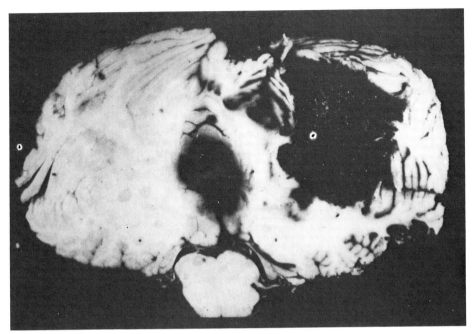

Figure 10. Coronal section through the cerebellum of a 59-year-old man with a cystic astrocytoma invading the vermis and left hemisphere. The patient complained of intermittent vertigo and progressive gait difficulty for 5 months. Headache, vomiting, and increasing instability in the left arm prompted the investigation that revealed the tumor. The patient died immediately after surgery from hemorrhage into the tumor bed.

lin and eosin staining are scattered between fascicles of coarsely fibrillated bipolar cells. The masses are called Rosenthal fibers and probably represent degenerated astrocytic processes.[60] The presence of these masses also is a benign feature.

Most cerebellar astrocytomas are extensively cystic, and some appear as little more than a mural nodule in a fluid filled cyst[60] (Fig. 10). Only 20 percent of these tumors are grossly solid.[35] Solid tumors occur primarily in the vermis[23] and typically are present only in childhood cases.[60] Cerebellar cysts presenting in adult life with no mural tumor nodules may represent the final stage of degeneration of highly cystic cerebellar astrocytomas.[60] These cysts become symptomatic in middle age; the average age at the onset of symptoms is 34 years. Clearly they are not ependymal cysts arising from the fourth ventricle. The cyst wall is composed of dense astroglial cells with no lining epithelium and it is surrounded by many Rosenthal fibers. If this is the endpoint of astrocytoma degeneration in the cerebellum, radiation to partly resected astrocytomas may be both unnecessary and hazardous. The irradiation might account for some cases of malignant transformation in cerebellar astrocytomas.

Seventy-nine percent of truly malignant astrocytomas occur in the lateral portions of the cerebellum.[14] Most affected patients are adults; two-thirds of cerebellar "glioblastoma multiforme" cases appear in individuals with a median age of 47 years. Most adult cases and virtually all childhood cases of cerebellar glioblastoma develop from tumor originating outside the cerebellum. Substantial evidence of glioblastoma arising as a primary cerebellar tumor has appeared in the reports

349

of only 11 cases.[21] Anaplastic progression of a brainstem glioma to a highly malignant astrocytoma is not at all unusual in children, but progression of an intrinsic cerebellar astrocytoma to glioblastoma multiforme is rare.[35] Malignant transformation of the cerebellar tumor is signaled by hypercellularity, frequent mitoses, areas of necrosis, pseudopalisading of bipolar cells about necrotic zones, and a diffusely infiltrating growth pattern.[21] Median survival with these highly anaplastic astrocytomas is only one year.[14]

In a series of 132 children with various gliomas of the cerebellum, excluding medulloblastomas, all but 10 percent could be characterized by two sets of features, designated *A* and *B*.[63] *A* features were microcysts, Rosenthal fibers, foci of oligodendroglia, and leptomeningeal deposits. *B* features were perivascular pseudorosettes, necrosis, high cell density, frequent mitoses, and calcification. These features have considerable significance in prognosis, as described below.

Symptoms and Signs

The clinical history in cases of cerebellar astrocytoma is longer than that for patients with medulloblastoma or ependymoma.[6] Headache and vomiting appear 4 to 5 months before the appearance of other symptoms such as gait difficulty and clumsiness.[23] Staggering, impaired running, and difficulty turning are the complaints usually prompting medical attention. This is true for both benign and malignant astrocytoma. By the time a disorder of gait develops, there is evidence of longstanding increased intracranial pressure.[23] Progressive limb ataxia appears as the tumor grows, especially if it involves a hemisphere. As with medulloblastomas, the signs and symptoms of the neoplasm reflect the site of disease.[16] More than half of all cerebellar astrocytomas occur in the midline.[23] Obstructive hydrocephalus develops with this tumor, but at a later stage of growth than with ependymomas and medulloblastomas, which are more likely to fill and obstruct the fourth ventricle. Papilledema is present commonly as a sign of the increased intracranial pressure, and when skull films show separation of the sutures, papilledema invariably is present.[23]

Therapy

Cerebellar astrocytomas often are cured by resection. If complete resection is impossible, partial resection of the tumor may provide years or decades of symptom-free life.[4] In most cases, if symptoms are going to recur, they appear within a few years after surgery. A patient apparently free of disease for five years is likely to remain free of tumor symptoms indefinitely. If the astrocytoma extends along the ventricle, toward the aqueduct, or into the cerebellar peduncle, complete resection is not feasible.[6] When resection of the tumor is complete, as it usually is, the survival at 5 years with no other treatment is as high as 93 percent after the immediate postoperative period.[25, 37] With incomplete resection, survivals ranging from 12 to 39 years after surgery have been documented, even if no irradiation or chemotherapy is given to these children.[23] Survival is not altered by irradiation.[25] One of the causes of increased mortality with medulloblastoma and with ependymoma is subarachnoid or ventricular seeding with tumor cells. This is a notably uncommon occurrence with cerebellar astrocytomas.[56] Even in the rare cases where there has been seeding, survival has not been foreshortened.[56]

350

Prognosis

As mentioned earlier, certain histologic features in cerebellar astrocytomas have strong prognostic significance. In a recent study, patients with astrocytomas having strictly type *A* features had a 10 year survival of 94 percent after surgery.[63] Patients with type *B* astrocytomas had a 10 year survival of only 29 percent. Some features had greater prognostic significance than others. Calcification alone was associated with a high mortality, but not if it occurred with other type *A* features. All children with macrocysts had a low mortality and the 10 year survival for a group based on this one feature was 85 percent. These survivals were considered strictly postsurgical survivals since radiation therapy given to some patients and not to others had no effect on survival in the group with either type *A* or type *B* features.[63] Some impressive differences appear if type *A* tumors are subdivided into those with strongly fibrillated areas separated by loosely packed nonfibrillated astrocytes and microcysts and those with uniform cells and evenly distributed glial fibers.[25] The former type, termed "juvenile cerebellar astrocytoma," has a 94 percent survival rate at 25 years, whereas the latter type, termed "diffuse benign astrocytoma," has a 38 percent survival rate at 25 years postoperatively.[25] These studies also indicated an improved prognosis with cystic, as opposed to solid, tumors. The juvenile type has the onset of signs from 0 to 14 years of age with no striking peak, while the diffuse benign form occurs primarily in the 10- to 14-year-old age group. Thus, although these are both histologically benign tumors, they are substantially different in morphology, onset, and prognosis.

The overall survival of patients with cerebellar astrocytomas has improved during recent years, an observation which may reflect changes in the tumor as much as advances in neurosurgery and postoperative care. The incidence of foci of oligodendroglia, a good prognostic sign, has increased steadily from the early 1950s to the present.[22] Indeed, all group *A*[63] features have been increasing in incidence over the past two decades,[22] a change in tumor character inexplicable in terms of current understanding of tumor pathogenesis. Such changes in the basic character of a tumor place considerable constraints upon the interpretation of the effectiveness of new treatments. If historical controls are used, any agent introduced in the 1970s would appear to be improving survival. Any trials of chemotherapeutic agents or radiotherapy regimens in the treatment of cerebellar astrocytomas must include a sample of patients simultaneously left untreated, except for surgery.

Case Presentation

The following patient illustrates the typical onset and progression in cases of cerebellar astrocytoma.

A 20-year-old woman developed morning headaches centering about the occiput or over the frontal area. Within a few months, the headaches increased in severity and were accompanied by vomiting. After the headaches and vomiting had persisted for about six months, she developed double vision on looking to the left. Coincident with diplopia, her gait deteriorated. Staggering and frequent falling started about one month before hospital admission.

On examination, she was alert and cooperative and her speech was normal. She was unable to walk at all because of a tendency to fall. Bilateral papilledema with hemorrhages was associated with a left abducens palsy. She had no nystagmus, but there was left facial weakness. Rebound was excessive and check was impaired in both arms, with the right side affected more severely than the left. Dysmetria also was more prominent on the right than the left, and her arms were more affected than her legs. Rapid alternating movements were impaired similarly. The arms were hypotonic and the deep tendon reflexes were symmetric.

A ventriculogram revealed significant displacement of the fourth ventricle from right to left. Cerebrospinal fluid protein was 60 mg/dl. Suboccipital craniectomy revealed a cystic astrocytoma replacing the inferior vermis. A macrocyst containing 40 ml of fluid filled the fourth ventricle and infiltrated the vermis. Although the cyst pressed laterally into both hemispheres, there was no apparent infiltration of tumor into either hemisphere, and it was resected completely.

Immediately after surgery, check and rebound were greatly improved, but a left VIth and a left VIIth nerve palsy persisted. Radiotherapy was administered to the posterior fossa to a total dose of 4600 rads over six weeks. Two months after surgery her gait was entirely normal and no dysmetria was evident. She was readmitted eight years later with ulcerative colitis and was free of all neurologic deficits at that time.

This patient had the slow progression of symptoms and signs referable to the posterior fossa commonly observed with cerebellar astrocytoma. Her favorable response to surgical therapy was typical, but she was unusual in showing such a complete reversal of symptoms and signs.

Metastatic Disease

Metastatic tumors involving the cerebellum are common in most series of cerebellar neoplasms[1] and were the most common type of pathology in the series of Lechtenberg and Gilman (see Table 2). Metastatic tumors occur chiefly in adults, principally after the third or fourth decade of life. Solitary lesions in the cerebellum occur more often than multiple tumors.[42, 57] Twenty-five percent of solitary metastases in the brain develop in the cerebellum.[42] The common sources of metastases include the lung (Fig. 11), breast, gastrointestinal tract, skin, and kidney.[57] Bronchogenic carcinoma is the most frequent source of metastases in all patients,[57] but breast carcinoma is responsible for many cerebellar tumors in women.

The symptoms and signs of cerebellar disease may be the first evidence that the patient has a tumor, the primary lesion remaining occult until the metastasis is advanced. Headache is by far the most common presenting symptom, although gait difficulty appears early and further evidence of cerebellar dysfunction becomes more prominent as the lesion expands. Arteriography, computerized tomography, and skull radiographs help to establish the nature of the lesion in most cases, but a diagnosis of metastatic disease in a patient with no extracranial evidence of metastases should be held suspect until tissue is available. Even when a primary lesion already has been identified, biopsy of a cerebellar lesion will spare the patient the misfortune of an improperly diagnosed benign cerebellar lesion occurring coincidentally with a tumor elsewhere in the body.

The treatment of solitary cerebellar metastases is controversial. In our view, there are clear advantages to operating on these lesions if the patient's overall condition is sufficiently stable to permit the risks of surgery. Radiation of the cerebellar lesion may produce considerable relief of signs if the neoplasm is radio-

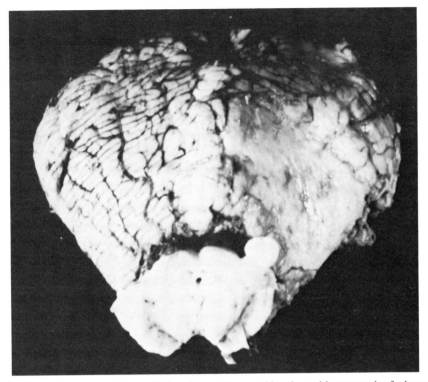

Figure 11. Superior aspect of the cerebellum from a 47-year-old patient with metastasis of a broncho-genic carcinoma to the left cerebellar hemisphere. The patient had headache, nausea, and vomiting for 3 months prior to developing gait difficulty and diplopia. The tumor could not be resected and radio-therapy was administered, but survival was limited to 5 months from the initial diagnosis.

sensitive.[49] The prognosis is poor for patients with metastatic disease to the cerebellum; both the quality and duration of survival are worse than with meta-static disease to supratentorial structures.[57] The tumor type is the most important factor determining the length of survival.

The mean survival with metastatic lung carcinoma is about three months, whereas paients with breast metastases survive on the average a year. Malignant melanoma has as grim a prognosis as lung carcinoma and the outlook with gas-trointestinal carcinoma is even poorer.[57] Part of the limited prognosis with these metastases is attributable to their inclination to bleed.[41] Even without a terminal hemorrhage, tumors metastatic to the cerebellum eventually will compress vital brainstem structures if the patient lives long enough to allow substantial tumor growth.[16]

Case Presentation

The following patient illustrates the onset and progression of symptoms with a metastatic cerebellar neoplasm.

A 59-year-old woman complained of an occipital headache lasting days at a time and recurring several times over the course of a month. She had vertigo, nausea, and vomiting initially associated with the headaches and after three weeks she developed progressive gait difficulty. Her mentation also changed over the weeks prior to admission, changes best characterized as confusion. She was disoriented and argumentative. On examination, her speech was normal. Papilledema appeared in both fundi and nystagmus was evoked on right lateral gaze. Heel-to-shin and finger-to-nose tests revealed ataxia on the right more than on the left. Rapid alternating movements were intact and rebound was not excessive. Muscle strength was intact but she was unable to walk alone. Her unsteady gait worsened with attempted turning.

Electroencephalography and echoencephalography were normal initially, but a subsequent electroencephalogram revealed bilateral temporal slowing. A radionuclide brain scan demonstrated right posterior fossa uptake. Cerebrospinal fluid protein was 90 mg/dl and the opening pressure was 280 mm H_2O. Ventriculography confirmed the presence of a mass displacing the right cerebellar hemisphere, and on surgical exploration this proved to be a metastatic carcinoma nodule measuring 4 cm × 3 cm. It was found subsequently to have originated in the gastrointestinal tract. The mass was resected from the inferior aspect of the lateral part of the right hemisphere. Postoperatively, the patient's mentation became more clear and appropriate and her gait improved, but the previous level of ataxia persisted in both arms.

She was stable after surgery for only two months at which time her primarily frontal headaches recurred in association with increasing stupor. On readmission nine weeks after surgery, she was unable to walk and had bilateral abducens palsies. She had a kinetic tremor on finger-to-nose testing, especially on the left. The deep tendon reflexes were increased on the left and the right pupil was larger than the left. Repeat arteriography demonstrated a right frontal intracerebral mass. After whole brain irradiation and chemotherapy she failed to improve. Within a few weeks she worsened: she had nystagmus on both horizontal and vertical gaze; dysmetria was prominent bilaterally; and kinetic tremor was present, worse on the left than the right. Additional radiotherapy and chemotherapy were administered but the patient continued her deterioration and died 20 months after her first admission to the hospital.

The relentless deterioration observed in this case exemplifies the inadequacy of current therapy in the management of most metastatic lesions to the cerebellum. The primary tumor must be dealt with effectively by chemotherapy. Until such treatment is available, resection of cerebellar metastases will be palliative in most instances. Many patients still do profit considerably from resection of individual nodules and patients with potentially fatal cerebellar metastases have survived years after the resection of a metastatic nodule.[57]

Ependymoma

Incidence

Intracranial ependymomas comprise 3.2 percent of all brain tumors[55] and about 12 percent of primary intracranial neoplasms of children.[39] They occur much less often in children than infratentorial astrocytomas and medulloblastomas, but still rank as the third most common infratentorial tumor of childhood.[55] Sixty-five percent of brain ependymomas are in the posterior fossa.[39]

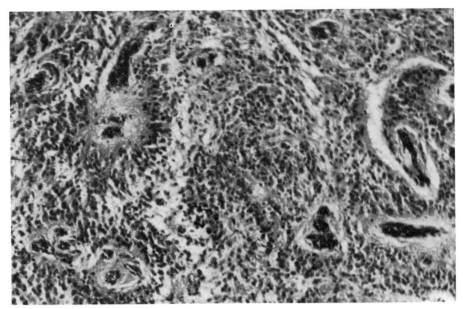

Figure 12. Histologic section of a recurrent fatal ependymoma of the cerebellum and medulla in a 3-year-old child. The patient presented at age 28 months with complaints of vomiting and frequent stumbling of 3½ months duration. On examination the patient had a broad based gait with falling to either side, papilledema, extensor plantar responses, and unsustained clonus at the ankles. In this section, the tumor is composed of ependymal cells often radiating by their processes from vessels or clustered in groups. In other places, the tumor cells form long ependymal cavities. There is a moderately high mitotic rate in many parts of the growth (phosphotungstic acid hematoxylin stain).

Pathology

The infratentorial ependymoma is not truly a cerebellar tumor; it is a posterior fossa tumor which occasionally damages the cerebellum. Ependymomas arise from the lining of the fourth ventricle or the choroid plexus and develop into tumors often compressing, if not actually invading, the cerebellum. Ependymomas invariably have more than one characteristic cell type or tissue arrangement (Fig. 12); the tumors develop as a mixture of neoplastic forms. The three major forms are papillary, glandular, and cellular.[39] The choroid plexus papilloma may be included as a fourth form because it is similar in cell type to well differentiated ependymomas. The choroid plexus papilloma has an outer layer of well differentiated stratified or columnar cells overlying a highly branched connective tissue core rich with blood vessels. The tumor morphology is reminiscent of normal choroid plexus, even to the point of not invading brain tissue. The base of the papilloma may have less well differentiated cells. Viewed in this way, the choroid plexus papilloma is a form of ependymoma slightly better differentiated than the papillary ependymoma.[39]

The *papillary* form of ependymoma has villi covered with tumor cells which range from cuboidal at the base to multipolar superficially. This type of tumor is not at all anaplastic. It may be referred to as myxopapillary when individual papillae are distended by accumulations of a mucinous substance in the tumor stroma. The *glandular* form of ependymoma is the least common type, but it may appear

355

interspersed with the more common papillary form.[39] The cells of the glandular tumor are also well differentiated, but they are termed glandular because of the arrangement of columnar cells around glandular spaces of various size. The columnar cells form ependymal rosettes with cilia filling the minute central lumens formed by the radially oriented cells. The *cellular* form of ependymoma is the most common type. The cells of this tumor have elongated processes drawn to blood vessel walls and perivascular pseudorosettes occur typically. The arrangement of cells in the cellular type is less orderly than in either the papillary or glandular form, but the cells still have uniform ovoid nuclei. This type of ependymoma may be confused with astrocytomas because of the nuclear appearance and random cell arrangement, but the principal cells of the ependymoma do not demonstrate glial fibers on phosphotungstic acid-hematoxylin stain, as found with astrocytomas. The ependymoma cells also have blepharoplasts, the intracellular base plates for their cilia, stained by the PTAH method.[15] Areas resembling astrocytoma or oligodendroglioma are intermingled with these other tissue types, thereby further complicating the identification of the tumor. Recurrent waves of palisading cells may appear in the cellular type of ependymoma, a histologic appearance much more typical of medulloblastoma. This apparent palisading is probably from obliquely sectioned perivascular pseudorosettes. Necrosis and hemorrhage are common, but cysts and mucin are rare.[59]

The ependymoblastoma is not typically an infratentorial tumor.[15] It is a highly anaplastic form of ependymoma with closely packed, hyperchromatic cells with scanty cytoplasmic processes. The usual site of tumor extension is about the lateral ventricles.

Dividing ependymomas into three grades, A, B, and C, on the basis of differentiation[39] and irrespective of tumor type, provides a fairly reliable basis for predicting tumor behavior. Grade A is the most well differentiated tumor, regardless of whether it shows one or several histologic patterns. Grade C ependymoma has bizarre giant cells, hyperchromaticism, and other signs of anaplastic change. Grade B is an intermediate form. Infratentorial ependymomas are largely grade A, thereby providing a good prognosis for survival if the tumor is resected completely.[39] Resection is not always possible, however; 90 percent of infratentorial ependymomas arise in the lateral recesses of the fourth ventricle or in the floor of the ventricle.[59] Extirpation from the floor of the ventricle is dangerous, resulting in an operative mortality reaching as high as 40 percent.[55]

As with medulloblastomas, seeding from the tumor may result in spread of the lesions and reduce the likelihood of recovery after removal of the original ependymoma. The five year survival with subarachnoid spread of the tumor despite posterior fossa irradiation in one series of 32 patients was 16.7 percent as opposed to 51.3 percent in patients with local irradiation and no spread.[34] Seeding from ependymomas is apparent clinically in only 3 percent of all cases, whether infratentorial or supratentorial.[55] Forty percent of patients have tumor cells that can be collected from the spinal fluid on lumbar or cisternal puncture.[18] Spinal implants are more likely with infratentorial than supratentorial ependymomas, especially if they are poorly differentiated.[34] The clinical manifestations of seeding are rarer than the documented instances of seeding,[2, 18] indicating that not all of these tumor cells can proliferate in the subarachnoid space or in the ventricle. Nonetheless, estimates of spinal metastases ranging up to 47 percent with posterior fossa ependymomas[34] are weighty arguments for total craniospinal axis irradiation after the discovery of an infratentorial ependymoma.

Symptoms and Signs

The most common age for the onset of symptoms from an ependymoma is between one and two years.[39] The mean age for diagnosis is five years. The presentation in patients with ependymoma is not substantially different from that seen with medulloblastomas and astrocytomas.[1] Headache, nausea, vomiting, gait difficulty, and obtundation are likely to dominate the clinical picture, not as a result of cerebellar damage, but rather from the obstructive hydrocephalus likely to develop with this usually intraventicular tumor.[59] More focal signs of cerebellar damage such as kinetic tremor, limb dysmetria, and unilateral deficits of rapid alternating movements may be absent or appear only late in the course of the disease.

Therapy

Effective treatment requires both surgical resection and postoperative irradiation.[2] Complete resection should be attempted whenever feasible. Irradiation to a wide area about the operative site may be adequate when full resection is possible. With residual tumor or a high grade malignancy, 5000 rads to the posterior fossa over 60 days and 3000 to 4000 rads to the remainder of the craniospinal axis is advisable.[34] Repeated surgery may be necessary when the tumor recurs. Repeated radiotherapy is limited by the allowable tissue dose. No chemotherapy has yet proved useful, other than the use of high dose steroids to limit edema.

Prognosis

The prognosis with ependymoma depends upon several factors, including the site of the tumor, the type of histology, the age of the patient at the onset, and the type of therapy. The prognosis for ependymoma is generally better than that for medulloblastoma, but poorer than that for astrocytoma. The prognosis in ependymoma is poorest when the tumor is in the fourth ventricle and is characterized histologically as grade C. Tumors in the fourth ventricle appear in the youngest of the ependymoma patients, and these patients may have rapidly growing tumors which are not necessarily invasive.

Survival with optimal treatment varies greatly in different studies.[2, 15, 55] Five year survival figures range from 12 percent to 51 percent and much of the discrepancy in survival rates between series derives from combining both infratentorial and supratentorial tumors[15] and the inclusion of choroid plexus papillomas[39] as a form of ependymoma in some series. Supratentorial ependymomas have a better prognosis than infratentorial lesions,[15] and choroid plexus papillomas may be cured with resection alone.[28] The recurrence rate of resected ependymomas, excluding choroid plexus papillomas, is about 71 percent even with irradiation and various efforts at chemotherapy.[18] Radiation therapy is an important factor in outcome. The two year survival is only 17 percent for those operated upon but not irradiated whereas survival increases to 35 percent at two years when irradiation is given after surgery.[15] The apparent advantage of treating with irradiation disappears by five years after the surgery. Survival with irradiation at that time is 12 percent and without irradiation is 17 percent. Series with better survival figures contain older patients with more well differentiated tumors.[34] Although the ependymoma may recur whether it is supratentorial, infratentorial, or spinal, the fourth ventricle tumor has the shortest symptom free period if the tumor is to recur.[59]

357

Case Presentation

The following patient shows a characteristic history of onset and progression of symptoms resulting from a cerebellar ependymoma.

A 3-year-old boy complained of headaches and was noticed to be unstable on his feet. At age $2\frac{1}{2}$, after several weeks of slight unsteadiness, he developed a waddling gait and had clumsy arm movements. These symptoms progressed over the next six months until he became unable to walk without holding onto objects. Immediately prior to admission, he had difficulty sitting up without assistance. His parents noticed that when the child was younger he seemed to be right handed, whereas at the time he was admitted to the hospital, he was clearly left handed.

Neurologic examination revealed papilledema bilaterally and an abnormal gait. He waddled on a wide base and could not walk on his heels or run. A slight body tilt to the left was noted. The finger-to-nose test was performed poorly bilaterally with the right side more impaired than the left. He had significant past-pointing on the right. The deep tendon reflexes were generally decreased. During the hospitalization he had morning vomiting, coincident with headaches which were localized about the occiput.

Skull x-ray revealed a calcification in the posterior fossa, an electroencephalogram was normal, and a radionuclide brain scan was positive. There was increased uptake of mercury isotope on the left side of the posterior fossa. An arteriogram suggested a large mass filling the fourth ventricle and computerized tomography confirmed the presence of a mass in the fourth ventricle extending into the left cerebellopontine angle. Suboccipital craniectomy revealed an ependymoma extending from the posterior fossa into the spinal canal to the level of C_3. The tumor extended under the left lateral medulla and appeared to arise from the left lateral recess of the fourth ventricle. The tumor was resected incompletely.

Immediately after surgery, the patient had a transient gaze palsy, persistent left facial weakness, and mild right sided weakness. Two weeks after the surgery, he had not returned to his normal level of consciousness. He was still quite irritable, appeared apathetic, and had an obvious left VIth nerve weakness. Radiotherapy was administered to the posterior fossa, as well as the whole brain and spinal axis. Within three weeks of the irradiaion he was more vocal and alert. Two-and-a-half months after surgery, he continued to show no new signs except for a head tilt to the left and nystagmus on left lateral gaze. His gait did not improve after surgery and he could walk only with assistance.

This patient showed the progressive disorder of cerrebellar function characteristic of ependymomas in this location as well as the development of symptoms and signs resulting from obstruction to the fourth ventricle. The definite but incomplete improvement after both surgical resection and radiotherapy is also characteristic.

Hemangioblastoma

Incidence

Hemangioblastoma is a benign tumor occurring only in the nervous system. It accounts for 7 to 12 percent of posterior fossa neoplasms and occurs most often in the cerebellum.[30] Retinal angiomas, vascular tumors with histologic features of the hemangioblastoma, develop with this cerebellar tumor in the von Hippel-Lindau syndrome. The tumor usually becomes symptomatic in the fourth decade of life, although with this neoplasm, more than with other cerebellar tumors, there is a broad range of ages at which the patient may become symptomatic.

Pathology

The tumor presents the appearance of a fine mesh of blood channels on light microscopy (Fig. 13).[31] Endothelial cells lining the vessels and forming the capillaries are entirely benign. A normal basement membrane appears on reticulin staining and stromal cells between the blood vessels have no mitoses. The interstitial cells are small and round, large and slightly polygonal, or large and distended by mucin. Based on the histologic appearance and the pattern of basement membranes, these tumors can be divided into capillary, cellular, or cavernous.[31] These designations refer to the most prominent tissue features. Based upon cell morphology, these tumors segregate into three types, type A or juvenile with no mucin-distended (clear) cells, type B or transitional with few mucin-distended cells, and type C with virtually all interstitial cells of the clear type. Although the clear cells probably arise from the small round cells, this latter classification does correlate with some behavioral characteristics of the hemangioblastoma. Type A tumors occur in the younger age group and are not associated with an elevated serum hemoglobin. Erythropoietin is found in cyst fluid of B and C tumors but not in A. Other tumor characteristics have prognostic value. Patients with cystic tu-

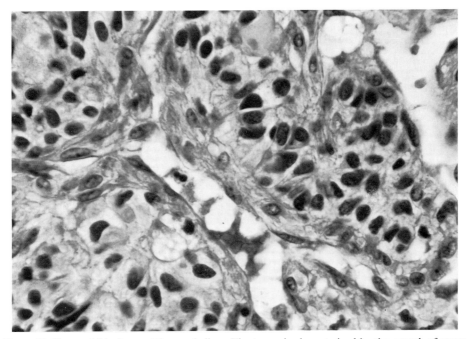

Figure 13. Hemangioblastom⸻ ⸻ the cerebellum. The tumor is characterized by the growth of many small vessels among which are numerous islands of large polygonal cells, often closely packed (trichrome stain).

mors, which account for 72 percent of the hemangioblastomas,[30] have a better postoperative course than patients with solid tumors. None of these tumors spread by metastasis and none are highly invasive.

Symptoms and Signs

More than 80 percent of hemangioblastomas present with frontotemporal or occipital headache.[12, 46] Headache is followed by vertigo, vomiting, diplopia, tinnitus, and other symptoms of intracerebellar mass enlargement in most of these patients. Papilledema, gait or limb ataxia, and nystagmus usually are evident on the initial examination. About 12 to 25 percent of patients with hemangioblastoma have a family history of such tumors or of the von Hippel-Lindau syndrome.[30, 31] Hematologic signs are helpful in recognizing the patients with hemangioblastoma. Forty-two percent of patients with this tumor have a serum hemoglobin in excess of 16 gm/dl and 18 percent have hemoglobins over 18 gm/dl.[30]

The tumor can be seen easily on enhanced computerized tomography. Arteriography may better define the vascular supply of the tumor, but these lesions usually are discrete enough to allow adequate preoperative localization with computerized tomography alone. Arteriography is helpful in the diagnosis of the tumor type because hemangioblastomas usually have a prominent vascular blush.[24] Radionuclide brain scan also is often positive with these tumors.

Therapy and Prognosis

Surgical resection is the most effective treatment. In 10 percent of patients the tumors are multiple and in 15 percent resected tumors recur.[30] Multiple resections over the course of decades may be necessary. Postoperative radiotherapy does not improve survival. The prognosis with treatment is good unless hemorrhage into an undetected tumor produces a large cerebellar hematoma.[12]

Case Presentation

The following patient shows the history characteristic of cerebellar hemangioblastoma, including the onset in middle age, the occurrence of symptoms and signs referable to the cerebellum, and recurrence despite complete resection.

A 55-year-old right handed woman had frontal and occipital headaches for three weeks prior to developing gait difficulty. She staggered and tended to fall backward or to the right. Within a month of the gait difficulty she developed vomiting and sought medical attention. On examination she was mildly lethargic. Papilledema was observed bilaterally and there was mild left facial weakness and a decreased right corneal reflex. Her gait was cautious and staggering, and she was unable to walk in tandem. She fell backward when unassisted and had obvious titubation. A kinetic tremor developed terminally on finger-to-nose movements with the left arm. Past-pointing was obvious with the left arm and rapid alternating movements were slowed on the left. She had good strength but slight downward drift of the right arm when extended with her eyes closed. The deep tendon reflexes were increased on the right and the plantar responses were unreactive.

An echoencephalogram showed no abnormality, but a vertebral angiogram revealed a flattened basilar artery and ventriculography suggested a superior cerebellar mass in the midline. Suboccipital craniectomy demonstrated a well circumscribed hemangioblastoma on the superior aspect of the medial left hemisphere. The tumor was in contact with the subpial surface and extended 3.5 cm below the surface as a fairly round mass. It was resected completely and the vermis was split to search for the midline component suggested by the ventriculogram. No tumor mass was found in the vermis.

After surgery she had both ocular and limb dysmetria, as well as nystagmus in the primary position of gaze and on lateral gaze. This subsided over the next few days, but three days after surgery, she became overtly psychotic. She had vivid delusions, at times seeming to merge with frank hallucinations. This behavior was transient also, but persisted for more than a week. Subsequently radiotherapy was given to the posterior fossa and within three months of surgery she was virtually asymptomatic. The only deficits were mild dysmetria in the arms, more on the right than on the left. She could walk in tandem fairly well, but had difficulty stopping when walking normally. She continued to improve over the ensuing months and three years after surgery she was asymptomatic except for slight unsteadiness on tandem walking.

Five years later she presented again with gait ataxia and a tendency to fall to the right. On examination she was alert, but depressed and anxious, weeping and talking incessantly. A kinetic tremor appeared terminally on finger-to-nose testing bilaterally, especially on the right. Rapid alternating movements were slowed on the left and heel-to-shin testing revealed an impairment on the left. A radionuclide brain scan showed increased uptake in the left posterior fossa. A vertebral angiogram again revealed a 6 cm vascular tumor on the left side of the posterior fossa. She was re-explored and another hemangioblastoma appeared at the site of the original tumor. This was 6 to 7 cm in diameter and replaced much of the left cerebellar hemisphere with no apparent extension. The tumor was resected completely and the posterior fossa was irradiated after the surgery.

Within five months of the surgery the patient again was asymptomatic except for slight dysmetria in the left arm and mild gait ataxia. She was followed for seven years after the second operation and at the end of that time had persistent dysmetria of the left arm, a broad-based gait, and inability to walk in tandem. She was otherwise free of neurologic deficits. A computerized tomogram of the posterior fossa revealed no evidence of tumor.

Other Tumors

The cerebellum may be the site of several rare brain tumors and semineoplastic tissue abnormalities. Some of these tumors, such as dysplastic gangliocytomas, probably are variants of the more common cerebellar tumors. Others, such as lymphoma, are common extracranially, appearing only rarely as primary intracranial tumors. Some tumors such as cerebellar hemangiomas behave like neoplasms without clear evidence of neoplasic growth.[61]

Neuroblastoma

This tumor appears similar to medulloblastoma on light microscopy, but it has a level of differentiation never seen in medulloblastomas. The neuroblastoma has numerous synaptic vesicles in the majority of cell processes and occasionally complete synapses are apparent. This tumor has been described in the cerebellum of children,[58] manifesting uniform, round tumor cells, aligned in rows or groups, all with scanty cytoplasm. The tumor cells are reminiscent of the external granule cells which descend through the parallel fiber layer during development.[51] The tumor may have no glial elements or Purkinje cell involvement. Necrosis does not appear in the tumor substance proper.

Dysplastic Gangliocytoma

The dysplastic gangliocytoma is a rare disorder that probably represents a congenital malformation rather than a neoplasm.[50] The cells comprising the malformation are probably derived from granule cells. This lesion presents in the adult as any other mass lesion does, but the cerebellar folia are found to be hypertrophied with abnormally large axons in the cortex and absent central white matter underlying the folia. There may be calcific deposits, but there are few of the characteristics of a neoplasm.

Lymphoma

Lymphoma arises in the cerebellar hemispheres only rarely,[62] although it may be more common than recognized because of the similarity between lymphoma cells and medulloblastoma cells. Lymphoma is not at all uncommon in the central nervous system, but it is usually disseminated from sites elsewhere in the body. Intracranial meningeal involvement is well recognized. Intraparenchymal cerebral lymphoma usually affects the cerebral hemispheres.

Capillary Hemangioma

This is not strictly a neoplastic lesion, although its organization and character may change with age and lesions in the cerebellum may evolve as a mass. A capillary hemangioma can enlarge with focal hemorrhages or with increased blood flow through relatively vestigial channels. In one series of non-neoplastic lesions of the cerebellum presenting as rapidly evolving tumors, 9 of 12 patients had capillary-cavernous hemangiomas.[61] These lesions are borderline between neoplasms and arteriovenous malformations.

EXTRAPARENCHYMAL TUMORS

Meningioma

Meningioma is an insidiously growing, but usually benign, tumor that may involve the posterior fossa (Figs. 14 through 16). Posterior fossa meningiomas cause cerebellar dysfunction through pressure rather than invasion. Adults are affected primarily. Posterior fossa meningiomas occur infrequently, representing only 7.7 percent of intracranial meningiomas.[54] About 2.5 to 3.7 percent of intracranial meningiomas attach to the tentorium cerebelli, but most grow from the superior surface and do not extend inferiorly.[5] Other sites providing a base for growth are the clivus, the cerebellopontine angle (Figs. 14, 16), and the squamous portion of the occipital bone.

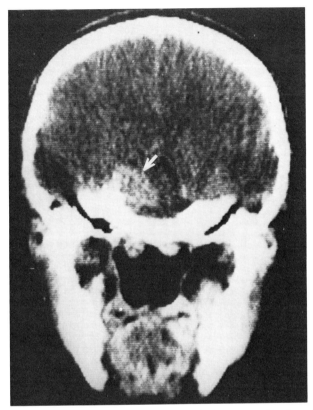

Figure 14. CT scan in coronal section demonstrating a meningioma extending from the cerebellopontine angle on the right. The tumor is indicated by the white arrow.

Symptoms and Signs

The slow growth pattern and meningeal attachment of the tumor may result in little more than chronic headache as a major symptom.[11] Unless the tumor develops in a relatively sensitive area such as the cerebellopontine angle, the tumor mass may be very large before the patient comes to medical attention. Eighty percent of patients presenting with clivus meningiomas have papilledema on initial examination, reflecting the large size of the tumor rather than an early obstructive hydrocephalus.[11] As with other tumors, when cerebellar dysfunction occurs, the signs of this dysfunction reflect the area of cerebellum impinged upon.[16] Distinguishing between a clivus meningioma and a chordoma usually is facilitated by the high incidence of ocular motor palsies and chiasmal compression seen with the chordoma.[11]

The tumor may be located easily with computerized tomography, especially if calcification in the tumor outlines a solid, high density lesion. The highly vascular character of the tumor should provide good visualization with contrast enhancement, even if the tumor is uncalcified. Arteriography is the most definitive means of characterizing the tumor prior to the biopsy. The vascular supply to the menin-

363

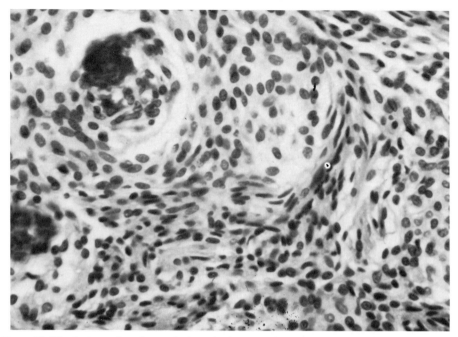

Figure 15. Histologic section of a meningioma in the cerebellopontine angle of a 67-year-old woman. The patient complained of weakness of the left limbs, slurred speech, and difficulty swallowing. Examination revealed weakness of the left lower face, dysarthria, a decreased gag reflex, a left hemiparesis, generally hyperactive deep tendon reflexes, and extensor plantar responses. At operation a large vascular meningioma lying anterior to the brainstem was removed partially but the patient expired 4 days postoperatively. The tumor is composed of arachnoid cells arranged in whorls and sheets (hematoxylin and eosin stain).

gioma develops from blood vessels to the meninges of the posterior fossa. Both internal and external carotid branches usually are involved. The clivus is supplied by recurrent branches from the cavernous portion of the internal carotid,[54] and the posterior aspect of the petrous temporal bone obtains its supply from the middle meningeal artery. The dura mater about the cerebellopontine angle is supplied by an accessory meningeal branch arising from the ascending pharyngeal artery.[54] Hypertrophy of this vessel as it courses into the skull by way of the foramen lacerum and prominent branching of the vessel in the posterior fossa is good evidence that a cerebellopontine angle tumor is a meningioma. The more posteriorly placed meningiomas developing off the squamous portion of the occipital bone will be supplied by the vertebral arteries medially and the occipital arteries laterally. Angiography also may reveal whether the transverse sinus is involved. More than half of all tentorial meningiomas extend to the transverse sinuses, making complete resection impossible.[5]

Therapy and Prognosis

Treatment of this tumor is strictly surgical. Complete cure is possible with complete resection but, if complete resection requires sacrifice of a major venous

364

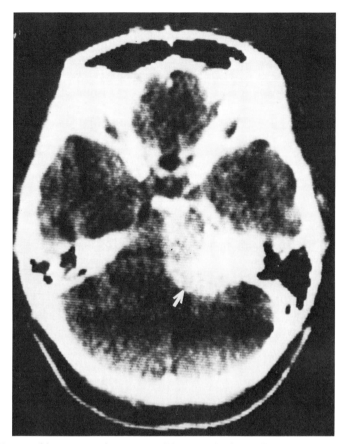

Figure 16. CT scan with contrast enhancement of the posterior fossa of a 46-year-old woman with progressive hearing loss, right facial numbness, and blurred vision. A large cerebellopontine angle meningioma is seen overlying the petrous portion of the temporal bone. (White arrow indicates the tumor.) This tumor extended supratentorially along the dorsum sellae and displaced the suprasellar cistern to the left.

sinus, part of the tumor must be left. With partial resection, about 50 percent will regrow to preoperative size in four years.[5] Irradiation is of no additional value in the treatment of meningiomas.

Case Presentation

The following case history illustrates one of the many types of presentation that can occur with posterior fossa meningiomas. In this patient the history began with headaches, as frequently occurs, but the duration of symptoms was unusually short.

A 33-year-old, left handed woman noticed a 20 lb weight loss over three months preceding the onset of occipital headaches. After three weeks of daily headaches, she developed difficulty with gait and balance, occasionally falling to the right. Rarely, she had episodes of transient double vision. When nausea and vomiting

365

developed she sought medical attention. On examination she had no papilledema and was alert and oriented. Her mentation and speech were normal. Nystagmus was evoked by right lateral gaze. Finger-to-nose and heel-to-shin testing demonstrated slight dysmetria in the right arm and leg, but there was no past-pointing or excessive rebound. Rapid alternating movements were normal. She walked on a broad base and fell to the right. Motor, sensory, and reflex activities were normal.

Computerized tomography demonstrated a large right cerebellar mass and slightly enlarged lateral ventricles. An arteriogram indicated that this was a highly vascular mass in the right cerebellar hemisphere. At operation a meningioma was found arising from the tentorium cerebelli near the right transverse sinus. The right cerebellar hemisphere was largely displaced and compressed by the tumor, especially along the inferior and lateral aspects of the hemisphere. Complete resection of the tumor was attempted and after the surgery the patient had no new deficits.

Cerebellopontine Angle Schwannoma

Incidence

Most tumors of the cerebellopontine angle arise from Schwann cells of the eighth nerve and thus bear the term "acoustic neuroma" or "acoustic schwannoma" (Figs. 17,18). A variety of other tumors and malformations occurs in the cerebellopontine angle, including meningiomas, ependymomas, lipomas, hemangiomas, arteriovenous malformations, metastases, and choroid plexus papillomas.[13] Giant aneuryms of the vertebral artery may be indistinguishable clinically from cerebellopontine angle tumors.[26]

Acoustic neuroma occurs often in patients with von Recklinghausen's neurofibromatosis; it is the most common intracranial tumor in adults with this disease.[9] Acoustic neuromas occur bilaterally in 5 percent of cases.[26] Although the age of clinical onset of disease in patients with acoustic neuromas varies from the second to the eighth decade, bilateral acoustic neuromas in a child are virtually pathognomonic of neurofibromatosis.[9]

Symptoms and Signs

Patients with acoustic neuromas usually have unilateral sensorineural hearing loss and tinnitus. These patients are predominantly women[40] with an insidiously progressive hearing loss characterized by loss of high tone discrimination and poor speech discrimination.[26] Only 8 percent of patients with schwannomas have dysphagia, and only 10 percent have signs of corticospinal tract dysfunction.[11] Vertigo and gait ataxia may develop as the tumor expands into the cerebellum, but the signs of cerebellar dysfunction may be limited to slight dysmetria or kinetic tremor in one arm.

Definitive diagnosis rests heavily on radiographic studies.[13] Skull radiograms alone may provide substantial evidence of a cerebellopontine angle schwannoma. About 90 percent of eighth nerve tumors cause enlargement of the internal auditory canal on the involved side and at least 11 percent have erosion of the petrous pyramids.[26] Polytomography through this area can clarify equivocal changes, but usually it is unnecessary. Computerized tomography may reveal an enhancing le-

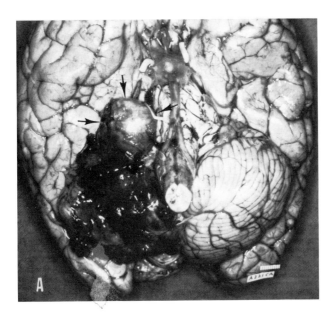

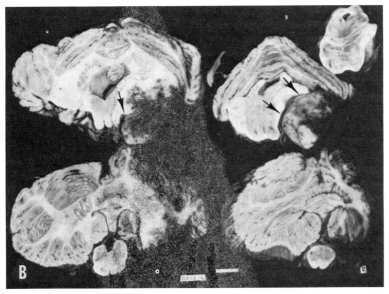

Figure 17. The gross neuropathology of a 55-year-old woman with an acoustic neuroma. The patient had intermittent nausea and vomiting for 3 years, tinnitus, a hearing loss on the right, and numbness on the right side of her face for 1 year and frequent falls for 6 months. Examination revealed papilledema, absent sensation on the right side of the face, an absent corneal reflex on the right, and complete deafness on the right. A gag reflex could not be detected. Movements of the right leg were ataxic and tandem walking evoked a mild ataxia. An occipital craniotomy was performed, the lateral one-third of the cerebellum was removed and the acoustic neuroma was partially resected, but the patient expired about two weeks postoperatively with an aspiration pneumonia. A, A ventral view of the brain showing a large portion of the acoustic neuroma remaining in situ (arrows). B, Coronal sections through the cerebellum and brainstem showing compression of the brainstem by the partially excised tumor (arrows).

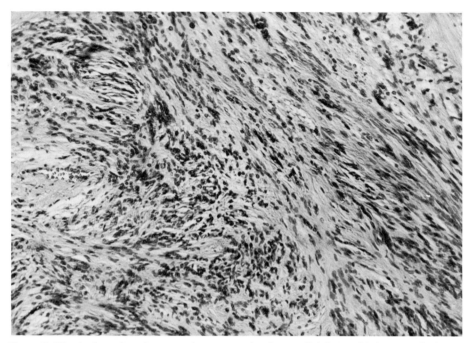

Figure 18. Histologic section of an acoustic neuroma showing parallel sheets of Schwann cells densely packed (hematoxylin and eosin stain).

sion (Fig. 19) displacing the brainstem of the cerebellum, but a fairly high resolution instrument is needed to find tumors projecting only a few millimeters from the porus acusticus. Essentially all tumors larger than 2 cm in diameter will be found with computerized tomography and contrast enhancement.[13] Only 20 percent of the acoustic neuromas overall will be overlooked with this technique.[13]

Contrast studies are helpful. Arteriography occasionally shows an avascular area about the cerebellopontine angle or an elevated anterior inferior cerebellar artery. Pneumoencephalography indicates whether the cerebellopontine angle is devoid of air or whether the fourth ventricle is shifted. Radionuclide brain scan with Tc 99m pertechnetate frequently is positive, but the most unambiguous radiographic test for a small acoustic schwannoma is a posterior fossa myelogram.[13] Lumbar puncture during this procedure also is useful, since cerebrospinal fluid protein almost invariably is increased.[26] If the myelographic dye enters the internal auditory canal and does not outline a mass, it is unlikely that there is a tumor. Metrizamide cisternography with hypocycloidal tomography probably is the best of the currently available myelographic techniques to demonstrate masses in this region.[13] Auditory evoked potential studies are of some use in identifying the type of lesion. If the tumor is a schwannoma of the eighth cranial nerve, the latency of wave V of the brainstem evoked response is prolonged.[26] This does not occur with other lesions, such as meningiomas or epidermoids.

Therapy

The treatment of most cerebellopontine angle lesions, including schwannomas, meningiomas en plaque,[26] or choroid plexus papillomas,[28] requires surgical inter-

368

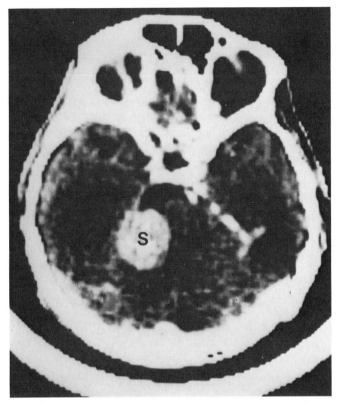

Figure 19. CT scan of the posterior fossa in a 68-year-old man complaining of progressive hearing loss and tinnitus over the course of 5 years. Neurologic investigations were prompted by episodes of syncope, diplopia, and urinary frequency. At the time of this study the patient was unable to walk unless assisted. A large cerebellopontine angle schwannoma (S) was resected from the left side of the posterior fossa. Contrast enhancement accounts for the apparent density of the tumor.

vention. Several approaches are used with equal success, some entailing transaural surgery and other suboccipital approaches. About 80 percent of cerebellopontine angle tumors can be removed completely.[26] Considerations in resecting the tumor include extension of the tumor to other structures and the feasibility of avoiding the facial nerve. In a series of 132 patients with acoustic neuromas, only 50 had intact facial nerve function after surgery.[40] In another series facial nerve function was preserved in over 80 percent of patients operated upon. Twenty-two percent of patients developed cerebrospinal fluid leakage after surgery, and 7 percent developed meningitis in association with the leak.[26] About 5 percent of patients die as a result of the surgery with complications including hemorrhage, cardiac arrest, and brainstem compression.[40]

Case Presentation

The following case illustrates a typical history of onset and progression in a man with an acoustic neuroma.

A 68-year-old, right handed man lost much of the hearing in his left ear over the course of five years. He had occasional ringing in his ears. Four months prior

369

to hospitalization, he developed syncope, which occurred infrequently, but repeatedly. He lost 50 pounds of weight and noticed fine tremors in his hands and clumsiness on attempting fine tasks. Although he had occasional headaches, they were not substantially different from similar headaches he had had throughout his life. Gait became increasingly more difficult over the three weeks prior to his hospitalization and he developed transient double vision, urinary frequency, and urgency. On admission he could walk only with assistance. In addition to substantial hearing deficits on the left, he had slight left facial weakness and coarse nystagmus, evoked primarily on left lateral gaze. Minor nystagmus developed on right lateral gaze, but none occurred with vertical gaze. He was confused and disoriented and his responses to questions often were tangential and inappropriate. Slight decomposition of movement was detectable in the left arm.

A technetium brain scan indicated a dense area of uptake in the posterior fossa on the left and computerized tomography revealed a mass in the left cerebellopontine angle, associated with marked hydrocephalus and displacement of the brainstem. An acoustic schwannoma was found in the cerebellopontine angle on posterior fossa exploration. With microsurgical techniques the tumor was resected in toto with no resection of cerebellar tissue. No substantial improvement was observed after the operation.

REFERENCES

1. AMICI, R., AVANZINI, G., AND PACINI, L.: *Cerebellar Tumors.* Monographs in Neural Sciences, Vol. IV. Karger, Basel, 1976.

2. BARONE, B. M., AND ELVIDGE, A. R.: *Ependymomas.* J. Neurosurg. 33:428, 1970.

3. BERGER, E. C., AND ELVIDGE, A. R.: *Medulloblastomas and cerebellar sarcomas.* J. Neurosurg. 20:139, 1963.

4. BUCY, P. C., AND THIEMAN, P. W.: *Astrocytomas of the cerebellum.* Arch. Neurol. 18:14, 1968.

5. CAREY, J. P., FISHER, R. G., AND POLOFSKY, S.: *Tentorial meningiomas.* Surg. Neurol. 3:41, 1975.

6. CARMEL, P.: *Cerebellar tumors in childhood.* Dev. Med. Child. Neurol. 14:809, 1972.

7. CARMEL, P.: Personal communication.

8. CAMERON, S. J., AND DOIG, A.: *Cerebellar tumors presenting with clinical features of phaeochromocytoma.* Lancet 1:492, 1970.

9. CHALHUB, E. G.: *Neurocutaneous syndromes in children.* Ped. Clin. North Amer. 23:499, 1976.

10. CHATTY, E. M., AND EARLE, K. M.: *Medulloblastoma. A report of 201 cases with emphasis on the relationship of histologic variants to survival.* Cancer 28:977, 1971.

11. CHERINGTON, M., AND SCHNECK, S. A.: *Clivus meningiomas.* Neurology 16:86, 1966.

12. CRAMER, F., AND KIMSEY, W.: *Cerebellar hemangioblastomas.* Arch. Neurol. Psychiat. 67:237, 1952.

13. DAVIS, K. R., PARKER, S. W., NEW, P. F. J. ET AL.: *Computed tomography of acoustic neuroma.* Radiol. 124:81, 1977.

14. DOHRMANN, G. J., AND DUNSMORE, R. H.: *Glioblastoma multiforme of the cerebellum.* Surg. Neurol. 3:219, 1975.

15. DOHRMANN, G. J., FARWELL, J. R., AND FLANNERY, J. T.: *Ependymomas and ependymoblastomas in children.* J. Neurosurg. 45:273, 1976.

16. DOW, R. S., AND MORUZZI, G.: *The Physiology and Pathology of the Cerebellum.* University of Minnesota Press, Minneapolis, 1958.

17. ECKER, A.: *Upward transtentorial herniation of the brainstem and cerebellum due to tumor of the posterior fossa.* J. Neurosurg. 5:51, 1948.

18. ENZMANN, D. R., NORMAN, D., LEVIN, V., ET AL.: *Computed tomography in the follow-up of medulloblastomas and ependymomas.* Radiology 128:57, 1978.

370

19. FARWELL, J. R., DOHRMANN, G. J., AND FLANNERY, J. T.: *Intracranial neoplasms in infants.* Arch. Neurol. 35:533, 1978.

20. FAUST, D. S., TATEM, H. R., III, BRADY, L. W., ET AL.: *Radiation therapy in the management of medulloblastoma.* Neurology 20:519, 1970.

21. FRESH, C. B., TAKEI, Y., AND O'BRIEN, M. S.: *Cerebellar glioblastoma in childhood.* J. Neurosurg. 45:705, 1976.

22. FULCHIERO, A., WINSTON, K., LEVITON, A., ET AL.: *Secular trends in cerebellar gliomas in children.* J. Nat. Cancer Inst. 58:839, 1977.

23. GEISSINGER, J. D., AND BUCY, P. C.: *Astrocytomas of the cerebellum in children.* Arch. Neurol. 24:125, 1971.

24. GESCHWIND, N.: *Case records of the Massachusetts General Hospital: case 15-1975.* N. Engl. J. Med. 292:852, 1975.

25. GJERRIS, F., AND KLINKEN, L.: *Long-term prognosis in children with benign cerebellar astrocytoma.* J. Neurosurg. 49:179, 1978.

26. GLASSCOCK, M. E., III: *The diagnosis and management of cerebellopontine angle tumors.* J. Otolaryngol. 7:125, 1978.

27. GRIGGS, R. C., MOXLEY, R. T., III, LAFRANCE, R. A., ET AL.: *Hereditary paroxysmal ataxia: response to acetazolamide.* Neurology 28:1259, 1978.

28. HAMMOCK, M. K., MILHORAT, T. H., AND BRECKBILL, D. L.: *Primary choroid plexus papilloma of the cerebellopontine angle presenting as brainstem tumor in a child.* Child's Brain 2:132, 1976.

29. HOPE-STONE, H. F.: *Results of treatment of medulloblastomas.* J. Neurosurg. 32:83, 1970.

30. JEFFREYS, R.: *Clinical and surgical aspects of posterior fossa haemangioblastoma.* J. Neurol. Neurosurg. Psychiat. 38:105, 1975.

31. JEFFREYS, R.: *Pathological and haematological aspects of posterior fossa haemangioblastoma.* J. Neurol. Neurosurg. Psychiat. 38:112, 1975.

32. KESCHNER, M., AND GROSSMAN, M.: *Cerebellar symptomatology evaluation on the basis of intracerebellar and extracerebellar lesions.* Arch. Neurol. Psychiat. 19:78, 1928.

33. KESSLER, L. A., DUGAN, P., AND CONCANNON, J. P.: *Systemic metastases of medulloblastoma promoted by shunting.* Surg. Neurol. 3:147, 1975.

34. KIM, Y. H., AND FAYOS, J. V.: *Intracranial ependymomas.* Radiol. 124:805, 1977.

35. KLEINMAN, G. M., SCHOENE, W. C., WALSHE, T. M., III, ET AL.: *Malignant transformation in benign cerebellar astrocytoma.* J. Neurosurg. 49:111, 1978.

36. LASSMAN, L. P.: *Diagnosis and management of skeletal metastases from cerebellar medulloblastoma.* Child's Brain 2:38, 1976.

37. LEIBEL, S. A., SHELINE, G. E., WARA, W. M., ET AL.: *The role of radiation therapy in the treatment of astrocytomas.* Cancer 35:1551, 1975.

38. LEWIS, M. B., NUNES, L. B., POWELL, D. E. ET AL.: *Extra-axial spread of medulloblastoma.* Cancer 31:1287, 1973.

39. LIU, H. M., BOGGS, J., AND KIDD, J.: *Ependymomas of childhood. I.* Child's Brain 2:92, 1976.

40. MACCARTY, C. S.: *Acoustic neuroma and the suboccipital approach.* Mayo Clin. Proc. 50:15, 1975.

41. MANDYBUR, T. I.: *Intracranial hemorrhage ccused by metastatic tumors.* Neurology 27:650, 1977.

42. MASUCCI, E. F.: *Posterior fossa metastases simulating primary tumors.* Acta Neurol. Scand. 42:589, 1966.

43. MATAKAS, F., CERVÓS-NAVARRO, J., AND GULLOTA, F.: *The ultrastructure of medulloblastomas.* Acta Neuropathol. (Berl.) 16:271, 1970.

44. MAURICE-WILLIAMS, R. S.: *Mechanism of production of gait unsteadiness by tumors of the posterior fossa.* J. Neurol. Neurosurg. Psychiat. 38:143, 1975.

45. MILES, J. AND BHANDARI, Y. S.: *Cerebellar medulloblastoma in adults: review of 18 cases.* J. Neurol. Neurosurg. Psychiat. 33:208, 1970.

46. MILLER, R. G., PORTER, R. J., NIELSEN, S. L. ET AL.: *Von Hippel-Lindau's disease.* Can. J. Neurol. Sci. 3:29, 1976.

47. OJEMANN, R. G.: *Case records of the Massachusetts General Hospital: case 36-1976.* N. Engl. J. Med. 295:553, 1976.

48. OPPENHEIMER, D. R.: *The effect of irradiation on medulloblastoma.* J. Neurol. Neurosurg. Psychiat. 32:94, 1969.

49. POSNER, J. B., AND SHAPIRO, W. R.: *Brain tumor: current status of treatment and its complications.* Arch. Neurol. 32:781, 1975.

50. PRITCHETT, P. S., AND KING, T. I.: *Dysplastic gangliocytoma of the cerebellum—an ultrastructural study.* Acta Neuropathol. (Berl.) 42:1, 1978.

51. RENOU, G., FONCIN, J. F., PRADAT, P., ET AL.: *Formes latéro-cérébelleuses des médulloblastomes de l'adulte.* Neuro-Chirurgie (Paris) 17:191, 1971.

52. RINGERTZ, N., AND TOLA, J. H.: *Medulloblastoma.* J. Neuropathol. Exp. Neurol. 9:354, 1950.

53. RUBINSTEIN, L. J., AND NORTHFIELD, D. W. C.: *The medulloblastoma and the so-called "arachnoidal cerebellar sarcoma."* Brain 87:379, 1964.

54. SALAMON, G. M., COMBALBERT, A., RAYBAUD, C., ET AL.: *An angiographic study of meningiomas of the posterior fossa.* J. Neurosurg. 35:731, 1971.

55. SALAZAR, O. M., RUBIN, P., BASSANO, D., ET AL.: *Improved survival of patients with intracranial ependymomas by irradiation: dose selection and field extension.* Cancer 35:1563, 1975.

56. SHAPIRO, K., AND SHULMAN, K.: *Spinal cord seeding from cerebellar astrocytomas.* Child's Brain 2:177, 1976.

57. SHARR, M. M., AND GARFIELD, J. S.: *Management of intracranial metastases.* Br. Med. J. 1: 1535, 1978.

58. SHIN, W., LAUFER, H., LEE, Y., ET AL.: *Fine structure of a cerebellar neuroblastoma.* Acta Neuropathol. (Berl.) 42:11, 1978.

59. SHUMAN, R. M., ALVORD, E. C., JR., AND LEECH, R. W.: *The biology of childhood ependymomas.* Arch. Neurol. 32:731, 1975.

60. SILVERBERG, G. D.: *Simple cysts of the cerebellum.* J. Neurosurg. 35:320, 1971.

61. SUNDBÄRG, G., BRUN, A., EFSING, H. O. ET AL.: *Non-neoplastic expanding lesions of the vermis cerebelli.* J. Neurosurg. 37:55, 1972.

62. WHITE, B. E., AND ROTHFLEISCH, S.: *Primary cerebellar lymphoma.* Neurology 18:582, 1968.

63. WINSTON, K., GILLES, F. H., LEVITOU, A., ET AL.: *Cerebellar gliomas in children.* J. Natl. Cancer Inst. 58:833, 1977.

64. ZUMPANO, J.: *Spinal intramedullary metastatic medulloblastoma.* J. Neurosurg. 48:632, 1978.

CHAPTER 18

Cerebellar Stimulation

In 1972, Cooper[11] initiated in humans the procedure of chronic electrical stimulation of the cerebellar surface through implanted electrodes in attempts to activate the inhibitory output of the cerebellar cortex for treating intractable epilepsy and certain disorders of posture and movement.[12-22, 48] When this work began, evidence from animal experiments indicated that a number of motor functions could be altered by electrical stimulation of the cerebellum. These experiments originated with the demonstration by Sherrington[66] and Loewenthal and Horsley[46] that decerebrate rigidity was reversed by electrical stimulation of the cerebellar anterior lobe. Cerebellar stimulation subsequently was shown to reduce the limb rigidity resulting from the crossed extensor reflexes in decerebrate animals[31] and to decrease the muscular response and after-discharge from electrical stimulation of the pericruciate region of the cerebral cortex.[50, 51] Later, cerebellar stimulation was found to interfere with seizure activity induced by electrical stimulation of the pericruciate cortex[9, 10] and the hippocampus.[44] Moreover, cerebellar stimulation interrupted the seizures resulting from the chronic effects of cobalt applied to the rodent brain,[32] although this effect could not be duplicated in the cat[61] or monkey.[37] Many of the inhibitory effects resulting from stimulation of the cerebellar surface have been attributed to the activation of Purkinje cells, which inhibit neurons in the deep cerebellar and vestibular nuclei.[42, 43]

Since the introduction of cerebellar stimulation to treat patients with epilepsy and disorders of posture and movement, a number of problems with the procedure has arisen. These problems have led to sharp controversies concerning the efficacy of the procedure, the types of disorders that respond to the procedure, the safety of the implantation of electrodes over the cerebellar surface and stimulation through these electrodes, and the mechanisms by which the procedure may affect patients with neurologic disorders. Thus far, most of these controversies have not been resolved. Moreover, the introduction of cerebellar stimulation as a therapy for emotional disorders has provided a new field for controversy.[40]

CEREBELLAR STIMULATION FOR EPILEPSY

Small numbers of patients with epilepsy intractable to medical therapy have been treated with cerebellar stimulation, with conflicting results. Three series of cases have been reported in the literature and only one of these series has been studied with double blind cross-over techniques. The results in the largest series of cases, reported by Cooper and coworkers,[20] were favorable. The series consisted of 32 patients with convulsive disorders unresponsive to prolonged treatment with commonly used anticonvulsant drugs in therapeutic doses. Seizure frequency was established from records maintained by the patients' families, hospital records, and from interviews with the patients and their families. No attempts were made to conduct blinded control studies systematically without stimulation after implantation in these patients. Eighteen of the 32 patients showed a good clinical response to chronic cerebellar stimulation, with a reduction of seizure frequency of at least 50 percent. Among the remaining patients, 9 were rated as failures and 5 died. The seizure types among the patients who benefited from chronic cerebellar stimulation included 3 patients with type I (partial seizures or seizures beginning locally); 9 with type II (generalized, bilateral, and symmetrical seizures); and 6 with mixed types I and II. The 9 who did not benefit from the procedure consisted of 2 with type I epilepsy, 3 with type II, 3 with mixed types I and II, and 1 with type III (unilateral seizures).

In addition to the beneficial effects upon seizure frequency, chronic cerebellar stimulation was reported to cause many subjective changes in this series.[20] Virtually all patients stated that they were more alert, better able to concentrate, and more effective in performing the functions of daily living. They also noted reduced depression, improved fluency of speech, and reduced anger or aggression.

In the same series of cases, 5 patients died after electrode implantation.[20] One patient died as a result of a postoperative extradural hematoma. Stimulation of the cerebellum was never begun. The other 4 patients probably died from seizures. One of these patients died during a nocturnal seizure at age 25 after 17 months of chronic electrical stimulation of the cerebellum. This patient's seizures had not been improved by cerebellar stimulation. Another patient, a 30-year-old man, died in his sleep 6 weeks after implantation. He had been free of his grand mal and petit mal seizures during the brief postoperative period. A 23-year-old man with severe psychomotor seizures died 26 months postoperatively after a series of grand mal seizures. The cerebellar electrodes had been removed several months earlier because they had failed to improve his seizure disorder. The fourth patient, a 19-year-old man with a history of grand mal and akinetic epilepsy, died 28 months after chronic cerebellar stimulation was begun. A series of nocturnal seizures in this patient also preceded death. It is unclear whether cerebellar implantation and stimulation was related to these four deaths, since patients with seizures are known to die suddenly, probably as a result of a cardiac disorder or hypoxia during a seizure.

The results of chronic cerebellar stimulation for epilepsy in the remaining two series of cases have not been as favorable as those in the series of Cooper and colleagues,[20] although many of the same types of subjective improvement occurred. Gilman and associates[36] reported the results of this procedure in 7 patients. The patients were referred by neurologists who had treated them with a variety of anticonvulsant medications, monitoring treatment with frequent determinations of serum drug levels. Despite careful management, these patients were incapacitated almost completely by the seizure disorder. Four patients required constant observation by family members to avoid injury from frequent seizures. The other three patients were able to work: two functioned ineffectively in a protective environment or family business and the third could do only volunteer work for limited periods of time.

In the first 4 patients of this series, 1 electrode array was placed over the ante-

374

rior lobe of the arachnoidal surface of the cerebellum and a second over the posterior lobe. In the first 2 patients, an 8 electrode array was used for the anterior lobe and a 16 electrode array for the cerebellar hemisphere. In subsequent patients, all arrays had only 8 electrodes. Details of the stimulation procedure are described elsewhere.[36] Records of seizure frequency were kept by the patients and their families. Single blind control studies were performed with the patients in their home environment by substituting induction coils that did not transmit current to subcutaneous antennae. These studies were carried out in 4 patients without the direct knowledge of the patients but with the prior consent of the patients and their families. The duration of treatment ranged from 7 months to 2 years.

The results in these patients were remarkable. Five of the 7 patients showed a change in the character or frequency of their seizures, although the degree of improvement allowed only 2 of the patients to undergo appreciable vocational rehabilitation. In Case 1 (KH), there was a substantial decrease in the frequency and duration of both grand mal and psychomotor seizures. Case 2 (RM) showed a decrease in frequency and duration of psychomotor seizures. Case 3 (RB) had no change in the frequency of focal motor and grand mal seizures, a clinical impression corroborated by a single blind control study. Case 4 (LB) showed no change in the frequency or intensity of her incapacitating psychomotor seizures. There was a decrease in the frequency of her grand mal seizures, however. In Case 5 (AR) there was no change in frequency or intensity of the epilepsia partialis continua or grand mal seizures. Case 6 (JW) ceased having grand mal seizures for several months from the time stimulation was begun, but disabling psychomotor akinetic attacks did not change. Subsequently, grand mal seizures recurred in this patient. Case 7 (JP) showed no change in the frequency or intensity of his psychomotor seizures. Unfortunately, the two patients who showed the best results from cerebellar stimulation (KH and RM) refused to cooperate for double blind control studies.

Van Buren and coworkers[75] reported the only double blind cross-over study of epileptic patients treated with cerebellar stimulation. The series consisted of 5 patients with medically intractable seizures. All of these patients had an average of over one seizure per day when observed in the hospital and by history. The patients had combinations of partial and generalized seizures with focal and/or bilaterally synchronous epileptiform activity. One patient had nearly continuous myoclonic activity. The investigators adjusted the serum levels of phenytoin, primidone, and phenobarbital to therapeutic ranges. Three patients had additional medication consisting of diazepam and ethosuximide.

After implantation of cerebellar stimulating electrodes, Van Buren and others[75] evaluated seizure frequency with the patients hospitalized. The patients were admitted to the hospital three or four times over the ensuing 15 to 21 months, with each admission lasting for 4 to 6 weeks. Seizure frequency was measured by trained observers carrying out constant surveillance in the hospital. They found no improvement or deterioration in seizure frequency over this period of time. Also, they found no significant differences in seizure frequency when they compared intervals of about 7 days in which the cerebellar stimulator was turned on or off as determined both in the double blind and unblinded paradigms. There were no changes in EEG or intelligence and memory quotients except for those attributable to variations in the serum levels of antiepileptic drugs. Despite the lack of objective improvement, the patients and their families indicated a positive to enthusiastic acceptance of the effects of cerebellar stimulation.

Apart from the three series reviewed above, the only published report of the effects of chronic cerebellar stimulation on seizures concerns a single additional patient described by Fenton and coworkers.[33] This 29-year-old woman developed generalized seizures, including an episode of status epilepticus, and had transient drop attacks and brief petit mal absences. Cerebellar stimulation was associated with no appreciable change in frequency of the major seizures, but there was a significant reduction in both drop attacks and petit mal seizures. Cognitive function improved as evidenced by better performance of tasks involving the learning of new material, both verbal and nonverbal. The patient was described as more alert and socially more competent, showing a greater degree of maturity in dealing with other people.

To summarize the above, the published studies have shown a decrease of seizure frequency in some patients treated with cerebellar stimulation. These studies have not demonstrated, however, whether the response to stimulation represents a valid increase of seizure threshold or a placebo effect. The single rigorous study involving double blind cross-over techniques has cast serious doubt on the true efficacy of the procedure.

CEREBELLAR STIMULATION FOR CEREBRAL PALSY

Chronic cerebellar stimulation has been performed in three large series and two small series of patients with postural and movement disorders, most of whom carried a diagnosis of cerebral palsy. Despite the large number of patients studied, however, the results remain controversial. The controversy results in part from the difficulties in measuring motor function objectively in patients with complex disorders of posture and movement. Cooper and colleagues[22] described the results of this procedure in 141 patients with a diagnosis of cerebral palsy. The population consisted of 76 males and 65 females with a mean age of 23.3 years and a range of 7 to 55 years. In about 90 percent of the patients, the motor disturbances were related to injury at birth or in the immediate postnatal period. Anoxia and prematurity were the most common disturbances cited. In most of the patients, severe spasticity was the major sign of neurologic disability. Sixty-two percent of the patients were rated as having moderate to marked spasticity. Athetosis of moderate to marked degree was present in 52 percent of the patients. In 70 percent and 80 percent of the patients there was a moderate to marked degree of disturbance in balance and gait, respectively.

Most of the patients in Cooper's series were treated with implantation of stimulating electrodes bilaterally over the anterior lobe of the cerebellum.[22] One death occurred in the series; a patient died in the first postoperative day from a cardiac air embolus and a subdural hematoma. Of the remaining 140 patients, 16 were not seen for followup examinations. Among the 124 patients seen for at least one followup examination, 41 percent were rated as having moderate or marked improvement in spasticity. Athetosis was improved in many patients, but to a lesser degree than the spasticity. Twenty-four percent were rated as moderately to markedly improved in the degree of athetosis. Twenty-six percent were rated as showing marked to moderate improvement in both ambulation and activities of daily living. The investigators reported a cumulative therapeutic effect of chronic stimulation during the first six months. Neither single nor double blind control studies were carried out.

A second large series of patients treated with cerebellar stimulation for postural and movement disorders was described by Davis and others,[27-30] but these patients also were evaluated only by clinical observation, without the benefit of single or double blind controlled observations. The population consisted of 214 patients with movement disorders categorized in the following fashion: cerebral palsy, 194 cases; cerebral vascular disease, 4; head injuries, 7; anesthetic arrests, 3; carbon monoxide poisoning, 1; drowning, 3; dystonia musculorum deformans, 2; Huntington disease, 2. No deaths occurred in these series, but one morbidity was reported: a 64-year-old woman developed a transient hypotensive episode in the recovery room resulting in a cerebral infarction with hemiparesis. Local infections occurred at the receiver site in 5 patients with cerebral palsy, necessitating removal of part or all of the stimulating system. One case of meningitis was reported. Patients were treated with cerebellar stimulation if they had moderate to severe spasticity associated with functional disability. The youngest patient was 3 years of age and the oldest was 64. Seventy percent of the cases were below the age of 20 years.

The patients were evaluated by clinical examination and the results were tabulated at six month intervals or, in some cases, yearly. Some data were collected from the patients or their families by telephone inquiries. The authors reported that chronic cerebellar stimulation reduced spasticity to some extent in all of the patients. These effects were noted within minutes after the stimulator was turned on and were maintained over months and years. Ninety-seven percent of the patients have continued to use their stimulators. In three patients, spasticity was decreased for several weeks but then returned. In 78 percent of patients with athetosis, this disorder was improved during the first week. At six months, essentially all patients with athetosis showed improvement of the symptoms referable to this movement disorder. The patients with Huntington disease treated with cerebellar stimulation showed a reduction of involuntary movements.

The investigators found that voluntary motor abilities improved, and they attributed this improvement to a decrease in spasticity and involuntary movements.[27, 30] Hand coordination was affected in 85 percent of the group with cerebral palsy. Ninety-two percent of these patients improved in the first week after the onset of cerebellar stimulation and improved further at six months. Complex voluntary movement associated with feeding and dressing showed major improvement at six months and continued to improve thereafter. Speech and drooling generally improved in the first week. Independent mobility was improved in 56 percent of the patients with cerebral palsy. Two-thirds showed marked to moderate improvement as exemplified by the fact that 24 patients initially were confined to a wheelchair but only 6 remained so after cerebellar stimulation was instituted.

Larson and associates[45] reported the third large series of patients with postural and movement disorders treated with cerebellar stimulation. These patients also were evaluated clinically without blind control studies. The effects of cerebellar stimulation were studied in 62 patients with disturbances of posture and movement. Eight of the 48 patients with cerebral palsy were able to walk more normally after stimulation was begun. Three patients who were unable to walk prior to cerebellar stimulation could walk afterwards, and those who had been walking showed improvement. Three of the patients who were unable to speak at all prior to cerebellar stimulation began to speak afterwards, and the 32 who could speak prior to stimulation were able to do so more intelligibly afterwards. A patient with a midbrain infarction and a continuous tremor failed to improve, but two patients with multiple sclerosis and disabling intention tremor did improve. According to

Larson and coworkers,[45] the most prominent overall effect of cerebellar stimulation is a reduction in spasticity; improvement in dystonic postures and involuntary movements is less pronounced.

A fourth series of patients with cerebral palsy was reported by Penn and Etzel,[54] who noted that evaluating the effects of cerebellar stimulation in children with cerebral palsy is complicated by problems in categorizing these patients diagnostically. These problems result from the variety of CNS disorders included in the diagnosis of cerebral palsy and the difficulties in following changes in the patients' abnormalities during treatment. The etiology and locations of lesions are inconstant and consequently the manifestations of cerebral palsy are varied. In addition, the terms used to describe the clinical states are inadequate. In order to compensate for these problems, Penn and Etzel used the Milani-Comparetti developmental testing program for evaluating children by quantitating motor functions and reflexes in an age related manner. This testing program avoids use of terms such as rigidity, spasticity, dystonia, and paresis. They examined the effects of cerebellar stimulation on five patients with cerebral palsy and found that four of the five patients who underwent chronic anterior lobe cerebellar stimulation showed progressive improvement of the developmental reflexes.

Ratusnick and colleagues[59] evaluated speech in 7 spastic and athetoid cerebral palsy patients before and during cerebellar stimulation. They found no significant improvement in speech intelligibility or articulatory accuracy in the group with stimulation, although certain speech characteristics improved in 3 patients. They found no factors that might help them predict which patients might be improved by the procedure.

Thus far, only two studies have been carried out using double blind methods of determining the effects of chronic cerebellar stimulation in patients with cerebral palsy. Both of these studies have raised serious questions concerning the efficacy of this procedure. Whittaker[76] described studies in which 8 patients with cerebral palsy implanted with cerebellar stimulating electrodes were evaluated by 6 experienced clinicians. At the time of the evaluations, neither the clinicians nor the patients knew whether the power to the cerebellar stimulating electrode was turned on or turned off. His data demonstrated that the examiners could not predict by clinical examination whether the patients had their stimulators turned on or off. Essentially a random distribution of opinions occurred among examiners. Thus, in a total of 48 opinions (8 patients, 6 examiners), comparing real and sham periods of cerebellar stimulation, 25 opinions of no difference were obtained, while 12 opinions were that the patient was better with real stimulation, and 11 opinions were that the patient was better with sham stimulation. The patients themselves similarly gave a random distribution of responses about whether the power was turned on or off.

Russman and associates[63] reported the second double blind cross-over study of cerebellar stimulation in patients with cerebral palsy, which also failed to document any benefit objectively. Eight children were implanted with cerebellar stimulating electrodes and studied for several one month intervals. During each interval the external transmitter was set by random assignment to function or not to function. Before implantation and at the end of each month, under standard conditions the postures and movements of the children were recorded on videotape and evaluated by a neurologist, neurosurgeon, occupational therapist, physical therapist, and speech therapist. The individuals evaluating the patients were instructed to remain objective, indicating neither enthusiasm nor lack of enthusiasm during the assessment. Two of the eight children reported improvement in the form of lessened spasticity and greater mobility regardless of whether stimulation was being applied or not. Objective assessment did not reveal any improvement in these or any of the other six children. The investigators mention the possibility that careful avoidance of positive reinforcement during the study may have been responsible for the low percentage of patients who thought that they had improved.

The two studies utilizing double blind techniques of evaluating the effects of cerebellar stimulation indicate that, although a large percentage of patients with cerebral palsy have been reported to be improved, the improvement must be viewed with a high level of skepticism. The problems of subject and experimenter bias have not been managed adequately in the large series.[38, 39] In addition, the factors of maturation and normal growth and development must be taken into account in assessing the effects of this therapy when used in growing patients. An appropriate evaluation also requires that stimulus parameters employed in the study be adequate to evoke motor changes. Thus, additional well-designed clinical studies are required before further conclusions can be reached regarding the efficacy of cerebellar stimulation.

MORPHOLOGIC CHANGES IN THE CEREBELLUM OF PATIENTS WITH INTRACTABLE EPILEPSY

Degenerative changes in the cerebellum have been found in autopsy studies of patients with severe chronic epilepsy.[23, 47, 53, 67] Forty to 50 percent of these patients show cerebellar lesions,[47, 53] and these lesions often accompany neuropathologic disorders elsewhere in the central nervous system, particularly in the hippocampus. The latter is the site most frequently found to be abnormal in essentially all studies. In some epileptic patients the cerebellum is the only structure in the brain showing damage.[47]

The pathogenesis of the degenerative changes in the cerebellum of epileptic patients has not been established and, although unlikely, the possibility remains that the changes occur during agonal events. Implantation of electrodes over the surface of the cerebellum in patients with severe seizures provides the opportunity of taking biopsy specimens during operation, permitting the observation of neuropathologic changes uninfluenced by postmortem changes. Most investigators involved with cerebellar stimulation have taken advantage of this opportunity. Correlation of the findings in biopsy specimens with the clinical results of cerebellar stimulation also has practical value; positive stimulation effects may require a reasonably intact structure. Three groups of investigators have studied biopsy specimens from their patients and all have made similar observations.

Rajjoub and colleagues[58] examined cerebellar biopsies taken at the time of cerebellar electrode implantation in three epileptic patients. Cerebellar autopsy specimens also were examined for comparison from four epileptic patients and five patients without epilepsy or neurologic disease. All specimens from seizure patients showed isomorphic gliosis of the cerebellar cortex. Significantly lower Purkinje cell densities were found in epileptic patients than in nonepileptic control patients.

Salcman and others[64] reported the neuropathologic findings in small biopsies of the cerebellum obtained from five patients undergoing operative implantation of cerebellar stimulating electrodes for the treatment of epilepsy. Eight biopsy specimens were obtained from these patients. The biopsy site was immediately adjacent to the site of implantation of the stimulating electrodes. Cerebellar biopsy

379

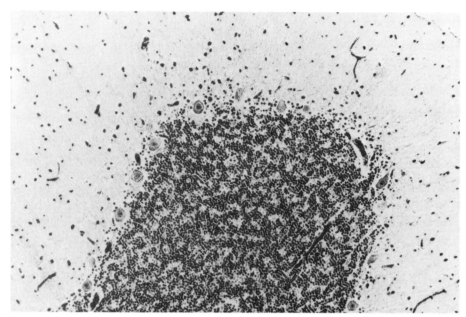

Figure 1. Control biopsy specimen of the cerebellar cortex from a 61-year-old patient, incidental to occipital craniotomy and surgical approach to a cerebellopontine angle nerve sheath tumor. The nerve cells and Bergmann astrocytes of the Purkinje cell layer are normally most numerous along the crest of the folium. (H & E; reduced 25% from × 110) (From Salcman et al.,[64] with permission.)

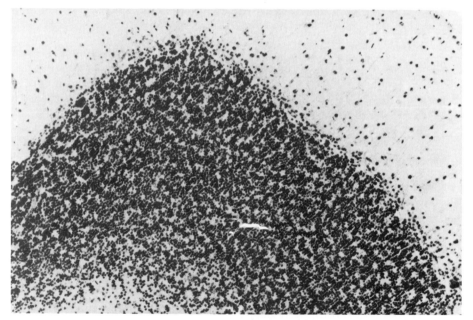

Figure 2. Cerebellar cortical biopsy specimen from a 26-year-old male with psychomotor seizures that began at age 17. The specimen shows marked loss of Purkinje cells and mild to moderate proliferation of Bergmann astrocytes. The remaining Purkinje cells are shrunken and hyperchromatic. (Cresyl violet; reduced 25% from × 110) (From Salcman et al.,[64] with permission.)

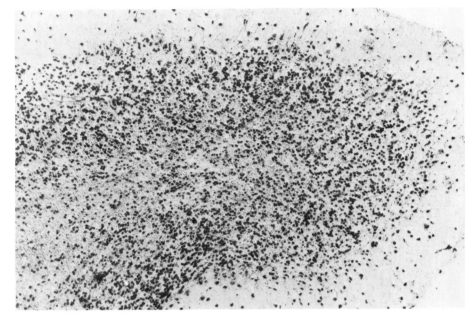

Figure 3. Cerebellar cortical biopsy specimen from a 49-year-old man with focal motor and grand mal seizures beginning at age 12. The specimen shows complete loss of Purkinje cells, atrophy of the molecular layer, moderately severe depletion of granular neurons, and rarefaction and astrocytosis of folial white matter. (H & E; reduced 25% from × 110) (From Salcman et al.,[64] with permission.)

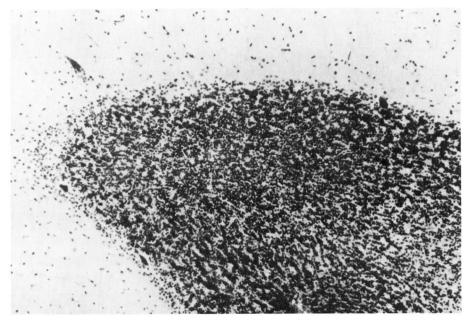

Figure 4. Cerebellar cortical biopsy specimen from a 14-year-old male with epilepsia partialis continua, grand mal, and psychomotor seizures since the age of 10. There is severe loss of Purkinje cells and moderate proliferation of Bergmann astrocytes. Scattered remaining Purkinje cells are shrunken and hyperchromatic. (H & E; reduced 25% from × 110) (From Salcman et al.,[64] with permission.)

381

specimens incidental to surgical exposure of acoustic neuromas served as controls (Fig. 1). All specimens from the patients with seizures showed moderately severe to severe degeneration of Purkinje cells with concomitant proliferation of Bergmann astrocytes as well as a variable degree of degeneration of other elements in the structure of the cerebellum (Figs. 2 through 4). Two of the patients with seizure disturbances had no history of grand mal status; nevertheless, these patients showed severe degeneration of Purkinje cells in the biopsy specimens. Among the other patients, the seizure disorders included epilepsia partialis continua, grand mal and psychomotor seizures, and psychomotor and focal motor seizures. Despite these findings in the biopsies, none of the patients had evidence of a cerebellar disorder on neurologic examinations, four vessel arteriography, pneumoencephalography, or, in two cases, CT scans. At surgery the superior surface of the cerebellum appeared normal to visual inspection in all cases. These findings provide evidence, obtained antemortem and thus uncomplicated by agonal changes, of severe degenerative processes in the cerebellum of some patients with intractable epilepsy.

Urich and coworkers[74] reported findings similar to those of the others. Biopsies were obtained from 12 of the patients with epilepsy operated upon for implantation of cerebellar stimulation electrodes. One of these biopsies showed no change in the number of Purkinje cells or of other elements. Three showed a patchy loss of Purkinje cells, four a subtotal loss, three a total loss, and one showed a total loss of Purkinje cells plus loss of granule cells. The one biopsy judged to be normal was small and perhaps unreliable.

Although the pathogenesis of the changes in the cerebellum of patients with severe epilepsy has not been determined, anoxia and the administration of anticonvulsant drugs have been viewed as the most likely causes. In attempting to differentiate between these factors, Dam counted Purkinje cells in sections from the cerebellum of 38 autopsied cases of idiopathic grand mal epilepsy of long duration. He classified the cases in terms of attack frequency and level of phenytoin intake. He found loss of Purkinje cells only in patients with severe epilepsy, that is, one or more attacks each week. There was no correlation between the occurrence of cerebellar damage and the dose of phenytoin. He concluded that cerebellar damage results from the epileptic process and not the medication.

Despite Dam's clear conclusions, the issue remains unresolved. In patients with at least three categories of epilepsy, episodes of grand mal status do not appear to be necessary for the development of degenerative changes in the cerebellum.[36] It is impossible, of course, to exclude the possibility of hypoxic damage to the cerebellum in these patients, even in individuals with psychomotor attacks. In addition, Dam's study correlated dosage administered and not serum drug levels.[23] Hence the possibility of drug effects, particularly those of phenytoin, still needs to be considered. It remains possible that phenytoin accounts for the degenerative changes in the cerebellum of severe epileptics.

NEUROPHYSIOLOGIC AND BIOCHEMICAL CHANGES DURING CEREBELLAR STIMULATION IN HUMANS

A number of neurophysiologic and biochemical determinations have been made in patients undergoing cerebellar stimulation in attempts to monitor the effects of stimulation and to understand the mechanisms of these effects. Upton[71] studied nine patients undergoing chronic cerebellar stimulation for the treatment of epilepsy. He found that cerebellar stimulation resulted in a depression of paroxysmal discharges in the EEG, a decrease in the amplitude of somatosensory potentials evoked by peripheral nerve stimulation, and a reduction in the amplitude of the H reflexes. In similar studies of patients with cerebral palsy, Upton[72] found a consistent decrease in the amplitude of somatosensory potentials evoked by peripheral nerve stimulation, a reduction in the amplitude of the H reflexes, and a decrease in the clinical signs of spasticity. He found no change in the amplitude of flash induced visual evoked potentials. Upton commented, however, that in studies on additional patients, he found some reduction in the amplitude of visual evoked potentials.

Contrary to the results of Upton,[71, 73] Van Buren and others[75] found no change in the H reflexes during the cerebellar stimulation of patients with epilepsy. They also found no change in the tendon vibratory responses during stimulation.[75]

Larson and collegues[45] studied somatosensory evoked potentials before, during, and after application of current to the cerebellum in 46 patients with postural and

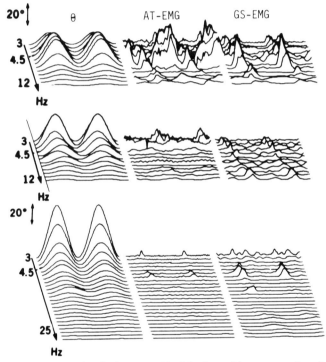

Figure 5. Recordings of the angular displacement (θ) of the foot with corresponding electromyographic (EMG) records. The frequency of oscillation was varied from 3 Hz (background) to 12 Hz (foreground); two cycles are shown. Upper traces: Prestimulation. Typical spastic pattern of maximum compliance at 5 to 6 Hz with coactivation of anterior tibial (AT) and gastrocnemius-soleus (GS) muscles and hyperactive stretch reflex activity. Center traces: Repeat test after the first 5 minutes of superior cerebellar stimulation. Note that maximum compliance shifts to the 3 to 4 Hz range and little coactivation or response to stretch is found. Lower traces: After 3 weeks of chronic stimulation the record becomes basically normal, with maximum displacement of 3 Hz and minimal response to stretch. These recordings were taken from a 16-year-old female with spastic quadriplegia. Unable to walk or crawl, the patient had hyperactive reflexes and bilateral Babinski signs with flexion posturing of the arms greater on the left than the right. (From Penn et al.,[55] with permission.)

383

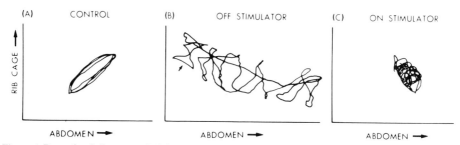

Figure 6. Records of rib cage and abdominal motion from magnetometers. *A*, The pattern of expansion during several consecutive breaths in a normal subject. *B*, The pattern in an 18-year-old girl with an athetoid type of cerebral palsy. Cerebellar stimulating electrodes were implanted but not turned on. *C*, The pattern in the patient with the stimulator turned on. (From Miyasaka et al.,[49] with permission.)

movement disorders. In 44 of these, application of current was followed by a reduction in amplitude of the evoked potential by at least 50 percent. They found that approximately the same amount of current was required to achieve a clinical effect such as reduced spasticity. They noted that the reduction in amplitude of evoked potentials was not uniformly immediate, sometimes developing over a period of 15 to 20 minutes.

Penn and associates[55] developed objective techniques to study the effects of chronic anterior lobe cerebellar stimulation on patients with cerebral palsy. Muscle rigidity and the stretch reflex were quantified by oscillating the ankle sinusoidally and measuring compliance at several frequencies (Fig. 5). The electromyographic activity of extensor and flexor muscles was recorded simultaneously. These studies demonstrated that cerebellar stimulation can reduce rigidity and coactivation of muscles immediately or slowly over days or months.

Miyasaka and others[49] studied the effects of chronic cerebellar stimulation on respiratory muscle coordination in a patient with cerebral palsy (Fig. 6). They used magnetometer recordings to determine whether expansion movements of the abdomen and rib cage were in phase. They found that cerebellar stimulation resulted in marked improvement of respiratory function, although normal values were not achieved.

Van Buren and coworkers[75, 77] examined cerebrospinal fluid (CSF), obtained by lumbar puncture, for gamma-aminobutyric acid (GABA) and norepinephrine (NE) levels in their epileptic patients. They found a rise in CSF-NE and a fall in CSF-GABA accompanying cerebellar stimulation. These changes were significant in comparison with levels observed after an interval without stimulation.

MORPHOLOGIC AND BIOCHEMICAL EFFECTS OF CEREBELLAR STIMULATION IN THE MONKEY

At the time that chronic stimulation of the cerebellum was initiated in humans, little was known about the effects of implantation of stimulating electrodes in the nervous system and of stimulation through these electrodes.[1, 6, 8, 38, 39, 52, 56, 57] Since that time, several investigations have been carried out to study the effects of chronic cerebellar stimulation in experimental animals.[35, 36, 41, 45, 65]

In the studies of Dauth and coworkers[24] and Tennyson and associates,[68] electrodes identical to those used in humans were implanted on the cerebellar surface of the monkey and stimulation was applied chronically with stimulation values similar to those used in humans (30 μC/cm^2, 2.4 μC/phase, 2.4 mA, 1 msec, capacity-coupled pulses at 10 Hz for 205 hrs). After 2 to 6 months of stimulation, operative exploration under general anesthesia revealed that the electrodes and wire leads were embedded in dense reactive fibrous tissue (Fig. 7). Only a single nonstimulated electrode in one animal appeared grossly free of meningeal reaction. Many of the electrodes and wire leads indented the cerebellar surface and, in several instances, the wire leads had burrowed into the surface of the cerebellum, forming deep channels. The stimulating electrodes usually were surrounded by thicker fibrous tissue than the electrodes that had not been used for stimulation, particularly at the interface between dura and electrode.

Neuropathologic changes in cerebellar tissue were related to the duration of stimulus trains. When stimulation was applied continuously for several hours daily through electrodes over the cerebellum, a severe loss of Purkinje cells was found beneath the stimulating electrodes. Many of the neurons remaining were shrunken and hyperchromatic. There was a variable attendant proliferation of Bergmann astrocytes. Purkinje cell changes were conspicuous in the immediate vicinity of the stimulating electrodes and diminished gradually in intensity away from the electrodes (Fig. 8). These changes remained readily apparent 12 to 17 millimeters from the cathode. The superficial folia were much more affected than the deeper folia. A control set of electrodes was placed over the opposite cerebellar hemisphere in these animals to determine the effects of implantation without stimulation. The pattern of pathologic changes was similar to that in the hemisphere stimulated but the changes were less marked.

In animals stimulated intermittently in 8 minute cycles, the histopathologic changes in the Purkinje cells were much less severe than in the continuously stimulated animals and were confined to the immediate vicinity of the electrode.[24, 68] Immediately adjacent to the stimulating site the tissue showed mild changes or no detectable changes. Animals in which electrodes had been implanted for a long duration (6 to 8 months) had more extensive and severe damage than animals with a short duration of implantation (51 to 57 days). Mechanical damage was found under the unstimulated electrodes, but this was more focal and less severe than that caused by stimulation.

Phase and electron microscopy revealed damage under all stimulating elec-

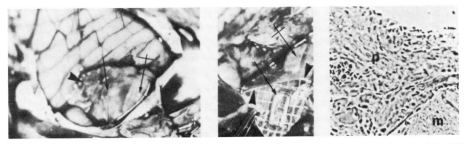

Figure 7. Left, electrodes over crus I of the cerebellar hemisphere of a monkey stimulated for 205 hours. The photograph was taken after the dura was opened with the animal under anesthesia. Note the marked meningeal proliferation (arrowhead) surrounding the site of the stimulating cathode (arrow) and anode (crossed arrow). Center, the electrodes elevated from the cerebellar surface with thickened pia-arachnoid (arrowheads) stripped from the cathode (arrow), but still adherent to the anode (crossed arrow). Right, phase micrograph of aldehyde-OsO$_4$ fixed tissue showing thickened pia-arachnoid (p) overlying molecular layer (m) of the area beneath the cathode. (Reduced 25% from × 260) (From Gilman et al.,[35] with permission.)

385

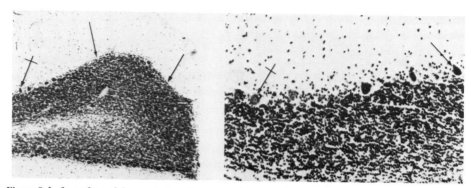

Figure 8. Left, surface of the cerebellum from a monkey stimulated for 205 hours. The section is about 17 mm caudal and ventral from the cathode and shows loss of Purkinje cells (arrows) and pyknotic cells (crossed arrow) at a depth of about 1 mm. (Cresyl violet; original magnification × 60) Right, section adjacent to folium depicted on the left of this illustration, at a depth of 1.5 mm from the cerebellar surface. Note the transition between shrunken pyknotic cells (arrow) and normal appearing Purkinje cells (crossed arrow) with moderately dense cytoplasm and vesicular nuclei. (Cresyl violet; reduced 25% from × 150) (From Gilman et al.,[35] with permission.)

trodes. In most animals, short term placement of electrodes and alternating periods of stimulation between them caused less severe damage than long term placement, regardless of the type of stimulation. Changes under the cathode consisted of a marked loss of Purkinje cells, a decrease in the height of the molecular layer, and a moderate amount of swelling of the neuropil. The surviving Purkinje cells showed marked swelling of the mitochondria. There was often an increase in fibrous glial processes and occasional phagocytes with lipofuscin granules. All layers beneath the anode, particularly the superficial molecular layer, exhibited swelling. This was especially prominent in glial and dendritic processes. There was a variable loss of Purkinje cells and a variable increase in fibrous glial processes. Despite the damage under both anode and cathode, some normal appearing synaptic terminals survived in all layers of the cerebellum, although they were more sparse in fibrotic areas. Placement of electrodes without stimulation resulted in mild to moderate swelling of the neuropil and often a decrease in height of the molecular layer. Purkinje cells usually were present but their organelles frequently were swollen.

Biochemical changes in specimens removed from beneath the stimulating electrodes showed good correlation with the morphologic changes. Tissue GABA levels were measured because of the high concentration of this substance in the molecular and Purkinje cell layers. Polyamine levels were determined to measure cellular degenerative changes and the production of fibrous glia. The findings were remarkable. GABA levels were decreased beneath the cathode in the animals with an observed loss of Purkinje cells. The decreased levels of GABA probably reflected damage to basket and stellate cells as well as Purkinje cells, since all of these elements have been shown to contain GABA. The results of examination of polyamine levels revealed no change in putrescine levels and an increase in spermidine and spermine levels. These findings were thought to reflect the histologic findings of tissue injury and increased glial activity in the damaged regions.

Brown and coworkers[7] performed essentially the same studies as Dauth and colleagues[24] with intermittent stimulation, but used five different charge densities ranging from 7.4 to 323 $\mu C/cm^2$. They found that both stimulating and nonstimulating electrodes become encapsulated and cause mechanical damage to the molecular layer and Purkinje cells. At the lowest level of charge density evaluated (7.4 $\mu C/cm^2$), no cerebellar damage was found that could be attributed to stimulation effects. When a charge density of 35 $\mu C/cm^2$ was used, equivocal damage appeared and 70 $\mu C/cm^2$ resulted in clear damage attributable to stimulation.

The results of these investigations lead to the conclusion that present techniques of electrical stimulation in humans may damage cerebellar tissue. Implantation of platinum electrodes over the arachnoidal surface of the cerebellum without stimulation leads to an intense leptomeningeal reaction and degenerative changes of the underlying Purkinje cells, probably from mechanical pressure effects. Chronic electrical stimulation through these electrodes enhances the meningeal reaction and results in considerably greater degrees of cerebellar damage which, under certain circumstances, may extend beyond the immediate vicinity of the stimulating electrodes. Intermittent stimulation appears to be less damaging than continuous stimulation.

MORPHOLOGIC EFFECTS OF CEREBELLAR STIMULATION IN THE HUMAN

The studies in animals described above have led to the expectation that implantation of electrodes over the cerebellum and stimulation through the electrodes in the human will lead to electrode encapsulation and injury to the surface of the cerebellum. These studies indicate that mechanical damage can result from the wire leads as well as the electrodes. Greater damage is anticipated from electrical stimulation than would result from mechanical effects alone. Thus far, autopsy findings have become available only from a few patients who received cerebellar stimulation, and these findings are controversial.

Cooper and others[16] published the autopsy examination of an epileptic patient with chronic implantation of electrodes and reported no evidence of encapsulation of these electrodes or of damage to the cerebellum underlying the electrodes. Subsequently, Urich and colleagues[74] reported on the autopsy findings in a patient with amyotrophic lateral sclerosis implanted with cerebellar stimulating electrodes for two years and showed that there was no encapsulation of these electrodes. The cerebellum showed a well defined lesion at the site of electrode implantation, 5 mm in diameter and 3 mm in depth. This area had complete loss of Purkinje cells and generally severe loss of granule cells and neurons of the molecular layer. There was an accompanying dense fibrillary gliosis. The cerebellar cortex adjacent to the site of implantation showed diffuse rarefaction of Purkinje cells extending up to 1 cm on each side. The areas remote from the electrodes had normal cerebellar cortical structure. Another case was illustrated as Figure 10 in the report of Urich and colleagues[74] but not described further. This was a patient with dystonia who died $2\frac{1}{2}$ months after installation of cerebellar stimulating electrodes. The illustration shows no fibrosis of the electrodes or the cerebellar hemisphere. Further information about this patient was not provided.

In a similar report, Larson and others[45] examined histologically the cerebellum of a patient who died of unrelated causes five months after implantation of cerebellar stimulating electrodes. During this time, current had been applied unilaterally to the cerebellum for several hours each day. The arachnoid was thickened beneath the implant but, in their opinion, not sufficiently to interfere with the application of current. They found on histologic examination no evidence of neuronal degeneration secondary to the application of current.

Observations contrary to those of Cooper and others,[16] Urich and coworkers,[74] and Larson and associates[45] have been recorded. Gilles[34] reported neuropathologic changes in an epileptic man in his mid-20s who died about 4 months after the implantation of cerebellar stimulation electrodes. The electrodes were surrounded by connective tissue that was at least half the thickness of the dura of the tentorium. The Purkinje cells were moderately depleted throughout the cerebellum, but this was particularly marked beneath the stimulating electrodes. Rayport and Harris[60] have made almost identical observations. Their patient was an 18-year-old man with psychomotor seizures owing to bitemporal independent foci. Stimulating electrodes had been implanted over the superior surface of the cerebellum bilaterally for 3 years and stimulation had been applied for about 1½ years. The procedure had not improved the patient's seizure frequency or severity and stimulation was discontinued by the patient about 1½ years before death. On the day of his death he had a seizure soon after awakening in the morning. Subsequently he got up and spoke with a family member, then returned to bed. He was found dead in bed about one hour later. Neuropathologic examination revealed that both stimulating electrodes contacted the cerebellum at each end of the electrode, but the central portions of the electrodes were out of contact with the cerebellar surface. The electrodes were partially encapsulated with dense fibrous connective tissue (Fig. 9). The encapsulation was denser about the central portions of the electrodes than about the ends. Cerebellar tissue beneath the electrodes and connecting wires was deeply indented and histologic examination revealed destruction of essentially all elements in the molecular, Purkinje cell, and granular layers. Areas of cerebellar cortex adjacent to the site of implantation showed damage to the Purkinje cells.

Robertson and others[62] described the histopathology associated with chronic cerebellar stimulation in three patients who received stimulation for 6½ to 15 months. The electrodes were completely encapsulated with loose connective tissue. Severe injury of the cerebellar cortex was found between 1 and 2 mm directly beneath the electrode array, and included thinning of the molecular layer and loss of most Purkinje cells, interneurons, and associated fibers (Figs. 10 and 11). Neuropathologic changes were also evident in the dentate nucleus and the medial accessory olivary nucleus.

With so little neuropathologic material available, it is difficult to reach conclusions concerning the discrepancies between the reports of the neuropathologic effects of cerebellar stimulation. The principal conclusion at this time, however, is that appreciable electrode encapsulation and marked damage beneath the stimulating electrodes can occur. Widespread cerebellar damage attributable to focal stimulation, however, has not been found in humans thus far.

THE EFFECTS OF CEREBELLAR SURFACE STIMULATION ON THE EXCITABILITY OF CEREBELLAR NEURONS

Cerebellar surface stimulation was used to treat epilepsy and movement disorders based on the assumption that this procedure would activate Purkinje cells, thereby reducing the excitability of neurons in cerebellar and brainstem nuclei. Present information shows, however, that it is impossible to predict the effects of cerebellar stimulation on the discharge of these neurons in any individual patient.

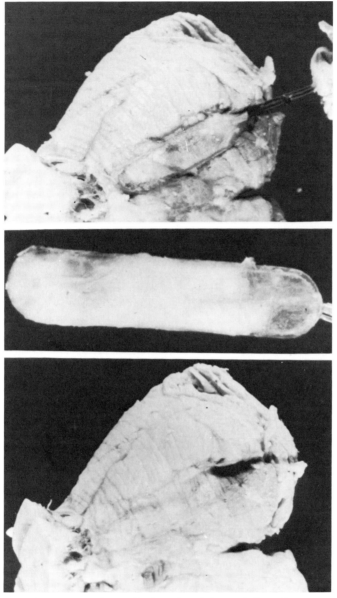

Figure 9. Upper panel, superior surface of the right side of the cerebellum of an 18-year-old man with psychomotor seizures implanted with cerebellar stimulating electrodes for 3 years. A stimulating electrode and its wires are embedded within the surface of the cerebellum. Middle panel, the stimulating electrode after removal from the cerebellar surface. The electrode is encapsulated with a dense layer of connective tissue. Lower panel, the cerebellar surface after removal of the electrode, showing the indentation from the electrode and wires. (Reproduced through the courtesy of Drs. Mark Rayport and James Harris.)

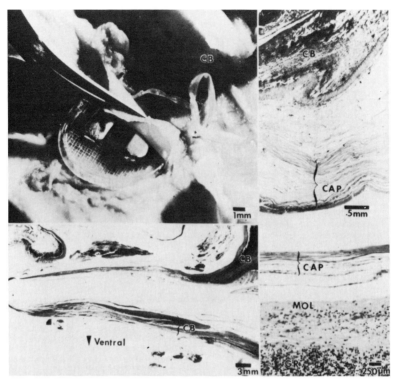

Figure 10. Tissue specimens taken from a 19-year-old man with a 16 year history of grand mal and psychomotor seizures who had received cerebellar stimulation for 15 months at 10 Hz with a voltage setting of 8V, 0.5 msec pulse width, and a stimulus program of 10 minutes on and off, day and night. Upper left, the ventral surface of the tentorium and the electrode array. The array is encased completely in a thick fibrous membrane that is tightly adherent to the tentorium and the cerebellar cortex. Pieces of cerebellar cortical tissue (CB) are still attached to the capsule. Lower left, a sagittal section through the dorsal and ventral layers of the most rostral area of the capsule. Pieces of isolated cerebellar cortex (CB) are found dorsal to the capsule and the ventral capsule is adherent to portions of the cerebellar cortex. Upper right, photomicrograph of the dorsal rostral area of the capsule (CAP). The isolated cerebellar cortex (CB) shows almost complete neuronal degeneration. (H & E) Lower right, photomicrograph of the ventral capsule (CAP) and a piece of the cerebellar cortex that had adhered to the capsule. The cortex shows a depression of the molecular layer (MOL), loss of Purkinje cells, and a decrease in granule cells (GR). (From Robertson et al.,[62] with permission.)

Moreover, recent studies have raised doubts about whether some patients with intractable epilepsy have substantial numbers of surviving Purkinje cells. In addition, many studies have shown that cerebellar surface stimulation evokes a potential in the cerebellar cortex, suggesting that at least some cerebellar output pathways are activated rather than suppressed by this procedure.

Recent studies have been concerned with the effects of cerebellar surface stimulation on neurons in both the cerebellar cortex and the deep nuclei of the cerebellum. One study focused on the effects of cerebellar stimulation on the discharge of Purkinje cells.[25] In cats lightly anesthetized with barbiturates, 17 percent of the Purkinje cells were unaffected by stimuli applied at frequencies of 0.5/sec. Thirty percent responded with an initial increase followed by a decrease in activity, and 53 percent responded only with an initial decrease in activity (Fig. 12A). When

390

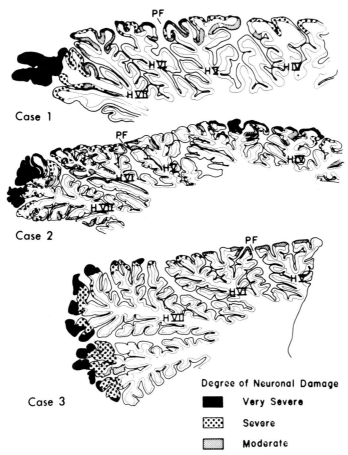

Figure 11. The effects of cerebellar stimulation on cellular morphology in the cerebellar cortex. Schematic reconstructions of parasagittal sections of the cerebellar cortex for three specimens showing the type and extent of neuronal damage beneath the electrode array. The array extended to the caudal pole of lobule HVI and the connecting wires traversed lobule HVII where very severe degenerative changes occurred. PF indicates the primary fissure. Case 1 was a 19-year-old man with grand mal and psychomotor seizures stimulated for 15 months. Case 2 was a 21-year-old woman with grand mal and focal seizures stimulated for 8 months. Case 3 was a 32-year-old man with psychomotor seizures stimulated for 6.6 months. Case 1 was stimulated with 10 minutes on and off cycles. Cases 2 and 3 were stimulated with 8 minute on and off cycles. (From Robertson et al.,[62] with permission.)

the stimulus rate was increased to 10 pulses/sec, most units, including some of those unaffected by stimulation at 0.5 pulse/sec, showed a decrease in firing rate (Fig. 12B). In this study, the need to use an artifact suppressing circuit made it impossible to observe the events occurring in the first 4 to 8 msec after each stimulus. Consequently, any initial activation of Purkinje cells by the stimulus could not be detected. Despite this reservation, the study shows that the effects of cerebellar surface stimulation on Purkinje cell activity are complex, including an increase, a decrease, or a complex sequence of excitability changes.

Other studies have been concerned with the effects of cerebellar stimulation on neuronal excitability in the cerebellar nuclei. One study showed that posterior

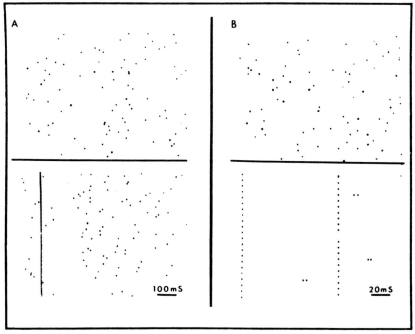

Figure 12. Dot raster displays of Purkinje cell activity in the anesthetized cat. Each dot represents the spike discharge of a Purkinje cell photographed from the face of an oscilloscope with the beam sweeping from left to right. The unit was recorded in the paramedian lobule 6.5 mm lateral to the cathode at a depth of 954 μ. Note the different time calibration bars in panels A and B. A, Spontaneous activity (upper panel) and the responses to 64 consecutive stimuli to the surface of the cerebellum (lower panel) at 2.5 mA with a pulse duration of 1.0 msec and a stimulus rate of 0.5 Hz. The vertical column in the lower panel results from the stimulus artifacts. The stimulus was delivered 100 msec after the beginning of each sweep. B, Spontaneous activity (upper panel) and responses to stimulation (lower panel) at 2.5 mA with a pulse duration of 1.0 msec and a stimulus rate of 10 Hz. The left vertical column of dots in the lower panel represents the stimulus artifacts for odd numbered stimuli. The right vertical column of dots in the lower panel represents the stimulus artifacts for even numbered stimuli. The final 30 msec following the even numbered stimuli are not shown. (From Dauth et al.,[25] with permission.)

vermal surface stimulation suppressed fastigial neuronal activity (Fig. 13).[26] This finding is compatible with the notion that each cerebellar surface stimulus initially activates Purkinje cells which exert inhibitory effects upon the output of the cerebellum via the deep nuclei. The initial activation of Purkinje cells was not detected in the earlier study[25] because of the artifact suppressor circuit. Another investigation showed that dentate neurons were activated by the collaterals of both mossy fibers and climbing fibers projecting to the cerebellar surface.[4] These collaterals are large diameter fibers that can be activated easily by the current densities employed clinically in cerebellar surface stimulation. In addition, axons of nuclear neurons projecting to the cerebellar cortex as nucleocortical fibers can be activated antidromically by stimulating the cerebellar surface.[70] Stimulation of both these groups of collateral fibers results in the direct activation rather than the suppression of cerebellar nuclear neuronal activity.

As a result of the many neuronal elements responsive to cerebellar surface stimulation, conclusions concerning the overall effects of cerebellar stimulation

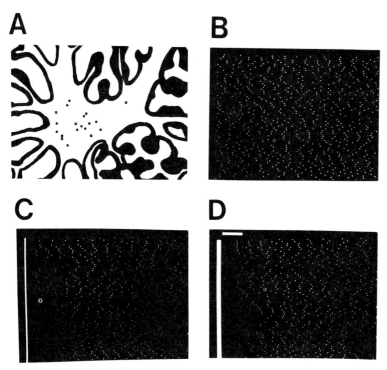

Figure 13. The responses of single neural units in the rostral fastigial nucleus to electrical stimulation of the posterior vermis in anesthetized cats. A, The location of units responding to stimulation at 0.3 Hz (filled squares), 200 Hz (open squares), and both 0.3 and 100 Hz (filled circles). B, Dot raster display of the spontaneous activity of a fastigial unit. C and D, Responses to stimulation at 0.3 Hz and 200 Hz, respectively. The vertical lines in C and D indicate the stimulus artifact. The horizontal calibration bar in D indicates 200 msec. (Unpublished record of Dauth, Yokoyama, and Gilman.)

will require statistical evaluation of the responses of large populations of the affected neurons. Already it is clear that the frequency and intensity of stimulation are important in determining the results of the procedure. For example, a recent study was concerned with the effects of cerebellar stimulation on the seizure activity in penicillin foci of unanesthetized cats.[3] A retrospective analysis of the data revealed an inverse relationship between the amplitude of the cortical potential evoked by stimulating the cerebellar surface and the number of seizures. The amplitude of the evoked potential was correlated with the intensity of the cerebellar surface stimulus. Consequently, the intensity of the cerebellar stimulus has a considerable effect on the number of seizures. These conclusions were confirmed recently in a prospective study with a similar animal model and a statistically designed blinded paradigm.[5]

The initial burst of enthusiasm for the clinical implementation of cerebellar stimulation resulted in the extensive use of this procedure before adequate laboratory studies could be accomplished. As a result, our knowledge about the mechanisms involved has lagged considerably. The basic studies available have shown that much more needs to be known about how this procedure affects neuronal activity in the cerebellum and elsewhere in the nervous system.

REFERENCES

1. AGNEW, W. F., YUEN, T. G. H., PUDENZ, R. H., ET AL.: *Electrical stimulation of the brain, IV. Ultrastructural studies.* Surg. Neurol. 4:438, 1975.

2. BABB, T. L., SOPER, H. V., LIEB, J. P., ET AL.: *Electrophysiological studies of long term electrical stimulation of the cerebellum in monkeys.* J. Neurosurg. 47:353, 1977.

3. BANTLI, H., BLOEDEL, J. R., ANDERSON, G., ET AL.: *The effects of stimulating the cerebellar surface on the activity in penicillin foci.* J. Neurosurg. 48:69, 1978.

4. BANTLI, H., BLOEDEL, J. R., AND TOLBERT, D. L.: *Activation of neurons in the cerebellar nuclei and ascending reticular formation by stimulation of the cerebellar surface.* J. Neurosurg. 45:539, 1976.

5. BANTLI, H.: Personal communication.

6. BARTLETT, J. R., DOTY, R. W., SR., LEE, B. B., ET AL.: *Deleterious effects of prolonged electrical excitation of striate cortex in macaques.* Brain Behav. Evol. 14:46, 1977.

7. BROWN, W. J., BABB, T. L., SOPER, H. V., ET AL.: *Tissue reactions to longterm electrical stimulation of the cerebellum in monkeys.* J. Neurosurg. 47:366, 1977.

8. BRUMMER, S. B., AND TURNER, M. J.: *Electrical stimulation of the nervous system: The principle of safe charge injection with noble metal electrodes.* Bio. Electrochem. Bio. Energet. 2:13, 1975.

9. COOKE, P. M., AND SNIDER, R. S.: *Some cerebellar effects on the electrocorticogram.* EEG Clin. Neurophysiol. 5:563, 1953.

10. COOKE, P. M., AND SNIDER, R. S.: *Some cerebellar influences on electrically-induced cerebral seizures.* Epilepsia 4:19, 1955.

11. COOPER, I. S.: *Two new neurosurgical techniques for spasticity and epilepsy in cerebral palsy.* Presented at the Annual Meeting of the Academy of Cerebral Palsy, St. Louis, Mo., December 1972.

12. COOPER, I. S.: *Chronic stimulation of paleocerebellar cortex in man.* Lancet 1:206, 1973.

13. COOPER, I. S.: *Effect of chronic stimulation of anterior cerebellum on neurological disease.* Lancet 1:1321, 1973.

14. COOPER, I. S., AMIN, I., AND GILMAN, S.: *The effect of chronic cerebellar stimulation upon epilepsy in man.* Trans. Am. Neurol. Assoc. 98:192, 1973.

15. COOPER, I. S., AMIN, I., GILMAN, S., ET AL.: *The effect of chronic stimulation of cerebellar cortex upon epilepsy in man,* in Cooper, I. S., Riklan, M., and Snider, R. S. (eds.): *The Cerebellum, Epilepsy and Behavior.* Plenum Press, New York, 1974, p. 119.

16. COOPER, I. S., AMIN, I., RIKLAN, M., ET AL.: *Chronic cerebellar stimulation in epilepsy.* Arch. Neurol. 33:559, 1976.

17. COOPER, I. S., AMIN, I., UPTON, A., ET AL.: *Safety and efficacy of chronic cerebellar stimulation.* Neurosurgery 1:203, 1977.

18. COOPER, I. S., AMIN, I., UPTON, A., ET AL.: *Safety and efficacy of chronic cerebellar stimulation.* App. Neurophysiol. 40:124, 1977/78.

19. COOPER, I. S., CRIGHEL, E., AND AMIN, I.: *Clinical and physiological effects of stimulation of the paleocerebellum in humans.* J. Am. Geriat. Soc. 21:40, 1973.

20. COOPER, I. S., RIKLAN, M., AMIN, I., ET AL.: *A long-term follow-up study of cerebellar stimulation for the control of epilepsy,* in Cooper, I. S. (ed.): *Cerebellar Stimulation in Man.* Raven Press, New York, 1978, pp. 19–38.

21. COOPER, I. S., RIKLAN, M., AMIN, I., ET AL.: *Chronic cerebellar stimulation in cerebral palsy.* Neurology 26:744, 1976.

22. COOPER, I. S., RIKLAN, M., TABADDOR, K., ET AL.: *A long-term follow-up of chronic cerebellar stimulation for cerebral palsy,* in Cooper, I. S. (ed.): *Cerebellar Stimulation in Man.* Raven Press, New York, 1978, pp. 39–99.

23. DAM, M.: *Number of Purkinje cells in patients with grand mal epilepsy treated with diphenylhydantoin.* Epilepsia 11:313, 1970.

24. DAUTH, G. W., DEFENDINI, R., GILMAN, S., ET AL.: *Long-term surface stimulation of the cerebellum in monkey. I. Light microscopic, electrophysiologic, and clinical observations.* Surg. Neurol. 7:377, 1977.

25. DAUTH, G. W., DELL, S., AND GILMAN, S.: *Alteration of Purkinje cell activity from transfolial stimulation of the cerebellum in cat.* Neurology 28:654, 1978.

26. DAUTH, G. W., YOKOYAMA, T., AND GILMAN, S.: *The effects of transfolial stimulation on fastigial neurons.* Neurology 29:597, 1979.

27. DAVIS, R., CULLEN, R. F., DUENAS, D., ET AL.: *Cerebellar stimulation for cerebral palsy.* J. Fla. Med. Assoc. 63:910, 1976.

28. DAVIS, R., CULLEN, R., DUENAS, D., ET AL.: *The effects of chronic cerebellar stimulation on cerebral palsy spasticity: A three year study.* Presented at the 45th Annual Meeting of the American Association of Neurological Surgeons, Toronto, Ontario, April 25, 1977.

29. DAVIS, R., CULLEN, R. R., FLITTER, M. A., ET AL.: *Control of spasticity and involuntary movements.* Neurosurgery 1:205, 1977.

30. DAVIS, R., CULLEN, R. F., JR., FLITTER, M. A., ET AL.: *Control of spasticity and involuntary movements — cerebellar stimulation.* Appl. Neurophysiol. 40:135, 1977/78.

31. DENNY-BROWN, D., ECCLES, J. C., AND LIDDELL, E. G. T.: *Observations on electrical stimulation of the cerebellar cortex.* Proc. Roy. Soc. Lond. 104:518, 1929.

32. DOW, R. S., FERNÁNDEZ-GUARDIOLA, A., AND MANNI, E.: *The influence of the cerebellum on experimental epilepsy.* EEG Clin. Neurophysiol. 14:383, 1962.

33. FENTON, G. W., FENWICK, P. B. C., BRINDLEY, G. S., ET AL.: *Chronic cerebellar stimulation in the treatment of epilepsy, a preliminary report,* in Penry, J. K. (ed.): *Epilepsy, the Eighth International Symposium.* Raven Press, New York, 1977, pp. 333–340.

34. GILLES, F.: *Discussion of "Morphological and biochemical effects of chronic cerebellar stimulation in monkey,"* by Gilman, S., Dauth, G. W., Tennyson, V. M. et al. Trans. Am. Neurol. Assoc. 100:9, 1975.

35. GILMAN, S., DAUTH, G. W., TENNYSON, V. M. ET AL.: *Chronic cerebellar stimulation in the monkey: preliminary observations.* Arch. Neurol. 32:474, 1975.

36. GILMAN, S., DAUTH, G. W., TENNYSON, V. M., ET AL.: *Clinical, morphological, biochemical, and physiological effects of cerebellar stimulation,* in Hambrecht, F. T., and Reswick, J. B. (eds.): *Functional Electrical Stimulation.* Marcel Dekker, New York, 1977, pp. 191–226.

37. GRIMM, R. S., FRAZEE, J. G., BELL, C. C. ET AL.: *Quantitative studies in cobalt model epilepsy: The effect of cerebellar stimulation.* Int. J. Neurol. 7:126, 1970.

38. HAMBRECHT, F. T.: *Functional electrical stimulation: an overview of the present and speculations on the future.* Electroenceph. Clin. Neurophysiol. Suppl. 34:369, 1978.

39. HAMBRECHT, F. T.: *Neural prostheses.* Ann. Rev. Biphys. Bioeng. 8:239, 1979.

40. HEATH, R. G.: *Modulation of emotion with a brain pacemaker. Treatment for intractable psychiatric illness.* J. Nerv. Ment. Dis. 165:300, 1977.

41. HEMMY, D. C., LARSON, S. J., SANCES, A., JR., ET AL.: *Effect of cerebellar stimulation on focal seizure activity and spasticity in monkeys.* J. Neurosurg. 46:648, 1977.

42. ITO, M.: *Neurophysiological aspects of the cerebellar motor control system.* Int. J. Neurol. 7:162, 1970.

43. ITO, M., AND YOSHIDA, M.: *The cerebellar-evoked monosynaptic inhibition of Deiters' neurones.* Experientia (Basel) 20:515, 1964.

44. IWATA, K., AND SNIDER, R. S.: *Cerebello-hippocampal influences on the electroencephalogram.* EEG Clin. Neurophysiol. 11:439, 1959.

45. LARSON, S. J., SANCES, A., JR., HEMMY, D. C., ET AL.: *Physiological and histological effects of cerebellar stimulation.* Appl. Neurophysiol. 40:160, 1977/78.

46. LOEWENTHAL, M. AND HORSLEY, V.: *On the relations between the cerebellar and other centers (namely cerebral and spinal) with special reference to the action of antagonistic muscles.* Proc. Roy. Soc. 61:20, 1897.

47. MARGERISON, J. H., AND CORSELLIS, J. A. N.: *Epilepsy and the temporal lobes: a clinical, electroencephalographic and neuropathological study of the brain in epilepsy, with particular reference to the temporal lobes.* Brain 89:499, 1966.

48. McCLELLAN, D. L., SELWYN, M., AND COOPER, I. S.: *Time course of clinical and physiological effects of stimulation of the cerebellar surface in patients with spasticity.* J. Neurol. Neurosurg. Psychiat. 41:150, 1978.

49. Miyasaka, K., Hoffman, H. J., and Froese, A. B.: *The influence of chronic cerebellar stimulation on respiratory muscle coordination in a patient with cerebral palsy.* Neurosurg 2:262, 1978.

50. Moruzzi, G.: *Sui rapporti fra cervelleto e corteccia cerebrale. II. Azione d'impulsi cerebellari sulle attivita motrici provocate dalla stimolazione faradica o chimica del giro sigmoideo nel gatto.* Arch. Fisiol. 41:157, 1941.

51. Moruzzi, G.: *Sui raporti fra cervelleto e corteccia cerebrale. III. Meccanismi e localizzazione delle azioni inibitrici e dinamogene del cervelletto.* Arch. Fisiol. 41:183, 1941.

52. Nielson, K. D., Watts, C., and Clark, W. K.: *Peripheral nerve injury from implantation of chronic stimulating electrodes for pain control.* Surg. Neurol. 5:51, 1976.

53. Norman, R. N., Sandry, S., and Corsellis, J. A. N.: *The nature and origin of pathoanatomical change in the epileptic brain,* in Vinken, P. J., Bruyn, G. W. (eds.): *Handbook of Clinical Neurology,* Vol. 15. North-Holland Publishing Company, Amsterdam, 1974, pp. 611–620.

54. Penn, R. D., and Etzel, M. L.: *Chronic cerebellar stimulation and developmental reflexes.* J. Neurosurg. 46:506, 1977.

55. Penn, R. D., Gottlieb, G. L., and Agarwal, G. C.: *Cerebellar stimulation in man, quantitative changes in spasticity.* J. Neurosurg. 48:779, 1977.

56. Pudenz, R. H., Bullara, L. A., Jacques, S., et al.: *Electrical stimulation of the brain. III. The neural damage model.* Surg. Neurol. 4:389, 1975.

57. Pudenz, R. H., Bullara, L. A., Dru, D., et al.: *Electrical stimulation of the brain. II. Effects on the blood-brain barrier.* Surg. Neurol. 4:265, 1975.

58. Rajjoub, R. K., Wood, J. H., and Van Buren, J. M.: *Significance of Purkinje cell density in seizure suppression by chronic cerebellar stimulation.* Neurology 26:645, 1976.

59. Ratusnik, D. L., Wolfe, V. I., Penn, R. D., et al.: *Effects on speech of chronic cerebellar stimulation in cerebral palsy.* J. Neurosurg. 48:876, 1978.

60. Rayport, M., Harris, J.: Personal communication, 1980.

61. Reimer, G. R., Grimm, R. J., and Dow, R. S.: *Effects of cerebellar stimulation on cobalt induced epilepsy in the cat.* EEG Clin. Neurophysiol. 23:456, 1967.

62. Robertson, L. T., Dow, R. S., Cooper, I. S., et al.: *Morphological changes associated with chronic cerebellar stimulation in the human.* J. Neurosurg. 51:510, 1979.

63. Russman, B. S., Gahm, N., Cerciello, R. L., et al.: *Chronic cerebellar stimulator in children with cerebral palsy—a controlled study.* Neurology 29:543, 1979.

64. Salcman, M., Defendini, R., Correll, J., et al.: *Neuropathological changes in cerebellar biopsies of epileptic patients.* Ann. Neurol. 3:10, 1978.

65. Sances, A. Jr., Larson, S. J., Myklebust, J., et al.: *Evaluation of electrode configurations in cerebellar implants.* Appl. Neurophysiol. 40:141, 1977/78.

66. Sherrington, C. S.: *Double (antidrome) conduction in the central nervous system.* Proc. R. Soc. (Lond.) 61:243, 1897.

67. Spielmeyer, W.: *The anatomic substratum of the convulsive state.* Arch. Neurol. Psychiat. 23:869, 1930.

68. Tennyson, V. M., Kremzner, L. T., Dauth, G. W., et al.: *Long-term surface stimulation of the cerebellum in the monkey. II. Electron microscopic and biochemical observations.* Surg. Neurol. 8:17, 1977.

69. Tennyson, V. M., Kremzner, L. T., Dauth, G. W., et al.: *Chronic cerebellar stimulation in the monkey: Electron microscopic and biochemical observations.* Neurology 25:650, 1975.

70. Tolbert, D. L., Bantli, H., and Bloedel, J. R.: *Anatomical and physiological evidence for a cerebellar nucleo-cortical projection in the cat.* Neurosci. 1:205, 1976.

71. Upton, A. R. M.: *Neurophysiological mechanisms in modification of seizures,* in Cooper, I. S. (ed.): *Cerebellar Stimulation in Man.* Raven Press, New York, 1978, pp. 39–57.

72. Upton, A. R. M.: *Neurophysiological aspects of spasticity and cerebellar stimulation,* in Cooper, I. S. (ed.): *Cerebellar Stimulation in Man.* Raven Press, New York, 1978, pp. 101–122.

73. Upton, A. R., and Cooper, I. S.: *Some neurophysiological effects of cerebellar stimulation in man.* Can. J. Neurol. Sci. 3:237, 1976.

74. Urich, H., Watkins, E. S., Amin, I., et al.: *Neuropathologic observations on cerebellar cortical lesions in patients with epilepsy and motor disorders,* in Cooper, I. S. (ed.): *Cerebellar Stimulation in Man.* Raven Press, New York, 1978, pp. 145–159.

75. VAN BUREN, J. M., WOOD, J. H., OAKLEY, J., ET AL.: *Preliminary evaluation of cerebellar stimulation by double blind stimulation and other biologic criteria in the treatment of epilepsy.* J. Neurosurg. 48:407, 1978.

76. WHITTAKER, K.: *Cerebellar stimulation for cerebral palsy.* J. Neurosurg. 52:648, 1980.

77. WOOD, J. H., GLAESER, B. S., HARE, T. A., ET AL.: *Cerebrospinal fluid GABA reductions in seizure patients evoked by cerebellar surface stimulation.* J. Neurosurg. 47:582, 1977.

Index